T0326337

Caring for the Female Cancer Patient-Gynecologic Considerations

Caring for the Female Cancer Patient - Gynecologic Considerations

Edited by

Laurie J. McKenzie, M.D.
University of Texas MD Anderson Cancer Center

Denise R. Nebgen, M.D., Ph.D.
University of Texas MD Anderson Cancer Center

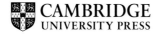
CAMBRIDGE
UNIVERSITY PRESS

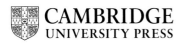

Shaftesbury Road, Cambridge CB2 8EA, United Kingdom

One Liberty Plaza, 20th Floor, New York, NY 10006, USA

477 Williamstown Road, Port Melbourne, VIC 3207, Australia

314–321, 3rd Floor, Plot 3, Splendor Forum, Jasola District Centre, New Delhi – 110025, India

103 Penang Road, #05–06/07, Visioncrest Commercial, Singapore 238467

Cambridge University Press is part of Cambridge University Press & Assessment, a department of the University of Cambridge.

We share the University's mission to contribute to society through the pursuit of education, learning and research at the highest international levels of excellence.

www.cambridge.org
Information on this title: www.cambridge.org/9781009279857

DOI: 10.1017/9781009279864

First published 2024

A catalogue record for this publication is available from the British Library.

A Cataloging-in-Publication data record for this book is available from the Library of Congress

ISBN 978-1-009-27985-7 Paperback

Contents

Contents

Contributors

Mary Katherine Anastasio, M.D.
Department of Obstetrics and Gynecology, Duke University Medical Center, Durham, NC

Maria Azhar, M.D.
Divisions of Critical Care, Pulmonary and Sleep Medicine, McGovern Medical School at UTHealth, Houston, TX

Lara Bashoura, M.D.
Department of Pulmonary Medicine, The University of Texas MD Anderson Cancer Center, Houston, TX

Samantha H. Batman, M.D., Ph.D.
Department of Gynecologic Oncology and Reproductive Medicine, The University of Texas MD Anderson Cancer Center, Houston, TX

Therese B. Bevers, M.D.
Department of Clinical Cancer Prevention, The University of Texas MD Anderson Cancer Center, Houston, TX

Kelly Bree, M.D.
Department of Urology, The University of Texas MD Anderson Cancer Center, Houston, TX

Donal Brennan, Ph.D.
UCD Gynaecological Oncology Group (UCD-GOG), School of Medicine, Mater Misericordiae University Hospital Group, Ireland

Sara Bresser, PA
Department of Leukemia, The University of Texas MD Anderson Cancer Center, Houston, TX

Sukhkamal B. Campbell, M.D.
Department of Obstetrics and Gynecology, Division of Reproductive Endocrinology and Infertility, University of Alabama at Birmingham, Birmingham, AL

Ana Ciurea, M.D.
Department of Dermatology, Division of Internal Medicine, M. D. Anderson Cancer Center, Houston, TX

Caitlin M. Coviello, M.D., M.B.A.
Department of Otolaryngology-Head and Neck Surgery, Baylor College of Medicine, Houston, TX

Molly S. Daniels, M.S.
Department of Gynecologic Oncology and Reproductive Medicine, University of Texas MD Anderson Cancer Center, Houston, TX

Kristina R. Dahlstrom, Ph.D.
Section of Epidemiology and Population Sciences, Department of Medicine, Baylor College of Medicine, Houston, TX

Sai Prasad Desikan, M.D.
Department of Leukemia, The University of Texas MD Anderson Cancer Center, Houston, TX

Jenifer Dinis Ballestas, M.D.
Department of Obstetrics and Gynecology, Baylor College of Medicine - Texas Children's Hospital, Pavilion for Women, Houston, TX

Fionán Donohoe, MB BCh
UCD Gynaecological Oncology Group (UCD-GOG), School of Medicine, Mater Misericordiae University Hospital Group, Ireland

Timothy Dunn, M.D.
Department of Obstetrics and Gynecology, Division of Reproductive Endocrinology and Infertility, Baylor College of Medicine, Houston, TX

Saadia A. Faiz, M.D.
Department of Pulmonary Medicine, The University of Texas MD Anderson Cancer Center, Houston, TX

Jordana Faruqi, M.D., M.P.H.
Division of Diabetes, Endocrinology, and Metabolism, Baylor College of Medicine, Houston, TX

Alessandra Ferrajoli, M.D.
Department of Leukemia, The University of Texas MD Anderson Cancer Center, Houston, TX

Austin B. Gardner, M.D.
Department of Obstetrics and Gynecology, Division of Reproductive Endocrinology and Infertility University of Alabama at Birmingham, Birmingham, AL

Valentina Grajales, M.D.
Department of Urology, The University of Texas MD Anderson Cancer Center, Houston, TX

Martha Hickey, Ph.D.
Department of Obstetrics and Gynaecology, University of Melbourne and the Royal Women's Hospital, Melbourne, Australia

Emma B. Holliday, M.D.
Department of Gastrointestinal Radiation Oncology, The University of Texas MD Anderson Cancer Center, Houston, TX

Rosa F. Hwang, M.D.
Department of Breast Surgical Oncology, The University of Texas MD Anderson Cancer Center, Houston, TX

Anuja Jhingran, M.D.
Department of Radiation Oncology, The University of Texas M. D. Anderson Cancer Center, Houston, TX

Nupur Kikani, M.D.
Department of Endocrine Neoplasia and Hormonal Disorders, University of Texas MD Anderson Cancer Center, Houston, TX

Christina Kraus, M.D.
Department of Dermatology, University of California, Irvine, CA

Suzanne Lange, M.D.
Department of Urology, The University of Texas MD Anderson Cancer Center, Houston, TX

Melissa Mauskar, M.D.
Department of Dermatology and Obstetrics and Gynecology, University of Texas Southwestern Medical School, Dallas, TX

Laurie J. McKenzie, M.D.
Division of Reproductive Endocrinology and Infertility, Baylor College of Medicine, Department of Gynecologic Oncology and Reproductive Medicine, University of Texas MD Anderson Cancer Center, Houston, TX

Craig Messick, M.D.
Department of Colon and Rectal Surgery, The University of Texas MD Anderson Cancer Center, Houston, TX

Melissa Mitchell, M.D., Ph.D.
Department of Breast Radiation Oncology, The University of Texas MD Anderson Cancer Center, Houston, TX

Jessica F. Moore, M.D.
The University of Miami Department of Obstetrics, Gynecology & Reproductive Science, Coral Gables, FL

Van Morris, M.D.
Department of Gastrointestinal Medical Oncology, The University of Texas MD Anderson Cancer Center, Houston, TX

Giancarlo Moscol, M.D.
Department of General Oncology, The University of Texas MD Anderson Cancer Center, Houston, TX

Denise R. Nebgen, M.D., Ph.D.
Department of Gynecologic Oncology and Reproductive Medicine, University of Texas MD Anderson Cancer Center, Houston, TX

Anna C. Nelson, APRN FNP-BC
Department of Clinical Cancer Prevention, The University of Texas MD Anderson Cancer Center, Houston, TX

Dawn Palaszewski, M.D.
Department of Obstetrics and Gynecology University of South Florida, Morsani College of Medicine, Tampa, FL

Anna Claire Reynolds, M.D.
Division of Reproductive Endocrinology and Infertility, Baylor College of Medicine, Houston, TX

Kristin E. Rojas, M.D.
Division of Surgical Oncology, The University of Miami Sylvester Comprehensive Cancer Center, Coral Gables, FL

Neil Ryan, MBChB, Ph.D.
Department of Gynaecology Oncology, Royal Infirmary of Edinburgh and The University of Edinburgh, Edinburgh, Scotland

Mila P. Salcedo, M.D., Ph.D.
Department of Gynecologic Oncology and Reproductive Medicine, University of Texas MD Anderson Cancer Center, Houston, TX

Kathleen M. Schmeler, M.D.
Department of Gynecologic Oncology and Reproductive Medicine, University of Texas MD Anderson Cancer Center, Houston, TX

Travis T. Sims, M.D., Ph.D.
Department of Gynecologic Oncology, The University of Texas MD Anderson Cancer Center, Houston, TX

Erich M. Sturgis, M.D., M.P.H.
Department of Otolaryngology-Head and Neck Surgery, Baylor College of Medicine, Houston, TX

Maryam Tetlay, M.D.
Division of Diabetes, Endocrinology, and Metabolism, Baylor College of Medicine, Houston, TX

Terri L. Woodard, M.D.
Division of Reproductive Endocrinology and Infertility, Baylor College of Medicine, Houston Texas, Department of Gynecologic Oncology and Reproductive Medicine, University of Texas MD Anderson Cancer Center, Houston, TX

Chapter

1

Fertility Assessment and Fertility Preservation Options

Anna Claire Reynolds, Terri L. Woodard, and Laurie J. McKenzie

Case Presentation

J.T. is a 38-year-old female P0 with a clinical stage IA, grade 2, left breast intraductal carcinoma ER + (65%), PR + (95%) HER2-, Ki-67 15% left breast intraductal carcinoma that presents two weeks after her initial diagnosis. Her treatment plan involves upfront surgery, with adjuvant therapy to be determined based on her intraoperative findings. She is referred for an oncofertility consultation to discuss the potential impact of her upcoming cancer treatment on her fertility, as she may be interested in having children in the future.

Introduction

Worldwide, approximately 9 million women were diagnosed with cancer in 2020, and 9.6% were under the age of 40 [1]. Younger patients with cancer commonly present with more advanced disease due to delays in diagnosis, higher uninsured rates, and higher prevalence of aggressive disease [2]. Fortunately, cancer mortality rates in adolescent and young adults (AYAs; typically defined as ages 15–39 years) and all age groups, have been declining since at least 1975. The AYA five-year relative survival rates are 94% or greater for many of the most common cancers such as thyroid, melanoma, and Hodgkin's lymphoma.

As survival rates improve, there is an increased focus on the complex issues surrounding cancer survivorship, particularly for younger women of reproductive age. Among young women diagnosed with cancer, concerns regarding future fertility are secondary only to concerns regarding survival [3, 4]. One study found that among childless cancer survivors, over 75% endorsed wanting children in the future, yet only 6% had undergone fertility treatment [5]. Guidelines from the American Society of Clinical Oncology (ASCO) and American Society for Reproductive Medicine (ASRM) state that healthcare providers should discuss the risk of infertility and fertility preservation options with all reproductive age patients diagnosed with cancer [6, 7]. While the majority of males diagnosed with cancer receive information regarding treatment impact on fertility, 40–62% of reproductive age women diagnosed with cancer have reported not receiving fertility counseling at diagnosis or report unmet fertility needs [8–11]. Unaddressed fertility concerns may significantly impact quality of life among reproductive-aged female cancer survivors [9]. One qualitative study exploring survivor preference surrounding fertility concerns asked women how they would like to learn about fertility issues, and one prevalent theme was that survivors wanted their doctors or another healthcare provider to initiate a discussion about their options [12]. Receipt of counseling regarding fertility preservation has been shown to reduce long-term regret and dissatisfaction amongst cancer survivors and may be associated with both improved physical and psychological quality of life [13–15].

Fortunately, current oncology care has evolved from a primary focus on cancer treatment to a comprehensive model that includes survivorship issues. With advancements in screening, diagnostic tools and effective treatments, life after cancer becomes increasingly important for optimizing patient care. The term oncofertility was coined in the early 2000s and represents an interdisciplinary approach to closing the information, data, and option gaps in the care of reproductive age cancer survivors [16]. Through oncofertility counseling, life-preserving treatments are balanced with fertility preservation options with a focus on reproductive survivorship care. The psychological, social, physical, and emotional changes that occur following cancer treatment are now a focus, as patients are expected to live well beyond their cancer treatment years.

Cancer treatment may include a combined approach of surgery, radiation therapy (proton and photon), and chemotherapy. These treatment modalities may have a detrimental effect on fertility based on the type of treatment and agent(s), number of treatment cycles, cumulative dosing, and timing between treatment cycles [17]. Additional factors such as patient age at time of cancer treatment and the patient's baseline fertility status also influence future reproductive capacity. The relative probability of a childhood female cancer survivor having a child is reduced by approximately 50% compared to siblings, and the 10-year cumulative postdiagnosis parenthood rate is only 14% among patients diagnosed with cancer at the age of 15–45 [18, 19]. Therefore, it is imperative that healthcare providers counsel patients about the impact of cancer treatment on future fertility and provide options for fertility preservation.

Fertility Assessment

A baseline fertility assessment includes obtaining a thorough history, targeted physical examination, bloodwork, and pelvic ultrasound. Comprehensive medical and surgical history should be obtained including gynecologic history such as a detailed menstrual history, date of last menstrual cycle, current contraception, menarche, cycle interval and length, ovulation and obstetric history (gravidity, parity, time to previous pregnancies, and mode of delivery). Prior fertility attempts, testing, and treatment history should be elicited. Physical examination should include basic vital signs, body mass index (BMI), thyroid, breast, and pelvic examinations with attention to uterine size, shape, position, adnexal masses, or tenderness.

While age remains the most important overall predictor of reproductive potential and live birth rates, laboratory and ultrasound evaluation to determine ovarian reserve is a key aspect of a baseline fertility evaluation in cancer patients (Table 1.1). Ovarian reserve represents the total number of healthy, immature oocytes available within the ovaries. Ovarian reserve testing includes both ultrasound imaging and hormonal measures to predict reproductive potential. Transvaginal ultrasound examination is performed to determine the antral follicle count (AFC), ovarian volume, and uterine characteristics. AFC describes the total number of small follicles that measure between 2 and 10 mm in diameter with transvaginal ultrasound [20]. Normal range for antral follicle count is broad, depending on the patient's history. For example, women with polycystic ovary syndrome may have an AFC of >40 on transvaginal ultrasound assessment, which would be normal for that disease physiology. AFC of at least 7 is considered normal. AFC of less than 5–7 is consistent with diminished ovarian reserve [20]. This value is especially important when considering treatment options for fertility preservation, as it correlates with expected oocyte recruitment during in vitro fertilization (IVF).

Table 1.1 Ovarian reserve assessment

Test	Values indicative of DOR[a]	Timing in menstrual cycle	Advantage	Effect of hormone therapies
AFC[b]	<5–7	Days 2–5	Good predictive value for response to ovarian stimulation	AFC levels may be slightly decreased
AMH[c]	<1 ng/mL	Any day	High sensitivity; good predictive value for response to ovarian stimulation; minimal variability during menstrual cycle	Levels decrease with GnRHa, but effect of other hormone therapies is low
FSH[d]	>10 IU/L	Days 2–5	High specificity for poor response to ovarian stimulation response; readily available	FSH serum levels decrease
Estradiol[e]	>60–80 pg/mL[d]	Days 2–5	Increases sensitivity of FSH in predicting diminished ovarian reserve	Levels may be altered

[a]DOR, diminished ovarian reserve; [b]AFC, antral follicle count, the number of follicles that are 2–10mm in both ovaries as assessed by transvaginal ultrasonography; [c]AMH, antimullerian hormone, can be used as an alternative to AMH in combination with estradiol; [d]FSH, follicle stimulating hormone; [e]Elevated estradiol levels can be indicative of DOR when abnormal FSH is masked, thereby increasing sensitivity for detecting DOR

Hormonal measures of ovarian reserve include serum follicle-stimulating hormone (FSH), estradiol, inhibin B, and anti-mullerian hormone (AMH). AMH is a glycoprotein product of small ovarian follicles. FSH, estradiol and inhibin B must be measured in the early follicular phase (typically days 2–5 of a menstrual cycle) to provide an accurate assessment of ovarian reserve. These tests are not reliable while taking combination oral contraceptive pills, and often require a several-week "wash out" before values can be interpretable. In contrast to these traditional markers of ovarian reserve, AMH levels are independent of menstrual cycle phase; although may be slightly reduced in women taking combined oral contraceptive pills [21]. A recent cross-sectional study that reviewed AMH levels in over 27,000 women found lower AMH levels with women utilizing oral contraceptive pills, as well as the vaginal ring, hormonal intrauterine device, implant and progesterone-only when compared to women not using any hormonal contraceptive [22]. An AMH greater than 1.0 ng/mL in an adult female indicates good ovarian reserve while values less than 1.0 ng/mL indicate diminished ovarian reserve. Individuals with higher AMH values before cancer treatment may be more likely to regain ovarian function following cancer treatment [23–26]. While AMH is the gold-standard marker of ovarian reserve and a valuable predictor of response to ovarian stimulation in women undergoing IVF, there is conflicting data on its ability to predict future live birth rates. Not surprisingly, AMH levels and live birth rates diminish remarkably at age 40 and beyond. However, for younger women (under age 35) AMH levels have little influence on live birth rate prediction [27]. Prospective data have also confirmed that there is no association with AMH and natural fecundity in the general population [28]. Thus, AMH must be interpreted in conjunction with other indices including age and AFC to provide a more informative assessment of ovarian reserve. Despite its limitations, baseline ovarian reserve testing is helpful to counsel patients regarding the expected success of oocyte/embryo banking and for comparison after cancer treatment.

Reproductive Effects of Treatment

Chemotherapy

Chemotherapy administration may result in permanent cessation of menses, and the risk is typically quantified as high (>80%), intermediate (20%–80%), or low (<20%). Patient-related factors such as age and baseline fertility, as well as cumulative dose and cycle schedule, affect this risk [29]. For traditional chemotherapies, the alkylating agents pose the highest risk for deleterious effects on fertility by inducing double-stranded DNA breaks in oocytes, resulting in direct ovarian toxicity [30, 31]. Alkylating agents with high ovarian toxicity include chlorambucil, cyclophosphamide, ifosfamide, melphalan B sulfate, nitrogen mustard, and procarbazine (Figure 1.1) [32, 33]. Platinum agents (cisplatin, carboplatin, oxaliplatin) also carry a moderate to high risk for oocyte/ovarian damage. In contrast, the antimetabolites and vinca alkaloids, such as vincristine and methotrexate, are classified as low risk for ovarian toxicity [30, 34]. Specific chemotherapy agents can also vary in their level of ovarian toxicity, based on patient age. For example, women older than 40 years of age receiving doxorubicin are at higher risk of ovarian toxicity, whereas those younger than 30 years are at lower risk [35].

Several methods can be utilized to assess ovarian function following treatment with systemic chemotherapeutic agents. Women with ovarian toxicity following chemotherapy will often present with menstrual irregularities (oligomenorrhea and amenorrhea) and

Class/Agent		Risk Level
Alkylating agents	Busulfan[a] > 500 mg/m^2	High risk, all ages
	Carboplatin[b]	Intermediate risk
	Chlorambucil[a] > 300 mg/m^2	High risk, all ages
	Cisplatin[b]	Intermediate risk
	Cyclophosphamide[c]	Low to high risk depending on age and regimen
		Age younger than 20 years with cumulative dose greater than 7.5 g/m^2, high risk
		Age 30-39 years with cumulative dose 5 g/m^2, intermediate risk
		Age older than 40 years with cumulative dose greater than 5 g/m^2, high risk
		Age 20-39 years as part of AC*/AC-T regimen for breast cancer, low risk
		Age 40 years and older as part of AC*/AC-T regimen for breast cancer, intermediate risk
		Age younger than 30 years as part of CAF, CEF, CMF x 6 cycles for breast cancer, low risk
		Age 30-39 years as part of CAF, CEF, CMF x 6 cycles for breast cancer, intermediate risk
		Age younger than 35 years as part of CHOP protocol for non-Hodgkin lymphoma, low risk (including dose-dense CHOP and CHOEP)
		All ages as part of a stem-cell transplant conditioning regimen, high risk
	Dacarbazine	Lower risk when combined with doxorubicin in ABVD regimen
	Ifosfamide[a] > 16 g/m^2	High risk, all ages
	Melphalan[a] > 100 mg/m^2	High risk, all ages
	Nitrosoureas[a] > 300 mg/m^2	High risk, all ages
	Procarbazine[a] > 5 g/m^2	High risk, all ages

Figure 1.1 Chemotherapy-induced ovarian toxicity [35] Reprinted by permission by Reynolds et al. JCO 2023 [35]

Antimetabolites	Fluorouracil	Low or no risk
	Mercaptopurine	Low or no risk
	Methotrexate	Low or no risk
Cytotoxic antibiotics	Bleomycin	Low or no risk
	Dactinomycin	Low or no risk
	Doxorubicin hydrochloride	Low to high risk depending on age Younger than 30 years, low risk
		Older than 30 to younger than 40 years, intermediate risk
		Older than 40 years, high risk
Vinka alkaloids	Vinblastine	Lower risk as part of ABVD regimen
	Vincristine	Low or no risk
	Vinorelbine	Low risk
Plant alkaloid	Taxanes	Intermediate risk
Miscellaneous agents		BCL-2 inhibitor (venetoclax), unknown risk
		Bevacizumab (anti-VEGF), intermediate risk[d]
		Immune checkpoint inhibitors (eg, anti–CTLA-4), unknown risk
		Microtubule depolymerizing agent (eg, eribulin mesylate), unknown risk
		Rituximab (anti-CD20), low risk
		Trastuzumab (anti-HER2), low risk
		Tyrosine kinase inhibitors, low risk[e]

Figure 1.1 (cont.)

vasomotor symptoms, including hot flushes and night sweats. However, regular menstrual cycles do not necessarily indicate normal fertility potential. Patients with diminished ovarian reserve may have regular menstrual cycles for a time period prior to experiencing

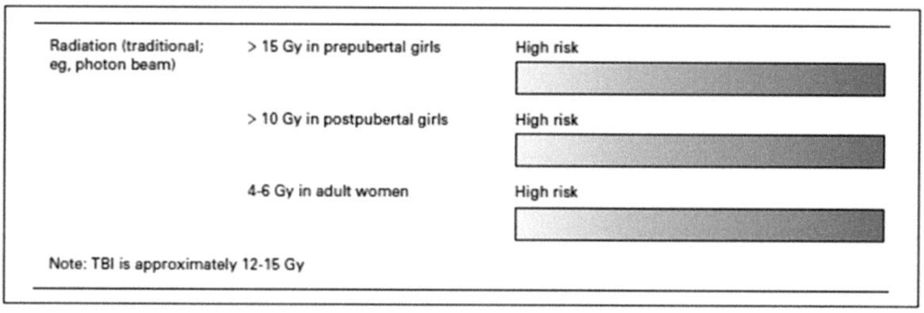

Figure 1.1 (cont.)

menstrual cycle changes. Diminished ovarian reserve may initially present as hormonal abnormalities such as an increase in FSH or decrease in AMH before progressing into clinical symptoms of irregular or absent menses [35]. Patients who have undergone gonadotoxic therapy may develop primary ovarian insufficiency (POI). POI (formerly known as premature ovarian failure) is a diagnosis defined by menstrual irregularity for at least three to four consecutive months and a FSH >40 IU/L on 2 separate measurements (spaced at least one month apart) prior to age 40 [30, 35, 36].

Proposed Mechanisms for Chemotherapy-Induced Ovarian Toxicity

It is difficult to predict the effect of chemotherapy on fertility, however, multiple mechanisms have been proposed regarding the underlying pathophysiology of chemotherapy-induced gonadotoxicity. Ovarian tissue ischemia may occur as a result of vasoconstriction or inhibition of angiogenesis [36]. DNA cross-linking/intercalation or inhibition of protein synthesis through DNA methylation inhibition leads to ovarian follicle apoptosis. Follicular death may also arise from a disruption in follicular cycling, as inhibition of microtubule assembly can arrest follicles in metaphase [34]. Destruction of larger follicles may decrease AMH, which is responsible for suppression of the primordial (early) follicular pool. With the drop in AMH, primordial follicles are then activated and subsequently recruited in an effort to replace the loss of growing follicles. The primordial follicular pool represents a finite, nongrowing population; therefore, once it is depleted, follicles are not replaced [35, 36].

Radiation

The human oocyte is exquisitely sensitive to radiation. It is estimated that the lethal dose of radiation required to eliminate 50% of oocytes (LD50) is 2 Gray (Gy) [37]. A radiotherapy dose of 45–50 Gy induces POI in greater than 90% of patients [31]. Prescribed radiation doses vary based on cancer type and stage at diagnosis. For example, in colorectal cancer (CRC) treatment, cumulative radiation doses can typically approximate 50 Gy [38]. For cancer that require treatment with total body irradiation, radiation doses can be estimated at 12–14 Gy. POI would be expected with both of these examples.

Pituitary or hypothalamic exposure to radiation can result in gonadotropin deficiency, precocious puberty and/or hyperprolactinemia. The degree of neurotoxicity depends on the total dose, fraction size and duration of radiation. Gonadotropin deficiency is typically a late complication of radiation administration with a cumulative incidence of approximately 20–30% during long term follow up, irrespective of childhood versus adulthood exposure [39]. Fortunately, however, gonadotropin(s) can be replaced exogenously and allow a pregnancy to occur. Proton beam as opposed to photon radiation may confer less neurotoxicity, although reproductive outcomes are lacking.

While the ovaries are much more susceptible to radiation-induced damage compared to the uterus, the uterus can also be negatively impacted. Histological changes following radiation include edema of the uterine serosa, uterine atrophy, and abnormal vascularity particularly in the prepubertal patient [40]. However, the adult uterus is susceptible as well. Uterine radiotherapy doses of more than 5 Gy in a postpubertal females confer a relative risk of 2.48 for infertility, increase in the incidence of premature births (OR = 3.5, 95% CI: 1.5–8.0), low birth weight (OR = 6.8, 95% CI: 2.1–22.2) and small for gestational age (OR = 4.0, 95% CI: 1.6–9.8) when compared to women with no history of radiotherapy [41]. Unfortunately, there is no consensus on the dose above which a pregnancy is not sustainable. It has been suggested that pregnancy is contraindicated with doses exceeding 45 Gy in adulthood and 25 Gy in childhood [40].

Immunotherapies/Other

Evidence of ovarian toxicity from immunotherapy and targeted agents, such as small-molecule inhibitors, is limited and mixed. Immunotherapies, particularly ipilimumab (either alone or in combination with other immune checkpoint inhibitors), have been linked to risk of hypophysitis, which can lead to menstrual cycle irregularity and infertility [42–44]. Small-molecule inhibitors, such as tyrosine kinase inhibitors and mammalian target of rapamycin (mTOR) inhibitors, have limited reproductive data in humans, but may have a negative impact on ovarian reserve. Tyrosine kinase inhibitors (TKI) specifically have shown varied ovarian effects; however, most clinical case series suggest that they cause reversible changes in ovarian function. A recent study assessing 361 childhood outcomes following TKI exposure in women at the time of conception, found twice the baseline incidence of teratogenicity. Clinical observational studies show an association of menstrual disorders and ovarian cysts during treatment with mTOR inhibitors, specifically sirolimus [45–47]. Reassuringly, normal menstrual cycles were restored within a few months after treatment cessation [35].

Monoclonal antibodies, such as the anti-angiogenic agent of bevacizumab, have unknown impact on long-term fertility. In 2011, the FDA required the addition of a revised package insert warning of detrimental fertility effects as a result of a study involving 179 colon cancer patients exposed to bevacizumab [42]. Those utilizing bevacizumab + FOLFOX (combination of leucovorin calcium, fluorouracil and oxaliplatin) experienced a 34% ovarian failure rate compared to 2% that did not utilize bevacizumab [43]. Ovarian function returned in approximately 20% of women after discontinuation of bevacizumab therapy. In contrast, trastuzumab, a monoclonal antibody targeting human epidermal growth factor receptor, has not been shown to increase risk of ovarian failure [44].

There is a notable increase in the use of immunomodulatory drugs, and the data regarding fertility impact is exceedingly scarce. Hopefully the next several years will yield data regarding reproductive outcomes in humans.

Fertility-Sparing Approaches for Gynecologic Malignancies

Endometrial Cancer

Endometrial cancer is the most common gynecologic cancer affecting women. While it more commonly affects postmenopausal women, the overall prevalence continues to rise among women younger than age 45. Standard-of-care approach includes surgical staging with hysterectomy, bilateral salpingo-oophorectomy (BSO) and pelvic and para-aortic lymph node assessment. Current society guidelines permit the consideration of fertility-sparing management with progestin therapy in patients with stage IA, grade 1 (well-differentiated) endometrioid type endometrial cancer. Pretreatment magnetic resonance imaging (MRI) should be obtained confirming no evidence of metastatic disease or myometrial invasion. In addition, if the initial diagnosis is based on an office endometrial biopsy, dilation and curettage should then be performed as it has been shown to have a better diagnostic performance in determining cancer grade [48]. Fertility-sparing treatment of grade 2 endometrioid endometrial cancer is only reported in very small case studies and should only be considered in highly selected individuals with a shared decision-making approach [49].

A progestin-containing regimen with or without hysteroscopic resection is the recommended fertility-sparing treatment of appropriately selected endometrial cancer patients. Regimens include the use of a levonorgestrel-releasing intrauterine system (LNG-IUS) alone and/or in combination with oral progestins (most commonly medroxyprogesterone acetate or megestrol acetate). Serial surveillance endometrial biopsies are obtained every three months to monitor treatment response. The majority of patients will respond with reported complete response rates ranging from 64–88% with median time to response two to nine months [50–53]. Risk of recurrence is 20–40% and once childbearing is complete, definitive standard-of-care surgical treatment should be strongly considered [51, 54].

In patients undergoing definitive surgical staging including hysterectomy and lymph node dissection, ovarian preservation is a reasonable option in patients with early-stage, low grade tumors. A large recent study reported that ovarian preservation in women under age 50 at time of endometrial cancer surgery was a safe option, and was associated with decreased risk of death due to cardiovascular disease and improved overall survival [55]. In patients wishing to pursue pregnancy, IVF could later be performed to produce embryos for transfer into a gestational carrier.

Endometrial cancer patients encompass a group of women who often have other baseline health and fertility challenges such as obesity, diabetes, hypertension, polycystic ovarian syndrome (PCOS), anovulation, and irregular menses. These same factors may also negatively impact one's ability to conceive and maintain a healthy pregnancy. Oral progestin therapy is associated with weight gain; therefore, for these women, a LNG-IUS may be a better first line treatment choice. Lifestyle counseling regarding diet, exercise, nutrition, and weight loss are important and patients may benefit from referral to a weight loss team and/or bariatric surgeon. Optimizing overall health and metabolic status increases the likelihood of conception and decreases the risk of miscarriage, fetal anomalies, and maternal morbidity during pregnancy [56].

Cervical Cancer

Cervical cancer is often diagnosed in reproductive age women, with 37% of new cervical cancer cases in women younger than age 45 [57]. Radical trachelectomy with lymph node assessment is an acceptable alternative in those who desire future fertility [58]. Potential candidates for a fertility-sparing surgical approach include the following: squamous or adenocarcinoma histology, lesion less than or equal to 2 cm, no deep stromal invasion, and no evidence of lymph node involvement or distant metastatic disease [59, 60]. Overall, oncologic outcomes are excellent for fertility-sparing surgery in cervical cancer with no reported difference in overall or disease-free survival rates [61, 62]. A large systematic review including 2,777 fertility-sparing procedures for cervical cancer and 944 pregnancies reported fertility, live birth, and prematurity rates of 55%, 70%, and 38%, respectively [63]. Routine completion hysterectomy is not recommended after childbearing is complete, but given lack of data, it may be considered based on individual patient factors.

It is important to stress that a radical trachelectomy procedure does not ensure future conception, and increased rates of preterm births have been reported. Infertility rates post-procedure range from 14–41%, and many patients will require insemination of sperm or IVF to conceive [64, 65]. Cervical stenosis is a major cause of post-trachelectomy infertility. Management of cervical stenosis can be challenging and require additional procedures to correct the issue, which are not always successful. If the stenosis is severe, hematometra may develop resulting in the need for chronic menstrual suppression and/or completion hysterectomy. With appropriate patient selection, radical trachelectomy in early-stage cervical cancer is safe with acceptable reproductive outcomes.

Ovarian Cancer

Most ovarian cancer cases are diagnosed in postmenopausal women, with only 12% of new cases arising in women under 45 years of age [66]. Ovarian cancer is the most lethal gynecologic cancer as it is often diagnosed at advanced stages, however younger women are more likely to present with earlier-stage disease and have a better prognosis [67]. For patients with tumors of low malignant potential, nonepithelial ovarian tumors and stage I epithelial ovarian cancer, fertility-sparing surgery is an acceptable option. A fertility sparing approach may include an ovarian cystectomy or unilateral salpingo-oophorectomy, omentectomy, peritoneal washings, pelvic and paraaortic lymphadenectomy, and peritoneal biopsies with preservation of the uterus and contralateral ovary. The extent of surgical staging varies depending on the individual ovarian tumor histology. Unlike endometrial and cervical cancer, the pathology of the tumor is typically unknown preoperatively. Patients must be counseled on the potential etiologies including benign, borderline, and malignant tumors as well as standard treatment options including both conventional and fertility-sparing treatment options. Intraoperative decision-making is required based on operative findings and frozen section pathology so it is essential to obtain as much information as possible preoperatively about a patient's desire to preserve fertility. It is also imperative that a patient understands that frozen section pathology may differ from final pathology and a two-step procedure may be necessary in some cases [68, 69].

Oncologic outcomes after fertility-sparing treatment in select patients with ovarian cancer are reassuring based on observational data. A prospective analysis of fertility sparing surgery in patients with nonepithelial ovarian cancer was not associated with worse oncologic outcomes and demonstrated equivalent five-year overall and progression free survival rates [70]. In epithelial ovarian cancer however, the safety of fertility sparing surgery in patients with high-risk features such as stage IC disease or other high grade histologies is debated [71, 72]. A large cohort study using the National Cancer Database demonstrated that fertility sparing surgery in stage IA or unilateral stage IC epithelial ovarian cancer was not associated with an increased risk of death when compared to conventional surgery; however, the total number of patients with high-risk histology was relatively low [73]. Patients with stage IC epithelial ovarian cancer or other high-risk features should be counseled with caution given the paucity of oncologic safety data. Completion hysterectomy and bilateral salpingo-oophorectomy should be considered after childbearing is complete based on individual tumor characteristics.

Fertility Preservation Options: Surgical Approaches

Ovarian Transposition

One surgical option for women undergoing pelvic radiation therapy who desire future fertility is ovarian transposition (oophoropexy). Ovarian transposition involves mobilizing one or both ovaries and attaching them to the sidewall of the abdomen at the pelvic brim. Ovarian transposition may be performed either open or laparoscopically, although the laparoscopic approach is increasingly preferred due to less postoperative pain, faster recovery, and shorter hospital stay [74, 75]. Even with oophoropexy, the ovaries are not without risk of damage, as they can still receive 8–15% of the prescribed dose of radiation due to scatter and transmission through a pelvic shield [76,77].

Methods to assess success of oophoropexy vary. Scant data exist regarding pregnancy rates and outcomes in those attempting pregnancy after oophoropexy and subsequent pelvic radiotherapy for CRC. Spontaneous pregnancies following ovarian transposition in patients with CRC have been reported, although the cases are exceedingly limited [78]. A series of 11 women who underwent ovarian transposition prior to pelvic radiotherapy for Hodgkin's lymphoma reported 14 pregnancies among the 11 women, with 12 live births [79]. Separate meta-analyses have reported that ovarian transposition in women younger than 40 years is associated with an 70–88.6% chance of fertility preservation [80, 81]. Once the ovaries are mobilized out of the pelvis, future conception may require an abdominal approach to access the ovaries for assisted reproductive technologies or a second surgery to restore the ovaries to their original anatomic position.

Uterine Transposition and Fixation

Ovarian transposition may move the ovaries out of the radiation field but still leave the uterus vulnerable to radiotoxicity. An emerging fertility-sparing technique is uterine transposition and fixation [82]. Uterine transposition involves repositioning the uterus into the upper abdomen to avoid radiation exposure and then repositioning it in the pelvis after treatment [83, 84]. This surgery can be performed laparoscopically and involves transecting the round ligament at the pelvic sidewall, separating the broad ligament, ligating the uterine arteries, and separating the cervix from the vagina. The uterus is then transposed to the upper abdomen and fixed to the anterior abdominal wall, followed by attaching the cervix to the fascia near an umbilical incision. While the technique for uterine transposition has been demonstrated, it is considered experimental and data regarding subsequent pregnancy outcomes are exceedingly limited.

Ovarian Suppression

Gonadotropin-releasing hormone (GnRH) agonists, such as leuprolide acetate, are often used as a means of fertility preservation in patients with cancer who are undergoing chemotherapy. Several mechanisms have been proposed by which GnRH agonists may be protective of fertility, including FSH suppression leading to a decreased number of primordial follicles entering development, hypoestrogenism causing a decrease in ovarian perfusion and therefore lower exposure of the ovaries to cytotoxic chemotherapeutic agents, and a direct effect on the ovary that protects the germline stem cells [85, 86]. Despite these proposed mechanisms, GnRH use has not been definitively shown to improve fertility outcomes and remains controversial [87]. A meta-analysis of 11 RCTs with 1,062 participants demonstrated a greater number of women treated with a GnRH agonist resumed menses after chemotherapy (pooled OR 2.57, 95% CI 1.65, 4.01), but subgroup analysis failed to show a difference in spontaneous pregnancy rates between those who did and did not receive GnRH agonist during chemotherapy (pooled OR 1.77, 95% CI 0.92, 3.40) [88]. Most of the research assessing GnRH agonists as a protective agent has been performed in women with breast cancer. Consequently, the most recent ASCO guidelines from 2018 recommend that patients be offered GnRH agonist treatment if there is high likelihood of chemotherapy-induced ovarian failure; however, patients should be extensively counseled regarding the conflicting data of its efficacy, and GnRH agonists should not be used to replace other proven fertility preservation methods [7].

Although GnRH agonists are most commonly employed for gonadal protection in this patient population, they (in addition to medroxyprogesterone or oral contraceptives) may be used for menstrual suppression during cancer treatments [89, 90]. For hematologic malignancies, avoiding menses is of central importance given the bleeding risks associated with thrombocytopenia. Importantly, menstrual suppression with GnRH agonist therapy is not a reliable form of contraceptive and additional protection against pregnancy should be administered throughout chemotherapy treatment. Multiple contraceptive options are available, depending on the type of malignancy and hormone sensitivity, including barrier contraception, intrauterine device with or without progestin, implants or oral medications (see Chapter 6 for further discussion).

GnRH agonist treatment ideally should begin before the initiation of chemotherapy for best efficacy [85, 86] and can be administered in monthly doses or every 12 weeks via intramuscular injections (Table 1.2). A moderate or heavy menses can occur approximately two weeks after the first injection. This can be alleviated by initiating combination oral contraceptive pills at the same time as the leuprolide. Patients with central nervous system tumors are recommended to avoid use of GnRH agonists due to alteration in the seizure threshold associated with this medication [89]. For patients with breast cancer, the initial administration of medication may result in worsening of cancer symptoms due to a transient increase in estradiol production (i.e. "flare effect") resulting in bone pain or

Table 1.2 Dosing of menstrual suppression therapies

Therapy	Dosage
Progestin only – Oral Therapy	
Medroxyprogesterone acetate	10–20 mg/day
Norethindrone acetate	5–15 mg/day
Drospirenone	4 mg/day
Norethindrone	0.35 mg/day
Gonadotropin-releasing hormone agonists – Injection Therapy	
Goserelin acetate	3.6 mg/28 days
Leuprolide acetate	3.75 mg/month or 11.25 mg/3 months

neuropathies. Patients with vertebral bone lesions should be monitored carefully for signs of spinal cord compression [89]. In patients with thrombocytopenia, the medication may be administered subcutaneously in lieu of the intramuscular injection. Platelet levels of $\geq 50,000$ are recommended for intramuscular administration [90]. GnRHa therapy induces a hypoestrogenic state within two weeks of initiation, and the most common adverse side effects are bone density loss with long-term use and vasomotor symptoms.

Fertility Preservation: Assisted Reproductive Technology (ART)

Oocyte and Embryo Cryopreservation

Current established methods of fertility preservation in postpubertal females include oocyte, embryo, and ovarian tissue cryopreservation. Oocyte and/or embryo cryopreservation are the most established, successful methods of preserving fertility and require an approximate two-week window prior to the initiation of cancer treatments. Typically, 8–12 days of recombinant FSH and luteinizing hormone (LH) are administered to facilitate oocyte recruitment and development followed by transvaginal oocyte harvest. Transvaginal aspiration of the oocytes is a thirty-minute outpatient procedure often performed under conscious sedation. Once the oocytes are harvested, they are assessed for maturity and either cryopreserved as oocytes, or fertilized, cultured and cryopreserved as embryos. Oocyte and/or embryo cryopreservation also allow the opportunity for preimplantation genetic testing (PGT) of embryos for monogenic disorders, which is particularly relevant for those with hereditary cancer.

Random-start IVF protocols allow a patient to initiate fertility treatment immediately regardless of menstrual cycle phase. Random start protocols have been shown to produce similar oocyte and embryo yields when compared to traditional follicular (early menstrual cycle) phase protocols [91]. A recent comparison of live birth rates between cryopreserved oocytes and embryos revealed a slightly lower survival rate for thawed oocytes than embryos (79.1% versus 90.1%), but similar fertilization rates (76.2% versus 72.8%), clinical pregnancy rates (26.5% versus 30%) and live birth rates (25% versus 25.1%) [92]. Given the high circulating estradiol levels that result from fertility medications, and the concern for stimulating estrogen-sensitive tumors, ovarian stimulation protocols have been developed that utilize anti-estrogenic drugs, such as letrozole, to minimize estradiol levels [93]. In addition, careful monitoring is required during ART to avoid complications such as ovarian hyperstimulation syndrome which could further delay cancer treatment.

Ovarian Tissue Cryopreservation

Despite the current use of random start protocols, women diagnosed with cancer who wish to preserve their fertility through embryo or oocyte cryopreservation still require a two-week timeframe to complete a treatment cycle. Ovarian tissue cryopreservation (OTC) exists as an option specifically for patients in whom oocyte harvest is unfeasible due to time constraints and/or for prepubertal females. Previously, OTC was considered an experimental fertility preservation option, but ASRM removed its experimental label in 2019.

Ovarian tissue cryopreservation typically involves laparoscopic removal of a portion of one or both ovaries and then the tissue is sectioned into strips of tissue less than 2 mm thick and cryopreserved [94]. This procedure can often be coordinated with other planned surgeries such as port or central line placement, tumor resection, or bone marrow aspiration, particularly in the prepubertal or pediatric population [95]. The ovarian tissue is then subsequently reimplanted to the patient following completion of treatment with gonado-toxic agents. Transplantation may be performed in an orthotopic manner by reimplantation into the pelvis which is preferable, or a heterotopic (extra pelvic) manner with transplantation to the forearm or abdominal wall [96].

In a 2017 review, just over 130 live births were documented from OTC and reimplantation [97–100]. A more recent study, published in 2021, reported an additional 95 healthy newborns from a cohort of 285 women who underwent OTC with ovarian tissue transplantation. In this same study by Dolmans et al. ovarian tissue transplantation restored endocrine function in 88.7% (181/204) of patients [101]. Ovarian function typically returns within 4.5 +/- 2.2 months post-tissue transplant and lasts an average of five years. Pregnancy success rates range from 23–40% in most reports [100–102]. Of the births and pregnancies where data was available, the conception rate is comparable between those who spontaneously conceived and those that underwent in vitro fertilization.

Although data is limited, there are concerns with the cost of OTC as a surgical option for fertility preservation. The incurred costs are often higher than oocyte cryopreservation, particularly when considering the additional costs of reimplantation of the previously cryopreserved tissue.

There are also specific ethical issues involved when completing fertility preservation in the prepubertal or pediatric population. Minors do not have the ability to truly "consent" for a procedure but instead can only "assent." Although parents most often have their child's best interest at heart, there can be discrepancy in future reproductive desires. Additional complex challenges with OTC are chain of custody for the tissue if the patient does not survive. The legal system in the United States has identified gametes as "property"; however, cryopreserved ovarian tissue is an organ rather than a gamete. This is a legal area which is largely unexplored and is currently being handled on an individual basis [103].

Another concern regarding ovarian tissue transplantation in oncology patients is the risk of reintroduction of malignant cells [104]. In patients with leukemia, ovarian tissue transplantation is not recommended as harvested ovarian tissue can demonstrate infiltration with leukemic cells. In patients with active leukemia, immunohistochemical and genetic markers have been utilized to determine the presence of malignant cells in cryopreserved ovarian tissue through polymerase chain reaction (PCR)-based platforms [105]. In other cancer types, such as breast cancer, PCR testing did not detect malignant cells in ovarian tissue [106]. These findings suggest that PCR testing of ovarian tissue prior to reintroduction may be an option. However, the presence of malignant cells through PCR testing in ovarian cortex tissue previously cryopreserved does not appear to fully determine the malignant potential of those cells when reimplanted. At a minimum, histological examination of the cryopreserved ovarian tissue prior to reimplantation is recommended [107]. To avoid the risk of reimplantation of occult tumor cells, in vitro maturation (IVM) techniques hold future promise in the ability to mature oocytes from ovarian tissue ex vivo. In vitro maturation would avoid the need for a reimplantation procedure, however, such technology is not yet widely available [101].

Third Party Reproduction and Adoption

For those unable to conceive with their own oocytes, third party reproductive options, such as oocyte donation, embryo donation, gestational surrogacy, or child adoption, should be offered. Patients can work with a fertility specialist or adoption agency to pursue their desired options for family-building. Donor and gestational carrier agencies can help patients access donor oocytes, embryos, or gestational carriers based on their needs with regard to family-building. Fertility specialists can facilitate gamete donation using known or anonymous donors. There are specific FDA-regulated requirements for all third-party reproduction, including infectious disease testing of donors and quarantine of certain donor samples. Over 60% of cancer survivors state a willingness to adopt if they could not have a biological child; adoption agencies assist with child adoption and foster-to-adopt programs [5]. Counseling with a mental health professional with expertise in third-party reproduction is recommended. In addition to addressing the psychosocial impact associated with cancer-related infertility, this counseling can help patients process the family-building options available to them if they are unable to have a genetic child or carry a pregnancy.

Safety of Assisted Reproductive Technology in Patients with Cancer

Ovarian Stimulation

To develop multiple oocytes during oocyte or embryo banking cycles, recombinant FSH and LH are administered for approximately 8–12 days. During this 8–12-day window, estradiol levels are supraphysiologic often peaking in the range of 1500–3000 pg/ml. For patients with hormonally sensitive or responsive tumors, this supraphysiologic estradiol exposure has presented concerns for increased tumor recurrence/growth. However, adjuncts can be utilized to decrease plasma levels of estradiol throughout fertility treatment. Most commonly, aromatase inhibitors such as letrozole, are given throughout the stimulation to suppress estrogen levels. In the setting of fertility preservation, adding letrozole to gonadotropins during ovarian stimulation decreases serum estradiol levels to a physiologic range without compromising oocyte or embryo outcomes [108]. Other alternatives include natural cycle IVF (no exogenous gonadotropin exposure), which has high cancellation rates and low oocyte yield, or tamoxifen with or without gonadotropins exposure.

Ovarian stimulation for purposes of oocyte or embryo cryopreservation takes approximately two weeks, specifically with random-start protocols. Patients have expressed concern that fertility preservation would negatively impact their outcomes due to delaying the start of treatment, and providers often lack knowledge on the length of time required for fertility preservation. When assessing time to chemotherapy initiation in breast cancer patients, those that underwent fertility preservation started chemotherapy at the same time interval as those that declined fertility preservation [109]. Understanding that each cancer diagnosis is unique with regard to time to treatment, with few exceptions, the time required for fertility preservation treatment is often allowable.

Safety of Gonadotropin Exposure and Timing of Subsequent Pregnancy

There does not appear to be an increased risk of cancer recurrence in those who receive fertility medication before, during, or after their cancer treatment, although long-term data are limited [110]. Patients are often counseled to wait at least two years following cancer diagnosis to attempt conception as the vast majority of recurrences will occur within the first two years of diagnosis and treatment [111]. For patients with hormonally responsive breast cancer, adjuvant endocrine therapy, such as tamoxifen, GnRH agonists, and aromatase inhibitors are often recommended for up to 10 years. For women who would like to conceive prior to the completion of endocrine therapy, many clinicians have recommended a "drug holiday" after completion of two years to allow for conception efforts. Recent results of the POSITIVE study (Pregnancy Outcome and Safety of Interrupting Therapy for Women with Endocrine Responsive Breast Cancer) demonstrated that women with early-stage breast cancer who interrupted endocrine therapy had the same breast cancer free interval as women that did not [112]. The median age for this patient sample was 37 years and all received endocrine therapy for at least 18 months but no more than 30 months. Other considerations when planning subsequent conception include overall risk of recurrence, health status including cardiovascular risk profile, adjuvant treatment length, residual fertility, and patient age at delivery.

Resources for Fertility Preservation

There are a variety of resources for patients seeking more information regarding cancer related fertility preservation. The Oncofertility Consortium website (https://oncoferti lity.msu.edu) provides a resource browser with over 300 patient facing materials on fertility preservation options for both men and women. Additionally, the website also offers access to a clinical navigator through their FertLine in order to locate the closest medical program that can offer fertility services for the patient. Oncofertility Consortium also sponsors SaveMyFertility (www.savemyfertility.org) – an online fertility toolkit for patients and providers. This website provides patient and provider pocket guides with counseling information on fertility preservation resources. Further, these materials are available in multiple languages and the brochures can be downloaded for reading and distribution.

Livestrong Fertility (www.livestrong.org/) provides patients with supportive measures such as access to community programs that discuss the daily struggles cancer patients may face and day-to-day concerns of survivors. Additionally, Livestrong Fertility has a dedicated program to provide financial support for patients pursuing fertility preservation and offers a guidebook to help patients and survivors navigate both emotional and physical needs throughout their cancer journey.

The Young Survival Coalition (https://youngsurvival.org) is a resource targeted to the unique needs of young women with breast cancer; specifically postdiagnosis fertility concerns. This platform offers patients a rich online community of support groups and discussion boards as well as educational materials for survivors. The American Society for Clinical Oncology (ASCO) shares its detailed guidelines and recommendations via its online platform at Cancer Net (www.cancer.net). This resource provides educational materials and support to cancer patients and their caregivers to help them make informed decisions on their therapy and future fertility. Other useful organizations include Chick Mission (www.thechickmission.org), Alliance for Fertility Preservation (www.allianceforfer tilitypreservation.org), American Society for Reproductive Medicine (www.reproductive facts.org) and Stupid Cancer (https://stupidcancer.org).

Conclusion

Approximately 10% of women diagnosed with cancer are of reproductive age, and future childbearing is a significant survivorship issue for many of them. Discussing their risk of cancer-related infertility as well as fertility preservation options will improve reproductive decision making and quality of life, while decreasing distress and long-term regret.

Case Resolution

J.T. reports regular menses with no prior fertility evaluation or treatment. She is not currently in a committed relationship and is inquiring about options for fertility preservation. Baseline ovarian reserve testing was obtained and found to be reassuring with an AMH of 1.2 ng/mL (normal 1.0–4.5 ng/mL) and an antral follicle count of 14 (normal greater than 7). In light of her advanced maternal age, treatment-related delay of pregnancy, and the potential for gonadotoxic adjuvant therapy, oocyte cryopreservation was recommended. Financial resources were provided and the logistics of a typical cycle were reviewed.

J.T. underwent a left lumpectomy with sentinel lymph node biopsy. Surgical pathology revealed an intraductal carcinoma measuring 2.5 cm, with mucinous and micropapillary features grade 2. Micrometastases noted in one of six lymph nodes. Adjuvant therapy with localized radiation was recommended, followed by Adriamycin and Cytoxan every two weeks (x 4 cycles) then weekly paclitaxel (x 12 cycles). Treatment plan included monthly Zoladex for menstrual suppression during adjuvant chemotherapy. Endocrine therapy for a minimum of five years was anticipated.

Two weeks postoperatively J.T. initiated a random start oocyte cryopreservation treatment cycle. She utilized recombinant gonadotropins (FSH and LH) for 10 days with concomitant letrozole to attenuate her estradiol levels. Peak estradiol level during her stimulation was 214 pg/ml and 16 mature oocytes were harvested transvaginally.

Although 16 cryopreserved oocytes does not guarantee her a live birth, it will provide her with an additional option for future conception. Conception is more difficult at maternal age 40 or 41 compared to 38 and dose-dense chemotherapy protocols may induce more ovarian toxicity compared to traditional dosing regimens. Menstrual suppression with a GnRH agonist may attenuate chemotherapy-induced ovarian toxicity but data is mixed in regards to degree of benefit.

Effective nonhormonal contraception is recommended and repeat ovarian reserve testing was scheduled for 18 months after completion of chemotherapy. J.T. expressed that she was very thankful she underwent fertility preservation prior to chemotherapy start, and stated she felt hopeful and better prepared to manage her cancer treatment journey.

Take Home Points

- Approximately 10% of women diagnosed with cancer are of reproductive age.
- Concerns regarding future fertility are secondary only to concerns regarding survival for many young adult women diagnosed with cancer.
- Undergoing fertility preservation via oocyte or embryo banking takes approximately two weeks, which is allowable for the majority of cancer patients prior to initiation of cancer therapy.
- For prepubertal girls or women in which a two-week delay in cancer therapy is not appropriate, ovarian tissue cryopreservation can be considered.
- For patients with a known germline variant in a hereditary cancer gene, preimplantation genetic testing with IVF can be utilized to decrease the chance of an affected child.
- Aromatase inhibitors (letrozole) are recommended in conjunction with gonadotropin administration in women with endocrine responsive tumors undergoing fertility preservation.

- Baseline AMH and antral follicle counts correlate with number of oocytes procured with fertility preservation and can be employed for post-treatment assessment of ovarian reserve.

Reference

1. World Health Organization (WHO). Global Health Estimates 2020: Deaths by Cause, Age, Sex, by Country and by Region, 2000–2019. WHO; 2020. Accessed December 11, 2020. who.int/data/gho/data/themes/mortality-and-global-health-estimates/ghe-leading-causes-of-death

2. Miller, K. D., Fidler-Benaoudia, M., Keegan, T. H., et al. Cancer statistics for adolescents and young adults, 2020. *CA Cancer J Clin.* 2020;**70**:443–59. https://doi.org/10.3322/caac.21637

3. Loscalzo M. J., Clark K. L. The psychosocial context of cancer-related infertility. *Cancer Treat Res.* 2007;**138**:180–90.

4. Carvalho B. R., Kliemchen J., Woodruff T. K. Ethical, moral and other aspects related to fertility preservation in cancer patients. *JBRA Assist Reprod.* 2017;**21**:45–8.

5. Schover L. R., Rybicki L. A., Martin B. A., Bringelsen K. A. Having children after cancer. A pilot survey of survivors' attitudes and experiences. *Cancer.* 1999;**86**:697–709.

6. Ethics Committee of the American Society for Reproductive Medicine. Fertility preservation and reproduction in cancer patients. *Fertil Steril.* 2005;**83**:1622–8.

7. Oktay K., Harvey B. E., Partridge A. H., et al. Fertility preservation in patients with cancer: ASCO Clinical Practice Guideline Update. *J Clin Oncol.* 2018;**36**:1994–2001.

8. Chin H. B., Howards P. P., Kramer M. R., Mertens A. C., Spencer J. B. Which female cancer patients fail to receive fertility counseling before treatment in the state of Georgia? *Fertil Steril.* 2016;**106**:1763–71.e1.

9. Benedict C., Thom B., Friedman D., et al. Young adult female cancer survivors' unmet information needs and reproductive concerns contribute to decisional conflict regarding posttreatment fertility preservation. *Cancer.* 2016;**122**:2101–9.

10. Niemasik E. E., Letourneau J., Dohan D., et al. Patient perceptions of reproductive health counseling at the time of cancer diagnosis: a qualitative study of female California cancer survivors. *J Cancer Surviv.* 2012;**6**:324–32.

11. Armuand G. M., Rodriguez-Wallberg KA, Wettergren L, et al. Sex differences in fertility-related information received by young adult cancer survivors. *J Clin Oncol.* 2012;**30**:2147–53.

12. Gorman J. R., Bailey S., Pierce J. P., Su H. I. How do you feel about fertility and parenthood? The voices of young female cancer survivors. *J Cancer Surviv.* 2012;**6**:200–09.

13. Letourneau J. M., Ebbel E. E., Katz P. P., et al. Pretreatment fertility counseling and fertility preservation improve quality of life in reproductive age women with cancer. *Cancer.* 2012;**118**:1710–17.

14. Deshpande N. A., Braun I. M., Meyer F. L. Impact of fertility preservation counseling and treatment on psychological outcomes among women with cancer: a systematic review. *Cancer.* 2015;**121**:3938–47.

15. Benedict C., Thom B., Kelvin J. F. Young adult female cancer survivors' decision regret about fertility preservation. *J Adolesc Young Adult Oncol.* 2015;**4**:213–18.

16. Woodruff T., Snyder K. *Oncofertility: fertility preservation for cancer survivors.* Springer Science and Business Media. October 30, 2007.

17. American Cancer Society. How cancer treatments can affect fertility in women. June 28, 2017. www.cancer.org/treatment/treatments-and-side-effects/physicalside-effects/fertility-and-sexual-side-effects/fertility-andwomen-with-cancer/how-cancer-treatments-affect-fertility.html. Accessed March 24, 2018.

18. Madanat L. M., Malila N., Dyba T., et al. Probability of parenthood after early onset cancer: a population-based study. *International Journal of Cancer.* 2008;**123** 2891–8.

19. Magelssen H., Melve K. K., Skjaerven R., Fossa S. D. Parenthood probability and pregnancy outcome in patients with a cancer diagnosis during adolescence and young adulthood. *Hum Reprod.* 2008;**23**:178–86.

20. Infertility workup for the women's health specialist: ACOG Committee Opinion, Number 781. *Obstet. Gynecol* 2019;**133**: e377–84.

21. Landersoe S. K., Larsen E. C., Forman J. L., et al. Ovarian reserve markers and endocrine profile during oral contraception: is there a link between the degree of ovarian suppression and AMH? *Gynecol Endocrinol* 2020;**36**:1090–5.

22. Hariton E., Shirazi T. N., Douglas N. C., et al. Anti-Müllerian hormone levels among contraceptive users: evidence from a cross-sectional cohort of 27,125 individuals. *Am J Obstet Gynecol* 2021;**225**:515.e1–10.

23. Dezellus A., Barriere P., Campone M., et al. Prospective evaluation of serum anti-Müllerian hormone dynamics in 250 women of reproductive age treated with chemotherapy for breast cancer. *Eur J Cancer.* 2017;**79**:72–80.

24. Anderson R. A., Cameron D. A. Pretreatment serum anti-müllerian hormone predicts long-term ovarian function and bone mass after chemotherapy for early breast cancer. *J Clin Endocrinol Metab.* 2011;**96**:1336–43.

25. Rosendahl M., Andersen C. Y., la Cour Freieslesen N., et al. Dynamics and mechanisms of chemotherapy-induced ovarian follicular depletion in women of fertile age. *Fertil Steril.* 2010;**94**:156–66.

26. Dillon K. E., Sammel M. D., Prewitt M., et al. Pretreatment antimüllerian hormone levels determine rate of posttherapy ovarian reserve recovery: acute changes in ovarian reserve during and after chemotherapy. *Fertil Steril.* 2013;**99**:477–83.

27. Goswami M., Nikolaou D., Level IAMH. Is AMH level, independent of age, a predictor of live birth in IVF? *J Hum Reprod Sci* 2017;**10**:24–30.

28. Zarek S. M., Mitchell E. M., Sjaarda L. A., et al. Is anti-Müllerian hormone associated with fecundability? Findings from the EAGeR trial. *J Clin Endocrinol Metab* 2015;**100**:4215–21.

29. Nelson L. M. Clinical practice: primary ovarian insufficiency. *N Engl J Med* 2009;**360**:606–14.

30. De Vos M., Devroey P., Fauser B. C. Primary ovarian insufficiency. *Lancet* 2010;**376**:911–21.

31. Schüring A. N., Fehm T., Behringer K., et al. Practical recommendations for fertility preservation in women by the FertiPROTEKT network: Part I: indications for fertility preservation. *Arch Gynecol Obstet.* 2018;**297**:241–55.

32. Wan J., Gai Y., Li G., Tao Z., Zhang Z. Incidence of chemotherapyand chemoradiotherapy-induced amenorrhea in premenopausal women with stage II/III colorectal cancer. *Clin Colorectal Cancer.* 2015;**14**:31–4.

33. Dolmans M. M. Recent advances in fertility preservation and counseling for female cancer patients. *Expert Rev Anticancer Ther.* 2018;**18**:115–20.

34. Bedoschi G., Navarro P. A., Oktay K. Chemotherapy-induced damage to ovary: mechanisms and clinical impact. *Future Oncol* 2016;**12**:2333–44.

35. Reynolds A. C., McKenzie L. J. Cancer treatment-related ovarian dysfunction in women of childbearing potential: management and fertility preservation options. *J Clin Oncol.* 2023;JCO2201885. doi: 10.1200/JCO.22.01885.

36. Mauri D., Gazouli I., Zarkavelis G., et al. Chemotherapy associated ovarian failure. *Front Endocrinol (Lausanne)* 2020;**11**:572388.

37. Arian S. E., Goodman L., Flyckt R. L., Falcone T. Ovarian transposition: a surgical option for fertility preservation. *Fertil Steril.* 2017;**107**:e15.

38. Shandley L. M., McKenzie L. J. Recent advances in fertility preservation and counseling for reproductive-age women with colorectal cancer: a systematic review. *Dis Colon Rectum* 2019;**62**:762–71.

39. Darzy K. H., Shalet S. M. Hypopituitarism following radiotherapy revisited. *Endocr Dev.* 2009;**15**:1–24.

40. Teh W. T., Stern C., Chander S., Hickey M. The impact of uterine radiation on subsequent fertility and pregnancy outcomes. *Biomed Res Int.* 2014;**2014**:482968.

41. Barton S., Najita J., Ginsburg E., et al. Infertility, infertility treatment, and achievement of pregnancy in female survivors of childhood cancer: a report from the Childhood Cancer Survivor Study cohort. *Lancet Oncol* 2013;**14**:873–81.

42. Azem F., Amit A., Merimsky O., Lessing J. B. Successful transfer of frozen-thawed embryos obtained after subtotal colectomy for colorectal cancer and before fluorouracil-based chemotherapy. *Gynecol Oncol.* 2004;**93**:263–5.

43. WHO Drug Information, Safety and Efficacy Issues. Safety and Efficacy Issues, 2011:364–5.

44. U.S. BL 125085 Supplement, *AVASTIN (bevacizumab). AVASTIN (bevacizumab).* Genentech, Inc; 2011.

45. Kerr J. B., Hutt K. J., Cook M., et al. Cisplatin-induced primordial follicle oocyte killing and loss of fertility are not prevented by imatinib. *Nat Med.* 2012;**18** (8):1170–72; author reply 1172–4.

46. Salem W., Ho J. R., Woo I., et al. Long-term imatinib diminishes ovarian reserve and impacts embryo quality. *J Assist Reprod Genet.* 2020;**37**(6):1459–66.

47. Braun M., Young J., Reiner C. S., et al. Low-dose oral sirolimus and the risk of menstrual-cycle disturbances and ovarian cysts: analysis of the randomized controlled SUISSE ADPKD trial. *PLoS One.* 2012;**7**(10):e45868.

48. Leitao M. M., Kehoe S., Barakat R. R., et al. Comparison of D&C and office endometrial biopsy accuracy in patients with FIGO grade 1 endometrial adenocarcinoma. *Gynecol Oncol* 2009;**113**:105–08.

49. Falcone F., Leone Roberti Maggiore U., Di Donato V., et al. Fertility-sparing treatment for intramucous, moderately differentiated, endometrioid endometrial cancer: a Gynecologic Cancer Inter-Group (GCIG) study. *J Gynecol Oncol* 2020;**31**:1–13.

50. Obermair A., Janda M., Baker J., et al. Improved surgical safety after laparoscopic compared to open surgery for apparent early stage endometrial cancer: results from a randomised controlled trial. *Eur J Cancer* 2012;**48**:1147–53.

51. Gunderson C. C., Fader A. N., Carson K. A., et al. Oncologic and reproductive outcomes with progestin therapy in women with endometrial hyperplasia and grade 1 adenocarcinoma: a systematic review. *Gynecol Oncol* 2012;**125**: 477–82.

52. Ushijima K., Yahata H., Yoshikawa H., et al. Multicenter phase II study of fertility-sparing treatment with medroxyprogesterone acetate for endometrial carcinoma and atypical hyperplasia in young women. *J Clin Oncol* 2007;**25**:2798–803.

53. Simpson A. N., Feigenberg T., Clarke B. A., et al. Fertility sparing treatment of complex atypical hyperplasia and low grade endometrial cancer using oral progestin. *Gynecol Oncol* 2014;**133**:229–33.

54. Ramirez P. T., Frumovitz M., Bodurka D. C., et al. Hormonal therapy for the management of grade 1 endometrial adenocarcinoma: a literature review. *Gynecol Oncol* 2004;**95**:133–8.

55. Matsuo K., Machida H., Shoupe D., et al. Ovarian conservation and overall survival in young women with early-stage low-

grade endometrial cancer. *Obstet Gynecol* 2016;**128**:761–70.

56. Prepregnancy counseling: ACOG Committee Opinion Number 762; *Obstet Gynecol* 2019;**133**:e78–89.

57. Cervical cancer – cancer STAT facts, (n.d.). https://seer.cancer.gov/statfacts/html/cervix.html. Accessed October 13, 2020.

58. Koh W. J., Abu-Rustum N. R., Bean S., et al. Cervical cancer, version 3.2019, JNCCN J. *Natl. Compr. Cancer Netw* 2019;**17**: 64–84.

59. Machida H., Iwata T., Okugawa K., et al. Fertility-sparing trachelectomy for early-stage cervical cancer: a proposal of an ideal candidate. *Gynecol Oncol* 2020;**156**:341–8.

60. Sonoda Y., Abu-Rustum N. R., Gemignani M. L., et al. A fertility-sparing alternative to radical hysterectomy: how many patients may be eligible? *Gynecol Oncol* 2004;**95**:534–8.

61. Zhang Q., Li W., Kanis M. J., et al. Oncologic and obstetrical outcomes with fertility-sparing treatment of cervical cancer: a systematic review and meta-analysis. *Oncotarget* 2017;**8**:46580–92.

62. Prodromidou A., Iavazzo C., Fotiou A., et al. Short- and long-term outcomes after abdominal radical trachelectomy versus radical hysterectomy for early stage cervical cancer: a systematic review of the literature and meta-analysis. *Arch Gynecol Obstet* 2019;**300**:25–31.

63. Bentivegna E., Maulard A., Pautier P., et al. Fertility results and pregnancy outcomes after conservative treatment of cervical cancer: a systematic review of the literature. *Fertil Steril* 2016;**106**:1195–211.

64. Plante M., Gregoire J., Renaud M.-C., et al. The vaginal radical trachelectomy: an update of a series of 125 cases and 106 pregnancies. *Gynecol Oncol* 2011;**121**: 290–97.

65. Shah J. S., Jooya N. D., Woodard T. L., et al. Reproductive counseling and pregnancy outcomes after radical trachelectomy for early stage cervical cancer. *J Gynecol Oncol* 2019;**30**:1–10.

66. Ovarian cancer – cancer STAT facts, (n.d.). https://seer.cancer.gov/statfacts/html/ovary.html. Accessed October 18, 2020.

67. Hanatani M., Yoshikawa N., Yoshida K., et al. Impact of age on clinicopathological features and survival of epithelial ovarian neoplasms in reproductive age. *Int J Clin Oncol* 2020;**25**:187–94.

68. Shah J. S., Mackelvie M., Gershenson D. M., et al. Accuracy of intraoperative frozen section diagnosis of borderline ovarian tumors by hospital type. *J Minim Invasive Gynecol* 2019;**26**:87–93.

69. Park J. Y., Lee S. H., Kim K. R., et al. Accuracy of frozen section diagnosis and factors associated with final pathological diagnosis upgrade of mucinous ovarian tumors. *J Gynecol Oncol* 2019;**30**:1–10.

70. Johansen G., Dahm-Kähler P., Staf C., et al. Fertility-sparing surgery for treatment of non-epithelial ovarian cancer: oncological and reproductive outcomes in a prospective nationwide population-based cohort study. *Gynecol Oncol* 2019;**155**:287–93.

71. Sinno A. K., Fader A. N., Roche K. L., et al. A comparison of colorimetric versus fluorometric sentinel lymph node mapping during robotic surgery for endometrial cancer. *Gynecol Oncol* 2014;**134**:281–6.

72. Fruscio R., Ceppi L., Corso S., et al. Long-term results of fertility-sparing treatment compared with standard radical surgery for early-stage epithelial ovarian cancer. *Br J Cancer* 2016;**115**:641–8.

73. Melamed A., Rizzo A. E., Nitecki R., et al. All-cause mortality after fertility-sparing surgery for stage I epithelial ovarian cancer. *Obstet Gynecol* 2017;**130**:71–9.

74. Ben-Aharon I., Granot T., Meizner I., et al. Long-term follow-up of chemotherapy-induced ovarian failure in young breast cancer patients: the role of vascular toxicity. *Oncologist.* 2015;**20**:985–91.

75. Kye B. H., Cho H. M. Overview of radiation therapy for treating rectal cancer. *Ann Coloproctol.* 2014;**30**:165–74.

76. Tulandi T., Al-Took S. Laparoscopic ovarian suspension before irradiation. *Fertil Steril.* 1998;**70**:381–3.

77. Wo J. Y., Viswanathan A. N. Impact of radiotherapy on fertility, pregnancy, and neonatal outcomes in female cancer patients. *Int J Radiat Oncol Biol Phys.* 2009;**73**:1304–12.

78. Farber L. A., Ames J. W., Rush S., Gal D. Laparoscopic ovarian transposition to preserve ovarian function before pelvic radiation and chemotherapy in a young patient with rectal cancer. *MedGenMed.* 2005;7:66.

79. Terenziani M., Piva L., Meazza C., Gandola L., Cefalo G., Merola M. Oophoropexy: a relevant role in preservation of ovarian function after pelvic irradiation. *Fertil Steril.* 2009;**91**:935.e15–935.e16.

80. Bisharah M., Tulandi T. Laparoscopic preservation of ovarian function: an underused procedure. *Am J Obstet Gynecol.* 2003;**188**:367–70.

81. Iwase A., Nakamura T., Nakahara T., Goto M., Kikkawa F. AntiMüllerian hormone and assessment of ovarian reserve after ovarian toxic treatment: a systematic narrative review. *Reprod Sci.* 2015;**22**:519–26.

82. Köhler C., Marnitz S., Biel P., Cordes T. Successful delivery in a 39-year-old patient with anal cancer after fertility-preserving surgery followed by primary chemoradiation and low antiMullerian hormone level. *Oncology.* 2016;**91**:295–8.

83. Mossa B., Schimberni M., Di Benedetto L., Mossa S. Ovarian transposition in young women and fertility sparing. *Eur Rev Med Pharmacol Sci.* 2015;**19**:3418–25.

84. Nezhat F., Falik R. Cancer and uterine preservation: a first step toward preserving fertility after pelvic radiation. *Fertil Steril.* 2017;**108**:240–41.

85. Harada M., Osuga Y. Fertility preservation for female cancer patients. *Int J Clin Oncol.* 2019;**24**:28–33.

86. Chen H., Li J., Cui T., Hu L. Adjuvant gonadotropin-releasing hormone analogues for the prevention of chemotherapy induced premature ovarian failure in premenopausal women. *Cochrane Database Syst Rev.* 2011;(**11**): CD008018.

87. Bildik G., Akin N., Senbabaoglu F., et al. GnRH agonist leuprolide acetate does not confer any protection against ovarian damage induced by chemotherapy and radiation in vitro. *Hum Reprod.* 2015;**30**:2912–25.

88. Shen Y. W., Zhang X. M., Lv M., et al. Utility of gonadotropin releasing hormone agonists for prevention of chemotherapy induced ovarian damage in premenopausal women with breast cancer: a systematic review and meta-analysis. *Onco Targets Ther.* 2015;**8**:3349–59.

89. Coccia P. F., Pappo A. S., Beaupin L., et al. Adolescent and young adult oncology, version 2.2018, NCCN clinical practice guidelines in oncology. *J Natl Compr Canc Netw* 2018;**16**:66–97.

90. Primary ovarian insufficiency in adolescents and young women. ACOG Committee Opinion Number 605. *Obstet Gynecol* 2014;**124**:193–7.

91. Cakmak H., Rosen M. P. Random-start ovarian stimulation in patients with cancer. *Curr Opin Obstet Gynecol* 2015;**27**:215–21.

92. Ho J. R., Woo I., Louie K., et al. A comparison of live birth rates and perinatal outcomes between cryopreserved oocytes and cryopreserved embryos. *J Assist Reprod Genet* 2017;**34**:1359–66.

93. Oktay K., Buyuk E., Libertella N., et al. Fertility preservation in breast cancer patients: a prospective controlled comparison of ovarian stimulation with tamoxifen and letrozole for embryo cryopreservation. *J Clin Oncol* 2005;**23**:4347–53.

94. Practice Committee of American Society for Reproductive Medicine. Fertility preservation in patients undergoing gonadotoxic therapy or gonadectomy: a committee opinion. *Fertil Steril.* 2019;**112**:1022–33.

95. Smith K. L., Gracia C., Sokalska A., Moore H. Advances in Fertility Preservation for Young Women With Cancer. *American*

Society of Clinical Oncology Educational Book 38. 2018. 27–37.

96. Fritz MA, Speroff L. *Clinical Gynecologic Endocrinology and Infertility*. 8th ed. Wolters Kluwer Health; 2011.

97. Kihara K., Yamamoto S., Ohshiro T., Fujita S. Laparoscopic ovarian transposition prior to pelvic irradiation in a young female patient with advanced rectal cancer. *Surg Case Rep*. 2015;**1**:113.

98. Donnez J., Dolmans M. M. Fertility preservation in women. *N Engl J Med*. 2017;**377**(17):1657–65.

99. Wallace W. H., Smith A. G., Kelsey T. W., Edgar A. E., Anderson R. A. Fertility preservation for girls and young women with cancer: population-based validation of criteria for ovarian tissue cryopreservation. *Lancet Oncol*. 2014;**15**:1129–36.

100. Gellert S. E., Pors S. E., Kristensen S. G., et al. Transplantation of frozen-thawed ovarian tissue: an update on worldwide activity published in peer-reviewed papers and on the Danish cohort. *J Assist Reprod Genet*. 2018;**35**:561–70.

101. Dolmans M. M., von Wolff M., Poirot C., et al. Transplantation of cryopreserved ovarian tissue in a series of 285 women: a review of five leading European centers. *Fertil Steril*. 2021;**115**(5):1102–15. doi: 10.1016/j.fertnstert.2021.03.008. PMID: 33933173.

102. Fisch B., Abir R. Female fertility preservation: past, present and future. *Reproduction*. 2018;**156**:F11–F27.

103. Resetkova N., Hayashi M., Kolp L. A., Christianson M. S. Fertility preservation for prepubertal girls: update and current challenges. *Curr Obstet Gynecol Rep*. 2013;**2**(4):218–25. doi: 10.1007/s13669-013-0060-9. PMID: 25110617; PMCID: PMC4125124.

104. Dolmans M. M., Luyckx V., Donnez J., Andersen C. Y., Greve T. Risk of transferring malignant cells with transplanted frozen-thawed ovarian tissue. *Fertil Steril*. 2013;**99**:1514–22.

105. Rosendahl M., Andersen M. T., Ralfkiær E., et al., Evidence of residual disease in cryopreserved ovarian cortex from female patients with leukemia. *Fertility and Sterility* 2010;**94**(6):2186–90.

106. Rosendahl M., Wielenga V. T., Nedergaard L., et al. Cryopreservation of ovarian tissue for fertility preservation: no evidence of malignant cell contamination in ovarian tissue from patients with breast cancer. *Fertility and Sterility* 2011;**95**(6): 2158–61.

107. Rosendahl M., Greve T., Andersen C. Y. The safety of transplanting cryopreserved ovarian tissue in cancer patients: a review of the literature. *J Assist Reprod Genet*. 2013;**30**(1):11–24. doi: 10.1007/s10815-012-9912-x. Epub 2012 Dec 22. PMID: 23263841; PMCID: PMC3553351.

108. Cakmak H., Rose M. P. Ovarian stimulation in cancer patients. *Fertility and Sterility* 2013;**99**(6):1476–84.

109. Kitano A, Shimizu C, Yamauchi H, et al. Factors associated with treatment delay in women with primary breast cancer who were referred to reproductive specialists. *ESMO Open*. 2019;**4**(2):e000459. doi: 10.1136/esmoopen-2018-000459. PMID: 30962960; PMCID: PMC6435250.

110. Practice Committee of the American Society for Reproductive Medicine. Fertility preservation in patients undergoing gonadotoxic therapy or gonadectomy: a Committee opinion. *Fertil Steril* 2019;**112**:1022–33.

111. Srikanthan A., Amir E., Bedard P., et al. Fertility preservation in post-pubescent female cancer patients: a practical guideline for clinicians. *Mol Clin Oncol*. 2018;**8**:153–8.

112. Partridge A., Niman S., Ruggeri M., et al. Interrupting endocrine therapy to attempt pregnancy after breast cancer. *N Engl J Med* 2023;**388**:1645–56.

Chapter 2

Abnormal Uterine Bleeding

Denise R. Nebgen and Dawn Palaszewski

Case Presentation

A 32-year-old G0P0 woman is newly diagnosed with acute myelogenous leukemia (AML) and is being admitted to the inpatient leukemia service for initial workup and treatment. She had menarche at age 13 and reports normal monthly menses lasting four to five days of light to moderate flow until now. Her last menstrual period (LMP) started eight days ago and she is currently experiencing heavy abnormal uterine bleeding (AUB). She was evaluated by her gynecologist who obtained a complete blood count (CBC). Hemoglobin is 7.0 gram (g)/deciliter (dL), platelet count is 22 thousand (K)/microliter (μL), and white blood cell count is 0.5 K/μL, which led to her diagnosis. The patient desires fertility. How do you counsel and treat this patient?

Epidemiology of Abnormal Uterine Bleeding

Introduction and Background

Abnormal uterine bleeding is a common problem worldwide, with a prevalence of approximately 3%–30% in healthy premenopausal nonpregnant women [1]. Symptoms include heavy menstrual bleeding, intermenstrual bleeding, or irregular menstrual bleeding and contribute to work disruption, increased personal and health-care costs, and decreased quality of life [2].

FIGO-AUB Classification

In order to standardize the terminology used for AUB, the International Federation of Gynecology and Obstetrics (FIGO) published the FIGO-AUB system of terminology in 2011, which was updated in 2018 and implemented worldwide. The FIGO system divides causes of AUB into structural (PALM: Polyp, Adenomyosis, Leiomyoma, Malignancy and hyperplasia) and nonstructural (COEIN: Coagulopathy, Ovulatory dysfunction, Endometrial, Iatrogenic, Not otherwise classified) [1]. Abnormal uterine bleeding can also be described as acute or chronic. Chronic AUB in nonpregnant premenopausal women is defined as bleeding that is abnormal in duration, volume, frequency, and/or regularity and has been present most of the preceding six months [3]. Acute AUB is defined as an episode of heavy bleeding, that in the opinion of the clinician, is of significant quantity to warrant immediate intervention to prevent further blood loss [3]. Acute AUB can occur without a history of bleeding, or in the context of ongoing chronic AUB.

Acknowledgments: The authors thank David Farris in the Research Medical Library at The University of Texas MD Anderson Cancer Center for his assistance.

Cancer Patients

Premenopausal women undergoing cancer treatment are at elevated risk of AUB, but the prevalence in cancer patients is uncertain. The most common occurrence of AUB in patients with nongynecological cancer occurs in premenopausal women with hematologic malignancies and prior to bone marrow or hematopoietic stem cell transplantation (HSCT) and will be the focus of our discussion. Patients with hematologic malignancies may present to the emergency department or gynecologist with new onset heavy menstrual bleeding as their chief complaint leading to their diagnosis [4]. Patients with hematologic malignancies have frequent bleeding due to thrombocytopenia. However, women receiving care for breast and other cancer can also present with AUB. Bleeding can occur due to their cancer treatments including chemotherapy, radiation therapy, or conditioning regimens prior to HSCT [5]. The disease process itself, in the case of hematologic malignancies, or the treatment regimens can induce myelosuppression leading to anemia, neutropenia, and thrombocytopenia.

The Normal Menstrual Cycle

A thorough understanding of the menstrual cycle is helpful for evaluating patients with AUB. The normal menstrual cycle lasts four to eight days and occurs approximately monthly or every 24–38 days with cyclical variation over the span of a year [6]. The average menstrual blood loss is 30–40 milliliters (mls), with the 95th percentile of 80 mls. Menstruation is the orderly shedding of the endometrium secondary to hormonal fluctuations produced in or by the ovaries, hypothalamus, and the pituitary. The menstrual cycle is divided into two phases, the follicular or proliferative phase (day one of bleeding to ovulation) and the luteal or secretory phase (ovulation to the start of bleeding, if no fertilization occurs) [7].

The follicular phase of the menstrual cycle occurs when follicle-stimulating hormone (FSH) triggers the ovarian follicles to produce estrogen, which leads to formation of a dominant follicle. The dominant follicle leads to further estrogen rise and growth of the endometrium. The rise in estrogen creates a surge in luteinizing hormone (LH), which triggers ovulation, and creates a negative feedback to FSH. The corpus luteum produces progesterone, which creates a secretory endometrium ready for implantation. If fertilization does not occur, both estrogen and progesterone levels drop, resulting in sloughing of the endometrium. Blood loss during menstruation is limited by having the appropriate number of functioning platelets along with clotting factors. Estradiol production in the next primordial follicle heals the blood vessels, stops the bleeding, and the cycle resets [8].

When this system is disrupted in premenopausal patients, heavy and/or prolonged menstrual bleeding can occur. Abnormal uterine bleeding is the preferred term, however menorrhagia (heavy menstrual bleeding) and menometrorrhagia (heavy and irregular menstrual bleeding) are used as descriptors of the type of bleeding.

Etiology and Risk Factors

Premenopausal patients with hematologic malignancies are often diagnosed with thrombocytopenia which leads to abnormal bleeding of mucous membranes including the nasopharynx, eyes, rectum, uterine cavity, and cuts/injuries. These women are often treated with high-dose chemotherapy, myeloablative conditioning regimens prior to HSCT, or total body irradiation (TBI) which can also exacerbate thrombocytopenia and bleeding. High-dose chemotherapy leads to an iatrogenic sloughing of mucous membranes including the lining of the endometrium leading to heavy bleeding and bleeding outside of the normal cycle. In preparation for HSCT, myeloablative chemotherapy or conditioning regimens with or without TBI destroy the patient's bone marrow leading to pancytopenia. These conditioning regimens, administered one to two weeks prior to the HSCT, are administered to allow repopulation or recovery with stem cell or bone marrow transplanted cells (60–90 days) [9]. However, the resulting thrombocytopenia contributes to heavy menstrual bleeding. The conditioning regimens also lead to premature ovarian insufficiency or early menopause in 65–84% of patients, with age < 30 years associated with the lowest risk [10].

Diagnosis and Workup

Signs and Symptoms

Women with a history of normal menstrual cycles often present with new onset heavy menstrual bleeding which is significantly heavier than their normal flow and often accompanied by menstrual clotting. This bleeding can occur either before a diagnosis of cancer or with initiation of chemotherapy. Other presenting symptoms of hematologic malignancies include fatigue, shortness of breath, bruising or petechiae, and fever [4].

Physical Exam Findings

Women with AUB undergoing cancer treatment should be interviewed to determine their normal menstrual history and any history of heavy menstrual bleeding or known uterine fibroids. Most women will have normal physical and pelvic exams other than persistent bleeding. The use of an intrauterine system (IUS) should be noted, as these may be removed due to the theoretical concern for infection in some patients prior to transplant. However, in women with a levonorgestrel IUS (LNG-IUS) due to a history of heavy menstrual bleeding, consideration for retention of the LNG-IUS should be made, or bleeding may become worse after removal.

Imaging Studies

As a large percentage of premenopausal women with AUB and cancer have normal anatomy, it is often not necessary to initially obtain imaging. If they have a history of heavy menstrual bleeding, uterine fibroids, endometrial polyps, or endometrial hyperplasia, imaging with transvaginal ultrasound can be performed if bleeding persists.

Laboratory Tests

The workup for heavy menstrual bleeding in cancer patients includes a CBC with differential and pregnancy test. Often this information is already known and demonstrates pancytopenia. Platelet counts below 20–40 K/μL and hemoglobin levels below ~ 8 g/dL are considered severe and require transfusion support from the hematologic oncology team. Patients with thrombocytopenia with platelet counts below 20 K/μL have an increased risk of spontaneous bleeding from mucous membranes.

Postmenopausal Bleeding

Postmenopausal women are less likely to have bleeding secondary to thrombocytopenia or chemotherapy. Women presenting with postmenopausal bleeding in the setting of hematologic or other cancer should be evaluated for the signs and symptoms of endometrial cancer. Transvaginal ultrasound is used to measure the thickness of the endometrium to determine if endometrial sampling is indicated. If this is her first episode of postmenopausal bleeding and the ultrasound images reveal a thin endometrial echo of less than or equal to 4 millimeters (mm) then endometrial sampling is not necessary, given that an endometrial thickness of 4 mm or less has a greater than 99% negative predictive value for endometrial cancer [11]. However, if she has experienced repetitive bleeding, endometrial sampling is indicated. If hematologic counts are stable, perform pelvic examination, rectal examination, and endometrial biopsy if indicated.

Treatment Options

In adolescents and young adults, preventative menstrual suppression is recommended for many types of cancer, however oncology providers may not feel comfortable providing this care [5, 12]. Obstetrician-gynecologists are often consulted to induce menstrual suppression prior to cancer treatment or for the control of AUB during cancer treatment [9]. Recommendations should be implemented in coordination with the oncologist caring for the patient.

A retrospective chart review at a single tertiary pediatric institution between 2008–19 assessed patterns of care for 52 patients aged 15–39 years at diagnosis with new or relapsed lymphoma, AML, or sarcoma treated with chemotherapy with or without radiation. This study concluded that most patients (79%) were prescribed hormonal agents for menstrual suppression with the most prevalent options being depo-medroxyprogesterone acetate (DMPA) (49%) and combined oral contraceptive pills (OCPs) (39%). The initiation of a menstrual suppressive agent varied from prior to (20%), simultaneous with (25%), or after initiating (44%) chemotherapy. Ongoing research is evaluating these patterns in a larger cohort, aiming to understand differences in management [13].

Several algorithms for the prevention and treatment of AUB in cancer patients are published or available online and can facilitate care of these patients [5, 14]. The MD Anderson Cancer Center's Abnormal Uterine Bleeding algorithm includes the predominant use of leuprolide, OCPs, progestin-only options, and tranexamic acid (TXA) depending on specific scenarios, and includes alternatives for women with contraindications to OCPs (Figure 2.1) [15].

Medical Treatments

Most medical treatment options in premenopausal patients are hormonal and include the use of OCPs, gonadotropin-releasing hormone (GnRH) agonists, and progestin-only options including oral, injectable, and the levonorgestrel-intrauterine system (LNG-IUS) [16]. Intravenous conjugated equine estrogen (CEE) and a nonhormonal option of TXA may be considered as well.

Treatment regimens for acute bleeding were originally designed to mimic the hormonal changes of the menstrual cycle by initiating treatment with high-dose estrogen to stimulate cell proliferation and stabilize the endometrium. High-dose progestin was then added to

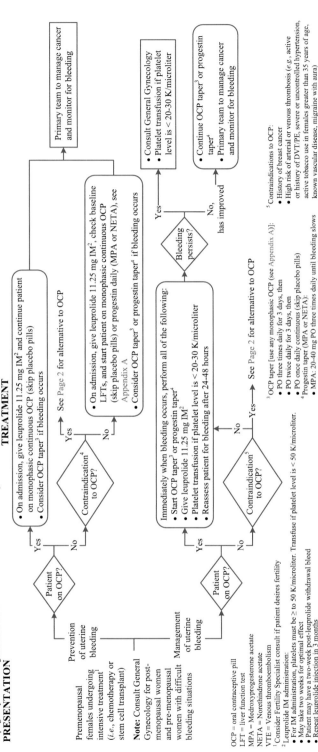

Figure 2.1 Abnormal Uterine Bleeding algorithm (for the complete algorithm see online) [15]

Abnormal Uterine Bleeding (AUB)

THE UNIVERSITY OF TEXAS
MD Anderson
Cancer Center
Making Cancer History

Disclaimer: This algorithm has been developed for MD Anderson using a multidisciplinary approach considering circumstances particular to MD Anderson's specific patient population, services and structure, and clinical information. This is not intended to replace the independent medical or professional judgment of physicians or other health care providers in the context of individual clinical circumstances to determine a patient's care. This algorithm should not be used to treat pregnant women.

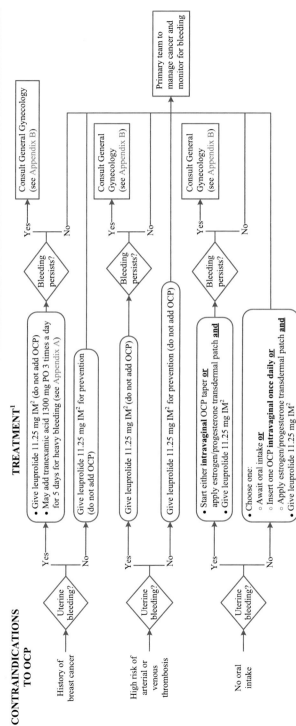

CONTRAINDICATIONS TO OCP

TREATMENT[1]

[1] See Appendix A - Dosing Recommendations
[2] Leuprolide IM administration:
- For IM administration, platelets must be ≥ 50 K/microliter. Transfuse if platelets < 50 K/microliter.
- Repeat leuprolide injection in 3 months
- May take two weeks for optimal effect
- Patients planned for stem cell transplant should receive injection 1 month prior to procedure
- Contraception should be recommended in women of childbearing potential as it is not ensured with leuprolide
- Contraindicated in women who are pregnant or breastfeeding

Copyright 2023 The University of Texas MD Anderson Cancer Center

Department of Clinical Effectiveness V4
Approved by the Executive Committee of the Medical Staff on 03/21/2023

Figure 2.1 (cont.)

cause secretory changes and shedding of the endometrium. However, the high-dose estrogen may increase the amount of progestin needed to transform the endometrium and may eventually result in more bleeding compared to treatment with progestin alone. Many progestin-only protocols have been shown to be at least as effective in stopping acute bleeding as protocols using high-dose estrogen and progestin combinations and there are often fewer side effects [17].

The World Health Organization (WHO) established medical eligibility criteria for contraceptive use, and these criteria have been regularly updated over time, adapted by the Center for Disease Control (CDC), and are described using four categories in the US Medical Eligibility Criteria for Contraceptive use (US MEC) guidelines [18]: Category 1 – the contraceptive can be used safely with no restriction; Category 2 – the benefits of using the contraception generally outweigh the risks; Category 3 – the risks of using the contraception generally outweigh the benefits; and Category 4 – the method should not be used.

Combined Oral Contraceptives

Patients who are taking OCPs on presentation can be changed from a cyclical to a continuous regimen to suppress menses and produce amenorrhea [19, 20]. Continuous OCP regimen implies taking the active pill daily and skipping the nonactive or "sugar pill" week. If the OCP is a triphasic formulation, consider changing to a monophasic OCP before changing to a continuous regimen to provide a steady state of hormone. For patients without contraindications to OCPs, consider starting a continuous OCP regimen. A 30 microgram (mcg) OCP can be used initially. The US MEC states that when OCPs are used as therapy as opposed to contraception, even in patients where combined contraceptives would lead to elevated risk such as in cancer patients, the benefits may outweigh the risks for therapeutic purposes [18]. If a patient is unable to tolerate oral pills or prefers to take fewer pills, the contraceptive intravaginal ring or contraceptive patch may be used in place of an OCP, but these formulations may be less effective for acute bleeding [21]. An OCP taper (one pill orally three times daily for three days then one pill twice daily for three days then one pill once daily continuously) can be used to control acute bleeding (Figure 2.1). Common contraindications to OCP use in the cancer population include breast cancer, venous thromboembolism (VTE), uncontrolled hypertension, migraine with aura, and oral mucositis leading to lack of oral intake. For patients with oral mucositis, consider placing the OCP tablet intravaginally until able to swallow pills, as absorption does occur at this site [22]. As patients with cancer have an elevated risk of VTE, it is important to have shared medical decision-making with the patient, her family, and care team regarding the risks and benefits of OCP use.

Gonadotropin-Releasing Hormone Agonists

Leuprolide is the most common GnRH agonist used for the prevention and treatment of AUB in cancer patients. Leuprolide can be administered as a subcutaneous (SC) or intramuscular (IM) injection. Patients require platelet values of ≥ 50 K/μL to receive an IM injection to avoid intramuscular hematoma formation and may require transfusion of platelets prior to IM injection to achieve this level. Longer (three-month) dosing regimens can be used to help avoid repetitive IM injections at a time of thrombocytopenia [5]. Leuprolide IM given monthly (3.75 mg) or every three months (11.25 mg) is effective in the prevention of menstrual bleeding in premenopausal patients prior to HSCT, with efficacy rates between 73–96% if given approximately 30 days in advance of the HSCT or 15 days before the conditioning regimen [23–25]. Additionally, GnRH agonists do not increase thrombotic risk.

After injection of a GnRH agonist, an initial flare effect causes a transient increase in circulating gonadotropins (LH and FSH) followed by sex steroids but then leads to a hypoestrogenic state in two weeks [26]. Withdrawal bleeding may occur for two to three weeks after the first injection until endometrial proliferation stops [27]. Leuprolide alone is used for the acute treatment of AUB but due to the two weeks of withdrawal bleeding it is often used in conjunction with another method such as an OCP or progestin taper to help control the acute bleeding. Leuprolide is not officially contraceptive. If used for menstrual suppression, leuprolide can cause vasomotor symptoms and bone density loss (with long-term use) related to the low estrogen state. OCPs also provide contraception and add back estrogen therapy for vasomotor symptoms and protection against bone loss. Add back therapy with a progestin, such as norethindrone acetate (NETA) 5 mg once daily, has also been shown to decrease vasomotor symptoms and provide protection against bone loss, although it is not contraceptive [28, 29].

Premenopausal patients treated with high-dose chemotherapy, such as alkylating agents, are also at risk of premature ovarian insufficiency (POI) or early menopause. Leuprolide given prior to chemotherapy in premenopausal cancer patients may also preserve ovarian function, but with conflicting data. Twelve randomized controlled trials were included in a Cochrane review which showed that GnRH agonists were more effective than controls in protecting the ovaries during chemotherapy, for return of menstruation, POI, and ovulation. However, evidence for rates of fertility and pregnancy was insufficient and needed further investigation [30]. It is important to remember that leuprolide should not be considered contraceptive as ovulation may occasionally occur. Several oral GnRH antagonists (elagolix, relugolix) have been developed for the treatment of endometriosis in recent years and would avoid the two-week flare effect and withdrawal bleed, however there are currently no studies or guidelines for their use in the prevention or treatment of AUB in patients with cancer.

Progestin-Only Hormone Therapy

Progestin-only therapy can stop acute bleeding and/or control long-term bleeding. Many progestin-only protocols are at least as effective in stopping acute bleeding as protocols using high dose estrogen/progestin combinations and have fewer side effects. All progestin-only medications are listed as Category 2 (benefits generally outweigh the risks) in patients with a history of VTE according to the US MEC [18]. However, a recent study of 21,405 patients of reproductive age showed NETA and MPA were significantly associated with increased odds of acute VTE, whereas use of oral progesterone, oral norethindrone, LNG-IUS, and etonogestrel implants were not [31]. The risk level of progestin-only medications in patients who have cancer depends on the type of cancer. There are no restrictions for use of this method for patients with ovarian cancer, but it is contraindicated in patients with current breast cancer [18].

Numerous progestin regimens are available. Oral progestins can be prescribed in multiple-dose regimens, such as two tablets orally three times per day, and even at high doses do not typically induce nausea [32]. To control AUB, oral MPA can be prescribed as 5–10 mg every one to two hours to total 60–120 mg/daily or until bleeding slows or stops, followed by 20 mg daily thereafter [32]. An alternative regimen includes oral MPA 20 mg three times per day for seven days tapering to 20 mg daily [33]. The MD Anderson regimen lists MPA 20–40 mg three times per day until bleeding slows or stops, tapering to 10–20 mg daily (Figure 2.1) [15]. To stop acute bleeding, NETA may be prescribed as 20 mg three times per day until bleeding stops, tapering to 5–15 mg/day [34]. MPA has a strong progestational effect as it is not converted into ethinyl estradiol and therefore may have an advantage in terms of bleeding cessation over NETA. NETA is partially converted to ethinyl estradiol with a 5 mg tablet of NETA producing about 10 mcg of ethinyl estradiol. While NETA has not been shown to have contraceptive efficacy, it can be used for bleeding control, as hormone therapy (HT), and bone protection in patients with POI or early menopause [17]. The high dose drosperinone (4 mg/day) contraceptive pill and norethin-drone "mini-pill" (0.35 mg/day) are other oral progestin-only options that provide contra-ception but are not as likely to achieve amenorrhea.

DMPA (150 mg) administration every three months can lead to cessation of bleeding with 70% of users becoming amenorrhoeic after two years of use [17]. Initial irregular bleeding limits its effectiveness for rapid menstrual suppression as a single agent [27]. However, it is a good option for patients unable to take pills. A subcutaneous formulation (104 mg) is available and can be used if hematoma formation is a concern in patients with severe thrombocytopenia.

The LNG-IUS has been shown in multiple studies to suppress bleeding in women with normal cycles and in those with heavy menstrual bleeding. A Cochrane review found that the 52 mg LNG-IUS reduced heavy menstrual bleeding more effectively than the combined OCP [17]. The LNG-IUS is a good option for long-term manage-ment. The literature on IUS use in immunocompromised women exists mainly in the HIV-infected population. A prospective cohort study of 649 women that examined use of copper intrauterine devices among HIV-1 infected and noninfected women showed no increase in overall infections in the HIV-infected women [35]. Also, the LNG-IUS was shown to reduce menstrual blood loss, with a slight increase in hemoglobin and with no occurrence of pelvic inflammatory disease in 12 HIV-infected women during a 12-month follow-up [36]. Another study using the LNG-IUS in renal transplant recipients showed no incidence of pelvic infections in 11 patients with a mean duration of use of 38 (range 1–84) months [37].

Based on these studies and others, IUSs are considered a viable treatment option for immunocompromised women who need contraception or menstrual suppression [38]. Based on studies in HIV-positive patients, the WHO and the CDC state that IUSs can be used safely by patients with immunosuppression due to cancer treatment [39]. The CDC's US MEC lists LNG-IUS as a possible treatment for menorrhagia in women with severe thrombocytopenia and lists it as Category 2 (benefits generally outweigh risks) [18]. However, there is little to no data on IUS use in hematologic cancer patients.

The etonogestrel single-rod contraceptive implant has limited usefulness for acute menstrual suppression in cancer patients due to irregular bleeding patterns. However, if a patient already has an implant before her cancer diagnosis and it is successfully managing her bleeding, then continuation of this contraceptive device is acceptable. If the implant is already present and there is bothersome bleeding, NETA or MPA could be given to improve bleeding [5]. Removal can be considered if bleeding persists.

Intravenous Conjugated Equine Estrogen

IV estrogen can be used for the acute treatment of AUB. In one randomized controlled trial of 34 patients, IV CEE was shown to stop bleeding in 72% of participants within 8 hours of administration compared with 38% of patients treated with a placebo [3]. CEE can be administered as 25 mg IV every 6 hours for 24 hours or until bleeding slows or stops, followed by an OCP taper. Antiemetics can be given with high dose estrogen. The need to acutely stop bleeding must be balanced against the risk of VTE in cancer patients.

Antifibrinolytics: Tranexamic Acid

Either oral or IV TXA can be used to treat acute AUB due to its antifibrinolytic properties. TXA oral dosing is 1.3 g orally three times daily for five days. The FDA has approved TXA for short-term use to reduce or prevent hemorrhage in individuals with heavy menstrual bleeding. The main contraindication of TXA is history of or active arterial or venous thromboembolic disease. Another contraindication is OCPs use, however clinical experience in Sweden showed no increased VTE risk with combined TXA and OCP use [40].

Surgical Management

For premenopausal patients who have not completed childbearing, surgical procedures are considered a last resort. For women who have completed childbearing and for whom hormonal options fail, surgical management is reasonable. Surgical options include balloon tamponade using a 26 French Foley catheter infused with 30 mL of saline solution, dilation and curettage, endometrial ablation, uterine artery embolization, and hysterectomy [3].

Special Considerations

Venous Thromboembolism (VTE)

Cancer patients are known to have an increased risk of VTE including deep venous thrombosis (DVT) and pulmonary embolus (PE), with incidence highest in patients with metastatic disease, aggressive cancer, and hematological cancer [41]. In HSCT patients, VTE is usually catheter-related [42]. Many of the medications (hormonal and TXA) which are used to prevent or treat AUB can also increase risk of VTE [31, 43]. The benefits of OCP use for cessation of AUB and prevention of unintended pregnancy often outweigh the risks of VTE. For those with a history of VTE, the LNG-IUS may be a good option to provide bleeding control and contraception. The entire care team including the patient and her family should participate in shared decision-making regarding risks and benefits of these treatment options.

Need for Contraception

Contraceptive counseling is important when patients are undergoing cancer treatment. There may be a misperception among providers that cancer patients are too ill to engage in or be interested in sexual activity. However, patients with cancer have been found to engage in sexual behaviors at similar rates as their cancer-free peers [17]. Even though fertility may be impacted, it is not universal or absolute during or after cancer treatment. Several studies suggest survivors are at a higher risk for unintended pregnancy than the general population as they are often unaware of their fertility status or assume that they are infertile. Pregnancy risks are substantial for patients during active cancer therapy. It is important to address the need for contraception with all patients, which can be taken into consideration when choosing a method for prevention or treatment of AUB. The US MEC restricts their recommendations to only four cancers including breast, ovary, cervix, and endometrium. They categorize use of all hormonal contraceptive methods for women with breast cancer as Category 3 or 4 (risks usually outweigh the benefits or unacceptable health risk). The copper IUS is a Category 1 (no risk). The US MEC categorizes use of all hormonal contraceptive methods for women with ovarian, cervical, and endometrial cancer as Category 1 or 2 (no risk or the benefits generally outweigh the risks). Exceptions include IUS placement in cervical and endometrial cancer patients due to concern for cancer seeding with insertion [18]. A Cochrane Review regarding HT states that available evidence does not suggest significant harm if HT is used after surgical treatment for early-stage endometrial cancer, but cautions use in more advanced (FIGO Stages II–IV) cancer as there is no data available [44]. See Chapter 6 for more information. This information may be extrapolated to consideration of contraceptive options in these patients.

Case Resolution

This case describes a common occurrence in a busy cancer hospital or on a transplant service of a young patient with AML about to undergo high-dose chemotherapy. The oncofertility team was urgently consulted, however it was determined that there was not enough time to cryopreserve oocytes due to her cancer severity. Treatment included leuprolide 11.25 mg IM injection after platelet transfusion to achieve a platelet count of $\geq$50 K/μl. OCP taper was also initiated utilizing one pill three times daily for three days followed by one pill twice daily for three days and lastly one pill daily for add back therapy and contraception. Her OCPs were prescribed in a continuous fashion (one tablet daily continuous avoiding placebo pills, please fill four packs in three months). Her menstrual bleeding ceased approximately one week after leuprolide injection, but she had a two-week withdrawal bleed before complete cessation of menses. She received a second leuprolide 11.25 mg IM injection three months after the first and after obtaining complete remission underwent HSCT while still amenorrheic from the leuprolide. Leuprolide was discontinued after the second injection, but her menses did not return. She was treated with HT thereafter.

Take Home Points

- Obtain a CBC when young women present with new onset prolonged and/or heavy menstrual bleeding. If leukocytosis, leukopenia, or thrombocytopenia are present, consult hematology.
- Common hormonal treatment options for AUB in premenopausal patients include the use of OCP tapers, continuous OCPs, GnRH agonists, and progestin-only options including oral formulations, injectables, and the LNG-IUS.
- Leuprolide given prior to chemotherapy in premenopausal cancer patients may also preserve ovarian function but it does not provide contraception.
- Several algorithms for the prevention and treatment of AUB are published or available on-line and can facilitate care of these patients.
- Many of the hormonal medications or TXA used to prevent or treat AUB can also increase risk of VTE. Shared decision making is necessary.

References

1. Munro M. G., Critchley H. O. D., Fraser I. S. The two FIGO systems for normal and abnormal uterine bleeding symptoms and classification of causes of abnormal uterine bleeding in the reproductive years: 2018 revisions. *Int J Gynaecol Obstet.* 2018;**143** (3):393–408.

2. Liu Z., Doan Q. V., Blumenthal P., Dubois R. W. A systematic review evaluating health-related quality of life, work impairment, and health-care costs and utilization in abnormal uterine bleeding. *Value Health.* 2007;**10**(3):183–94.

3. ACOG Committee Opinion No. 557. Management of acute abnormal uterine bleeding in nonpregnant reproductive-aged women. *Obstet Gynecol.* 2013;**121** (4):891–6.

4. Nebgen D. R., Rhodes H. E., Hartman C., Munsell M. F., Lu K. H. Abnormal uterine bleeding as the presenting symptom of hematologic cancer. *Obstet Gynecol.* 2016;**128**(2):357–63.

5. ACOG Committee Opinion No. 817. Options for prevention and management of menstrual bleeding in adolescent patients undergoing cancer treatment. *Obstet Gynecol.* 2021;**137**(1):e7–e15.

6. Munro M. G., Critchley H. O., Broder M. S., Fraser I. S. FIGO classification system (PALM-COEIN) for causes of abnormal uterine bleeding in nongravid women of reproductive age. *Int J Gynaecol Obstet.* 2011;**113**(1):3–13.

7. Reed B., Carr B. The normal menstrual cycle and the control of ovulation. 2000. [Updated August 5, 2018]. In *Endotext [Internet]*. South Dartmouth, MA: MDText.com, Inc. www.ncbi.nlm.nih.gov/books/NBK279054/.

8. Jones K. P. Uterine bleeding during high-dose chemotherapy and hematopoietic stem cell transplantation: A perfect storm. *Obstet Gynecol.* 2013;**121**(2 Pt 2 Suppl 1):419–21.

9. Chang K., Merideth M. A., Stratton P. Hormone use for therapeutic amenorrhea and contraception during hematopoietic cell transplantation. *Obstet Gynecol.* 2015;**126**(4):779–84.

10. Joshi S., Savani B. N., Chow E. J., et al. Clinical guide to fertility preservation in hematopoietic cell transplant recipients. *Bone Marrow Transplant.* 2014;**49** (4):477–84.

11. ACOG Committee Opinion No. 734. The role of transvaginal ultrasonography in evaluating the endometrium of women with postmenopausal bleeding. *Obstet Gynecol.* 2018;**131**(5):e124–e9.

12. Close A. G., Jones K. A., Landowski A., et al. Current practices in menstrual management in adolescents with cancer: A national survey of pediatric oncology providers. *Pediatr Blood Cancer.* 2019;**66** (12):e27961.

13. Thompson E., Wolfson J., Owen J., Arbuckle J. Menstrual suppression in the myelosuppressed: A retrospective chart review. *J Pediatr Adolesc Gynecol.* 2021;**34** (Poster Presentation Abstracts 2):264.

14. Ely J. W., Kennedy C. M., Clark E. C., Bowdler N. C. Abnormal uterine bleeding: A management algorithm. *J Am Board Fam Med.* 2006;**19**(6):590–602.

15. University of Texas MD Anderson Cancer Center. Abnormal Uterine Bleeding (AUB) Clinical Practice Algorithm. 2023. www.mdanderson.org/for-physicians/clinical-tools-resources/clinical-practice-algorithms/clinical-management-algorithms.html.

16. Kirkham Y. A., Ornstein M. P., Aggarwal A., McQuillan S. No. 313-menstrual suppression in special circumstances. *J Obstet Gynaecol Can.* 2019;**41**(2):e7–e17.

17. Shoupe D. The progestin revolution: Progestins are arising as the dominant players in the tight interlink between contraceptives and bleeding control. *Contracept Reprod Med.* 2021;**6**(1):1–9.

18. Curtis K. M., Tepper N. K., Jatlaoui T. C., et al. U.S. medical eligibility criteria for contraceptive use, 2016. *MMWR Recomm Rep.* 2016;**65**(3):1–103.

19. Miller L., Hughes J. P. Continuous combination oral contraceptive pills to eliminate withdrawal bleeding: A

randomized trial. *Obstet Gynecol.* 2003;**101**(4):653–61.

20. Bradley L. D., Gueye N. A. The medical management of abnormal uterine bleeding in reproductive-aged women. *Am J Obstet Gynecol.* 2016;**214**(1):31–44.

21. Milroy C. L., Jones K. P. Gynecologic care in hematopoietic stem cell transplant patients: A review. *Obstet Gynecol Surv.* 2010;**65**(10):668–79.

22. Coutinho E. M., da Silva A. R., Carreira C., Rodrigues V., Gonçalves M. T. Conception control by vaginal administration of pills containing ethinyl estradiol and dl-norgestrel. *Fertil Steril.* 1984;**42**(3):478–81.

23. Chiusolo P., Salutari P., Sica S., et al. Luteinizing hormone-releasing hormone analogue: Leuprorelin acetate for the prevention of menstrual bleeding in premenopausal women undergoing stem cell transplantation. *Bone Marrow Transplant.* 1998;**21**(8):821–3.

24. Meirow D., Rabinovici J., Katz D., et al. Prevention of severe menorrhagia in oncology patients with treatment-induced thrombocytopenia by luteinizing hormone-releasing hormone agonist and depo-medroxyprogesterone acetate. *Cancer.* 2006;**107**(7):1634–41.

25. Poorvu P. D., Barton S. E., Duncan C. N., et al. Use and effectiveness of gonadotropin-releasing hormone agonists for prophylactic menstrual suppression in postmenarchal women who undergo hematopoietic cell transplantation. *J Pediatr Adolesc Gynecol.* 2016;**29**(3):265–8.

26. Bedaiwy M. A., Mousa N. A., Casper R. F. Aromatase inhibitors prevent the estrogen rise associated with the flare effect of gonadotropins in patients treated with GnRH agonists. *Fertil Steril.* 2009;**91**(4 Suppl):1574–7.

27. Quaas A. M., Ginsburg E. S. Prevention and treatment of uterine bleeding in hematologic malignancy. *Eur J Obstet Gynecol Reprod Biol.* 2007;**134**(1):3–8.

28. Hornstein M. D., Surrey E. S., Weisberg G. W., Casino L. A. Leuprolide acetate depot and hormonal add-back in endometriosis: A 12-month study. *Lupron Add-Back Study Group. Obstet Gynecol.* 1998;**91**(1):16–24.

29. Surrey E. S., Judd H. L. Reduction of vasomotor symptoms and bone mineral density loss with combined norethindrone and long-acting gonadotropin-releasing hormone agonist therapy of symptomatic endometriosis: A prospective randomized trial. *J Clin Endocrinol Metab.* 1992;**75**(2):558–63.

30. Chen H., Xiao L., Li J., Cui L., Huang W. Adjuvant gonadotropin-releasing hormone analogues for the prevention of chemotherapy-induced premature ovarian failure in premenopausal women. *Cochrane Database Syst Rev.* 2019;**3**(3):Cd008018.

31. Cockrum R. H., Soo J., Ham S. A., Cohen K. S., Snow S. G. Association of progestogens and venous thromboembolism among women of reproductive age. *Obstet Gynecol.* 2022;**140**(3):477–87.

32. Aksu F., Madazli R., Budak E., Cepni I., Benian A. High-dose medroxyprogesterone acetate for the treatment of dysfunctional uterine bleeding in 24 adolescents. *Aust N Z J Obstet Gynaecol.* 1997;**37**(2):228–31.

33. Munro M. G., Mainor N., Basu R., Brisinger M., Barreda L. Oral medroxyprogesterone acetate and combination oral contraceptives for acute uterine bleeding: A randomized controlled trial. *Obstet Gynecol.* 2006;**108**(4):924–9.

34. ACOG Committee Opinion No. 785. Screening and management of bleeding disorders in adolescents with heavy menstrual bleeding. *Obstet Gynecol.* 2019;**134**(3):e71–e83.

35. Sinei S. K., Morrison C. S., Sekadde-Kigondu C., Allen M., Kokonya D. Complications of use of intrauterine devices among HIV-1-infected women. *Lancet.* 1998;**351**(9111):1238–41.

36. Heikinheimo O., Lehtovirta P., Suni J., Paavonen J. The levonorgestrel-releasing intrauterine system (LNG-IUS) in HIV-infected women: Effects on bleeding patterns, ovarian function and genital

shedding of HIV. *Hum Reprod.* 2006;**21**(11):2857–61.

37. Ramhendar T., Byrne P. Use of the levonorgestrel-releasing intrauterine system in renal transplant recipients: A retrospective case review. *Contraception.* 2012;**86**(3):288–9.

38. Browne H., Manipalviratn S., Armstrong A. Using an intrauterine device in immunocompromised women. *Obstet Gynecol.* 2008;**112**(3):667–9.

39. Patel A., Schwarz E. B. Cancer and contraception: Society of Family Planning Guideline #20121 Contraception. *Contraception.* 2012;**86**(3):191–8.

40. Thorne J. G., James P. D., Reid R. L. Heavy menstrual bleeding: Is tranexamic acid a safe adjunct to combined hormonal contraception? *Contraception.* 2018;**98**(1):1–3.

41. Wun T., White R. H. Epidemiology of cancer-related venous thromboembolism. *Best Pract Res Clin Haematol.* 2009;**22**(1):9–23.

42. Gerber D. E., Segal J. B., Levy M. Y., et al. The incidence of and risk factors for venous thromboembolism (VTE) and bleeding among 1514 patients undergoing hematopoietic stem cell transplantation: Implications for VTE prevention. *Blood.* 2008;**112**(3):504–10.

43. Mohammed K., Abu Dabrh A. M., Benkhadra K., et al. Oral vs transdermal estrogen therapy and vascular events: A systematic review and meta-analysis. *J Clin Endocrinol Metab.* 2015;**100**(11):4012–20.

44. Edey K. A., Rundle S., Hickey M. Hormone replacement therapy for women previously treated for endometrial cancer. *Cochrane Database Syst Rev.* 2018;**5**(5):Cd008830.

Chapter 3

Hereditary Gynecologic Cancer Predisposition Syndromes

Molly S. Daniels, Denise R. Nebgen, and Neil Ryan

Key terminology

Somatic: Relating to a genome that cannot be inherited, or the genome of the cancer

Germline: Relating to a genome that can be inherited as it is transmitted via the gametes (oocytes and sperm)

Pathogenic variant: A change in the DNA sequence of a specific gene, or its associated epigenetic controls, that leads to an abnormal functioning protein and (potentially) a disease phenotype

Epigenetic change: A change in gene function due to behavior(s) and environment. Unlike genetic changes, epigenetic changes are reversible and do not alter your DNA

Case Presentation

A 42-year-old G2P2 female requests risk-reducing bilateral salpingo-oophorectomy. Her 50-year-old sister was recently diagnosed with ovarian cancer (see Figure 3.1), and she is worried that she is at high risk for ovarian cancer. She is distressed by what her sister is currently experiencing and would like to decrease her risk. How should she be counseled regarding her risk of ovarian cancer and appropriate management of that risk?

Introduction

Cancer is a common, multifactorial disease. According to the American Cancer Society, approximately 40% of Americans will be diagnosed with cancer at some point between birth and death [1]. In most cases, a cancer diagnosis cannot be traced to one specific cause, but rather is due to a combination of random chance and risk factors such as age, medical history, family history, and environmental exposures. The primary risk factor for cancer is age; the older a person is, the more time has passed during which somatic (non hereditary) genetic changes can randomly accumulate in cells, ultimately leading to a cancer diagnosis.

A small but important fraction of cancers are primarily due to a hereditary cancer predisposition caused by a germline pathogenic variant (PV) in a tumor suppressor gene. The role of tumor suppressor genes is to help prevent cancer, therefore if an individual inherits a PV that disrupts the function of that gene, that individual will be at increased risk for the cancer(s) associated with that gene. Each of us has two copies of these tumor suppressor genes, one inherited from our mother and the other from our father. Most hereditary cancer predispositions are inherited in an autosomal dominant manner, meaning that a PV in just one of the two copies of the gene in question is enough to cause the hereditary cancer predisposition. Each child, irrespective of gender, of a person who has

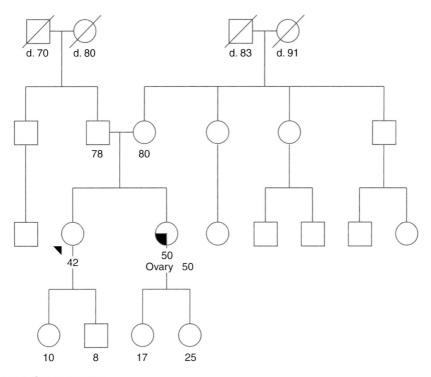

Figure 3.1 Case presentation

a PV has a 50% chance to have inherited it. Autosomal dominant conditions do not skip generations.

Overall, approximately 5% to 10% of cancer are attributable to a hereditary cancer predisposition, however the hereditary proportion varies based on the cancer type. Some cancer, such as lung cancer and cervix cancer, are very rarely due to a hereditary predisposition. Other cancer have a significantly higher likelihood to be hereditary; up to 23% of epithelial ovarian cancer (including fallopian tube and primary peritoneal cancer) are due to germline PVs [2], predominantly in *BRCA1* and *BRCA2*. Given both this high prevalence and the significant implications for patients with ovarian cancer as well as for their families when a PV is identified, genetic testing is recommended for all women with a diagnosis of epithelial ovarian cancer.

To accurately assess an individual's likelihood of having a hereditary cancer predisposition, several factors should be considered. Factors pointing towards a higher likelihood of a hereditary cancer predisposition include cancer diagnosed at an earlier age than is typical for that cancer; multiple primary cancers; and family history of the same or related types of cancer (e.g. family history of both breast cancer and ovarian cancer can be suggestive of a germline *BRCA1/BRCA2* PV). History of nonhereditary risk factors should also be considered. For example, an individual may have a personal and family history of lung cancer, but if this is in the context of tobacco exposure, this would not be suggestive of a hereditary predisposition. Other examples of cancer for which significant risk accrues due to non hereditary risk factors include melanoma and history of sunburn (particularly blistering sunburns in childhood) [3], and endometrial cancer and obesity [4]. Endometrial cancer is also associated with the hereditary cancer predisposition Lynch syndrome, as discussed later in this chapter.

Overview of Hereditary Cancer Genetic Testing

Consideration of whether hereditary cancer genetic testing may be indicated is an important component of oncology care. Genetic test results, both somatic and germline, are playing an ever-increasing role in treatment selection. Accordingly, hereditary cancer genetic testing is now recommended for all individuals diagnosed with certain cancer, including epithelial ovarian cancer and exocrine pancreatic cancer. For other cancers, such as non-metastatic, non triple negative breast cancer, whether genetic testing is recommended would depend upon additional factors including age at diagnosis and family history [5]. For common cancer with a well-defined hereditary component, Table 3.1 outlines criteria for genetic testing and associated genes.

Identifying patients with a hereditary cancer syndrome (HCS) associated with gynecological malignancy is important to fully counsel patients regarding their risks and options for risk-reducing strategies. These risks may include breast, colorectal, and gynecological cancer and complications beyond the female reproductive tract. Therefore, if a HCS is correctly identified by a clinician, a patient can benefit from a referral to a multidisciplinary team for comprehensive care and risk reduction. In a patient with a known gynecological cancer, the individual may be cured of their malignancy, but if the HCS is missed, the patient may go on to acquire extra-gynecological disease that could have been prevented.

In addition, family members of patients found to have a HCS (the index case) can be referred for genetic testing, a process known as cascade testing, which on average identifies three healthy carriers [6]. These healthy carriers are typically diagnosed with a HCS before they develop cancer. An early HCS diagnosis could allow Enrollment in screening programs, if applicable, and risk reduction strategies that could prevent cancer from ever developing.

The advent of high-throughput next generation DNA sequencing has led to a wide range of possible genetic tests, including panel genetic tests of varying size and scope. The effect of PVs on cancer risk varies by gene; this is referred to as penetrance. In the hereditary cancer context, "high penetrance" generally refers to a relative cancer risk ≥ 4, whereas "moderate penetrance" genes confer a lower risk. For example, there are high penetrance hereditary breast cancer predisposition genes such as *BRCA1* and *BRCA2* that cause a 50% to 85% lifetime risk of breast cancer, whereas the general population lifetime risk of breast cancer is 12%. Moderate penetrance hereditary breast cancer genes such as *ATM* and *CHEK2* cause a 20% to 40% risk of breast cancer. Panel genetic testing can include well characterized high penetrance hereditary cancer predisposition genes, low to moderate penetrance genes, and genes whose effect on cancer risk is not well characterized. Appropriate genetic test selection requires clinical judgement and ideally balances the priorities of including all clinically relevant genes while minimizing the likelihood of unclear or otherwise unhelpful results. A targeted testing panel that includes genes relevant to the patient's personal and family history of cancer but excludes nonrelated genes is an appropriate way to achieve this balance. Many clinical genetic testing laboratories offer disease-specific panel genetic testing and allow for further customization by including or excluding additional genes as needed. "Pan cancer" panel genetic testing of 80+ genes are also clinically available. Bigger, however, is not necessarily always better, and these larger panel genetic testing often include genes for which identification of a PV has no

Table 3.1 Common indications for hereditary cancer genetic testing

Primary Site of Cancer Diagnosis	Criteria for Consideration of Genetic Testing	Associated Genes	Prevalence of PV
Breast	All diagnosed <= 50 years All triple negative (ER- PR- Her2neu-) All metastatic and/or otherwise needed for adjuvant treatment decisions All individuals with multiple primary breast cancer diagnoses All breast cancer diagnoses in individuals of Ashkenazi Jewish ancestry If none of the above criteria are met, then genetic testing recommendation is dependent on family history of cancer	ATM, BARD1, BRCA1, BRCA2, CDH1, CHEK2, PALB2, PTEN, RAD51C, RAD51D, STK11, TP53	5% to 10%
Colorectal	All diagnosed < age 50 All with deficient mismatch repair phenotype consistent with Lynch syndrome All with a second primary Lynch syndrome-associated cancer All colorectal cancer accompanied by significant polyp burden (e.g. >=10 adenomatous polyps) If none of the above criteria are met, then genetic testing recommendation is dependent on family history of cancer	Lynch syndrome (EPCAM, MLH1, MSH2, MSH6, PMS2), various polyposis syndromes if clinically indicated	5% to 10%

Table 3.1 (cont.)

Primary Site of Cancer Diagnosis	Criteria for Consideration of Genetic Testing	Associated Genes	Prevalence of PV
Endometrial	All diagnosed < age 50 All with deficient mismatch repair phenotype consistent with Lynch syndrome All with a second primary Lynch syndrome-associated cancer If none of the above criteria are met, then genetic testing recommendation is dependent on family history of cancer	Lynch syndrome (EPCAM, MLH1, MSH2, MSH6, PMS2), PTEN	2% to 3%
Ovarian	All high grade nonmucinous epithelial ovarian, fallopian tube, and primary peritoneal cancer	ATM, BRCA1, BRCA2, BRIP1, Lynch syndrome (EPCAM, MLH1, MSH2, MSH6, PMS2), PALB2, RAD51C, RAD51D	15% to 20%
Pancreatic	All exocrine pancreatic cancer	ATM, BRCA1, BRCA2, CDKN2A, Lynch syndrome (EPCAM, MLH1, MSH2, MSH6, PMS2), PALB2, STK11, TP53	5% to 10%

clear clinical significance. Some germline variants, particularly missense variants and variants that may or may not impact splicing, are of uncertain clinical significance; these are referred to as variants of uncertain significance (VUS). Larger genetic testing panels increase the likelihood of identifying VUS in genes that may not be related to the personal and family history of cancer, leading to potential confusion that could have been avoided with a more targeted panel. Another possible source of confusion is clonal hematopoiesis of indeterminate potential (CHIP), in which somatically derived mutations in hematopoietic stem cells can appear to be consistent with a germline PV [7, 8]. Further workup including genetic testing of fibroblasts cultured from skin punch biopsy may be necessary to clarify the compartment of origin (hematopoietic somatic versus germline). CHIP becomes more frequent with advancing age and history of chemotherapy. Inclusion of CHIP-prone genes such as *TP53* and *NF1* on panels for patients for whom these genes are not clinically indicated increases the likelihood of unnecessarily confusing genetic test results.

Polygenic risk scores (PRS) use many single nucleotide polymorphisms (SNPs) to estimate cancer risk, and this is an area of active research. For example, more than 300 breast cancer-associated SNPs have been identified. As this research area continues to develop, PRS may evolve into a helpful tool for determining or refining risk of breast and/or other cancer. At this time, however, the clinical utility of PRS for cancer risk determination has not been established. While PRS are offered by some clinical genetic testing laboratories, given these current limitations, their use in the clinical setting is not recommended at this time [9, 10].

Often patients with a cancer diagnosis, particularly those with advanced cancer, will have undergone tumor genetic testing whose primary objective is to identify somatic mutations within the tumor that may help in treatment selection. Given significant overlap between genes of interest in the somatic and germline realms, identification of a mutation in a tumor could inform hereditary cancer risk assessment [11]. For example, most but not all *BRCA1/BRCA2* PVs identified in tumors are of germline origin, and thus consideration of germline testing is recommended anytime a PV is detected in the tumor [12, 13]. For other genes, such as *TP53*, somatic mutations are much more common than germline PVs, therefore identifying a *TP53* mutation in a tumor would not necessarily prompt consideration of germline *TP53* testing unless the individual has a personal and/or family history suggestive of Li Fraumeni syndrome. It is also important to recognize that tumor-focused genetic testing should never be considered a substitute for germline testing. Germline PVs can be missed on tumor-focused testing, therefore patients who are otherwise eligible for germline testing should still be offered germline testing even if a tumor focused genetic test did not find any mutations in the relevant genes [14].

Genetic Testing for Women with Ovarian Cancer

Given both high mutation prevalence and significant clinical implications for patients and their families, all women with high grade nonmucinous epithelial ovarian cancer should be offered hereditary ovarian cancer genetic testing including *BRCA1* and *BRCA2*.

Hereditary Breast and Ovarian Cancer (HBOC)

Incidence

The incidence of *BRCA1/BRCA2* PVs in the general population is estimated at 1:300 to 1:500 [15] with an increased incidence in high risk populations such as Ashkenazi Jewish women

(1:40) due to three known founder mutations [16]. Around 10–15% of women with epithelial ovarian cancer are found to have an underlying germline BRCA1/BRCA2 PV with high grade serous histotypes most closely associated (17).

Etiology

HBOC is a syndrome of elevated risk of breast and ovarian cancer caused by a germline PV in the BRCA1 or BRCA2 gene. These genes are autosomal dominant tumor suppressor genes involved in DNA damage repair before replication. The mechanism of DNA repair is known as homologous recombination in which cells repair double stranded DNA breaks [18]. Therefore, pathogenic variants in these key DNA repair genes lead to nonfunctional proteins which in turn leads to failure in double strand DNA repair and carcinogenesis through somatic mutation.

HBOC Associated Cancer

As the name would suggest, HBOC is most closely associated with breast and ovarian cancer; BRCA1 PV carriers are associated with triple negative breast cancer (estrogen/ progesterone receptor negative and weak HER2 expression) which classically are poorly differentiated infiltrating ductal carcinomas [19]. BRCA2 PV carriers more commonly develop breast cancer that express estrogen and progesterone receptors although triple negative cancer have been reported in these women [20]. Both BRCA1 and BRCA2 are associated with high grade serous ovarian cancer [21]. Ovarian cancer patients found to have BRCA1 or BRCA2 PVs are exquisitely sensitive to Poly (ADP-ribose) polymerase (PARP) inhibitors [22, 23]. HBOC associated cancer commonly demonstrate aberrant p53 immunohistochemistry (IHC) [19, 21]. In addition, HBOC associated ovarian cancer are thought to arise from a pre-cancerous tubal lesion referred to as a serous tubal intraepithelial carcinoma (STIC). Patients that have STIC lesions incidentally found on pathology, are offered germline BRCA1/BRCA2 testing due to the close association, with consideration of every-six-month surveillance including CA-125 and/or HE4 and pelvic ultrasound [24].

It is unclear if uterine cancer are associated with HBOC. Some case series have reported an association primarily with BRCA1, whereas others have failed to demonstrate any relationship [25, 26]. Where this association has been shown, there is a suggestion of an increased incidence of serous endometrial cancer [27, 28]. However, there is still a large degree of uncertainty as to the strength of this association and as such it is not currently recommended by any national guideline that women with HBOC undergo risk-reducing hysterectomy. PVs in BRCA2 in particular are also associated with pancreatic cancer, prostate cancer, and possibly melanoma [29].

Screening and Risk-Reducing Surgery for Gynecological Cancer

The lifetime risk of ovarian cancer is approximately 44% in BRCA1 and 17% in BRCA2 PV carriers [30]. As such, consensus management recommendations are for risk-reducing salpingo-oophorectomy (RRSO) between the ages of 35 and 40 years for BRCA1, and waiting until the age of 40–45 years for BRCA2, as ovarian cancer occurs approximately 8–10 years later for BRCA2 carriers [31]. Where there is a family history of earlier onset ovarian cancer, this should be taken into consideration as to inform shared decision making when planning timing of RRSO. Risk of ovarian cancer is greatly reduced by RRSO but cannot be reduced to zero given that microscopic ovarian tissue could remain and approximately 3% of ovarian cancer are in fact primary peritoneal cancer [32]. RRSO for women with *BRCA1/BRCA2* germline PVs meets the gold standard of mortality benefit: a multi-center prospective study demonstrated that RRSO resulted in an 80% reduction in the risk of ovarian, fallopian tube, or peritoneal cancer in *BRCA1* or *BRCA2* carriers and a 77% reduction in all-cause mortality [33].

Patients who have premenopausal RRSO will undergo surgical menopause and as such can experience deeply troubling vasomotor and sexual dysfunction symptoms. They are prematurely exposed to the medical sequelae of menopause including possible increased risk of cardiovascular, metabolic, bone density, and neurological disorders [34, 35]. To help prevent these sequelae, women who undergo RRSO should be offered hormone therapy (HT) if there are no contraindications, and this is typically facilitated by a provider knowledgeable in this area. Of concern is the increased risk of breast cancer in patients taking combined HT. Estrogen-alone HT does not appear to increase breast cancer risk, but is associated with increased risk with the use of systemic progesterone combined HT [36, 37]. Therefore, women need to be counseled on an individual basis and could choose the use of systemic estrogens with either micronized progesterone which may have a lower risk of breast cancer compared to synthetic progestins or a progesterone eluting intra-uterine system for endometrial protection [38]. The levonorgestrel intrauterine system (LNG-IUS) has shown minimal systemic absorption [39]. Two recent meta-analysis on LNG-IUS showed different results; one with slight relative increased breast cancer risk with the other showing no increased breast cancer risk [40, 41]. In addition, researchers are currently exploring the benefits of a two-step procedure in which women with *BRCA1/ BRCA2* PVs are offered a salpingectomy upon completion of childbearing and then oophorectomy five years later than the current recommended age for oophorectomy, when they are closer to the natural age of menopause [42–44]; due to the theory that ovarian cancer in *BRCA1/BRCA2* PV carriers originates in the fallopian tube. However, currently salpingectomy with delayed oophorectomy should not be offered outside of a research study.

For patients who have not elected RRSO, transvaginal ultrasound combined with serum CA-125 for ovarian cancer screening can be considered starting at age 30–35 years, although ovarian cancer screening has not been shown to be effective [45]. In women who carry a *BRCA1/BRCA2* PV, there is insufficient evidence that surveillance is effective in detecting ovarian cancer earlier or leads to an improvement in survival [46–48]. There is limited evidence that in high risk groups, ovarian cancer surveillance can lead to a stage shift [48], however this result needs to be interpreted with a degree of caution, as demonstrated by the large prospective randomised controlled trial United Kingdom Collaborative Trial of Ovarian Cancer Screening (UKCTOCS): detecting disease at an earlier stage did not translate into a survival benefit [45]. Therefore, women should be educated about the symptoms of ovarian cancer and empowered to seek expert medical attention early if they are concerned. Symptoms of ovarian cancer can be taught using the pneumonic BEACH: Bloating, Early satiety, Abdominal pain or abdominal girth increase, Changes in bowel or bladder habits, and Heightened fatigue, as recommended by an ovarian cancer patient advocacy group (https://ovarcome.org).

Other Considerations

Women with *BRCA1/BRCA2* PVs are at an increased lifetime risk of breast cancer (72% *BRCA1*, 69% *BRCA2*) and therefore need to be referred for increased breast surveillance [5, 30, 31]. This surveillance is comprised of annual breast magnetic resonance imaging (MRI) from the age of 25–29 years, then annual MRI alternating every 6 months with annual mammography from 30–75 years [5, 31]. Risk-reducing mastectomy should be discussed as this reduces breast cancer risk by 90% [49], however the timing of this should be directed by a specialist breast surgeon as the decision-making is nuanced and complex [50]. Chemoprophylaxis for breast cancer has also shown to be of benefit in high-risk women and can be considered under the direction of a breast medical oncologist [51, 52] however, it should be noted these studies were not specifically performed in *BRCA1/BRCA2* populations.

Other Hereditary Ovarian Cancer Predisposition Genes

There are also moderate penetrance ovarian cancer risk genes including *BRIP1*, *PALB2*, *RAD51C*, and *RAD51D*, which confer varying degrees of risk [32]. Patients found to have these germline PVs may also be offered RRSO between 45–50 years, as ovarian cancer risk rises after age 50 [32]. For patients with *ATM* PVs there is insufficient evidence to offer RRSO, unless positive family history of ovarian cancer [32]. Ovarian cancer risk is also elevated in women with Lynch syndrome.

Genetic Testing for Women with Endometrial Cancer

Endometrial cancer is the most common gynecologic malignancy in the developed world. The incidence and mortality of endometrial cancer continues to rise, primarily due to increasing rates of obesity which drives the disease and hinders its treatment [53]. Approximately 3% of all endometrial cancer, and 9% of endometrial cancer diagnosed under age 50 are attributable to a hereditary predisposition, nearly all of which is Lynch syndrome [53]. In many women, their endometrial cancer will be the first sign that they have an underlying hereditary cancer predisposition [54].

Lynch Syndrome

Incidence

Lynch syndrome is thought to be more common than HBOC, affecting up to 1:200 to 1:400 of the general population with 95% unaware that they have the condition [55]. This incidence can vary between populations because of founder mutations such as seen in Iceland [56]. In an unselected population of women with endometrial cancer or ovarian cancer, approximately 3% and 1% respectively will have Lynch syndrome [57, 58].

Etiology

Lynch syndrome arises due to a germline PV in one of the mismatch repair (MMR) genes (*MLH1*, *MSH2*, *MSH6*, and *PMS2). MSH2* can also be silenced by a mutation in the nearby gene *EPCAM (59).* The mismatch repair system maintains DNA fidelity by identifying and repairing base-base mismatches and insertion/deletion of mis-pairs during DNA replication. There is growing evidence that this system supresses homologous recombination and is involved in apoptosis signaling [60]. Therefore, once a heterozygotic carrier of a PV in an MMR gene develops a "second hit" leading to a homozygous MMR deficient cell, mutations accumulate rapidly during normal DNA replication. As a result, cells become hypermutated increasing the risk of carcinogenesis. Regions of DNA with repetitive sequences of code, known as microsatellites, are more commonly affected, termed microsatellite instability

(MSI) [55]. When microsatellite instability accumulates the term "MSI high" is commonly used. Since the epithelium of the endometrium and colorectum is regularly replaced requiring increased DNA synthesis, these tissues are particularly susceptible in mismatch repair deficiency [55]. The phenotypical features of mismatch repair deficient cancer lend themselves to diagnostic testing. Immunohistochemistry (IHC) for the mismatch repair proteins can be used to screen cancer for mismatch repair deficiency and therefore Lynch syndrome [57]. In addition, polymerase chain reaction (PCR)-based testing for microsatellite instability can also be used to detect errors in microsatellite tandems, although IHC is the preferred approach for endometrial cancer [61].

Lynch syndrome associated gynecologic cancers are biologically distinct. They tend to be highly immunogenic and often demonstrate many infiltrating immune cells [62, 63]. Ovarian cancer in Lynch syndrome is often detected at an earlier stage and seems less likely to metastasize [64]. This is thought to be because of Lynch syndrome related cancer being highly immunogenic as a result of the production of cancer antigens. In cancer lacking a functioning mismatch repair system, the hypermutated phenotype leads to an abundance of mutated proteins or neo-peptides which act as antigens and lead to either immune destruction or control of the cancer, limiting metastatic spread [63].

Lynch Syndrome Associated Cancer

Lynch syndrome is associated with a constellation of cancer but namely malignancies of the colorectum, endometrium, and ovary. The lifetime risk of these cancer varies depending on the gene that is affected and are summarized in Table 3.2. In addition, patients with Lynch syndrome are at risk of developing cancer of the stomach, urothelial tract, small bowel, pancreas, biliary tract, and sebaceous neoplasms of the skin although these are less common [55]. An individual's risk of different cancer, based on patient age, can be calculated with the use of the Prospective Lynch Syndrome Database (www.plsd.eu) which enables informed conversations around a patients' actual cancer risk. This resource benefits from being prospectively maintained and includes thousands of proven carriers with many thousands of observational years [65]. The Prospective Lynch Syndrome Database continues to grow and is sourced from across Europe.

Diagnosis

The diagnosis of Lynch syndrome can only be established by definitive germline testing and the identification of a PV in one of the known MMR genes. Populations can be enriched for Lynch syndrome with the use of predictive scoring models such as PREMM$_5$, MMRPro, or MMRpredict; however, these are not diagnostic [66].

Tumors can be screened for Lynch syndrome with the use of IHC or MSI testing. Traditionally using IHC, all four proteins are stained for, however, as the proteins are dimers (or working pairs), there is now evidence that two protein staining (MSH6 and PMS2) is accurate and could save time and money [67]. These methods aim to identify a tumor with MMR deficiency through the detection of an absent protein by IHC or through the phenotype of MSI high by PCR [55]. Tumors commonly lose a functional mismatch repair system due to a somatic event in which the promotor region of *MLH1* is hypermethylated. This hypermethylation (epigenetic change) silences the *MLH1* gene within the cancer, and it appears absent on IHC [57]. As this is not due to a germline genetic change such as Lynch syndrome, it is important to identify cancer caused by this process to prevent unnecessary referrals to clinical genetics and increased patient worry. Those cancer with

Table 3.2 Lynch syndrome cancer risk by age 70 [1]

Gene	Colorectal Cancer Risk	Average Age at Diagnosis	Endometrial Cancer Risk	Average Age at Diagnosis	Ovarian Cancer Risk	Average Age at Diagnosis
MLH1	44% – 53%	44	35%	47–50	11%	46
MSH2	42% – 46%	44	46%	47–50	17%	43
MSH6	12% – 20%	42–69	41%	53–55	11%	46
PMS2	3%	61–66	13%	47–50	3%	51–59
EPCAM	75%	43	12%	49	Unknown	

1.Idos G., Valle L. Lynch Syndrome. 2004 Feb 5 [updated 2021 Feb 4]. In: Adam M. P., Feldman J., Mirzaa G. M., Pagon R. A., Wallace S. E., Bean L. J. H., Gripp K. W., Amemiya A., editors. GeneReviews® [Internet]. Seattle (WA): University of Washington, Seattle; 1993–2023. PMID: 20301390.

MLH1 hypermethylation can be identified by reflex testing for hypermethylation in MSI high endometrial cancer or endometrial cancer with absent MLH1, MLH1/PMS2 staining on IHC. In patients whose cancer have hypermethylation, Lynch syndrome germline testing is not required unless there is a very high degree of clinical suspicion [6]. Patients whose cancer display microsatellite instability and/or IHC loss of staining for any of the mismatch repair proteins (not explained by hypermethylation) should be offered germline Lynch syndrome testing.

Screening and Risk-Reducing Surgery for Lynch Syndrome Gynecological Cancer

Endometrial cancer is often diagnosed at an early stage due to symptoms such as abnormal uterine bleeding, particularly in postmenopausal women for whom any uterine bleeding is abnormal. Women with Lynch syndrome should be informed of the symptoms of endometrial cancer and the importance of reporting any such symptoms to their healthcare provider. Women with Lynch syndrome who report any symptoms consistent with endometrial cancer should undergo urgent endometrial sampling.

Endometrial biopsy every one to two years for screening in the absence of symptoms can also be considered. Surveillance options are included in the European Society of Medical Oncology (ESMO) and the American Society of Clinical Oncology (ASCO) national guidelines, which include the option of annual endometrial ultrasound and consideration of annual endometrial biopsies starting from age 30–35. These surveillance options however are based on expert opinion and are not currently supported by the evidence [68, 69].

While there is not a demonstrated mortality benefit to risk-reducing hysterectomy for women with Lynch syndrome, surgery eliminates the risk of endometrial cancer and is therefore reasonable to consider if childbearing is complete [70]. Given moderate risk of ovarian cancer for women with Lynch syndrome, concomitant RRSO can also be considered.

Data do not support routine ovarian cancer screening for Lynch syndrome [71]. A large prospective, ideally randomized, study is therefore needed to definitively address this question. Currently, women are advised to visit their gynecologist annually so as to review red flag symptoms for endometrial cancer including abnormal uterine bleeding or postmenopausal bleeding, symptoms of ovarian cancer as previously described, and to discuss fertility and the timing of risk-reducing surgery [71].

Women should be counseled by a gynecologist with a special knowledge in Lynch syndrome as to the benefits, risks, and timing of surgery. When to perform the surgery can be individualized by considering the patient's wishes, their family history, and the type of pathogenic MMR mutation they carry [71, 72]. However, risk-reducing hysterectomy and bilateral salpingo-oophorectomy is generally offered between the ages of 40 to 45 with preference closer to 45 and childbearing complete. Surgery earlier than age 40 should generally be reserved for those with a family history of early onset endometrial cancer after shared decision making regarding risks and benefits. Where possible, risk-reducing surgery should be performed by a laparoscopic or robotic approach so as to reduce hospital stay and morbidity [73]. If risk-reducing surgery is performed before menopause, women should be offered estrogen-only HT up until the natural age of menopause assuming no contraindications exist [35, 71]. HT has a protective effect against colorectal cancer [71] and is helpful for the treatment of menopausal symptoms.

Other Considerations

Lynch syndrome is associated with a wide range of cancer including colorectal, endometrial, ovarian, renal and/or ureteral, and gastric. Therefore, women found to have Lynch syndrome need to be managed by a multidisciplinary team.

Colonoscopy is highly effective as both a screening test and as cancer prevention, in that precancerous colon adenomas are removed during the procedure. The mortality benefit of screening colonoscopy for individuals with Lynch syndrome has been known for decades [74, 75]. Screening colonoscopy is typically recommended every one to two years beginning ages mid-20s. This recommendation may vary based on gene and family history. In addition, aspirin chemoprophylaxis has been shown to reduce the risk of colorectal cancer and improve survival in patients who have Lynch syndrome and should therefore be offered if not contraindicated [76]. The exact doses of aspirin that should be prescribed is yet to be established and forms the central question at the heart of the CAPP3 study (www.capp3.org/), still ongoing at the time of this writing. Patients with Lynch syndrome have an increased risk of gastric cancer along with colorectal cancer, and international guidelines recommend upper GI surveillance with esophogastroduodenoscopy (EGD) in coordination with colonoscopy along with biopsies for the prophylactic eradication of *helicobacter pylori* [77, 78].

Rare Hereditary Gynecologic Cancer Predisposition Syndromes

Due to the rarity of most of these syndromes and the complexities of diagnosis and management, referral to a specialty team is recommended.

PTEN Hamartoma Tumor Syndrome (PHTS)

PHTS is a variety of disorders caused by a germline PV in *PTEN* (phosphatase and tensin homolog) [79, 80]. Cowden syndrome, although rare, is the main disorder in this spectrum and has an incidence of 1:200,000 [79, 80]. Cowden syndrome causes increased risks for breast, thyroid, and endometrial cancer and benign hamartomas of various tissues [79, 80].

Cowden syndrome is associated with a lifetime risk of endometrial cancer between 2–28%; however these estimates are based on small datasets [79, 80]. These endometrial cancer can develop at a very early age, therefore adolescents who develop endometrial cancer should be screened for *PTEN* PVs [79, 80]. Endometrial cancer surveillance does not have proven benefits, however endometrial biopsy is highly sensitive and specific and thus may be a consideration. Hysterectomy can be considered after completion of childbearing. European guidelines, however, do not encourage surveillance unless performed within a clinical trial [79, 80].

Rhabdoid Tumor Predisposition Syndrome

Rhabdoid Tumor Predisposition Syndrome is a rare autosomal dominant cancer predisposition syndrome of an unknown incidence in the general population [81]. The condition is due to germline PVs in the *SMARCB1* and *SMARCA4* genes. Most individuals are diagnosed by adolescence due the development of multiple rhabdoid tumors.

Small cell carcinoma of the ovary, hypercalcemic type (SCCOHT) is a rare form of ovarian neoplasm that is closely associated with PVs in the *SMARCA4* gene [82]. Furthermore, *SMARCA4* is associated with undifferentiated uterine sarcomas [83]. Diagnosis of Rhabdoid Tumor Predisposition Syndrome (RTPS) in the index case may be of limited utility to the index case, as both cancer have a poor prognosis, however cascade testing may help relatives who can benefit from intensive surveillance.

Due to the rarity of RTPS, current guidelines are based on expert opinion with limited evidence. Current consensus is that adults with the condition should have whole body MRI scans every six months [81]. In addition, female carriers could be offered pelvic ultrasounds every six months to exclude ovarian pathology; however it should be noted the value of these scans are not clear [81]. Risk-reducing hysterectomy with bilateral-salpingo-oophorectomy (with gamete preservation) has been performed in young women with *SMARCA4* PVs, however there is insufficient evidence to make this a recommendation [84].

Peutz-Jeghers Syndrome

Peutz-Jeghers syndrome (PJS) is a rare cancer predisposition that arises due to germline PVs in the *STK11* (serine threonine kinase 11) tumor suppressor gene affecting approximately 1:100,000 people in the general population [85]. A clinical diagnosis of PJS can be made with two or more of the following features: (1) two or more Peutz-Jeghers-type hamartomatous polyps of the GI tract, (2) mucocutaneous pigmentation in the oral mucosa, lips, nose, eyes, genitalia, or fingers, or (3) a family history of PJS (85). Clinical genetic testing is recommended for patients meeting the clinical diagnosis of PJS but diagnosis is not dependent on germline testing. Linked registry data has found an association between *STK11* and uterine, cervical, and ovarian cancer. By age 50 years, female carriers have a gynecological cancer risk eight times that of the general population; approximating 10–20% [86, 87]. The histology of uterine cancer is not well reported. Ovarian cancer seen in PJS seem to have a varied histology with reports of borderline, malignant sex cord stromal tumors with annular tubules (SCTAT) and invasive epithelial ovarian cancer; although SCTAT is most closely associated [88]. SCTAT is not detected with CA-125. With regard to cervical cancer, there is a strong association between *STK11* and a rare histological subtype: minimal deviation adenocarcinoma also known as adenoma malignum [85]. This subtype is independent of high-risk human papillomavirus (HPV) which drives oncogenesis in the vast majority of cervical cancer in the general population [89]. This could be problematic given the move towards HPV cervical cancer screening, as patients with Peutz-Jeghers syndrome who have developed adenoma malignum cervical cancer could be missed by HPV-only screening protocols. Therefore, international guidelines recommend annual cervical screening with cytology regardless of HPV status, as well as annual pelvic exam, annual pelvic ultrasound, and endometrial biopsy for abnormal bleeding [85]. Hysterectomy can be considered upon completion of childbearing. Counseling should be performed by an expert who can explain the degree of uncertainty within the data. Women should be counseled regarding the pathognomonic symptoms of gynecological cancer [85].

DICER1 Syndrome

The *DICER1* gene is central to the control of protein translation and is regarded as a tumor suppressor gene [90]. Patients who carry a germline PV in *DICER1* are known to develop numerous benign and malignant neoplasms [91]. Approximately 1:11000 people carry a *DICER1* PV (84). DICER1 syndrome is associated with cystic nephroma, multinodular goiter, thyroid cancer, lung cysts, and ovarian sex-cord stromal tumors [91].

There is a well-established connection between *DICER1* and Sertoli-Leydig cell tumor (SLCT) [91], which are usually unilateral and early-stage, with the majority occurring in adolescence. There is a suggestion that *DICER1* is also associated with gynandroblastoma and sarcomas of the ovary [90]. Young patients with gynandroblastomas and SLCTs often present with virilization or amenorrhea. By the age of 60 years it is thought the risk of SLCT is 7% with the other types of gynecological cancer only being documented rarely in *DICER1* PV carriers [90]. Gynecologists need to be mindful of *DICER1* in individuals diagnosed with SLCT, especially patients who are below the age of 20 years. Clinical guidance places emphasis on clinical examination as a means of surveillance with annual pelvic ultrasounds between 8–40 years only offered after expert consultation [91]. Risk-reducing surgery is not addressed in the current guidelines [91].

Hereditary Cancer Risk Assessment for Women with a Family History of Cancer

As illustrated in the case presentation, women who have never had cancer themselves but have a family history of cancer may express concern regarding cancer risk. Thorough assessment of family history of cancer will determine whether hereditary cancer genetic testing is indicated and will help to clarify next steps.

Whenever possible, the optimal first step is for the relative who has had cancer to undergo hereditary cancer genetic testing. By testing the affected family member first, the question of whether that cancer has an identifiable hereditary cause will be answered for the entire family. If the affected individual tests negative, then unaffected relatives can be reassured that it is not necessary for them to undergo genetic testing related to that family history. However, if the affected relative tests positive for a hereditary cancer predisposition, then relatives can undergo predictive genetic testing for the known familial PV. Both positive and negative results of predictive genetic testing for a known familial PV have clear interpretations. Testing positive for a known familial PV indicates increased risk for the cancer related to the gene in question. Testing negative for a known familial PV is a "true negative" result that in most cases allows for a high level of reassurance that the individual is not at significantly increased risk for the cancer(s) in question.

In some situations, there is not a living affected relative to test first, or the affected relative may be unwilling or unable to undergo hereditary cancer genetic testing. In this case it is reasonable for the unaffected individual to undergo hereditary cancer genetic testing including all genes that could be reasonably associated with the family history of cancer. If a hereditary cancer predisposing PV is identified, this is still an informative result indicating that the individual is at increased risk for the cancer related to the gene in question. However, negative genetic test results in the absence of a known familial PV are less clear and do not provide the same level of reassurance as the "true negative" result described above. As we would not know whether or to what extent the family history of cancer was due to the genes that were tested, the possibility that the individual may still be at increased risk for cancer due to the family history cannot be excluded.

For common cancer such as breast cancer and colorectal cancer, an additional ~10% to 15% of diagnoses may have a familial component that is multifactorial in nature rather than attributed to a single gene hereditary cancer predisposition. Thus, even in the absence of an identified hereditary cancer predisposition, empiric risk assessment based on both personal and family history can be helpful for those with a family history of breast and/or colorectal cancer. For example, an individual who has a family history of breast cancer and has undergone hereditary breast cancer genetic testing with negative results, may still be at increased risk of breast cancer. Models such as Gail [92] and Tyer-Cuzick [93] can be used to estimate breast cancer risk, and those estimates can then inform decisions about screening (such as whether or not to consider breast MRI in addition to mammogram) and chemo-prevention (such as tamoxifen). For those with a family history of colorectal cancer and uninformative negative genetic test results, screening colonoscopy starting at a younger age than is recommended for those at general population risk may still be recommended [94].

Interpretation of Genetic Test Results: Additional Considerations

Variants of Uncertain Significance

Benign germline variants (polymorphisms) are common and are generally excluded from genetic test results. Some germline variants, particularly missense variants and variants that may or may not impact splicing, are of uncertain clinical significance. Often these variants of uncertain significance (VUS) are included on germline genetic test reports. Many clinical genetic testing laboratories periodically revisit variant classification, and VUS result reports may later be amended once the variant has been definitively classified as either benign/likely benign, or, more rarely, upgraded to pathogenic or likely pathogenic. As there is no known clinical significance to a VUS result, it should not be used as the sole or primary basis for recommending any medical or surgical management. Instead, VUS results should be treated as normal, negative results, unless or until later proven otherwise. Providers who are ordering genetic tests should have procedures in place for the disposition of amended VUS genetic test results, including notifying patients of clinically significant changes in interpretation in a timely manner.

Risk of Autosomal Recessive Conditions

Many hereditary cancer predisposition PVs are also associated with autosomal recessive conditions. In the rare circumstance where an individual inherits a PV in the same gene from each of their parents, this can result in a serious medical condition, often with childhood onset. Such conditions include ataxia telangiectasia (*ATM*), Fanconi anemia (*BRCA1, BRCA2, PALB2, BRIP1, RAD51 C*), and CMMRD constitutional mismatch repair deficiency (Lynch syndrome). Individuals with childbearing potential who are found to have a PV in a gene also associated with an autosomal recessive condition, should be informed of the family planning implications, including the advisability of partner genetic testing. If her partner is also a carrier for the same PV, fertility treatment with genetic testing of embryos will markedly reduce the likelihood of an affected offspring.

Case Resolution

The patient's sister underwent hereditary ovarian cancer genetic testing and was found to have a germline *BRCA2* PV (see Figure 3.2). The patient then underwent predictive genetic testing and tested negative for the familial *BRCA2* PV. This is a true negative result indicating that the patient is not at increased risk for ovarian cancer. In addition, the patient's children are not at risk to have inherited this *BRCA2* PV.

However, the patient's niece did test positive for the familial *BRCA2* PV and is now undergoing annual breast MRI. She is attempting conception with in vitro fertilization with pre-implantation genetic testing of her embryos to reduce the chance of transmitting a *BRCA2* PV to her child. She intends to obtain a risk-reducing bilateral salpingo-oophorectomy when she is between the ages of 40 to 45 and has completed childbearing.

Molly S. Daniels, Denise R. Nebgen, Neil Ryan

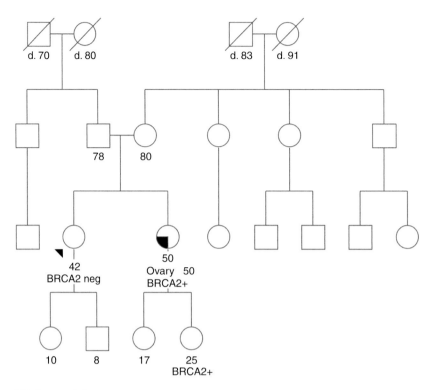

Figure 3.2 Case resolution

Take Home Points

- Hereditary ovarian cancer genetic testing including *BRCA1/BRCA2* should be offered to all women with high grade nonmucinous epithelial ovarian cancer, due to high mutation prevalence, treatment implications, and family implications.
- As 2% to 3% of women with endometrial cancer have Lynch syndrome, further assessment for Lynch syndrome (assessment of tumor mismatch repair status and/or germline testing) should be offered to all women with endometrial cancer.
- Genetic testing of the patient with cancer allows for the most accurate predictive genetic testing of family members.
- Risk reduction strategies for women with *BRCA1/BRCA2* mutations and for individuals with Lynch syndrome have proven mortality benefit.

References

1. Siegel R. L., Miller K. D., Fuchs H. E., Jemal A. Cancer statistics, 2022. *CA Cancer J Clin.* 2022 Jan;**72**(1):7–33. doi: 10.3322/caac.21708. Epub 2022 Jan 12. PMID: 35020204.

2. Walsh T., Casadei S., Lee M. K., et al. Mutations in 12 genes for inherited ovarian, fallopian tube, and peritoneal carcinoma identified by massively parallel sequencing. *Proc Natl Acad Sci U S A.* 2011;**108**(44):18032–7.

3. Henrikson N. B., Morrison C. C., Blasi P. R., et al. Behavioral counseling for skin cancer prevention: Evidence report and systematic review for the US Preventive Services Task Force. *JAMA*. 2018;**319**(11):1143–57.

4. Aune D., Navarro Rosenblatt D. A., Chan D. S., et al. Anthropometric factors and endometrial cancer risk: a systematic review and dose-response meta-analysis of prospective studies. *Ann Oncol*. 2015;**26**(8):1635–48.

5. Petrucelli N., Daly M. B., Pal T. BRCA1- and BRCA2-Associated Hereditary Breast and Ovarian Cancer. In: Adam M. P., Everman D. B., Mirzaa G. M., et al., editors. *GeneReviews((R))*. GeneReviews® [Internet]. Seattle (WA): University of Washington, Seattle; 1993–2023. PMID: 20301425.

6. Ryan N. A. J., McMahon R., Tobi S., et al. The proportion of endometrial tumours associated with Lynch syndrome (PETALS): A prospective cross-sectional study. *PLoS Med*. 2020;**17**(9):e1003263.

7. Chao E. C., Astbury C., Deignan J. L., et al. Incidental detection of acquired variants in germline genetic and genomic testing: A points to consider statement of the American College of Medical Genetics and Genomics (ACMG). *Genet Med*. 2021;**23**(7):1179–84.

8. Joo L., Bradley C. C., Lin S. H., Scheet P. A., Nead K. T. Causes of clonal hematopoiesis: A review. *Curr Oncol Rep*. 2023; **25**(3):211–20.

9. Shah P. D. Polygenic risk scores for breast cancer: Can they deliver on the promise of precision medicine? *JAMA Netw Open*. 2021;**4**(8):e2119333.

10. Wynn J., Levinson E., Koval C., Ernst M. E., Chung W. K. Questioning the validity of clinically available breast cancer polygenic risk scores: Comparison of two labs reveals discrepancies. *Fam Cancer*. 2022;**21**(2):125–7.

11. Cobain E. F., Wu Y. M., Vats P., et al. Assessment of clinical benefit of integrative genomic profiling in advanced solid tumors. *JAMA Oncol*. 2021;**7**(4):525–33.

12. Mandelker D., Donoghue M., Talukdar S., et al. Germline-focussed analysis of tumour-only sequencing: Recommendations from the ESMO Precision Medicine Working Group. *Ann Oncol*. 2019;**30**(8):1221–31.

13. Meric-Bernstam F., Brusco L., Daniels M., et al. Incidental germline variants in 1000 advanced cancer on a prospective somatic genomic profiling protocol. *Ann Oncol*. 2016;**27**(5):795–800.

14. Lincoln S. E., Nussbaum R. L., Kurian A. W., et al. Yield and utility of germline testing following tumor sequencing in patients with cancer. *JAMA Netw Open*. 2020;**3**(10):e2019452.

15. Group ABCS. Prevalence and penetrance of BRCA1 and BRCA2 mutations in a population-based series of breast cancer cases. *British Journal of Cancer*. 2000;**83**(10):1301–8.

16. Maxwell K. N., Domchek S. M., Nathanson K. L., Robson M. E. Population frequency of germline BRCA1/2 mutations. *Journal of Clinical Oncology*. 2016;**34**(34):4183–5.

17. Pal T., Permuth-Wey J., Betts J. A., et al. BRCA1 and BRCA2 mutations account for a large proportion of ovarian carcinoma cases. *Cancer*. 2005;**104**(12):2807–16.

18. Thompson L. H., Schild D. Homologous recombinational repair of DNA ensures mammalian chromosome stability. *Mutation Research/Fundamental and Molecular Mechanisms of Mutagenesis*. 2001;**477**(1):131–53.

19. Honrado E., Benítez J., Palacios J. Histopathology of BRCA1- and BRCA2-associated breast cancer. *Crit Rev Oncol Hematol*. 2006;**59**(1):27–39.

20. De Talhouet S., Peron J., Vuilleumier A., et al. Clinical outcome of breast cancer in carriers of BRCA1 and BRCA2 mutations according to molecular subtypes. *Scientific Reports*. 2020;**10**(1):7073.

21. Lakhani S. R., Manek S., Penault-Llorca F., et al. Pathology of ovarian cancer in BRCA1 and BRCA2 carriers. *Clinical Cancer Research*. 2004;**10**(7):2473–81.

22. Moore K., Colombo N., Scambia G., et al. Maintenance Olaparib in patients with newly diagnosed advanced ovarian cancer. *New England Journal of Medicine.* 2018;**379**(26):2495–505.

23. Tattersall A., Ryan N., Wiggans A. J., Rogozińska E., Morrison J. Poly(ADP-ribose) polymerase (PARP) inhibitors for the treatment of ovarian cancer. *Cochrane Database of Systematic Reviews.* 2022;**2**(2).

24. Weinberger V., Bednarikova M., Cibula D., Zikan M. Serous tubal intraepithelial carcinoma (STIC): Clinical impact and management. *Expert Rev Anticancer Ther.* 2016;**16**(12):1311–21.

25. Gasparri M. L., Bellaminutti S., Farooqi A. A., Cuccu I., Di Donato V., Papadia A. Endometrial cancer and BRCA mutations: A systematic review. *J Clin Med.* 2022;**11**(11).

26. Kitson S. J., Bafligil C., Ryan N. A. J., et al. BRCA1 and BRCA2 pathogenic variant carriers and endometrial cancer risk: A cohort study. *Eur J Cancer.* 2020;**136**:169–75.

27. de Jonge M. M., de Kroon C. D., Jenner D. J., et al. Endometrial cancer risk in women with germline BRCA1 or BRCA2 mutations: Multicenter cohort study. *J Natl Cancer Inst.* 2021;**113**(9):1203–11.

28. Smith E. S., Paula A. D. C., Cadoo K. A., et al. Endometrial cancer in BRCA1 or BRCA2 germline mutation carriers: Assessment of homologous recombination DNA repair defects. *JCO Precis Oncol.* 2019(3):1–11.

29. Mersch J., Jackson M. A., Park M., et al. Cancer associated with BRCA1 and BRCA2 mutations other than breast and ovarian. *Cancer.* 2015;**121**(2):269–75.

30. Kuchenbaecker K. B., Hopper J. L., Barnes D. R., et al. Risks of breast, ovarian, and contralateral breast cancer for BRCA1 and BRCA2 mutation carriers. *JAMA.* 2017;**317**(23):2402–16.

31. PDQ® Cancer Genetics Editorial Board. PDQ BRCA1 and BRCA2. Bethesda, MD: National Cancer Institute. Updated September 3, 2023. www.cancer.gov/about-cancer/causes-prevention/genetics/brca-genes-hp-pdq. Accessed April 4, 2023.

32. Liu Y. L., Breen K., Catchings A., et al. Risk-reducing bilateral salpingo-oophorectomy for ovarian cancer: A review and clinical guide for hereditary predisposition genes. *JCO Oncol Pract.* 2022;**18**(3):201–09.

33. Finch A. P., Lubinski J., Moller P., et al. Impact of oophorectomy on cancer incidence and mortality in women with a BRCA1 or BRCA2 mutation. *J Clin Oncol.* 2014;**32**(15):1547–53.

34. Kingsberg S. A., Larkin L. C., Liu J. H. Clinical effects of early or surgical menopause. *Obstet Gynecol.* 2020;**135**(4):853–68.

35. Nebgen D. R., Domchek S. M., Kotsopoulos J., et al. Care after premenopausal risk-reducing salpingo-oophorectomy in high-risk women: Scoping review and international consensus recommendations. *BJOG.* 2023;**130**(12):1437–50.

36. Kotsopoulos J., Gronwald J., Karlan B. Y., et al. Hormone replacement therapy after oophorectomy and breast cancer risk among BRCA1 mutation carriers. *JAMA oncology.* 2018;**4**(8):1059–65.

37. Ross R. K., Paganini-Hill A., Wan P. C., Pike M. C. Effect of hormone replacement therapy on breast cancer risk: Estrogen versus estrogen plus progestin. *JNCI: Journal of the National Cancer Institute.* 2000;**92**(4):328–32.

38. Asi N., Mohammed K., Haydour Q., et al. Progesterone vs. synthetic progestins and the risk of breast cancer: a systematic review and meta-analysis. *Systematic Reviews.* 2016;**5**(1):1–8.

39. Mørch L. S., Skovlund C. W., Hannaford P. C., Iversen L., Fielding S., Lidegaard Ø. Contemporary hormonal contraception and the risk of breast cancer. *New England Journal of Medicine.* 2017;**377**(23):2228–39.

40. Conz L., Mota B. S., Bahamondes L., et al. Levonorgestrel-releasing intrauterine system and breast cancer risk: A systematic review and meta-analysis. *Acta Obstet Gynecol Scand.* 2020;**99**(8):970–82.

41. Silva F. R., Grande A. J., Lacerda Macedo A. C., et al. Meta-analysis of breast cancer risk in levonorgestrel-releasing intrauterine system users. *Clin Breast Cancer.* 2021;**21**(6):497–508.

42. Lu K. H., Nebgen D. R., Norquist B., et al. TUBectomy with delayed oophorectomy in high risk women to assess the safety of prevention (TUBA-WISP-II) NCT04294927 2019 [22]. Available from: https://clinicaltrials.gov/ct2/show/NCT04294927.

43. Harmsen M. G., Arts-de Jong M., Hoogerbrugge N., et al. Early salpingectomy (TUbectomy) with delayed oophorectomy to improve quality of life as alternative for risk-reducing salpingo-oophorectomy in BRCA1/2 mutation carriers (TUBA study): A prospective non-randomised multicentre study. *BMC Cancer.* 2015;**15**(1):593.

44. Gaba F., Goyal S., Marks D., et al. Surgical decision making in premenopausal BRCA carriers considering risk-reducing early salpingectomy or salpingo-oophorectomy: A qualitative study. *Journal of Medical Genetics.* 2022;**59**(2):122.

45. Menon U., Gentry-Maharaj A., Burnell M., et al. Ovarian cancer population screening and mortality after long-term follow-up in the UK Collaborative Trial of Ovarian Cancer Screening (UKCTOCS): A randomised controlled trial. *Lancet.* 2021;**397**(10290):2182–93.

46. Evans D. G., Gaarenstroom K. N., Stirling D., et al. Screening for familial ovarian cancer: Poor survival of BRCA1/2 related cancer. *Journal of Medical Genetics.* 2009;**46**(9):593.

47. Hogg R., Friedlander M. Biology of epithelial ovarian cancer: Implications for screening women at high genetic risk. *Journal of Clinical Oncology.* 2004;**22**(7):1315–27.

48. Olivier R. I., Lubsen-Brandsma M. A. C., Verhoef S., van Beurden M. CA-125 and transvaginal ultrasound monitoring in high-risk women cannot prevent the diagnosis of advanced ovarian cancer. *Gynecologic Oncology.* 2006;**100**(1):20–26.

49. Rebbeck T. R., Friebel T., Lynch H. T., et al. Bilateral prophylactic mastectomy reduces breast cancer risk in BRCA1 and BRCA2 mutation carriers: The PROSE study group. *Journal of Clinical Oncology.* 2004;**22**(6):1055–62.

50. Domchek S. M. Risk-reducing mastectomy in BRCA1 and BRCA2 mutation carriers: A complex discussion. *JAMA.* 2019;**321**(1):27.

51. Cuzick J., Sestak I., Forbes J. F., et al. Anastrozole for prevention of breast cancer in high-risk postmenopausal women (IBIS-II): An international, double-blind, randomised placebo-controlled trial. *The Lancet.* 2014;**383**(9922):1041–08.

52. Cuzick J., Forbes J. F., Sestak I., et al. Long-term results of Tamoxifen Prophylaxis for breast cancer: 96-month follow-up of the randomized IBIS-I trial. *JNCI: Journal of the National Cancer Institute.* 2007;**99**(4):272–82.

53. Lu K. H., Broaddus R. R. Endometrial cancer. *N Engl J Med.* 2020;**383**(21):2053–64.

54. Lu K. H., Dinh M., Kohlmann W., et al. Gynecologic cancer as a "sentinel cancer" for women with hereditary nonpolyposis colorectal cancer syndrome. *Obstet Gynecol.* 2005;**105**(3):569–74.

55. Ryan N. A. J., McMahon R. F. T., Ramchander N. C., Seif M. W., Evans D. G., Crosbie E. J. Lynch syndrome for the gynaecologist. *The Obstetrician & Gynaecologist.* 2021;**23**(1):9–20.

56. Haraldsdottir S., Rafnar T., Frankel W. L., et al. Comprehensive population-wide analysis of Lynch syndrome in Iceland reveals founder mutations in MSH6 and PMS2. *Nature Communications.* 2017;**8**(1):1–11.

57. Ryan N. A. J., Glaire M. A., Blake D., Cabrera-Dandy M., Evans D. G., Crosbie E. J. The proportion of endometrial cancer associated with Lynch syndrome: A systematic review of the literature and meta-analysis. *Genet Med.* 2019;**21**(10):2167–80.

58. Atwal A., Snowsill T., Dandy M. C., et al. The prevalence of mismatch repair

deficiency in ovarian cancer: A systematic review and meta-analysis. *Int J Cancer.* 2022;**151**(9):1626–39.

59. Tutlewska K., Lubinski J., Kurzawski G. Germline deletions in the EPCAM gene as a cause of Lynch syndrome: Literature review. *Hereditary Cancer in Clinical Practice.* 2013;**11**(1):9.

60. Li G.-M. Mechanisms and functions of DNA mismatch repair. *Cell Research.* 2008;**18**(1):85–98.

61. Vikas P., Messersmith H., Compton C., et al. Mismatch repair and microsatellite instability testing for immune checkpoint inhibitor therapy: ASCO endorsement of College of American Pathologists guideline. *J Clin Oncol.* 2023;**41**(10):1943–8.

62. Ryan N. A. J., Walker T. D. J., Bolton J., et al. Histological and somatic mutational profiles of mismatch repair deficient endometrial tumours of different aetiologies. *Cancer (Basel).* 2021;**13**(18).

63. Glaire M. A., Ryan N. A., Ijsselsteijn M. E., et al. Discordant prognosis of mismatch repair deficiency in colorectal and endometrial cancer reflects variation in antitumour immune response and immune escape. *The Journal of Pathology.* 2022; **257**(3):340–51.

64. Ryan N. A. J., Evans D. G., Green K., Crosbie E. J. Pathological features and clinical behavior of Lynch syndrome-associated ovarian cancer. *Gynecologic Oncology.* 2017;**144**(3):491–5.

65. Møller P. The Prospective Lynch Syndrome Database: Background, design, main results and complete MySQL code. *Hereditary Cancer in Clinical Practice.* 2022;**20**(1):37.

66. Mercado R. C., Hampel H., Kastrinos F., et al. Performance of PREMM1,2,6, MMRpredict, and MMRpro in detecting Lynch syndrome among endometrial cancer cases. *Genetics in Medicine.* 2012;**14**(7):670–80.

67. Aiyer K. T. S., Doeleman T., Ryan N. A., et al. Validity of a two-antibody testing algorithm for mismatch repair deficiency testing in cancer: A systematic literature review and meta-analysis. *Modern Pathology.* 2022;**35**(12):1775–83.

68. Paluch-Shimon S., Cardoso F., Sessa C., et al. Prevention and screening in BRCA mutation carriers and other breast/ovarian hereditary cancer syndromes: ESMO Clinical Practice Guidelines for cancer prevention and screening. *Ann Oncol.* 2016;**27**(suppl 5):v103–v10.

69. Stoffel E. M., Mangu P. B., Gruber S. B., et al. Hereditary colorectal cancer syndromes: American Society of Clinical Oncology Clinical Practice Guideline Endorsement of the Familial Risk–Colorectal Cancer. *European Society for Medical Oncology Clinical Practice Guidelines. Journal of Clinical Oncology.* 2014;**33**(2):209–17.

70. Schmeler K. M., Lynch H. T., Chen L. M., et al. Prophylactic surgery to reduce the risk of gynecologic cancer in the Lynch syndrome. *N Engl J Med.* 2006;**354**(3):261–9.

71. Crosbie E. J., Ryan N. A. J., Arends M. J., et al. The Manchester International Consensus Group recommendations for the management of gynecological cancer in Lynch syndrome. *Genet Med.* 2019;**21**(10):2390–400.

72. Dominguez-Valentin M., Seppala T. T., Engel C., et al. Risk-reducing gynecological surgery in Lynch syndrome: Results of an international survey from the Prospective Lynch Syndrome Database. *J Clin Med.* 2020;**9**(7).

73. Garry R., Fountain J., Mason S., et al. The eVALuate study: Two parallel randomised trials, one comparing laparoscopic with abdominal hysterectomy, the other comparing laparoscopic with vaginal hysterectomy. *BMJ.* 2004;**328**(7432):129.

74. de Jong A. E., Hendriks Y. M., Kleibeuker J. H., et al. Decrease in mortality in Lynch syndrome families because of surveillance. *Gastroenterology.* 2006;**130**(3):665–71.

75. Jarvinen H. J., Aarnio M., Mustonen H., et al. Controlled 15-year trial on screening for colorectal cancer in families with hereditary nonpolyposis colorectal cancer. *Gastroenterology.* 2000;**118**(5):829–34.

76. Burn J., Sheth H., Elliott F., et al. Cancer prevention with aspirin in hereditary colorectal cancer (Lynch syndrome), 10-year follow-up and registry-based 20-year data in the CAPP2 study: A double-blind, randomised, placebo-controlled trial. *The Lancet*. 2020;**395**(10240):1855–63.

77. Seppälä T. T., Latchford A., Negoi I., et al. European guidelines from the EHTG and ESCP for Lynch syndrome: An updated third edition of the Mallorca guidelines based on gene and gender. *Br J Surg*. 2021;**108**(5):484–98.

78. Gupta S., Provenzale D., Llor X., et al. NCCN Guidelines Insights: Genetic/familial high-risk assessment: Colorectal, Version 2.2019: Featured updates to the NCCN Guidelines. *Journal of the National Comprehensive Cancer Network J Natl Compr Canc Netw*. 2019;**17**(9):1032–41.

79. Pilarski R., Burt R., Kohlman W., et al. Cowden syndrome and the PTEN hamartoma tumor syndrome: Systematic review and revised diagnostic criteria. *J Natl Cancer Inst*. 2013;**105**(21):1607–16.

80. Tischkowitz M., Colas C., Pouwels S., Hoogerbrugge N., Group PGD, European Reference Network G. Cancer Surveillance Guideline for individuals with PTEN hamartoma tumour syndrome. *Eur J Hum Genet*. 2020;**28**(10):1387–93.

81. Nemes K., Bens S., Bourdeaut F., et al. Rhabdoid tumor predisposition syndrome. GeneReviews®[Internet]. 2017.

82. Auguste A., Blanc-Durand F., Deloger M., et al. Small cell carcinoma of the ovary, hypercalcemic type (SCCOHT) beyond SMARCA4 mutations: A comprehensive genomic analysis. *Cells*. 2020;**9**(6).

83. Lin D. I., Allen J. M., Hecht J. L., et al. SMARCA4 inactivation defines a subset of undifferentiated uterine sarcomas with rhabdoid and small cell features and germline mutation association. *Modern Pathology*. 2019;**32**(11):1675–87.

84. Kostov S., Watrowski R., Kornovski Y., et al. Hereditary gynecologic cancer syndromes: A narrative review. *Onco Targets Ther*. 2022;**15**:381–405.

85. Wagner A., Aretz S., Auranen A., et al. The management of Peutz-Jeghers Syndrome: European Hereditary Tumour Group (EHTG) guideline. *J Clin Med*. 2021;**10**(3).

86. Giardiello F. M., Brensinger J. D., Tersmette A. C., et al. Very high risk of cancer in familial Peutz-Jeghers syndrome. *Gastroenterology*. 2000;**119**(6):1447–53.

87. Resta N., Pierannunzio D., Lenato G. M., et al. Cancer risk associated with STK11/LKB1 germline mutations in Peutz-Jeghers syndrome patients: Results of an Italian multicenter study. *Dig Liver Dis*. 2013;**45**(7):606–11.

88. van Lier M. G. F., Wagner A., Mathus-Vliegen E. M. H., et al. High cancer risk in Peutz–Jeghers Syndrome: A systematic review and surveillance recommendations. *Official journal of the American College of Gastroenterology | ACG*. 2010;**105**(6):1258–64.

89. Zhao F.-H., Lin M. J., Chen F., et al. Performance of high-risk human papillomavirus DNA testing as a primary screen for cervical cancer: A pooled analysis of individual patient data from 17 population-based studies from China. *The Lancet Oncology*. 2010;**11**(12):1160–71.

90. González I. A., Stewart D. R., Schultz K. A. P., et al. DICER1 tumor predisposition syndrome: an evolving story initiated with the pleuropulmonary blastoma. *Modern Pathology*. 2022;**35**(1):4–22.

91. Bakhuizen J. J., Hanson H., van der Tuin K., et al. Surveillance recommendations for DICER1 pathogenic variant carriers: A report from the SIOPE Host Genome Working Group and CanGene-CanVar Clinical Guideline Working Group. *Fam Cancer*. 2021;**20**(4):337–48.

92. The Breast Cancer Risk Assessment Tool. https://bcrisktool.cancer.gov/index.html.

93. Online Tyrer-Cuzick Model Breast Cancer Risk Evaluation Tool. https://ibis.ikonopedia.com/.

94. Force U. S. P. S. T., Davidson K. W., Barry M. J., et al. Screening for colorectal cancer: US Preventive Services Task Force Recommendation Statement. *JAMA*. 2021;**325**(19):1965–77.

Managing Sexual Health Through Treatment and Survivorship

Jessica F. Moore and Kristin E. Rojas

Case Presentation

Celia is a 54-year-old patient diagnosed with AJCC Stage II estrogen receptor-positive, Her2-negative invasive ductal carcinoma of the left breast at age 50. She received neoadjuvant chemotherapy, followed by lumpectomy and sentinel node biopsy, adjuvant whole breast radiation, and has been on an aromatase inhibitor for almost three years. She presents to the clinic to discuss worsening vaginal dryness and painful sex. She describes any sexual activity as "burning," and any penetration feels "like papercuts". She reports these symptoms started during chemotherapy but have worsened over time. She now avoids any sexual activity with her partner, and this makes her anxious. During her visit, she endorses very low desire since starting the aromatase inhibitor, and she explains that this is very distressing for her.

Etiology of Sexual Health Concerns in Female Cancer Patients

By 2026, more than 10 million US cancer survivors will be women, and at least half of those women will experience life-altering disruptions in sexual function as a sequela of their diagnosis or treatment [1]. While sexual function concerns have common themes, the diverse presentation of these patients depends on preexisting health conditions, stage at diagnosis, and treatments received. Each patient's perception of these issues is also variable and affected by cultural norms, societal acceptance, and even hygiene traditions passed down within families.

The spectrum of sexual health concerns ranges from psychological to physical effects. The diagnosis itself can lead to shame, distress, and patients' confrontation with their own mortality. The physical manifestations include those arising from estrogen suppression which can be due to anti-estrogen medication, ovarian suppression during treatment, ovarian injury from cytotoxic chemotherapy, or bilateral oophorectomy. The likelihood of resolution of these symptoms is directly proportional to the availability of evidence-based patient education including mitigation strategies but also the familiarity of their providers with addressing these concerns.

Genitourinary syndrome of menopause (GSM), formerly known as vaginal atrophy, is a well-known but understudied effect of induced menopause or estrogen blockade, which are two treatment strategies in the pre- or postoperative setting. GSM is an inclusive term that describes changes to the female vulva, vestibule, vagina, and pelvic floor. Prolonged estrogen suppression or receptor modulation, either by ovarian suppression or anti-estrogen therapy, systemic therapies influencing ovarian function, and surgical ovarian resection may lead to GSM. The sexual sequelae include vaginal dryness, painful sex, recurrent urinary tract infections, and incontinence. In a South Florida sexual health after cancer program at a National Cancer Institute (NCI)-designated cancer center, patients presenting for care reported: 53% vaginal dryness, 45% painful sex, 10% urinary symptoms, and 5% problems with orgasm. These chief complaints are reported by more than 80% of patients found to have severe atrophy-related disruptions in their urogenital exams, and almost half were found to have a narrowed vaginal introitus precluding penetrative sexual intercourse [2]. With evolving targeted therapies and improved cancer survival, inadequate treatment of these quality-of-life and relationship-altering sequelae may lead to poor therapy compliance, tempering the field's progress in long-term oncologic outcome improvements [3].

During treatment, women diagnosed with cancer may put their intimate lives on hold, indefinitely. The psychosocial hit of the diagnosis is quickly followed by rapid-fire diagnostic, staging, and subspecialist appointments until treatment is started. Their multimodal treatment regimen, coupled with the ongoing demands of daily living, caretaker activities, and professional careers, often translates to a hiatus from sexual activity, partnered or unpartnered. Many women report that the diagnostic phase of their cancer journey does not include a discussion about the sexual side effects of treatment. This contrasts with a study that found that over 50% of male patients diagnosed with prostate cancer receive information about how treatment will impact their sexual function, and this information often plays into the therapeutic route chosen after a shared decision-making discussion [4]. This moment prior to or at the initiation of therapy represents an opportunity for preparation and a discussion of best practices moving through treatment that can prevent the most severe sequelae. Strategies for approaching this discussion will be reviewed in this chapter. An author-curated collection of online resources for patients and providers to assist in these discussions is shown in Figure 4.1.

Sexual Health Concerns During and After Treatment

The Effect of Anti-Estrogen Therapies in Women with Estrogen-Sensitive Cancer

Anti-estrogen medications are a common culprit of sexual health concerns for women with breast and gynecologic cancer, but women with other cancer types may experience similar symptoms through other mechanisms. Approximately 70–80% of all breast cancer are hormone receptor-positive. As such, most women will receive anti-estrogen therapy after surgery (adjuvant therapy) to reduce the risk of recurrence. Anti-estrogen therapy, also known as hormone or endocrine therapy, functions by blocking or degrading estrogen receptors in the breast and other tissues or by suppressing circulating estrogen through peripheral aromatase inhibition. These drugs include selective estrogen receptor modulators (SERMs), selective estrogen receptor degraders (SERDs), and aromatase inhibitors (AIs). Adjuvant anti-estrogen therapy has been shown in multiple large trials to improve disease-free survival for postmenopausal women with invasive breast cancer [5]. Aromatase inhibitors may also be used in the treatment of gynecologic malignancies such as endometrial cancer and some types of ovarian cancer [6].

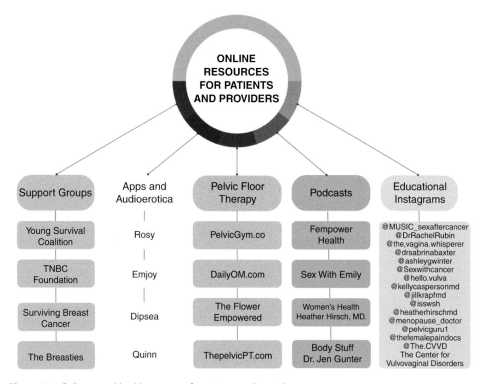

Figure 4.1 Online sexual health resources for patients and providers

Sexual Side Effects in Women on Anti-Estrogen Therapy

According to the North American Menopause Society, the normal postmenopausal estradiol (E2) range is likely lower than previously measured with conventional assays [7]. With the more accurate measurements, the Society postulates that normal postmenopausal E2 is < 10 pg/mL [8]. A recent study utilizing the ultra-sensitive liquid chromatography-mass spectrometry (LC-MS) method revealed that women on AIs may drive serum E2 levels as low as 0.16 pg/mL [9]. Prolonged estrogen deprivation can induce even more dramatic changes in vaginal architecture resulting in vaginal shortening, stenosis, and a complete inability to participate in penetrative sexual activity.

Anti-estrogen therapy is effective in both the preventive and adjuvant setting, but the side effect profile influences patient adherence [10, 11]. The gynecologic sequelae of anti-estrogen therapy lead to genitourinary syndrome of menopause (GSM) symptoms including vaginal dryness, irritation, pain with sexual intercourse, bleeding after sex, recurrent vaginal infections, increased urinary tract infections, and dysuria. Those receiving treatment with anti-estrogen therapy, the effects of which may be multiplied by prior cytotoxic chemotherapy, are put into a "supermenopause" and report even more frequent and severe adverse effects on the vulva and vagina that can significantly impact quality of life [12]. While natural menopause has been shown to increase the risk of hypoactive sexual desire disorder (HSDD) in women, this risk is more profound in women an on anti-estrogen therapy: approximately half of the women on aromatase inhibitors report decreased libido, and 74% report insufficient lubrication [3].

Symptoms of GSM and sexual dysfunction appear to be more common with aromatase inhibitor use when compared to tamoxifen use. In a survey study using the Female Sexual Function Index (FSFI) to evaluate sexual dysfunction among breast cancer survivors, women who had taken aromatase inhibitors were 1.6 times more likely to report sexual dysfunction when compared to the group that did not receive endocrine therapy [13].

Younger women may be more dramatically impacted by abrupt changes in sexual function and are more likely to receive a recommendation for prolonged (>5 years) anti-estrogen therapy [14]. Despite this recommendation, between 30–50% of breast cancer survivors are not compliant with their anti-estrogen medication, with >40% of women prescribed tamoxifen not adhering to therapy due to side effects, and 70% prematurely stopping anti-estrogen therapy before five years [10, 11]. Similarly, women who report severe side effects are five times more likely to stop taking their medication prematurely [15]. Better addressing these quality-of-life concerns including GSM and female sexual dysfunction has the propensity to improve treatment compliance.

Treatment of Genitourinary Syndrome of Menopause: Moisturizers

Avoiding Irritants

Vaginal or vulvar surgery, prolonged estrogen suppression, chemotherapy, or immunomo-dulating treatments may result in hypersensitivity of the delicate tissues of the vulva or vagina to certain product ingredients. Patients reporting the sensation of burning or irritation may have a worsening of their GSM symptoms from irritating products. For some, the onset of symptoms brings the temptation to apply a variety of drugstore feminine hygiene products including soaps and wipes, but this can lead to an exacerbation of symptoms. According to the American College of Obstetricians and Gynecologists (ACOG), common vulvar irritants include but are not limited to: cleansers, fragrances, lubricants, bodily fluids such as urine and sweat, and moisture. Studies estimate that between 20–40% of women still practice vaginal douching, which disrupts the vaginal flora and increases the pH of the vagina [16]. Exposure to fragranced products is associated with the development of contact dermatitis, and therefore patients with sensitive skin should avoid their use [17]. These irritants are prevalent in sanitary pads, tampons, toilet paper, and bubble baths. Similarly, patients should avoid intravaginal soap use, only wear undergarments made of 100% cotton, avoid laundry detergents with fragrance, and promptly change out of wet swimsuits after water activities.

For patients who present with GSM and report the use of potentially offending topicals or irritant exposure, complete cessation of topical products while substituting single-ingredient organic coconut oil to the external vulva is an effective first step in treatment. Nonpetroleum emollients such as bland oils protect the irritated skin from acidic urine, giving it a chance to heal before adding in a hyaluronic acid or hormone vaginal moisturizer as discussed in the following sections. Patients should also be encouraged to study ingredient lists for all vulvar moisturizers or sexual activity lubricants (and to select their own lubricant) to avoid irritating chemicals. For patients concerned about hygiene with the elimination of vaginal washes, a discussion regarding how cessation of vaginal washes and wipes can reconstitute the vaginal lactobacilli and decrease vaginal infections may be helpful [18]. The addition of a bidet toilet attachment may also help patients feel more comfortable moving away from this hygiene ritual.

Vaginal Moisturizers

The conversation between a patient with GSM and her provider should start with a discussion regarding the difference between moisturizers and lubricants. Moisturizers have a distinct role from lubricants. By reducing friction at the time of sexual activity or dilator use, lubricants lead to decreased discomfort during and after these activities. Lubricants are used "in the moment." Moisturizers, on the other hand, should be thought of similarly to moisturizers in the (nonintimate) skincare world: as part of a "maintenance" routine. The authors propose a vulvovaginal care algorithm that starts with irritant elimination and the regular use of nonhormonal moisturizers. The regimen may be weekly, two to three times weekly, or nightly, and may be adjusted according to symptom severity and evolution. Local hormone therapy can be added in the weeks or months after initiating a nonhormonal regimen if patients have persistent symptoms, as will be discussed later in this section.

Nonhormonal Vaginal Moisturizers

Oil-based therapies for vaginal moisturization include coconut oil, olive oil, and Vitamin E oil. While oils are commonly found in patients' pantries and may be seen as more "holistic" or "natural," data proving their effectiveness is limited, especially when compared to newer "higher-tech" nonhormonal moisturizers containing hyaluronic or lactic acid. However, they may be helpful when used as an emollient to protect irritated or radiated vulvovaginal epithelium, for periurethral protection from dysuria, or as a treatment "base" in which additional therapies can be added. Coconut oil is reported to have antimicrobial, antifungal, and antioxidant properties. In vitro studies have demonstrated growth inhibition of both *clostridium dificile* and several species of *candida* by virgin coconut oil [19, 20]. Limited evidence suggests that vitamin E vaginal suppositories may be a viable alternative to estrogen-based topical therapy in select patients, as its antioxidant properties may work to repair the vaginal epithelium [21]. Patients should be counseled against the use of petroleum jelly as a moisturizer or lubricant since incomplete refinement of petrolatum or petroleum jelly is associated with polycyclic aromatic hydrocarbons, which are possible carcinogens [22]. In sexually active patients, it is important to note that oil-based moisturizers may not be compatible with latex condoms.

Synthetic vaginal moisturizers containing hyaluronic acid (HLA) or lactic acid reduce GSM symptoms and improve sexual function. In healthy reproductive-aged women, the vaginal microbiome is characterized by the predominance of lactic-acid-producing *Lactobacillus* species. Lactic acid may suppress pathogenic bacteria, and therefore supplementation with exogenous lactic acid is thought to work the same way [23]. Hyaluronic acid is a polymer of disaccharides that has the unique capacity to retain water. The use of hyaluronic acid-based vaginal preparations three times per week for eight weeks improved patient symptoms and vaginal health indices as measured by the Vaginal Health Index (VHI) in 46 postmenopausal women with symptoms of GSM [24].

Hyaluronic acid vaginal suppositories may result in similar improvement in GSM symptoms when compared to vaginal estrogen. A randomized trial of 56 postmenopausal women received either vaginal conjugated estrogen (0.62 mg) or hyaluronic acid vaginal

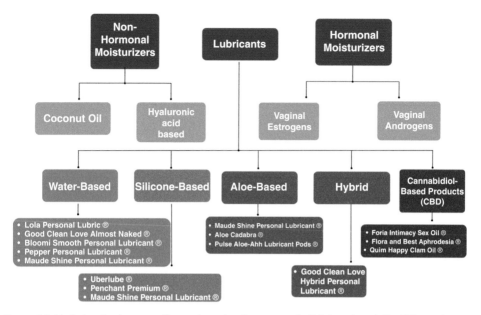

Figure 4.2 Vaginal moisturizer types (for regular use) and recommended lubricant brands (for PRN sexual activity or dilator use)

moisturizer as a tablet preparation. Both groups demonstrated improvement in GSM symptoms, vaginal pH, and dyspareunia [25]. The effectiveness of HLA was more recently demonstrated in partnered and unpartnered women with a history of estrogen-sensitive uterine cancer. Daily application of HLA for two weeks, then three to five times per week improved vulvovaginal health and sexual function [26]. Figure 4.2 outlines moisturizer types and detailed recommendations of lubricant brands, by type.

Vaginal Estrogen

Vaginal Estrogen in Women Without Estrogen-Sensitive Cancer

Hormonally unresponsive cancers proliferate independently of hormonal substrates due to a lack of hormone receptors. Vaginal estrogen therapy is not contraindicated, and instead, should be encouraged in women with GSM and hormone-unresponsive cancer. These cancers include cervical, vulvovaginal squamous, colorectal, and hematologic malignancies [27].

Vaginal Estrogen in Women With Estrogen-Sensitive Cancer

The most effective treatment for GSM is vaginal estrogen, but prior studies have shown that absorption of vaginal estrogen may temporarily increase circulating estradiol, which limits provider comfort with its use in women with a history of hormone-sensitive cancer [28]. A recent retrospective Danish study of patients treated for breast cancer between 1997–2004 suggested an increased risk of recurrence in certain breast cancer patients through an analysis of hormone users versus nonusers. Within this study, the only comparison suggesting an increased risk of recurrence in vaginal estrogen users was limited to those on aromatase inhibitors. Notably, the breast cancer treatment regimens predate modern guidelines in that Her2-targeted therapies were not used, and many with estrogen receptor positive tumors did not take endocrine therapy, therefore recurrence rates were higher than contemporary estimates. Furthermore, important confounders of recurrence including body mass index and physical inactivity were not accounted for [29]. Therefore, these data must be considered in light of the competing increased risk of recurrence associated with endocrine therapy noncompliance in patients whose GSM symptoms go untreated.

Studies examining vaginal estrogen use in women with gynecologic malignancies report rare adverse outcomes with comparable recurrence to those not prescribed vaginal estrogen. In a multicenter, retrospective cohort study, 244 women with a diagnosis of either endometrial, cervical, or ovarian cancer were prescribed vaginal estrogen. Overall adverse events were low, and recurrence rates were comparable to those of the general population. Despite the North American Menopause Society's (NAMS) endorsement that hormone therapy is safe for use in patients with early-stage, low-grade, surgically-treated-treated endometrial cancer, completely resected ovarian cancer, colorectal, and lung cancer, vaginal estrogen is still underutilized in these populations due to past dogma [30].

Treating GSM in women with estrogen-sensitive cancer represents a complex clinical challenge. While local hormone therapy applied to the vulvar and/or vaginal mucosa is distinct from "systemic" hormonal therapy given through oral or transdermal routes, increases in circulating estradiol may still occur, although temporary. For this reason, despite its proven superiority to nonhormonal moisturizers, some clinicians are still hesitant to prescribe low-dose vaginal estrogen to women on anti-estrogen therapy for fear of absorption-related increases in serum estradiol and the hypothetical increased risk of cancer recurrence [31].

There is no established threshold for the "safe" level of estradiol in women with a history of estrogen-sensitive cancer. The North American Menopause Society released a symposium report in 2020 that sought to establish normal postmenopausal estrogen ranges. They determined that estradiol levels were age-dependent and ranged from a mean of 8.2 pg/mL in women 40–45 to 3.5 pg/mL in women >70 years of age [8]. Absorption of vaginal estrogen is higher when the mucosa is atrophic and decreases with time, usually after two to four weeks. Lower doses of vaginal estradiol with less frequent dosing leads to smaller plasma estradiol increases. Santen et al. recently updated a prior review of the literature measuring systemic absorption of estradiol utilizing highly-specific LC-MS. Serum estradiol in women using low-dose (10 mcg) and ultralow-dose (4 mcg) estradiol suppositories ranged from 4.6–14.8 pg/mL for the 10 mcg dose to 3.6–3.9 pg/mL for the 4 mcg dose, and these increases resolved by the fourth day of treatment for those using the 4 mcg dose [9]. The authors concluded that systemic estrogen absorption with low-dose or ultralow-dose vaginal estrogen is minimal, suggesting that the US Food and Drug Administration's (FDA) "black box" warning linking estrogen and breast cancer is likely overstated given that there is not a significant increase in serum estradiol levels with very low dose vaginal estradiol formulations. According to a 2016 ACOG Committee Opinion, low-dose vaginal estrogen may be more appropriate in patients taking tamoxifen since this medication binds to receptors in breast tissue, blocking estrogen's downstream effects, and therefore its efficacy is not impacted by the potential absorption of vaginal estrogen [32].

In light of this ongoing controversy, for women with a history of estrogen-sensitive cancer, the authors recommend eliminating potential irritants and initiating a regimen of a nonhormonal moisturizer followed by the introduction of once- or twice-weekly low-dose vaginal estrogen for persistent symptoms (as opposed to the daily regimen utilized in the absorption studies). For patients with mild symptoms, starting with single-ingredient organic coconut oil may be sufficient, while a hyaluronic acid suppository may be better suited for those with severe symptoms. For women in whom symptoms persist at two months, once-weekly low-dose vaginal estrogen can be initiated and increased to twice weekly after two weeks. Oftentimes if regular sexual activity can be re-initiated, treatment with vaginal estrogen can eventually be tapered down to once weekly or stopped.

Vaginal Androgens

Recent studies have focused on the use of vaginal androgens to treat symptoms of GSM and sexual dysfunction. The tissues of the vulva and vagina have receptors for both androgens and estrogen, and the glands responsible for lubrication during arousal require androgens to function. Deficiencies of both hormones occur naturally during menopause, and patients with severe GSM are often found to have focal pain at specific points in the vulvar anatomy near the ostia of the Bartholin's glands (4:00 and 8:00 o'clock) and Skene's glands (1:00 and 11:00 o'clock), which are sites dependent on androgens [33]. This pain can culminate in severe penetrative dyspareunia and eventually chronic neuropathic pain.

DHEA or Prasterone

The androgens dehydroepiandrosterone sulfate (DHEA-S), DHEA, and androstenedione do not have androgenic activity unless they are converted to either testosterone or dihydro-testosterone (DHT), where they exert their action locally. In peripheral tissues, the prohor-mone DHEA is converted to the more active testosterone and DHT, exerting its action in the same cells where their synthesis takes place with minimal release into the circulation [34]. After their local formation and intracellular use, testosterone and DHT are inactivated and transformed into water-soluble glucuronide derivatives and eliminated through the circulation [35]. They may also be converted to estrogens by aromatase. Theoretically, an increase in serum testosterone may lead to increased serum estradiol, although this conversion may be at least partially inhibited by aromatase inhibitors.

In 2016, the Food and Drug Administration (FDA) approved the use of an androgen formulation for vaginal use, a 6.5 mg prasterone (synthetic DHEA) suppository for the use of dyspareunia in postmenopausal women. DHEA made within the body is generated and secreted from the zona reticularis of the adrenal glands, and its secretion frequency and quantity decreases with age [36]. Another notable function of DHEA is that it is a potent noncompetitive inhibitor of glucose-6-phosphate dehydrogenase which lowers the production of oxygen free radicals leading to decreased oxidative stress and inflammation, which mechanistically may also contribute to the symptoms seen in the vulva and vagina. Vaginal prasterone was found to improve GSM symptoms including painful sex in postmenopausal women, demonstrating improvement in both subjective and objective measures [37, 38].

DHEA was more recently studied in women with a history of breast cancer. The double-blind randomized Alliance for Clinical Trials in Oncology (NCCTG-N10C1) Trial compared compounded vaginal DHEA to a plain vaginal moisturizer [39]. Four hundred and sixty-four women with a history of breast or gynecologic cancer were randomized to either DHEA or plain moisturizer. Women on AIs who received DHEA experienced the same level of improvement in vaginal symptoms as those not on AIs without a subsequent change in serum estradiol. This finding supports that vaginal DHEA is not working through estrogenic means and may be an appropriate treatment for this population [40]. A Guideline

Summary released by the American Society of Clinical Oncology (ASCO) in 2018 recommended consideration of vaginal DHEA (prasterone) or vaginal estrogen in appropriately counseled women with breast cancer who did not respond to nonhormonal treatments [41]. The limitation to widespread uptake of this FDA-approved commercially available prasterone product is cost: it is expensive for some women without commercial insurance who are not eligible for the coupon program.

Vaginal Testosterone

Vaginal application of testosterone has not been FDA-approved for the treatment of vulvovaginal symptoms and/or sexual dysfunction related to women's cancer treatment, but its compounded form has been studied in women with breast cancer. In 2011, Witherby et al. treated 21 women on aromatase inhibitors with GSM symptoms with daily vaginal compounded testosterone cream for four weeks. Half of the study group received a dose of 150 mcg, and the other half 300 mcg. In both arms, serum estradiol levels remained well below the cutoff for the menopausal range (20 pg/mL) at <8pg/mL. The investigators also found symptom improvement in both arms that persisted more than a month after therapy [42]. A more recent study looked at global sexual functioning outcomes in 12 patients on aromatase inhibitors prescribed the same four weeks of therapy. Serum hormone levels were not measured but all domain scores of the FSFI were noted to significantly improve [43].

The efficacy of vaginal androgens compared to vaginal estrogen in women on AIs has been compared in two prospective trials. In 2016, Melisko et al. found that patients using a 1% testosterone cream (5000 mcg in 0.5 gm dose) every night for two weeks, then three times per week had similar improvements in vaginal symptoms and sexual interest compared to those who received an estradiol vaginal ring [44]. The large dose of vaginal testosterone utilized in this study (5000 mcg compared to 300 mcg in study by Witherby et al.) was based on data treating sexual desire disorders in postmenopausal women [45] but resulted in elevated serum total testosterone (greater than the postmenopausal range of 2 ng/dL to 45 ng/dL in 24 of 27 patients). A nested case-control cohort of women from the Women's Health Eating and Living (WHEL) study did not find an increased risk of breast cancer recurrence in women with higher baseline testosterone levels, but this question necessitates further study [46].

In summary, studies have demonstrated improvement in vaginal health and sexual function with large doses of vaginal testosterone (5000 mcg) that resulted in significant increases in serum testosterone, the significance of which is unknown in cancer survivors. Lower doses of vaginal testosterone (300 mcg) may produce improvement in vaginal health and potentially overall sexual satisfaction without the derangements in sex steroid hormone levels described in studies utilizing the larger testosterone dose (5000 mcg) or vaginal estrogen. However, the authors recommend initiating therapy with FDA-approved formulations instead of compounded hormones due to concerns regarding dose, purity, efficacy, and safety, which will be discussed further in the following section.

Bioidentical Hormones

Hormone prescriptions prepared by a compounding pharmacist may combine multiple hormones (estrogens, progesterone or synthetic progestins, and androgens) into unapproved mixtures and may be administered orally, transdermally, vaginally, or through untested routes such as subdermal implants or pellets. "Bioidentical" hormones are a marketing term, as both compounded and FDA-approved hormonal formulations can be "bioidentical." The difference between government-approved bioidentical estradiol, estrone, and medroxyprogesterone and their compounded versions is that the former are regulated and monitored for purity and efficacy. Furthermore, FDA-approved versions are sold with a package insert containing detailed patient and provider instructions, trial evidence of safety and efficacy, and government-mandated black box warnings if they exist [31].

Strategic marketing and the appeal of bespoke hormone recipes have led to an increase in the popularity of compounded hormonal formulations in recent years. The use of pelleted hormone therapy to treat menopausal symptoms is on the rise, and cancer patients may be particularly susceptible to this treatment touted as "safer" than FDA-regulated hormonal therapy. However, pelleted therapy leads to higher rates of side effects and supraphysiologic hormone levels. In 2021, Jiang et al. compared 539 postmenopausal women that received either pelleted hormonal therapy or FDA-approved therapy. The incidence of side effects was higher among those who received pelleted hormone therapy, and more than half of these patients with a uterus reported abnormal uterine bleeding. Mean and peak serum estradiol and testosterone levels were significantly higher in the pelleted hormone cohort, where peak estradiol reached 237.7 pg/mL (versus 93.45 pg/mL in the FDA products) and peak testosterone reached 194.04 pg/mL (versus 15.59 pg/mL). Notably, four women using pelleted therapy were found to have a serum estradiol >1000 pg/mL and nine women were found to have serum testosterone >400 ng/dL [47].

There is little to no evidence that hormone-containing products from compounding pharmacies are more safe or effective than FDA-approved hormone prescriptions. According to the NAMS, there is insufficient evidence to support the clinical use of compounded bioidentical hormone therapy for the treatment of menopausal symptoms, although there are serious concerns about the lack of safety data and government dosing regulation. If a patient cannot tolerate a government-approved therapy, prescribers choosing to utilize the services of compounding pharmacies should document the medical indication and provide the patient with the financial disclosures of the prescribers, pharmacists, and pharmacies. Lastly, compounding pharmacists should provide standardized content information including warnings of potential adverse effects and clearly stating that the preparation is not government-approved [31].

Vaginal Lasers

The perception of limited treatment options for sexual dysfunction has fostered an environment where patients with these quality-of-life impacting symptoms (and their providers) seek "alternative" therapies. Laser devices promising "vaginal rejuvenation" are being promoted to women in advertisements online, in spa windows, and in doctors' offices. Using lasers to treat skin conditions goes back as early as 1963 as a method for treating moles and warts [48]. In the years since, however, the medical aesthetics industry has gone beyond applying this technology on the external body to using it in the vagina, claiming it can treat a broad range of gynecologic and urologic conditions.

Patients with severe genitourinary changes related to cancer treatment-related estrogen deprivation or pelvic radiation may be susceptible to abnormal healing after treatment with energy-based devices, whose efficacy depends on the creation of microscopic injury and subsequent collagen formation. One of the most popular CO_2 lasers was cleared by the

FDA in 2014 "for use in general and plastic surgery and in dermatology." However, the 501(k) fast-tracking program is not an "approval" in the way the FDA approves medications to be safe for consumption, but more like a system of device registration for manufacturers.

Since granting the 510(k) registration for the CO2 laser, the FDA has issued a notice alerting providers and patients that the safety of these devices has not been established for cosmetic procedures on the vulva or in the vagina. The advisory warned consumers about "bad actors" who promote the "unapproved, deceptive product" and described how devices marketed as providing "vaginal rejuvenation" caused "numerous cases of vaginal burns, scarring, pain during sexual intercourse, and recurring or chronic pain." [49].

The argument against the use of CO2 laser devices in the medical aesthetics industry goes beyond questions of safety in patients treated for cancer: they may not even be effective. Two prospective randomized controlled trials found the device to be no better than a sham. In 2021, Li et al. reported the results of a sham-controlled, double-blinded, randomized clinical trial that included 90 women with postmenopausal vaginal symptoms treated with three treatments of a fractional microablative carbon dioxide laser four to eight weeks apart, or the same number of sham procedures where the device was placed in the vagina and turned on. There was no difference in symptom severity or histological comparisons between the laser and sham treatment groups [50]. A similar sham-controlled randomized trial including breast cancer patients did not find that treatments with the laser was superior to placebo [51].

Cancer patients may be particularly susceptible to the marketing messages of the companies of these devices, and providers should be aware of the lack of prospective data demonstrating efficacy, along with the potential dangers. The FDA has warned at least seven manufacturers to cease advertising their products for unapproved uses. Patients who have experienced adverse events are encouraged to report their experience to the FDA's Manufacturer and User Facility Device Experience (MAUDE) online database.

Dyspareunia

Lubricants

For pain with penetration, lubricants should be used with sexual activity and dilator use and should be distinguished from vaginal moisturizers. The optimal lubricant is one with minimal irritants that will minimize friction and therefore minimize intra- and postcoital spotting and burning. Patients should be encouraged to select their own lubricant for sexual activity instead of allowing their partner to select the lubricant. For patients that do not rely on condoms for pregnancy or infection protection, the authors recommend a silicone-based lubricant without parabens, glycerin, flavors, or other gimmicks. Water-based lubricants should be used with silicone toys or with condoms. Patients who report persistent burning after sexual activity may be irritated by an ingredient in the lubricant and they may benefit from selecting an alternative product. Oil-based lubricants are helpful for patients with persistent burning after sexual activity, but they are less slippery and will degrade latex condoms and silicone devices. Table 4.1 highlights nonhormonal moisturizer brands, hormonal moisturizer dosing, lubricant types (brands shown in Figure 4.1), and sexual devices.

Table 4.1 Nonhormonal moisturizers, hormonal moisturizer dosing, lubricant types, and sexual devices

Moisturizers, Lubricants, and Devices for Patients With Breast Cancer

FEATURES	NONHORMONAL MOISTURIZERS	HORMONAL MOISTURIZERS	RECOMMENDATIONS LUBRICANTS (SEE FIGURE 4.1 FOR BRANDS)	DEVICES
When to Use	Maintenance Use at night, after showering, nightly or 3x/week	Add 1–2x/week after >1 month of nonhormonal moisturizer Creams to introitus (external) or place on dilator for patients with stenosis Suppositories or tablets at night	Before all sexual activity With dilators and devices	Persistent pain with sexual activity Levator spasm Biofeedback for anticipatory anxiety
First-Line	Single-ingredient organic Coconut Oil Hyaluronic acid: Bonafide Revaree Suppositories Bionourish (CCL)	1% estradiol cream Estradiol tablet 4 mcg Estradiol tablet 10 mcg estradiol ring (7.5 mcg/day) Prasterone 6.5 mg (DHEA)	Silicone-based Water-based	Dilators Ohnut® Vibrators Milli Expanding Vaginal Dilator® Pelvic Wands
Second-Line	Lactic acid: Restore (CCL) Vitamin E suppositories	Compounded vaginal testosterone 300 mcg	Aloe-based Oil-based	

Vaginal Stenosis

Untreated GSM can lead to the shortening and narrowing of the vagina, known as vaginal stenosis. Vaginal stenosis (VS) is a subacute to late toxicity that was originally described in women undergoing pelvic radiation or radical surgery for gynecologic malignancies. There is currently no standard definition, but it has been described as the inability to insert two fingers in the vagina [52] and the shortening of the vagina to less than 8 cm [53]. Its prevalence in women with a history of pelvic radiation ranges from 13% to 88% [54].

Vaginal stenosis has been unexpectedly observed in women receiving treatment for GSM who were receiving anti-estrogen therapy, without a history of pelvic radiation. In the OVERcome (Olive Oil, Vaginal Exercise, and MoisturizeR) study, 11% of breast cancer survivors [55] that presented for enrollment were found to have VS and had to be excluded from the intervention. In a sexual health after-cancer program in South Florida, approximately half the women who presented for treatment after several years of anti-estrogen therapy were found to have VS making penetrative intercourse either impossible or extremely painful [56].

Vaginal stenosis may also prevent pelvic examinations necessary for cancer surveillance. Vaginal dilator use during cancer treatment can be particularly helpful for patients not sexually active by preserving the length and width of the vagina during periods of estrogen suppression. Dilator therapy improves elasticity but also provides biofeedback during pelvic floor relaxation exercises. Multiple studies have demonstrated that consistent use of a vaginal dilator during radiation treatment results in a reduced risk of VS [57, 58, 59], and published practice guidelines recommend having the patient use the dilator in the vagina with a lubricant three times per week for 10 minutes per dilation [60]. Dilators are ideally supplied at no cost to the patient by their medical providers, but could also be purchased through CMT medical (www.cmtmedical.com) or several other online vendors, including SoulSource®, IntimateRose®, and BioMoi® . Another sexual device helpful for patients with deep dyspareunia, termed a collision dyspareunia aid, is the Ohnut, which consists of soft, stackable rings that may be placed around the penis, dilator, or other sexual apparatus to limit the depth of penetration (Table 4.1).

Future work should focus on increasing provider and patient comfort with prescribing and utilizing dilator therapy. Patient adherence to a vaginal dilator regimen is reportedly very low. In one study, even after counseling and instruction, only 57% of patients had used the dilator at six months and only 14% dilated at the recommended three times per week [61]. However, when dilators are utilized, they are effective. In an observational study of 89 women who received pelvic radiation, median vaginal length increased from 6 to 9 cm over four months of dilator use. The addition of vaginal hormonal therapy as described above to dilator regimens may help further reverse the effects of vaginal stenosis through remodeling of the vaginal architecture [62].

Pelvic Floor Physical Therapy

In women with GSM, pelvic floor muscle training (PFMT), provided by pelvic floor-specific physical therapists, is indicated for those with the concomitant diagnosis of pelvic floor dysfunction. In a prospective cohort study undertaken by Mercier et al., thirty-two post-menopausal women underwent PFMT for 12 weeks with a significant reduction of GSM symptoms and improved sexual function [63]. These results suggest an important indication for PFMT beyond pelvic floor weakness and urinary incontinence. A detailed external pelvic floor muscle and internal pelvic assessment are performed at a first PMFT visit,

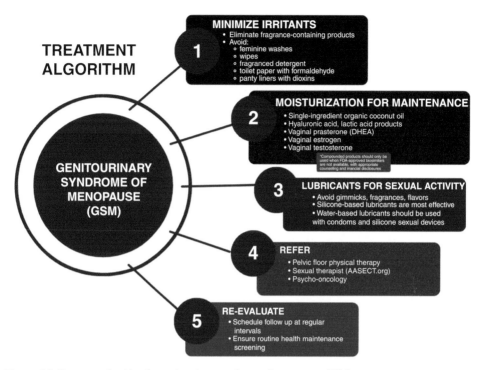

Figure 4.3 Treatment algorithm for genitourinary syndrome of menopause (GSM)

individualized to patient comfort. During this first visit, patients can expect that their pelvic floor therapist will take a detailed history, then perform both an external and internal pelvic exam, with additional orthopedic assessments as needed. Patients are usually sent home with educational materials and techniques that were taught in office to review and practice. Over the subsequent treatment visits, a personalized pelvic floor program is created, which may include continued education, yoga or stretching, biofeedback, electrical stimulation, diaphragmatic breathing, trigger point release, meditation, and with pelvic wand and dilator training, and intimate relationship preparation [64]. Figure 4.3 summarizes the authors' recommendations for the treatment of GSM including irritant minimization, moisturization, lubricants, and referrals.

Low Desire During and After Cancer Treatment: Hypoactive Sexual Desire Disorder

In female patients with a history of cancer reporting sexual dysfunction, 36% report low desire as their most significant concern [2]. Low desire is complex but may be a sequela of androgen suppression, the negative stimulus of painful sexual activity, or the result of the psychologic insult of enduring a cancer diagnosis and treatment. Treating dyspareunia, if present, is the first (and easiest) step to improving desire. Second, patients should be counseled about behavioral interventions. Regular physical activity, sleep hygiene (no screens in bed), and scheduled "date night" are appropriate recommendations. If there is relationship discord, this can be addressed with a referral to a couple's counselor or a sexual therapist. The American

Association of Sexuality Educators, Counselors, and Therapists (AASECT) website offers a search function for licensed practitioners by zip code (www.aasect.org).

There are two FDA-approved therapies for female hypoactive sexual desire disorder (HSDD): flibanserin and bremelanotide [65, 66]. Flibanserin, a post-synaptic 5-HT1a agonist, a partial D4 agonist, and a 5-HT2a antagonist, is a once-a-day pill that was originally developed as an antidepressant. It is effective in treating HSDD in premenopausal women but comes with a significant side effect profile. It was originally approved with the caveat that all providers must undergo specific risk management training related to hypotension and syncope when combined with alcohol. However, these regulations have since been lifted and now the formal recommendation is that women should discontinue drinking alcohol at least two hours prior to taking flibanserin or skip their dose that evening [67, 68]. Bremelanotide is a novel melanocortin receptor agonist given as a subcutaneous injection prior to sexual activity. Similar to flibanserin, bremelanotide is FDA-approved in premenopausal women with HSDD, and has demonstrated dose-responsive improvements in desire, arousal, and reductions in sexual-related distress. [69]. The most prevalent side effect is nausea, with 40% of patients in two randomized trials experiencing some level after medication administration [70]. Notably, both flibanserin and bremelanotide are FDA-approved to treat HSDD in premenopausal patients, although flibanserin has reported efficacy in postmenopausal patients as well [71].

While studies of patients taking both tamoxifen and flibanserin are ongoing, there is a dearth of evidence supporting their safety together in women with a history of cancer. However, both flibanserin and bremelanotide function centrally and are not sex hormone-dependent and therefore can be considered in certain situations with careful attention to drug-drug interactions.

Systemic testosterone as a treatment for HSDD was endorsed in 2019 through a Global Consensus Position Statement that included NAMS and other societies [72]. However, there is no universally accepted premenopausal serum concentration that predicts efficacy, and the safety of systemic androgens, particularly when some triple negative breast cancer are known to express an androgen receptor, is not known.

Case Resolution

Celia is a 54-year-old patient with estrogen receptor-positive breast cancer with worsening vaginal dryness, painful sex, and low desire. She received education about irritant minimization and initiated a three-times weekly hyaluronic acid suppository for vaginal moisturization. She was also given a medium-sized dilator and instructions to use with a silicone-based lubricant three times per week. After two months, she reported significant improvement in her symptoms and reinitiated weekly sexual activity with her partner.

Take Home Points

- Cancer treatment negatively impacts sexual health and is reported by more than half of female cancer survivors across disease sites, creating a high demand for both patient education and mitigation strategies.
- Genitourinary syndrome of menopause (GSM) is a common sequela of treatment and can result from surgery, chemotherapy, immunotherapy, radiation, and estrogen-suppressing therapies.

- Vaginal washes, irritating chemicals, and artificial fragrances can worsen symptoms of GSM and should be avoided.
- First-line treatment for GSM in women without a history of estrogen-sensitive cancer is vaginal estrogen. The regular use of nonhormonal moisturizers such as single-ingredient organic coconut oil or commercially available moisturizers with hyaluronic acid is an appropriate first step in women with estrogen-sensitive cancer, although vaginal prasterone or low-dose vaginal estrogen may be added once or twice weekly if symptoms persist.
- "Bioidentical hormones" is a marketing term, and compounded formulas should only be used when a biosimilar FDA-approved version with known dose and pharmacokinetics is not available.
- Dilators are underused but effective at decreasing dyspareunia and improving vaginal stenosis when used regularly. Patient education is important to ensure treatment adherence, and the recommendation is to place the dilator intravaginally three times weekly for ten minutes.
- Patients with a history of cancer with GSM should not be referred for treatment with energy-based devices including CO2 lasers. Patients experiencing adverse events should be encouraged to report their experience to the FDA's Manufacturer and User Facility Device Experience (MAUDE) online database.
- Low desire is complex, but treating dyspareunia and behavioral interventions may improve symptoms. Two FDA-approved medications for premenopausal patients with hypoactive sexual desire disorder (filbanserin and bremelanotide) have been shown to be safe and effective with caution to avoiding drug-drug interactions.

References

1. Dizon D. S., Suzin D., McIlvenna S. Sexual health as a survivorship issue for female cancer survivors. *Oncologist.* 2014;**19**(2):202–10. doi: 10.1634/ theoncologist.2013-0302. Epub 2014 Jan 6. PMID: 24396051; PMCID: PMC3926787.

2. Satish S., Pon F., Calfa C., Perez A., Rojas K. Characterizing genitourinary exam disruptions in women presenting to a sexual health after cancer program. *Journal of Clinical Oncology.* 2022;**40**:16_suppl, e24048–e24048

3. Baumgart J., Nilsson K., Evers A. S., Kallak T. K., Poromaa I. S. Sexual dysfunction in women on adjuvant endocrine therapy after breast cancer. *Menopause.* 2013;**20**(2):162–8. doi: 10.1097/gme.0b013e31826560da. PMID: 22990756.

4. Wells-Prado, D. R., Ross, M. W., Simon Rosser, B. R., et al. (2022). Prostate cancer disclosure and sexual orientation: Understanding outness to healthcare providers as a situational or consistent phenomenon. *Patient Education and Counseling*, **105**(7), 2033. https://doi.org/ 10.1016/j.pec.2021.11.017

5. Early Breast Cancer Trialists' Collaborative Group (EBCTCG). Effects of chemotherapy and hormonal therapy for early breast cancer on recurrence and 15-year survival: An overview of the randomised trials. *Lancet.* 2005;**365**(9472):1687–717. doi: 10.1016/S0140-6736(05)66544-0. PMID: 15894097.

6. Slomovitz B. M., Filiaci V. L., Walker J. L., et al. A randomized phase II trial of everolimus and letrozole or hormonal therapy in women with advanced, persistent or recurrent endometrial carcinoma: A GOG Foundation study. *Gynecol Oncol.* 2022;**164**(3):481–91. doi: 10.1016/j

.ygyno.2021.12.031. Epub 2022 Jan 19. PMID: 35063278.

7. Richardson, H., Ho, V., Pasquet, R., et al. Baseline estrogen levels in postmenopausal women participating in the MAP.3 breast cancer chemoprevention trial. *Menopause (New York, N.Y.).* 2020;27(6), 693. https://doi.org/10.1097/GME.0000000000001568

8. Pinkerton J. V., Liu J. H., Santoro N. F., et al. Workshop on normal reference ranges for estradiol in postmenopausal women: Commentary from The North American Menopause Society on low-dose vaginal estrogen therapy labeling. *Menopause.* 2020;27(6):611–13. doi: 10.1097/GME.0000000000001576 .PMID: 32459749.

9. Santen R. J., Mirkin S., Bernick B., Constantine G. D. Systemic estradiol levels with low-dose vaginal estrogens. *Menopause.* 2020;27(3):361–70. doi: 10.1097/GME.0000000000001463. PMID: 31794498; PMCID: PMC7050796.

10. Chlebowski R. T., Anderson G. L. Changing concepts: Menopausal hormone therapy and breast cancer. *J Natl Cancer Inst.* 2012;104(7):517–27. doi: 10.1093/jnci/djs014. Epub 2012 Mar 16. PMID: 22427684; PMCID: PMC3317878.

11. Fallowfield L., Cella D., Cuzick J., et al. Quality of life of postmenopausal women in the Arimidex, Tamoxifen, Alone or in Combination (ATAC) adjuvant breast cancer trial. *Journal of Clinical Oncology.* 2004;22(21):4261–71. doi:10.1200/jco.2004.08.029

12. Gandhi J., Chen A., Dagur G., et al. Genitourinary syndrome of menopause: an overview of clinical manifestations, pathophysiology, etiology, evaluation, and management. *Am J Obstet Gynecol.* 2016;215(6):704–11. doi: 10.1016/j.ajog.2016.07.045. Epub 2016 Jul 26. PMID: 27472999.

13. Gandhi C., Butler E., Pesek S., et al. Sexual dysfunction in breast cancer survivors: Is it surgical modality or adjuvant therapy? *Am J Clin Oncol.* 2019;42(6):500–06. doi: 10.1097/COC.0000000000000552. PMID: 31094713.

14. Burstein H. J., Lacchetti C., Griggs, J. J. Adjuvant endocrine therapy for women with hormone receptor–positive breast cancer: ASCO clinical practice guideline focused update. *Journal of Oncology Practice.* 2019;15(2):106–07. doi:10.1200/jop.18.00617

15. Bell S. G., Dalton L., McNeish B. L., et al. Aromatase inhibitor use, side effects and discontinuation rates in gynecologic oncology patients. *Gynecologic Oncology.* 2020;159(2):509. https://doi.org/10.1016/j.ygyno.2020.08.015

16. Arbour M., Corwin E. J., Salsberry, P. Douching patterns in women related to socioeconomic and racial/ethnic characteristics. *Journal of Obstetric, Gynecologic & Neonatal Nursing.* 2009;38(5):577–85. doi:10.1111/j.1552-6909.2009. 01053.x–

17. van Amerongen, C. A., Ofenloch, R. F., Cazzaniga, S., et al. Skin exposure to scented products used in daily life and fragrance contact allergy in the European general population: The EDEN Fragrance Study. *Contact Dermatitis.* 2021;84(6):385–94. https://doi.org/10.1111/cod.13807

18. Brotman, R. M., Ghanem, K. G., Klebanoff, M. A., et al. The effect of vaginal douching cessation on bacterial vaginosis: A pilot study. *American Journal of Obstetrics and Gynecology.* 2008;198(6):628.e1. https://doi.org/10.1016/j.ajog.2007.11.043

19. Ogbolu D. O., Oni A. A., Daini O. A., Oloko A. P. In vitro antimicrobial properties of coconut oil on Candida species in Ibadan, Nigeria. *J Med Food.* 2007;10(2):384–7. doi: 10.1089/jmf.2006.1209. PMID: 17651080.

20. Shilling M., Matt L., Rubin E., et al. Antimicrobial effects of virgin coconut oil and its medium-chain fatty acids on Clostridium difficile. *J Med Food.* 2013;16(12):1079–85. doi: 10.1089/jmf.2012.0303. PMID: 24328700.

21. Porterfield L., Wur N., Delgado Z. S., et al. Vaginal vitamin E for treatment of genitourinary syndrome of menopause: A systematic review of randomized controlled trials. *J Menopausal Med.*

2022;**28**(1):9–16. doi: 10.6118/jmm.21028. PMID: 35534426; PMCID: PMC9086347

22. International Agency for Research on Cancer. *Agents classified by the IARC monographs, volumes 1-112.* 2014. http://monographs.iarc.fr/ENG/Classification/. Accessed April 22, 2022.

23. Plummer, E. L., Bradshaw, C. S., Doyle, M., et al. (2020). Lactic acid-containing products for bacterial vaginosis and their impact on the vaginal microbiota: A systematic review. *PLoS ONE,* **16**(2). https://doi.org/10.1371/journal.pone.0246953

24. Nappi, R. E., Martella, S., Albani, F., et al. Hyaluronic Acid: A Valid Therapeutic Option for Early Management of Genitourinary Syndrome of Menopause in Cancer Survivors? *Healthcare.* 2022;**10**(8). https://doi.org/10.3390/healthcare10081528

25. Jokar A., Davari T., Asadi N., Ahmadi F., Foruhari S. (2016). Comparison of the hyaluronic acid vaginal cream and conjugated estrogen used in treatment of vaginal atrophy of menopause women: A randomized controlled clinical trial. *International Journal of Community Based Nursing and Midwifery.* 2016;**4**(1),69–78. https://www.ncbi.nlm.nih.gov/pmc/articles/PMC4709811/

26. Carter, J., Goldfarb, S., Baser, R. E., et al. A single-arm clinical trial investigating the effectiveness of a non-hormonal, hyaluronic acid-based vaginal moisturizer in endometrial cancer survivors. *Gynecologic Oncology.* 2020;**158**(2):366. https://doi.org/10.1016/j.ygyno.2020.05.025

27. Sinno A. K., Pinkerton J., Febbraro T., et al. Hormone therapy (HT) in women with gynecologic cancer and in women at high risk for developing a gynecologic cancer: A Society of Gynecologic Oncology (SGO) clinical practice statement: This practice statement has been endorsed by The North American Menopause Society. *Gynecol Oncol.* 2020;**157**(2):303–06. doi: 10.1016/j.ygyno.2020.01.035. Epub 2020 Feb 15. PMID: 32067815.

28. Santen R. J., Mirkin S., Bernick B., Constantine G. D. Systemic estradiol levels with low-dose vaginal estrogens. *Menopause (New York, N.Y.).*

2020;**27**(3):361–70. https://doi.org/10.1097/GME.000000000000146

29. Cold S., Cold F., Jensen M. B., et al. Systemic or vaginal hormone therapy after early breast cancer: A Danish observational cohort study. *Journal of the National Cancer Institute.* 2022;**114**(10):1347–54. https://doi.org/10.1093/jnci/djac112

30. Chambers L. M., Herrmann A., Michener C. M., Ferrando C. A., Ricci S. Vaginal estrogen uses for genitourinary symptoms in women with a history of uterine, cervical, or ovarian carcinoma. *International journal of gynecological cancer: official journal of the International Gynecological Cancer Society.* 2020;**30**(4):515–24. https://doi.org/10.1136/ijgc-2019-001034

31. "The 2022 Hormone Therapy Position Statement of The North American Menopause Society" Advisory Panel. The 2022 hormone therapy position statement of The North American Menopause Society. *Menopause.* 2022;**29**(7):767–94. doi: 10.1097/GME.0000000000002028. PMID: 35797481.

32. Biglia N., Bounous V. E., D'Alonzo M., et al. Vaginal atrophy in breast cancer survivors: Attitude and approaches among oncologists. *Clin Breast Cancer.* 2017;**17**(8):611–17. doi: 10.1016/j.clbc.2017.05.008. Epub 2017 May 19. PMID: 28655486.

33. Dew J. E., Wren B. G., Eden J. A. A cohort study of topical vaginal estrogen therapy in women previously treated for breast cancer. *Climacteric.* 2003;**6**(1):45–52. PMID: 12725664.

34. Traish A. M., Vignozzi L., Simon J. A., Goldstein I., Kim, N. N. (2018). Role of androgens in female genitourinary tissue structure and function: Implications in the genitourinary syndrome of menopause. *Sexual Medicine Reviews.* 2018;**6**(4):558–71. https://doi.org/10.1016/j.sxmr.2018.03.005

35. Labrie F. Intracrinology. *Mol Cell Endocrinol.* 1991;**78**(3):C113–18. doi: 10.1016/0303-7207(91)90116-a. PMID: 1838082.

36. Labrie F., Luu-The V., Bélanger A., et al. Is dehydroepiandrosterone a hormone? *J Endocrinol.* 2005;**187**(2):169–96. doi: 10.1677/joe.1.06264. PMID: 16293766.

37. Liu T. C., Lin C. H., Huang C. Y., Ivy J. L., Kuo C. H. Effect of acute DHEA administration on free testosterone in middle-aged and young men following high-intensity interval training. *Eur J Appl Physiol.* 2013;**113**(7):1783–92. doi: 10.1007/s00421-013-2607-x. Epub 2013 Feb 17. PMID: 23417481.

38. Schwartz A. G., Pashko L. L. Dehydroepiandrosterone, glucose-6-phosphate dehydrogenase, and longevity. *Ageing Res Rev.* 2004;**3**(2):171–87. doi: 10.1016/j.arr.2003.05.001. PMID: 15177053.

39. Labrie F., Archer D., Bouchard C., et al. Effect of intravaginal dehydroepiandrosterone (Prasterone) on libido and sexual dysfunction in postmenopausal women. *Menopause.* 2009;**16**(5):923–31. doi: 10.1097/gme.0b013e31819e85c6. PMID: 19424093.

40. Barton D. L., Sloan J. A., Shuster L. T., et al. Evaluating the efficacy of vaginal dehydroepiandosterone for vaginal symptoms in postmenopausal cancer survivors: NCCTG N10C1 (Alliance). *Supportive Care in Cancer: Official Journal of the Multinational Association of Supportive Care in Cancer.* 2018;**26**(2):643. https://doi.org/10.1007/s00520-017-3878-2

41. Carter J., Lacchetti C., Andersen B. L., et al. Interventions to address sexual problems in people with cancer: American Society of Clinical Oncology Clinical Practice Guideline Adaptation of Cancer Care Ontario Guideline. *J Clin Oncol.* 2018;**36**(5):492–511. doi: 10.1200/JCO.2017.75.8995. Epub 2017 Dec 11. PMID: 29227723.

42. Witherby S., Johnson J., Demers L., et al. Topical testosterone for breast cancer patients with vaginal atrophy related to aromatase inhibitors: a phase I/II study. *Oncologist.* 2011;**16**(4):424–31. doi: 10.1634/theoncologist.2010-0435. Epub 2011 Mar 8. PMID: 21385795; PMCID: PMC3228118.

43. Dahir M., Travers-Gustafson D. Breast cancer, aromatase inhibitor therapy, and sexual functioning: a pilot study of the effects of vaginal testosterone therapy. *Sex Med.* 2014;**2**(1):8-15. doi: 10.1002/sm2.22. PMID: 25356296; PMCID: PMC4184610.

44. Melisko M. E., Goldman M. E., Hwang J., et al. Vaginal testosterone cream vs estradiol vaginal ring for vaginal dryness or decreased libido in women receiving aromatase inhibitors for early-stage breast cancer: A randomized clinical trial. *JAMA Oncol.* 2017;**3**(3):313–19. doi: 10.1001/jamaoncol.2016.3904. Erratum in: JAMA Oncol. 2020 Sep 1;6(9):1473. PMID: 27832260.

45. El-Hage G., Eden J. A., Manga R. Z. A double-blind, randomized, placebo-controlled trial of the effect of testosterone cream on the sexual motivation of menopausal hysterectomized women with hypoactive sexual desire disorder. *Climacteric.* 2007;**10**(4):335–43. doi: 10.1080/13697130701364644. PMID: 17653960.

46. Rock C. L., Flatt S. W., Thomson C. A., et al. Effects of a high-fiber, low-fat diet intervention on serum concentrations of reproductive steroid hormones in women with a history of breast cancer. *J Clin Oncol.* 2004;**22**(12):2379–87. doi: 10.1200/JCO.2004.09.025. PMID: 15197199.

47. Jiang X., Bossert A., Parthasarathy K. N., et al. Safety assessment of compounded non-FDA-approved hormonal therapy versus FDA-approved hormonal therapy in treating postmenopausal women. *Menopause.* 2021;**28**(8):867–74.

48. Goldman L., Blaney D., Kindel D., et al. Pathology of the effect of the laser beam on the skin. *Nature.* 1963;**197**:91–14. https://doi.org/10.1038/197912b0

49. Statement from FDA Commissioner Scott Gottlieb, M.D., on Efforts to Safeguard Women's Health from Deceptive Health Claims and Significant Risks Related to Devices Marketed for Use in Medical Procedures for "Vaginal Rejuvenation." FDA, July 30, 2018, www.fda.gov/news-events/press-announcements/statement-fda-commissioner-scott-gottlieb-md-effort

s-safeguard-womens-health-deceptive-health-claims.

50. Li F. G., Maheux-Lacroix S., Deans R., et al. Effect of fractional carbon dioxide laser vs sham treatment on symptom severity in women with postmenopausal vaginal symptoms: A randomized clinical trial. *JAMA*. 2021;**326**(14):1381–9. doi: 10.1001/jama.2021.14892. PMID: 34636862; PMCID: PMC8511979.

51. Mension E., Alonso I., Anglès-Acedo S., et al. Effect of fractional carbon dioxide vs sham laser on sexual function in survivors of breast cancer receiving aromatase inhibitors for genitourinary syndrome of menopause: The LIGHT randomized clinical trial. *JAMA Netw Open*. 2023;**6**(2): e2255697. doi:10.1001/jamanetworkopen.2022.55697

52. Nunns D, Williamson K, Swaney L, Davy M. The morbity of surgery and adjuvant radiotherapy in the management of endometrial carcinoma. *Int J Gynecol Cancer*. 2000; **10**(3):233–8.

53. Flay L., Matthews J. H. L. The effects of radiotherapy and surgery on the sexual function of women treated for cervical cancer. *Int J Radiat Oncol Biol Phys*. 1995;**31**(2):399–440.

54. Miles T., Johnson N. Vaginal dilator therapy for women receiving pelvic radiotherapy. *Cochrane Database Syst Rev*. 2014;9:CD007291.

55. Juraskova I., Jarvis S., Mok K. et al. The acceptability, feasibility, and efficacy (phase I/II study) of the OVERcome (Olive Oil, Vaginal Exercise, and MoisturizeR) intervention to improve dyspareunia and alleviate sexual problems in women with breast cancer.*The Journal of Sexual Medicine*. 2013;**10**(10):2549–58. https://doi.org/10.1111/jsm.12156

56. Shields C., Kobiella E., Jeung L., et al. More than just *"vaginal dryness"*: Addressing an unmet need for sexual health intervention in female cancer survivors. 2022. Annual Sylvester Retreat. December 3, Miami FL.

57. Gondi V., Bentzen S. M., Sklenar K. L., et al. Severe late toxicities following concomitant chemoradiotherapy compared to radiotherapy alone in cervical cancer: an inter-era analysis. *Journal of Radiation Oncology, Biology, Physics*. 2012;**84**(4):973–82. [www.redjournal.org/article/S0360-3016(12)00137-X/abstract; PUBMED: www.ncbi.nlm.nih.gov/pubmed/22898381]

58. Bahng A. Y., Dagan A., Brunner D., Lin L. L. Determination of prognostic factors for long-term vaginal toxicity associated with intravaginal high-dose rate brachytherapy in patients with endometrial carcinoma. *International Journal of Radiation Oncology, Biology, Physics*. 2010;**78**(3 Suppl): S401–2. [www.redjournal.org/article/S0360-3016(10)01919-X/fulltext]

59. Law E., Kelvin J. F., Thom B., et al. Prospective study of vaginal dilator uses adherence and efficacy following radiotherapy. *Radiotherapy and Oncology: Journal of the European Society for Therapeutic Radiology and Oncology*. 2015;**116**(1):149. https://doi.org/10.1016/j.radonc.2015.06.018

60. Miles T., Johnson N. Vaginal dilator therapy for women receiving pelvic radiotherapy. *The Cochrane Database of Systematic Reviews* 2014;(**9**). https://doi.org/10.1002/14651858.CD007291.pub3

61. Schover L. R. Reduction of psychosexual dysfunction in cancer patients. In S. M. Miller, D. J. Bowen, R. T. Croyle, J. H. Rowland (Eds.), *Handbook of Cancer Control and Behavioral Science: A Resource for Researchers, Practitioners, and Policymakers* (pp. 379–89). American Psychological Association; 2009. https://doi.org/10.1037/14499-021

62. Velaskar S. M., Martha R., Mahantashetty U., Badakare J. S., Shrivastava S. K. Use of indigenous vaginal dilator in radiation-induced vaginal stenosis. *Indian Journal of Occupational Therapy*. 2007;**34**(1):3–6.

63. Mercier J., Morin M., Zaki D., et al. Pelvic floor muscle training as a treatment for genitourinary syndrome of menopause: A single-arm feasibility study. *Maturitas*. 2019;125:57–62. doi: 10.1016/j

.maturitas.2019.03.002. Epub 2019 Mar 29. PMID: 31133219.

64. Wallace S., Miller L., Mishra K. Pelvic floor physical therapy in the treatment of pelvic floor dysfunction in women. *Current Opinion in Obstetrics and Gynecology.* 2019;**31**(6):485–93. doi: 10.1097/GCO.0000000000000584.

65. Portman D. J., Brown L., Yuan J., Kissling R., Kingsberg S. A. Flibanserin in postmenopausal women with hypoactive sexual desire disorder: Results of the PLUMERIA study. *The Journal of Sexual Medicine.* 2017;**14**(6):834–42. https://doi.org/10.1016/j.jsxm.2017.03.258

66. English C., Muhleisen A., Rey J. A. Flibanserin (Addyi): The *first* FDA-*approved treatment* for *female sexual interest/arousal disorder* in *premenopausal women. P T.* 2017;**42**(4):237–41. PMID: 28381915; PMCID: PMC5358680.

67. Stevens D. M., Weems J. M., Brown L., Barbour K. A., Stahl S. M. The pharmacodynamic effects of combined administration of flibanserin and alcohol. *J Clin Pharm Ther.* 2017;**42**(5):598–606. doi: 10.1111/jcpt.12563. Epub 2017 Jun 13. PMID: 28608926.

68. Clayton A. H., Althof S. E., Kingsberg S., et al. Bremelanotide for female sexual dysfunctions in premenopausal women: A randomized, placebo-controlled

dose-finding trial. *Womens Health (Lond).* 2016;**12**(3):325–37. doi: 10.2217/whe-2016-0018. Epub 2016 May 16. PMID: 27181790; PMCID: PMC5384512.

69. Kingsberg S. A., Clayton A. H., Portman D., et al. Bremelanotide for the treatment of hypoactive sexual desire disorder: Two randomized phase 3 trials. *Obstetrics and Gynecology.* 2019.**134**(5), 899–908. https://doi.org/10.1097/AOG.0000000000003500

70. Simon J. A., Kingsberg S. A., Shumel B., Hanes V., Garcia M., Jr, Sand M. Efficacy and safety of flibanserin in postmenopausal women with hypoactive sexual desire disorder: results of the SNOWDROP trial. *Menopause (New York, N.Y.).* 2014;**21**(6):633–40. https://doi.org/10.1097/GME.0000000000000134

71. Katz M., DeRogatis L. R., Ackerman R., et al. Efficacy of flibanserin in women with hypoactive sexual desire disorder: Results from the BEGONIA trial. *The Journal of Sexual Medicine.* 2013;**10**(7):1807–15. https://doi.org/10.1111/jsm.12189

72. Davis S. R., Baber R., Panay N., et al. Global consensus position statement on the use of testosterone therapy for women. *J Clin Endocrinol Metab.* 20191;**104**(10):4660–6. doi:10.1210/jc.2019-01603.PMID: 31498871;PMCID:PMC6821450

Premature Ovarian Insufficiency

Austin B. Gardner and Sukhkamal B. Campbell

Case Presentation

A 34-year-old G0P0 with a history of stage IIIB cervical cancer treated with chemotherapy, external beam radiation, and vaginal brachytherapy one year ago presents to her gynecologic oncologist for a follow-up visit. She reports that she has not had a menstrual cycle in the past four months. Six months prior to her last menstrual period her cycles became progressively shorter until they stopped entirely. She denies any other medical problems or surgical procedures. She does not smoke and rarely drinks alcohol. Height and weight are within the normal ranges, and her breast and abdominal exams are unremarkable. Pelvic exam is consistent with changes due to radiation exposure. Laboratory analyses demonstrates a normal prolactin and thyroid-stimulating hormone (TSH). Estradiol levels are < 15 pg/mL and follicle-stimulating hormone (FSH) is 47 IU/L. At a subsequent visit one month later, the patient states she has random episodes of "feeling extremely hot" when she sleeps at night as well as fatigue, brain fog, and moodiness. Repeat serum FSH is 45 IU/L at that time. How do you best counsel this patient?

Epidemiology

Incidence and Long-Term Prognosis

Premature ovarian insufficiency (POI) is defined as loss of ovarian function prior to 40 years of age. Absence of ovarian function leads to a persistent state of hypergonadotropic hypogonadism with subsequent amenorrhea characteristic of menopausal women. FSH assessment greater than 40 IU/L on two measurements taken at least one month apart meet diagnostic criteria. If this clinical picture occurs between ages 40–45 years, then the patient is considered to have entered early menopause. A large study evaluating 11,652 women across the United States reported a spontaneous POI incidence of 1.1% [1]. Caucasian women were more likely to be affected whereas Asian women were significantly less so. Higher body mass index, use of female hormones (other than oral contraceptives), and smoking were independently associated with onset of POI. A recent meta-analysis of 31 studies suggests that the global prevalence of spontaneous POI is as high as 3.7% and women in countries scoring in the low or medium categories of the Human Development Index were more likely to have ovarian dysfunction [2].

Incidence of POI among patients who have undergone treatment for cancer varies based on several factors including age at treatment initiation and the specific treatment regimen. A study of approximately 900 patients treated for cancer at young ages found 11% of participants developed POI (median age of assessment 32 years) [3]. Thirty percent of patients treated with both abdominopelvic radiation and alkylating chemotherapeutic agents develop POI [4]. For those receiving high doses of alkylating agents, approximately 60% will subsequently develop POI [5]. Based on the increased prevalence of POI in patients undergoing cancer treatment relative to the general population, appropriate counseling prior to therapy is a critical aspect of care.

All-cause mortality in women with POI is higher than that of the general population, with some data indicating as high as a 10–20% increased risk [6]. Cardiovascular disease contributes to the majority of this risk. The absence of estrogen may induce additional sequelae such as osteoporosis, psychiatric comorbidities including dementia, and reduced quality of life through vasomotor symptoms, mood changes, and sexual dysfunction [6, 7]. Women with POI have a decreased life expectancy by 2 or more years when compared to women who experience menopause at 55 years of age or greater [8]. In light of the significant health implications of POI, accurate diagnosis and treatment is an important component of survivorship care for cancer patients.

Etiology, Risk Factors, and Health Consequences

A range of genetic, autoimmune, iatrogenic, environmental, and social factors can lead to POI. These risk factors have differing impact on ovarian function through either defective or abnormal development of ovarian follicles, follicular depletion, or auto-immune destruction of ovarian tissue. An underlying cause of POI may never be found, though recent studies are finding greater numbers of genetic mutations which may be significantly linked to the disease process [9]. To avoid overlooking an underlying factor, we will review the various etiologies of POI and summarize the recommended testing in Table 5.1 for non-iatrogenic causes. For cancer survivors however, the etiology of POI is typically iatrogenic.

Genetic

Up to 20–25% of non-iatrogenic POI cases may have a genetic cause and chromosomal abnormalities comprise half of those cases [10]. Approximately 10–15% of women with POI have a first-degree relative who is also affected. Turner Syndrome, or 45X (monosomy X), is the most common chromosomal abnormality associated with POI. Women with Turner Syndrome often have distinct phenotypic features including short stature and/or webbed necks, and many develop cardiovascular and renal anomalies, hepatic dysfunction, and autoimmune disorders [11]. Streak gonads contain minimal and poorly functioning antral follicles which may lead to lack of pubertal development and subsequent amenorrhea. Early mortality risk is approximately four-fold that of the general population, largely due to cardiac abnormalities predisposing to aortic dissection [11]. Karyotyping is important for these individuals, as up to 5% contain a portion of the Y chromosome which increases risk for developing gonadoblastoma and may require surgical management [12].

Table 5.1 Typical laboratory evaluation for confirmed POI with unexplained etiology

Potential etiology	Laboratory evaluation
Genetic	Fragile X screen (PCR of *FMR1*), karyotype
Autoimmune	Thyroid stimulating hormone, anti-thyroid peroxidase, anti-thyroglobulin, anti-21 hydroxylase/anti-17-alpha-hydroxylase

Swyer Syndrome is another chromosomal abnormality leading to streak gonads and hypergonadotropic hypogonadism, however the karyotype in these individuals is 46 XY. Patients appear phenotypically female as mutations in the gene encoding Sex-determining Region Y (*SRY*) protein lead to decreased anti-Mullerian hormone (AMH) and androgen production. Similar to those with Turner Syndrome, patients have delayed sexual maturation and primary amenorrhea. Gonadectomy should be performed early due to risk of gonadoblastoma or dysgerminoma [13].

Additional chromosomal abnormalities include mosaicism and Trisomy X. The supernummary X chromosome leads to tall stature, clinodactyly, speech and motor defects, as well as renal and genitourinary abnormalities which may ultimately predispose the individual to POI [14]. Variants in several different genes encoded on the X chromosome may play significant roles in the development of POI, including *DIAPH2* (diaphanous-related formin 2), *BMP15* (bone morphogenic protein 15), and *PGRMC1* (progesterone receptor membrane component 1) as some of the more prevalent [15]. Next-generation sequencing (NGS) is expanding current understanding of the genetic underpinnings of POI, with over 290 genes evaluated including those at loci other than the X chromosome [9, 16].

Perhaps the most recognized genetic cause of POI is carrier status of a Fragile X premutation. The Fragile X messenger ribonucleoprotein 1 (*FMR1*) gene resides on the X chromosome, and the normal gene contains less than 55 trinucleotide CGG repeats of DNA. This gene follows an inheritance pattern of anticipation, meaning that as it is passed to subsequent generations through the mother, the number of trinucleotide repeats may increase. The risk of acquiring a pre-mutation resulting in disease expression increases until the number of repeats surpasses 200, beyond which point it becomes a full mutation. The resulting hypermethylation and silencing of the gene causes little to no production of its product, fragile X mental retardation protein (FMRP), which normally functions as a translational regulator for many RNAs involved in neurologic function. Overexpression of various RNAs due to loss of FMRP functionality leads to neurotoxicity and the development of Fragile X Syndrome (FXS) [17]. FXS is characterized by intellectual disability as well as autism. Carriers of the premutation are also at risk for multiple medical, reproductive, cognitive, and psychiatric difficulties including fragile-X associated tremor/ataxia syndrome (primarily in males) and POI (in females). Nearly 15% of women who carry a *FMR1* premutation will be affected by POI [18]. Due to the high prevalence of POI in *FMR1* premutation carriers and its genetic implications for future generations, all women with unexplained POI should be offered fragile X premutation screening. Some reports suggest that women with FMR1 premutation alleles are also more prone to developing other endocrine abnormalities [19].

Autosomal defects related to POI exist although are rare in frequency. One such defect is galactosemia. Galactosemia is characterized by a deficiency in galactose-1-P uridylyltransferase (GALT) enzyme activity. GALT activity varies widely depending on the tissue in the body. The ovary has abundant enzymes involved with galactose metabolism, and deficiency in GALT leads to toxic accumulation of galactose and related metabolites within the ovary. The result is ovarian tissue destruction through apoptosis leading to POI [20].

Perrault syndrome involves both sensorineural loss and ovarian tissue destruction in a person with a 46 XX karyotype. The disorder is inherited in an autosomal recessive fashion and approximately half the cases are attributable to a mutation in one of eight specific genes [21].

Blepharophimosis, ptosis, epicanthus inversus syndrome is a form of eyelid malformation that can be associated with POI. It is secondary to a mutation in the forkhead transcription factor L2 (*FOXL2*) gene which plays a role in granulosa cell differentiation and maintenance [22]. The mutation causes a shortened, nonfunctional protein. Mutations in *FOXL2* also put women at risk for developing granulosa cell tumors, with over 95% of cases arising from defects in this gene [23].

Pseudo-hypoparathyroidism type 1a leads to hypocalcemia and hyperphosphatemia due to renal resistance to parathyroid hormone. Affected individuals are also resistant to thyroid-stimulating hormone, gonadotropins, and growth-hormone-releasing hormone. The etiology is a mutation in the *GNAS* gene which is involved in the activation cascade of FSH and LH receptors. Individuals will not appropriately respond to gonadotropins and may develop POI [24].

The examples of autosomal defects listed above not only lead to POI but are also associated with phenotypes that either require additional screening, medical intervention, or alterations in lifestyle habits for appropriate management. Genetic testing should be considered.

Autoimmune

Autoimmune etiologies contribute to approximately 5–30% of spontaneous POI cases and result in an autoimmune oophoritis. Antibodies against 21-hydroxylase, 17 alpha-hydroxylase, and side chain cleavage enzymes involved in steroidogenesis may be implicated in around 60–80% of these cases, and they classically damage the adrenal gland which is the primary site of steroid synthesis [25]. The immune system can also target the androgen-producing theca cells of the ovary. Loss of theca cell activity leaves the neighboring granulosa cells with depleted precursors with which to synthesize estrogen, leading to a hypoestrogenic state which causes menopausal symptoms and amenorrhea over time [26]. Interestingly, in many women with newly diagnosed POI and adrenal autoantibodies, AMH levels can be normal which suggests a functional follicle pool. However, the follicle count appears to decline rapidly over time and AMH ultimately becomes undetectable in the years following diagnosis [27].

The link between autoimmune adrenal and ovarian failure warrants screening for adrenal autoantibodies when POI is diagnosed. Ovarian biopsy to confirm oophoritis is generally avoided due to concern for potentially damaging antral follicles and further decreasing ovarian reserve [28]. A positive antibody serum test for 21-hydroxylase antibodies suggests an autoimmune etiology as the cause of POI. If adrenal antibodies are detected in a patient with POI, she should be evaluated for adrenal insufficiency with a morning serum cortisol and ACTH test. POI may precede onset to adrenal insufficiency by many years, so repeat screening tests may be warranted [29].

Autoimmune polyendocrine syndrome (APS) type I is an autosomal recessive disease which presents in childhood and is often characterized by adrenal insufficiency, hypoparathyroidism, and chronic candidiasis of the skin and mucosa. The underlying cause is a mutation in the autoimmune regulator (*AIRE*) gene [30]. APS type II presents in adulthood and similarly includes adrenal insufficiency as well as thyroid dysfunction and often type I diabetes. POI is associated with roughly 60% of APS type I cases and 10% of APS type II cases [31]. Women with either of these conditions require ongoing screening and management of multiple endocrinopathies throughout life.

POI may also be associated with isolated autoimmune conditions which may not lead to fulminant autoimmune oophoritis. For example, autoimmune thyroiditis (Hashimoto's disease) is common in those with POI and may be present in up to a third of POI cases at diagnosis [32]. Based on the prevalence of thyroid dysfunction in those with POI, the European Society of Human Reproduction and Embryology (ESHRE) recommends screening for thyroid peroxidase and thyroglobulin antibodies in all cases of POI [33]. If testing is positive, TSH can be monitored at regular intervals. Contrastingly, diabetes mellitus is associated with a rather small proportion of POI patients, hence routine screening is not recommended by the ESHRE.

Iatrogenic

Radiation therapy may be administered as a component of diagnostic studies or as localized and/or systemic therapy. The amount of radiation required to induce POI inversely correlates with age, as the ovaries of older women are far more susceptible to radiation induced gonadotoxicity. Destruction of 50% of oocytes has been postulated to occur at less than 2 Gray (Gy, which equals one joule of radiation energy per kilogram of matter) based on mathematical models [34]. At age 10, approximately 18 Gy to the ovaries are considered an effective sterilizing dose resulting in ovarian failure, while at age 30 only 14 Gy are required for the same effect [35]. Total body irradiation, which is often used prior to stem cell transplantation or in some cancer treatment regimens, may reach doses as high as 14 Gy. Women treated with radiation at younger ages also have a longer period of time until predicted ovarian failure than those treated at older ages, regardless of the dose of radiation [35]. Doses of at least 20 Gy to the ovaries have been demonstrated to ultimately cause POI in 70–100% of children and adolescents depending on the study [36, 37].

One method which may lower the total dose of radiation exposure to the ovaries is ovarian transposition. This method involves surgically relocating the ovaries higher in the abdominopelvic cavity, often at or above the level of the pelvic brim while maintaining original blood supply, and research has suggested that this procedure decreases the total dose of radiation that the ovaries may be exposed to during treatment. This decreases overall gonadotoxicity to ovarian follicles from pelvic radiation. Many women who undergo transposition will retain ovarian function despite receiving a dose of pelvic radiation which would otherwise sterilize them [38]. For further discussion please see Chapter 1 (Fertility Assessment and Fertility Preservation Options).

Chemotherapy administration may also induce POI. The likelihood of POI following treatment with chemotherapeutic drugs is dependent upon the age of the woman at the time of administration, baseline ovarian reserve (more damaging in those with diminished reserve), type of agent(s) used, number of cycles, and treatment schedule. A retrospective study of several thousand childhood cancer survivors found that those individuals treated at older ages were more likely to experience ovarian failure [39]. Cancer survivors treated with alkylating agents had higher rates of POI, with procarbazine associated with the highest risk. Cyclophosphamide was more likely to cause ovarian dysfunction if administered at ages 13–20 but is less damaging when given in prepubescent populations. Cumulative dose of agent is important in risk counseling. For example, procarbazine administered at a dose of 4.2 g/m^2 is not associated with a significant risk of POI, however, doubling the dose results in nearly a twenty-fold increase in POI risk [5]. For additional discussion regarding chemotherapy specific risks please see Chapter 1 (Fertility Assessment and Fertility Preservation Options).

Surgical management of certain cancer involves removal of the ovaries which can lead to POI. Depending on the type of tumor, ovarian cancer treatment requires unilateral or bilateral salpingo-oophorectomy (USO, BSO). Staging for endometrial cancer also includes BSO. Specific pathogenic variants carry high lifetime risk for epithelial ovarian cancer, and current guidelines recommend risk-reducing salpingo-oophorectomy (RRSO) for patients with many of these pathogenic variants and associated syndromes. The most well-known of these pathogenic variants are *BRCA1/2* and those involved in Lynch syndrome. The recommended age range for RRSO varies depending on the particular pathogenic variant or syndrome in question. For instance, patients with *BRCA1* are advised to undergo RRSO between ages 35–40 years, and POI would be inevitable in these individuals [40]. Patients with Lynch syndrome are advised to undergo hysterectomy/RRSO between ages 40–45 years, and early menopause would occur. Women who have USO, such as for desmoid tumors, may enter menopause on average two years earlier than individuals with both ovaries intact [41].

Environmental and Social

Environmental pollutants impact ovarian function through several mechanisms, specifically through endocrine disruption, oxidative stress, or epigenetic modifications [42]. Endocrine-disrupting chemicals (EDCs) interfere with hormonal function and have been linked to multiple health conditions including earlier onset of menopause. A study of over 30,000 women from the National Health and Nutrition Examination Survey evaluated 111 EDCs and focused specifically on those with over a one-year half-life. The authors found that women exposed to higher concentrations of these EDCs, particularly polychlorinated biphenyls (coolants) and phthalates (plasticizers), experienced menopause up to 4 years earlier than others in the cohort [43]. Many environmental chemicals lead to induction of reactive oxygen species from metabolic pathways, ultimately resulting in apoptosis within ovarian tissue. A study of approximately 100 women demonstrated increased markers of oxidative stress in those experiencing POI relative to unaffected individuals after controlling for multiple confounding variables such as age and family history [44]. Animal models have demonstrated inherited epigenetic changes through DNA methylation. One such study involved exposure of mice to compounds in pesticides and plastics as well as hydrocarbons. Specific regions of altered DNA methylation were identified in offspring of exposed mice, and the offspring were found to have decreased ovarian follicular counts compared to their unexposed counterparts [45]. Although these studies cannot be replicated in humans for ethical reasons, similar effects are possible and may contribute to POI in subsequent generations.

Incidence of spontaneous POI varies by ethnicity. Caucasian women are more likely to be affected and Asian women are less likely compared to Hispanic and Black women [1]. Social factors of higher body mass index and smoking are associated with development of POI [1]. On average, individuals who smoke enter menopause 1–2 years earlier than nonsmokers [46]. Greater rates of ovarian dysfunction have been seen in women from less developed countries [2].

Health Consequences

POI has been associated with a 10–20% increased risk of all-cause mortality, and women with POI have a life expectancy on average a few years shorter than that of women who enter menopause in the typical age range [6, 8]. Women with POI are predisposed to cardiac comorbidities due to lack of estrogen which has anti-atherosclerotic and vasodilatory effects in the cardiovascular system. They also develop abnormal lipid profiles which accelerate detrimental cardiac changes [47]. A cohort study of over 144,000 participants followed over a six-year timeframe found that those with POI were more likely to experience cardiovascular issues relative to women who experienced menopause within the average age range [48]. This risk was most pronounced in women who experienced a surgically induced POI, and was nearly double the risk of those that underwent natural menopause (even after controlling for hormone therapy (HT)). Given the link between POI and adverse cardiovascular outcomes, the American College of Cardiology recommends considering statin therapy in women with POI once they reach 40 years in age if other risk factors are also present [49]. Screening for hypertension, diabetes, and dyslipidemia should occur at regular intervals.

Estrogen stimulates factors involved in bone formation while inhibiting those which participate in resorption. As such, women with POI have decreased femoral neck and spine bone mineral density scores relative to similarly aged controls [50]. Patients require appropriate counseling on calcium and vitamin D intake in addition to regular weight-bearing exercise. HT should also be considered to mitigate bone loss and is discussed later in the chapter. There are current recommendations to order dual-energy X-ray absorptiometry (DXA) scanning in patients with POI within the first year, with suggestion of repeat screening every 1–2 years depending upon the results [51].

The effects of estrogen in the brain have been demonstrated in animal models and include improved cerebral blood flow and glucose metabolism, enhanced choline acetyltransferase activity, and decreased beta-amyloid formation [52]. Some research has suggested women who receive bilateral oophorectomy prior to menopause have nearly double the risk of developing neurocognitive dysfunction including Alzheimer's disease, and the likelihood further increases if the surgery is performed at younger ages [53]. However, intervention with HT within five years of surgery and through the average age of natural menopause mitigates the probability of neurocognitive decline. Women with POI experience higher rates of depression and perceived stress compared to the general population, hence mental health screening should be routinely incorporated into healthcare visits [54].

Women with POI may experience both physical and psychological components of sexual dysfunction. Loss of estrogen leads to atrophy of the urogenital tract and contributes to vaginal dryness and irritation. This physiologic change can lead to dyspareunia and recurrent urinary tract infections which may cause genital arousal disorder or avoidance of sexual practices. HT and lubricants can help alleviate these symptoms, with addition of vaginal estrogen to HT resulting in shorter interval to clinical improvement [55]. POI may also negatively impact a woman's self-esteem, body image, and sense of identity or femininity which could influence her relationship and intimacy with her partner. A survey study demonstrated women with POI were less likely to initiate or have intercourse, express sexual desires to their partner, and enjoy intercourse [56]. Psychosocial support and counseling should be a cornerstone of care for women with POI.

Anticipated Reproductive Impact

A diagnosis of POI may have devastating psychosocial implications particularly in regards to future childbearing. No current therapy has been shown to improve pregnancy rates with their own gametes, although spontaneous ovulation may occur. Traditional ovulation induction is often unsuccessful secondary to already elevated FSH and associated hypoestrogenism. Similar lack of success exists when attempting controlled ovarian stimulation with exogenous gonadotropins. The use of donor oocytes or embryos is the only established method to improve the chances of achieving a successful pregnancy.

Spontaneous pregnancies have been reported in women with POI, with pregnancy rates varying from 2.2–14%. Conception is more likely in women under age 30, recent diagnosis of POI and in those receiving cyclic estrogen and progesterone HT versus combination oral contraceptive pills [57]. HT creates the possibility of an escape ovulation cycle and conception which otherwise may not have occurred in these patients. The underlying cause of POI is also linked to the overall probability of a live birth. For instance, patients with idiopathic causes of POI or those with surgically induced POI after benign ovarian cystectomy had the highest likelihood of clinical pregnancies [58]. Future directions include in vitro activation of cryopreserved ovarian tissue with subsequent tissue grafting [59]. Other experimental methods, such as injection of platelet rich plasma into ovarian tissue, may offer potential to improve pregnancy rates in this population [60].

For women undergoing cancer therapy, the risk of POI if often not discussed and can further contribute to negative body image after treatment. Reproductive counseling is imperative, particularly for those women who have not completed childbearing.

Treatment

First line treatment for POI-related symptoms is HT. Women with POI are distinct from the typical postmenopausal population. Early loss of endogenous estrogen production leads to an increase in all-cause mortality largely due to coronary artery disease [2]. Estrogen supplementation mitigates bone loss, cognitive dysfunction, and vasomotor symptoms as well as mood irregularities [6, 7]. As such, physiologic HT is critical to preserve long-term health and is considered to be standard of care for an individual with POI. In other patient populations, such as postmenopausal women, it is often administered on a case-by-case basis.

The goal of HT in patients with POI is to replicate physiologic ovarian function. An important consideration is the addition of a progestogen to estrogen therapy if the patient still has a uterus in situ. Cyclic or daily progestogens protect the endometrial lining from persistent overgrowth, hyperplasia, and malignancy that can result from unopposed estrogen.

Estrogenic compounds are contraindicated in women with a history of hormone responsive tumors, such as breast cancer, advanced stage endometrial cancer, dermoid, and low grade ovarian serous tumors. See Chapter 6 for additional details. Further variables to consider are whether the patient has preexisting risk factors such as a history of stroke or a propensity for thrombosis.

Estrogen therapy can be administered through oral, transdermal, or vaginal routes. A small randomized trial in women with POI found that women with transdermal estrogen (0.1 mg/24 hr) delivery and vaginal progesterone (200 mg BID) had improved cardiovascular health and renal function compared to women treated with oral therapy consisting of ethinyl estradiol with norethisterone [61]. This benefit may be related to how transdermal preparations avoid first pass hepatic metabolism and the associated induction of hepatic proteins [62]. Women treated with transdermal estrogen for POI had greater improvements in bone density compared to those who received oral estrogen in a separate trial performed over a three-year period [63]. Current recommendations are to utilize hormone replacement until age 51, the age of typical menopause [64].

Case Resolution

The diagnosis is iatrogenic POI with chemoradiation as the underlying cause. Diagnosis was confirmed with two measurements of FSH >40 IU/L taken one month apart. Additional lab testing for TSH and prolactin was initially performed to rule out other frequent causes of amenorrhea. Further evaluation for other causes of POI could have been conducted with karyotyping, testing for antibodies against enzymes involved in steroidogenesis, and Fragile X screening, though this patient has a clear explanation for her POI based on her treatment history. She is counseled on use of HT to alleviate her vasomotor symptoms, eagerly agrees, and reports marked improvement in quality of life.

Take Home Points

- Premature ovarian insufficiency is a frequent consequence of cancer therapy.
- Symptoms of secondary amenorrhea and signs of estrogen deficiency should promptly be recognized and assessed to confirm the diagnosis of POI.
- Assuming no contraindications exist, early intervention with HT will help protect patients from complications later in life related to impaired cardiovascular, bone, and cognitive health.
- Non-iatrogenic causes of POI require additional screening and medical management of disease-specific sequelae.
- Unfortunately, options to use autologous oocytes are limited in individuals with POI, although spontaneous pregnancies do occur. Highest rates of successful pregnancies are achieved using donor oocytes or embryos.
- Consultation with a mental health provider experienced in reproductive counseling can address some of the psychosocial issues associated with the loss of fertility.

References

1. Luborsky J. L., Meyer P., Sowers M. F., Gold E. B., Santoro N. Premature menopause in a multi-ethnic population study of the menopause transition. *Hum Reprod.* 2003;**18**(1):199–206.

2. Golezar S., Tehrani F. R., Khazaei S., Ebadi A., Kashavarz Z. The global prevalence of primary ovarian insufficiency and early menopause: A meta-analysis. *Climacteric.* 2019;**22**(4):403–11.

3. Chemaitilly W., Li Z., Krasin M., Premature ovarian insufficiency in childhood cancer survivors: a report from the St. Jude lifetime cohort. *J Clin Endocrinol Metab.* 2017;**102**(7):2242–50.

4. Sklar C., Mertens A., Mitby P., et al. Premature menopause in survivors of childhood cancer: a report from the childhood cancer survivor study. *J Natl Cancer Inst.* 2006;**98**(13):890–6.

5. De Bruin M., Huisbrink J., Hauptmann M., et al. Treatment-related risk factors for premature menopause following Hodgkin lymphoma. *Blood.* 2008;**111**(1):101–08.

6. Huan L., Deng X., He M., Chen S., Niu W. Meta-analysis: Early age at natural menopause and risk for all-cause and cardiovascular mortality. *Biomed Res Int.* 2021 Mar **15**;2021.

7. Faubion S. S., Kuhle C. L., Shuster L. T., Rocca W. A. Long-term health consequences of premature or early menopause and considerations for management. *Climacteric.* 2015;**18**(4):483–91.

8. Ossewaarde M., Bots M., Verbeek Z., et al. Age at menopause, cause-specific mortality

and total life expectancy. *Epidemiology.* 2005;**16**(4):556–62.

9. Ruth K. Day F., Hussain J., et al. Genetic insights into biological mechanisms governing human ovarian ageing. *Nature.* 2021;**596**(7872):393–7.

10. Qin Y., Jiao X., Simpson J. L., Chen Z. J. Genetics of primary ovarian insufficiency: new developments and opportunities. *Hum Reprod Update.* 2015;**21**(6):787–808.

11. Hjerrild B. E., Mortensen K. H., Gravholt C. H. Turner syndrome and clinical treatment. *Br Med Bull.* 2008;**86**:77–93.

12. Kwon A, et al. Risk of gonadoblastoma development in patients with Turner syndrome with cryptic Y chromosome material. *Horm Cancer.* 2017;**8**(3):166–73.

13. Michala L., Stefanaki K., Loutradis D. Premature ovarian insufficiency in adolescence: A chance for early diagnosis? *Hormones (Athens).* 2020;**19**(3):277–83.

14. Tartaglia N. R., Howell S., Sutherland A., Wilson R., Wilson L. A review of trisomy X (47,XXX). *Orphanet J Rare Dis.* 2010;**5**:8.

15. Persani L., Rossetti R., Cacciatore C. Genes involved in human premature ovarian failure. *J Mol Endocrinol.* 2010;**45**(5):257–79.

16. Rossetti R., Moleri S., Guizzardi F. et al. Targeted next-generation sequencing indicates a frequent oligogenic involvement in primary ovarian insufficiency onset. *Front Endocrinol (Lausanne).* 2021;**12**:664645.

17. Man L., Lekovich J., Rosenwaks Z., Gerhardt J. Fragile X-associated diminished ovarian reserve and primary ovarian insufficiency from molecular mechanisms to clinical manifestations. *Front Mol Neurosci.* 2017;**10**:290.

18. Tassanakijpanich N., Hagerman R. J., Worachotekamjorn J. Fragile X premutation and associated health conditions: A review. *Clin Genet.* 2021;**99**(6):751–60.

19. Hoyos L. R., Thakur M. Fragile X premutation in women: Recognizing the health challenges beyond primary ovarian insufficiency. *J Assist Reprod Genet.* 2017;**34**(3):315–23.

20. Thakur M., Feldman G., Puscheck E. E. Primary ovarian insufficiency in classic galactosemia: Current understanding and future research opportunities. *J Assist Reprod Genet.* 2018;**35**(1):3–16.

21. Faridi R., Rea A., Fenollar-Ferrer C., et al. New insights into Perrault syndrome, a clinically and genetically heterogeneous disorder. *Hum Genet.* 2022;**141** (3–4):805–19.

22. Kim J., Bae J. Differential apoptotic and proliferative activities of wild-type FOXL2 and blepharophimosis-ptosis-epicanthus inversus syndrome (BPES)-associated mutant FOXL2 proteins. *J Reprod Dev.* 2014;**60**(1):14–20.

23. Pilsworth J., Cochrane D., Neilson S., et al. Adult-type granulosa cell tumor of the ovary: A FOXL2-centric disease. *J Pathol Clin Res.* 2021;**7**(3):243–52.

24. Rossetti R., Ferrari I., Bonomi M., Persani M. Genetics of primary ovarian insufficiency. *Clin Genet.* 2017;**91**(2):183–98.

25. Silva C. A., et al. Autoimmune primary ovarian insufficiency. *Autoimmun Rev.* 2014;**13**(4–5):427–30.

26. La Marca A., Brozzetti A., Sighinolfi G., et al. Primary ovarian insufficiency: Autoimmune causes. *Curr Opin Obstet Gynecol.* 2010;**22**(4):277–82.

27. Falorni A., Brozzetti A., Aglietti M. C., et al. Progressive decline of residual follicle pool after clinical diagnosis of autoimmune ovarian insufficiency. *Clin Endocrinol (Oxf).* 2012;**77**(3):453–8.

28. Kirshenbaum M., Orvieto R. Premature ovarian insufficiency (POI) and autoimmunity-an update appraisal. *J Assist Reprod Genet.* 2019; **36**(11):2207–15.

29. Carp H. J. A., Selmi C., Shoenfeld Y. The autoimmune bases of infertility and pregnancy loss. *J Autoimmun.* 2012;**38** (2–3):J266–74.

30. Bjorklund G., Pivin M., Hangan T., Yurkovskaya O., Pivina L. Autoimmune polyendocrine syndrome type 1: Clinical

manifestations, pathogenetic features, and management approach. *Autoimmun Rev.* 2022;**21**(8):103135.

31. Taylor H. S., Pal L., Seli E. *Speroff's Clinical Gynecologic Endocrinology and Infertility.* Ninth edition. Lippincott Williams & Wilkins; 2019.

32. Szeliga A., Calik-Ksepka A., Maciejewska-Jeske M., et al. Autoimmune diseases in patients with premature ovarian insufficiency: Our current state of knowledge. *Int J Mol Sci.* 2021;**22**(5):2594.

33. Webber L., Davies M., Anderson R., et al. ESHRE guideline: Management of women with premature ovarian insufficiency. *Hum Reprod.* 2016;**31**(5):926–37.

34. Wallace W. H. B., Thomson A. B., Kelsey T. W. The radiosensitivity of the human oocyte. *Hum Reprod.* 2003;**18**(1):117–21.

35. Wallace W. H. B., Thomson A. B., Saran F., Kelsey T. W. Predicting age of ovarian failure after radiation to a field that includes the ovaries. *Int J Radiat Oncol Biol Phys.* 2005;**62**(3):738–44.

36. Wallace W. H., Shalet S. M., Crowne E. C., Morris-Jones P. H., Gattamaneni H. R. Ovarian failure following abdominal irradiation in childhood: Natural history and prognosis. *Clin Oncol (R Coll Radiol).* 1989;**1**(2):75–9.

37. Green D., Sklar C., Boice J., et al. Ovarian failure and reproductive outcomes after childhood cancer treatment: Results from the Childhood Cancer Survivor Study. *J Clin Oncol.* 2009;**27**(14):2374–81.

38. Hilal L., Cercek A., Navilio J., et al. Factors associated with premature ovarian insufficiency in young women with locally advanced rectal cancer treated with pelvic radiation therapy. *Adv Radiat Oncol.* 2021;**7**(1):100801.

39. Chemaitilly W., Mertens A., Mitby P., et al. Acute ovarian failure in the Childhood Cancer Survivor Study. *Clin Endocrinol Metab.* 2006;**91**(5):1723–8.

40. Daly M., Pal T., Berry M., et al. Genetic/familial high-risk assessment: Breast, ovarian, and pancreatic, version 2.2021, NCCN clinical practice guidelines in oncology. *J Natl Compr Canc Netw.* 2021;**19**(1):77-102.

41. Rosendahl M., Simonsen M. K., Kjer J. J. The influence of unilateral oophorectomy on the age of menopause. *Climacteric.* 2017;**20**(6):540–44.

42. Vabre P., Gatimel N., Moreau J., et al. Environmental pollutants, a possible etiology for premature ovarian insufficiency: A narrative review of animal and human data. *Environ Health.* 2017;**16**:37.

43. Grindler N. M., Allsworth J., Macones G., et al. Persistent organic pollutants and early menopause in U.S. women. *PLoS One.* 2015; **10**(1): e0116057.

44. Tokmak A., Yıldırım G., Sarıkaya E., et al. Increased oxidative stress markers may be a promising indicator of risk for primary ovarian insufficiency: A cross-sectional case control study. *Rev Bras Ginecol Obstet.* 2015;**37**(9):411–16.

45. Manikkam M., Guerrero-Bosagna C., Tracey R., Haque M. M., Skinner M. K. Transgenerational actions of environmental compounds on reproductive disease and identification of epigenetic biomarkers of ancestral exposures. *PLoS One.* 2012;**7**(2):e31901.

46. Fleming L., Levis S., LeBlanc W., et al. Earlier age at menopause, work, and tobacco smoke exposure. *Menopause.* 2008;**15**(6):1103–08.

47. Knauff E., Westerveld H., Goverde A., et al. Lipid profile of women with premature ovarian failure. *Menopause.* 2008;**15**(5):919–23.

48. Honigberg M., Zekavat S., Aragam K., et al. Association of premature natural and surgical menopause with incident cardiovascular disease. *JAMA.* 2019;**322**(24):2411–21.

49. Grundy S., Stone N., Bailey A., et al. 2018 AAHA/ACC/AACVPR/AAPA/ABC/ACPM/ADA/AGS/APhA/ASPC/NLA/PCNA guideline on the management of blood cholesterol: a report of the American College of Cardiology/American Heart Association Task Force on clinical practice

guidelines. *Circulation.* 2019;**139**(25): e1082–e1143.

50. Uygur D., Sengül O., Bayar D., et al. Bone loss in young women with premature ovarian failure. *Arch Gynecol Obstet.* 2005;**273**(1):17–19.

51. Camacho P. M., Petak S., Binkley N., et al. American Association of Clinical Endocrinologists/American College of Endocrinology clinical practice guidelines for the diagnosis and treatment of postmenopausal osteoporosis: 2020 update. *Endocr Pract.* 2020;**26** (Suppl 1):1–46.

52. Rocca W. A., Grossardt B. R., Shuster L. T. Oophorectomy, menopause, estrogen treatment, and cognitive aging: Clinical evidence for a window of opportunity. *Brain Res.* 2011;**1379**:188–98.

53. Rocca W. A., Bower J., Maraganore D., et al. Increased risk of cognitive impairment or dementia in women who underwent oophorectomy before menopause. *Neurology.* 2007;**69**(11):1074–83.

54. Lambrinoudaki I., Paschou S., Lumsden M., et al. Premature ovarian insufficiency: A toolkit for the primary care physician. *Maturitas.* 2021;**147**:53–63.

55. Palacios S., Castelo-Branco C., Cancelo M. J., Vazquez F. Low-dose, vaginally administered estrogens may enhance local benefits of systemic therapy in the treatment of urogenital atrophy in postmenopausal women on hormone therapy. *Maturitas.* 2005;**50**(2):98–104.

56. Graziottin A., Basson R. Sexual dysfunction in women with premature menopause. *Menopause.* 2004;**11**(6)Pt 2:766–77.

57. Fraison E., Crawford G., Casper G., Harris V., Ledger W. Pregnancy following diagnosis of premature ovarian insufficiency: A systematic review. *Reprod Biomed Online.* 2019;**39**(3):467–76.

58. Ishizuka B., Furuya, Kimura M., Kamioka E., Kawamura K. Live birth rate in patients with premature ovarian insufficiency during long-term follow-up under hormone replacement with or without ovarian stimulation. *Front Endocrinol (Lausanne).* 2021;**12**:795724.

59. Suzuki N., Yoshioka N., Takae S., et al. Successful fertility preservation following ovarian tissue vitrification in patients with primary ovarian insufficiency. *Hum Reprod.* 2015;**30**(3):608–15.

60. Petryk N., Petryk M. Ovarian rejuvenation through platelet-rich autologous plasma (PRP)-a chance to have a baby without donor eggs, improving the life quality of women suffering from early menopause without synthetic hormonal treatment. *Reprod Sci.* 2020;**27**(11):1975–82.

61. Langrish J. P., Mills N., Bath L., et al. Cardiovascular effects of physiological and standard sex steroid replacement regimens in premature ovarian failure. *Hypertension.* 2009;**53**(5):805–11.

62. Chetkowski R. J., et al. Biologic effects of transdermal estradiol. *N Engl J Med.* 1986;**314**(25):1615–20.

63. Popat V. B., et al. Bone mineral density in young women with primary ovarian insufficiency: results of a three-year randomized controlled trial of physiological transdermal estradiol and testosterone replacement. *J Clin Endocrinol Metab.* 2014;**99**(9):3418–26.

64. Sullivan S. D., Sarrel P. M., Nelson L. M. Hormone replacement therapy in young women with primary ovarian insufficiency and early menopause. *Fertil Steril.* 2016;**106**(7):1588–99.

Hormone Therapy and Contraception Management

Fionán Donohoe, Donal Brennan, and Martha Hickey

Menopause and Hormone Therapy in Cancer Patients

Case Presentation

AB is a 39-year-old woman with a known *BRCA1* pathogenic variant. She has a previous history of triple negative breast cancer treated with bilateral mastectomy and adjuvant chemotherapy six years ago. Last year, she was diagnosed with stage 2B high grade serous ovarian cancer for which she had primary cytoreductive surgery. She had a complete macroscopic resection, which involved radical abdominal hysterectomy, bilateral salpingo-oophorectomy, omentectomy, pelvic peritonectomy, and recto-sigmoid resection with primary re-anastomosis followed by adjuvant carboplatin and paclitaxel chemotherapy for six cycles. She is now six months post-completion of chemotherapy and has started maintenance poly adenosine diphosphate-ribose polymerase (PARP) inhibitor therapy. She complains of debilitating hot flashes and night sweats, poor sleep, and recurrent urinary tract infections. She is seeking treatment to manage these symptoms as she feels they are "harder to cope with than the side effects of chemotherapy."

What advice and treatment should she be given?

Epidemiology

Menopause is the final menstrual period, but the term is commonly used to describe the menopause transition: the time from the onset of menstrual cycle changes to the final menstrual period (Menopause) [1]. For some women, the menopause transition might be accompanied by troublesome symptoms. The nature, severity, and impact of these symptoms varies considerably between women and within the same woman over time [2]. Some women experience very limited symptoms which do not impact on their quality of life; however, some women experience severe symptoms and request treatment.

Hot flashes and night sweats or vasomotor symptoms (VMS), as they are referred to collectively, are the most common symptoms of menopause in Caucasian populations affecting as many as 70% of women. Sleep and mood disturbance are also implicated in menopause [3]. Vaginal dryness affects around 60% of women and can impact on quality of life [4]. It is uncertain whether menopause leads to other symptoms, but joint aches are commonly reported in southeast Asian women [5].

The average age of menopause is approximately 51 years. Menopause occurring before the age of 40 is considered premature menopause and before 45 is considered early menopause. Once a woman has more than 12 months without a menstrual period, she is said to be postmenopausal.

Menopause and menopausal symptoms may be induced or exacerbated by cancer treatment in several ways:

- Surgical removal of the ovaries in a premenopausal woman will induce permanent menopause. This is relevant in many gynecologic cancer but also locally advanced colorectal cancer with ovarian or peritoneal metastasis. Women who undergo risk-reducing salpingo-oophorectomy (RRSO) to reduce their risk of ovarian cancer due to a genetic predisposition syndrome such as *BRCA* or Lynch syndrome will often experience surgical menopause.
- Radiotherapy to the pelvis often given to treat cervical, uterine, or rectal cancer will generally induce permanent menopause due to radiation damage to adjacent ovaries.
- Chemotherapy given for a wide range of malignancies can also be toxic to ovarian tissue and induce menopause. Depending on the woman's age and ovarian reserve and the type and dose of chemotherapy, this may be reversible in some cases and ovarian function may recover following completion of chemotherapy. In some cases, however, chemotherapy does induce permanent menopause. In general, the younger a woman is when she receives chemotherapy the more likely she is to regain ovarian function once the chemotherapy is completed. Anti-mullerian hormone (AMH) levels can help predict the likelihood of premature menopause [6].
- Endocrine therapy such as tamoxifen and aromatase inhibitors with or without gonadotropin releasing hormone (GnRH) analogues given as adjuvant therapy after breast cancer, function to reduce circulating estrogen to lower the risk of breast cancer recurrence and can induce menopausal symptoms – even in women who are postmenopausal.

Considerations Prior to Treatment

At the time of diagnosis, it is essential to counsel women about the possible effect that their treatment will have on their menopausal status. Where relevant and where possible, ovarian preservation techniques, particularly ovarian transposition, should be considered. Depending on the patient's age, tumor type, stage, and grade, ovarian preservation may be considered to prevent premature menopause. Clearly, this may not always be possible but is worth considering in cases where it is safe and feasible to do so such as locally advanced cervical cancer and rectal cancer with no obvious ovarian involvement.

Diagnosis

In the setting of cancer-induced menopause, the diagnosis may be clear based on the treatment the patient may have received, for example, pelvic radiotherapy for cervical or rectal cancer will reliably induce menopause. In some cases, the diagnosis can be more difficult to achieve. If the patient is aged 45 or older and describes typical menopause symptoms the diagnosis is clinical, and measurement of gonadotrophins or sex steroids is unlikely to be helpful. Under the age of 45, follicle stimulating hormone (FSH) testing may be helpful.

Treatment

Many women do not request treatment for menopausal symptoms, particularly when these are mild and do not impact on quality of life. Women experiencing menopause at the normal age (45+) do not require any treatment unless requested for symptom management.

However, if symptoms do impact on quality of life or if menopause occurs early or prematurely, then treatment should be considered. For VMS, hormone therapy (HT) is the most effective treatment [3]. However, it may not be suitable for all cancer patients depending on their tumor type. Growing evidence supports the efficacy of nonpharmacological options and nonhormonal pharmacotherapies for VMS [7]. It is important to discuss with patients that whatever form of treatment they pursue, it is unlikely to fully resolve their symptoms.

Hormone Therapy

HT consists of the administration of estrogen, primarily to manage troublesome VMS. For women with an intact uterus progestogen is given to prevent endometrial hyperplasia or malignancy. Older HT preparations contain conjugated equine estrogens whereas modern HT contains 17-beta estradiol which more closely resembles the endogenous estrogen produced by the premenopausal ovary. Estrogen can be given transdermally in a patch or a gel form, via vaginal ring, and can also be given orally. Where required, the progestogen component can be given orally or via the levonorgestrel releasing intrauterine system (LNG-IUS) where feasible or it may be included as part of the transdermal estrogen patch. HT is licensed for the management of VMS but may also benefit sleep, mood, and bone health.

Estrogen is started usually at a low or moderate dose and titrated for symptom control. If inadequate control is noted, then the estrogen dose can be increased. It is important to counsel women that HT is unlikely to treat all their menopausal symptoms.

Estrogen is also an effective treatment for maintaining bone density particularly in women experiencing premature menopause as it can have the dual benefit of improving their VMS while potentially reducing fracture risk. It is important to note that most data on the benefits of HT emanates from noncancer populations so caution must be taken in interpreting the results for an oncology cohort.

Testosterone is also produced by the ovary in premenopausal women. Many claims are made about testosterone's benefits on muscle mass, cognition, and wellbeing in postmenopausal women, however, reliable evidence only exists for its benefit in managing hypoactive sexual desire disorder in pre- or postmenopausal women [8]. Testosterone therapy in women with a history of hormone sensitive breast cancer is contraindicated as there are no data to support its safety in this population.

Cardiovascular disease (CVD) increases in women after menopause and is elevated after cancer treatment [9]. In the general population, surgical menopause before age 35 years is associated with an increased risk of CVD compared to natural menopause at the average age [10]. Treating surgical menopause with HT before the age of 50 years may be effective in reducing the risk of CVD [10]. Little is known about the role of HT in preventing CVD after cancer, but eligible women who experience menopause before age 40 years should be offered HT until the average age at menopause (45–50 years).

Venous thromboembolism (VTE) is commonly diagnosed in women with cancer and HT increases the risk of VTE, however, the risk appears to be related to the method of administration of HT. Transdermal estrogen appears to have a neutral effect on the risk of thromboembolism and should be considered first line in women at increased risk of VTE. However, there is a lack of randomized data to support this observation [11, 12].

Many patients will be concerned about the risk of breast cancer associated with HT and this can be particularly true in women who already have a cancer history. It appears that estrogen only HT may not increase the risk of breast cancer, however, combined HT, that is, with estrogen and progestogen in women with an intact uterus does increase the risk of breast cancer, rising with longer duration of use.

Duration of HT Use

In the setting of premature or early menopause, HT use should be considered until at least the natural age of menopause. Any decision to continue beyond this point should be made on an individual basis considering a woman's individual risk profile. It is important to inform women that they are likely to develop rebound symptoms on cessation of HT.

Nonpharmacological Treatments for Menopause Symptoms

Most nonpharmacological treatments are focused on treating VMS and in many cases are not exclusively studied in the setting of cancer-associated menopause. Treatments like hypnosis and acupuncture do have some randomized data to support their use and are unlikely to be harmful [13, 14].

Cognitive behavioral therapy (CBT) for VMS has level I data to support its use in a variety of settings including in groups and on a one-to-one basis in women with physiological menopause symptoms and induced menopause symptoms [15–18]. It is effective at reducing the degree to which the symptoms bother the woman or interfere with her day-to-day life and in some cases, it appears to reduce intensity and frequency of VMS also.

Nonhormonal Pharmacotherapy

There are several agents which have level I evidence to support their use in the management of VMS [19]. The most data exist for selective serotonin reuptake inhibitors (SSRIs) such as citalopram 10–30 mg, paroxetine 7.5 mg, and escitalopram 10–20 mg and serotonin nor-adrenaline reuptake inhibitors (SNRIs) such as venlafaxine 75–150 mg. These medications are normally used to treat anxiety or depression but have also been shown to be effective when compared to placebo for VMS with additional benefits on mood symptoms. These medications are mostly studied in women with a history of breast cancer. Very little data exists to support the use of these medications in women with other cancer types. Side effects may include nausea, appetite loss, and constipation.

Gabapentin which is an anti-epileptic drug and also used for the management of neuropathic pain is also useful for managing VMS with additional benefits on sleep [20, 21]. Effective doses are 900–2400 mg which can be given in divided doses or in a single dose at night if symptoms are predominantly nocturnal. If prescribed in a single dose at night regime, usual doses are 300–900 mg. Side effects of gabapentin include daytime somnolence, dizziness, and weight gain. Other agents include oxybutynin 2.5 mg–5 mg twice daily and clonidine 0.1 mg which can also be given as a patch, but are less commonly studied and less effective.

In practice, it can be a case of trial and error with patients to find which medication suits them best. Medications should be started at a low dose to ensure tolerance and then increased as required. It may take six to eight weeks before optimal effect can be demonstrated. Sometimes medications may need to be used in combination.

Newer agents called neurokinin receptor antagonists have shown very promising results in early studies for managing VMS with high response rates and rapid onset of action. Phase III studies in oncology populations are eagerly awaited [22].

Urogenital Symptoms

Urogenital symptoms of menopause may include vaginal dryness, itching, and discomfort. These symptoms may cause sexual dysfunction but also discomfort with day-to-day living. Vaginal estrogen has been shown to be effective in managing vaginal dryness, although the level of evidence is low [4]. Women taking systemic HT may also require vaginal estrogen for management of urogenital symptoms.

The use of vaginal estrogen after hormone sensitive cancer such as breast cancer is a much-debated topic. Observational data suggests no increased recurrence of breast cancer with the use of vaginal estrogen [23–27]. However, systemic absorption of estrogen does occur at low levels from vaginal estrogen, but still within the general postmenopausal range. Nevertheless, this raises concerns for its use in women on aromatase inhibitors where the goal of therapy is to lower estrogen levels as much as possible [28, 29]. A dearth of data exists for gynecological cancer [30]. Given the reassuring observational data in breast cancer survivors, it is reasonable to offer vaginal estrogen where required even in those for whom systemic HT is not recommended in discussion with the treating oncologist.

In practice, nonhormonal vaginal lubricants and moisturizers are commonly used first line for urogenital symptoms in the setting of hormone sensitive cancer despite uncertain evidence of benefit [31, 32]. Many oncologists prefer that nonhormonal options be considered first line in the setting of breast cancer, particularly in women using aromatase inhibitors.

Site Specific Considerations

When addressing cancer site specific considerations, the discussion tends to focus on which subgroups of people can consider HT if it is required. For simplicity, it is best to approach this from the point of view of which cancer subtypes should avoid HT, those in whom it is considered safe to use if it is required and those in whom it may be used in certain circumstances. It is important to note, that in many cases there may not be high quality evidence to guide decisions and, therefore, it is important that any discussion around the use of HT after a cancer diagnosis is multidisciplinary and involves treating oncologists, menopause specialists, and the patient herself.

Situations in Which HT Can Be Used to Manage VMS or in the Setting of Early or Premature Menopause

HT is considered safe to use if it is required to manage menopausal symptoms or if the woman is experiencing premature or early menopause, following cancer treatment including colorectal, cervical, vulvar squamous cell carcinoma (SCC), vaginal cancer, leukemia, and lymphoma.

Combined HT has been associated with a reduced risk of colorectal cancer and there is limited evidence to say its use may be associated with improved overall and colorectal cancer associated mortality [33, 34]. This is important as the rate of colorectal cancer is increasing amongst people under the age of 50 [35], making the management of menopausal symptoms more and more relevant in this population as neoadjuvant radiotherapy often given in the setting of rectal cancer will impact ovarian function in younger women.

Cervical, vulvar SCC, and vaginal cancer are all predominantly driven by human papillomavirus (HPV) and, thus, hormones are not implicated in their pathogenesis. Positive hormone receptor expression can sometimes be found in the setting of adenocarcinoma of the cervix, but this does not seem to affect survival and thus, HT can be safely used where required for these women [30]. Premenopausal women with cervical cancer managed surgically can be spared iatrogenic menopause through ovarian preservation which is preferable where possible. Vulvar and vaginal cancer are more common in postmenopausal women and thus, HT is rarely sought to manage symptoms, however, it can be safely considered.

Hematological malignancy such as leukemia and lymphoma are also not hormonally driven and iatrogenic menopause may be a result of stem cell transplantation. Administration of HT if required does not seem to increase recurrence in this setting [36].

Situations in Which HT Should Be Avoided

Breast cancer is the principal cancer in which HT should be avoided. A large randomized controlled trial (RCT) in Sweden demonstrated a significantly higher rate of recurrence of hormone receptor positive breast cancer in women randomized to receive HT to manage menopausal symptoms after being treated for hormone receptor positive breast cancer when compared with women randomized to placebo [37]. Another RCT, also in Sweden, the Stockholm trial, did not show an increased recurrence risk possibly because participants were mainly treated with estrogen-only HT. It did however show an increased risk of contralateral breast cancer in the combined HT group [38]. Both studies were terminated early following an interim analysis of the first. Tibolone is a synthetic steroid with estrogenic properties which is licensed for management of VMS. A large RCT demonstrated a higher risk of recurrence (HR1.4) in women with previous hormone receptor positive breast cancer when compared with placebo [39]. Thus, nonhormonal pharmacotherapy or nonpharmacological treatments should be first line for managing VMS in women with a history of breast cancer. For hormone receptor negative breast cancer and HER2 positive, hormone receptor negative breast cancer, little is known about the safety of HT in this population. In practice, most practitioners would consider nonhormonal therapy as first line and would carefully individualize decisions around use of HT in this population [40].

Other cancer subtypes in which HT should be avoided included low grade serous carcinoma of the ovary as it is almost always hormone sensitive and endocrine therapy can be used to treat it. For similar reasons, HT use is not recommended with desmoid tumors. Sex cord stromal tumors of the ovary, particularly granulosa cell tumors, often present with symptoms of hyperestrogenism and, therefore, HT should be avoided. Endometrial stromal sarcoma and adenosarcoma are also often hormone sensitive and while HT is rarely required as it is more commonly diagnosed in older women, in general, it should be avoided. For the same reason, adenocarcinoma of the vulva is a contraindication to HT as is Paget's disease of the vulva, given its status as a precursor lesion of vulvar adenocarcinoma [30]. See Table 6.1 for a summary of this information.

Table 6.1 Hormone therapy (HT) suitability by cancer type

Cancer site	HT use
Breast – hormone receptor positive	Avoid
Breast – hormone receptor negative	Avoid or carefully individualize decision
Colorectal	Permissible
Lung	Permissible
Hematological	Permissible
Malignant Melanoma	Appears safe in stage 1 disease, avoid in advanced disease
Desmoid tumors	Avoid
Endometrial	Appears safe in stage 1 disease, avoid in advanced disease
Uterine Sarcoma	Avoid
Endometrial Stromal Sarcoma/Adenosarcoma	Avoid
Cervical	Permissible
Vulvar/Vaginal	Permissible
Paget's Disease/Adenosarcoma of Vulva	Avoid
Epithelial ovarian	
High Grade Serous	Permissible
Low Grade Serous	Avoid
Clear Cell	Avoid
Endometrioid	Avoid
Mucinous	Permissible
Borderline	Permissible (Avoid if serous borderline)
Non-epithelial ovarian	
Sex Cord Stromal (Granulosa Cell, Germ Cell)	Avoid
Germ cell (Dysgerminoma, Yolk Sac Tumor, Embryonal Carcinoma, Immature Teratoma)	Permissible

Situations Where HT May Be Safe But With Certain Caveats

In endometrial cancer, based on limited data, HT appears safe in early-stage disease (stage 1) [41]. No data exists in the setting of advanced disease (stage 2, 3, or 4) and HT should not be used in this situation. Endometrial cancer is most often diagnosed in postmenopausal women and the management of menopausal symptoms may not be relevant, however, premenopausal endometrial cancer is increasing, due in part to rising rates of obesity worldwide. In women under the age of 45 with mismatch repair proficient, apparent stage

1, low grade endometrial cancer on preoperative imaging, ovarian preservation can be considered which will avoid menopause [42].

In ovarian, peritoneal, and fallopian tube cancer (collectively termed "ovarian cancer" here), histological subtype dictates suitability for HT. Ninety percent of ovarian cancer is epithelial in origin with three-quarters of cases the serous subtype. Limited data suggests short-term (up to four years) use of HT is safe and does not affect the risk of recurrence in ovarian cancer, however, it is important to note that all of the data is observational, more than 10 years old and comes from relatively small studies, therefore, it is important to discuss this with women when considering HT [43, 44]. As mentioned above, low grade serous ovarian cancer is a contraindication to HT. Clear cell ovarian cancer is associated with an increased risk of VTE which is a contraindication for the use of HT in this population [30].

Like with endometrial cancer, HT seems to be safe in early-stage (Stage 1) malignant melanoma based on a single study of 200 people. No data exists in advanced stage disease [45].

In the setting of lung cancer, the data is conflicting with prospective studies showing improved cancer outcomes [46, 47] and retrospective series showing poorer outcomes [48, 49]. Given the innate limitations of retrospective analyses, HT can be considered where necessary for woman with lung cancer.

Women with a diagnosis of Lynch syndrome or *BRCA* pathogenic variant will be recommended to undergo surgery to reduce their risk of gynecological cancer at a premenopausal age. We know that HT appears to be safe in women with a history of Lynch syndrome. For women with a BRCA diagnosis who do not have a personal history of breast cancer, short term (<4 years) HT use does not seem to affect risk of breast cancer [50, 51]. In women with a personal history of breast cancer, HT is contraindicated, and management of menopausal symptoms should be with nonhormonal pharmacotherapy or nonpharmacological treatments.

Case Resolution

Following consultation, AB identified her nocturnal symptoms as most troublesome, and she was started on a single nightly dose of gabapentin, starting at a dose of 300 mg and slowly increased to 900 mg. She was started on vaginal estrogen to try to prevent recurrent urinary tract infections.

At six-week follow-up, she reported a reduction in intensity and frequency of nocturnal VMS but persistent daytime symptoms which were affecting her ability to work. Her sleep was improved with fewer awakenings and less difficulty initiating sleep. She was reluctant to consider another medication for VMS so opted to enroll in a CBT group for VMS. At subsequent follow-up, ten weeks later, she reported less bother/interference of menopause symptoms, improved sleep, and no further urinary tract infections. Her symptoms were not eradicated but were much milder and less bothersome.

Take Home Points

- Young women should be counselled that cancer treatment may impact ovarian function and may cause infertility and/or menopausal symptoms.
- Treatment modalities for VMS of menopause may include HT, nonhormonal pharmacotherapy, and nonpharmacological options.

- The experience of menopause is highly variable between women. Women may request treatment for symptoms that impact on their quality of life. Women with menopausal symptoms happening at the average age (45+) that do not impact on quality of life do not require treatment.

Contraception in Cancer Patients

Case Presentation

CD is a 38-year-old G3P3 with 3 prior vaginal births who has been recently diagnosed with ER/PR positive breast cancer. She has been using a levonorgestrel containing IUS (LNG-IUS) for contraception since the birth of her youngest child three years ago. She comes to the office to discuss her contraceptive options considering this new diagnosis. She has found the LNG-IUS a very effective form of contraception and wishes to continue with it. How would you advise her?

Epidemiology

It is estimated that in the US in 2021, approximately 10 percent of new cancer diagnoses were made in women under the age of 45 [52]. For this cohort contraceptive considerations may be important. Pregnancy during cancer treatment is best avoided as cancer treatments can be teratogenic. For some women cancer treatment may induce health problems which make subsequent pregnancy higher risk such as cardiotoxic effects of some chemotherapy agents such as doxorubicin. For others the risk of recurrence of their cancer is highest in the first two years after treatment and it may be best to postpone pregnancy until after this time.

As mentioned previously, it can be hard to predict if and when fertility will return following cancer treatment and it also depends on the type of cancer treatment as the loss of fertility may be permanent in certain circumstances. AMH testing may help to predict this risk in the future [6]. However, for many women, fertility will return after completion of treatment and making appropriate contraceptive choices can be challenging. Indeed, data tells us that while cancer survivors do not have a higher rate of unintended pregnancy than the general reproductive age population, if they become pregnant it is more likely to be unintended [53], they are more likely to require emergency contraception, and less likely to use the most effective methods of contraception [54]. Furthermore, patients feel their reproductive care is suboptimal following cancer treatment [55].

The World Health Organization classifies suitability of contraception for women with a variety of health conditions including cancer [56]. The medical eligibility criteria for contraceptive use (MEC) are described in four categories. Category 1 means the method of contraception can be used safely in the context of the medical condition. Category 2 means the benefits of using the method outweigh the risks, category 3 means the risks of the method generally outweigh the benefits while category 4 identifies a situation in which the method should not be used. See Table 6.2.

Contraception is available in multiple forms – tablets, injectables, intrauterine devices, vaginal rings, transdermal patches, barrier methods – and in hormonal and nonhormonal forms.

Nonhormonal methods include the copper intrauterine system (Cu-IUS), condoms and diaphragms with or without spermicide. These methods are all MEC category 1 for women with a history of cancer as they do not contain hormones and thus do not affect prognosis of cancer.

Table 6.2 Contraceptive use in breast cancer

Cancer type	Contraceptive type	MEC category
Breast cancer (current)	Barrier methods	1
	Combined oral contraceptive pill/vaginal ring/patch	4
	Progestogen only pill	4
	Progestogen depot injectables	4
	Progestogen implants	4
	Copper IUS	1
	Levonorgestrel IUS	4
Breast cancer (no evidence of disease for 5 years)	Barrier methods	1
	Combined oral contraceptive pill/vaginal ring/patch	3
	Progestogen only pill	3
	Progestogen depot injectables	3
	Progestogen implants	3
	Copper IUS	1
	Levonorgestrel IUS	3*

*Available evidence suggests no increased risk of recurrence in women taking tamoxifen [57]
Medical Eligibility Criteria for Contraceptive Use (MEC)

Hormonal methods include combined (estrogen and progestogen) oral contraceptives, combined patches, or combined vaginal rings. Progestogen-only contraceptives include oral tablets, injectables, and implants. The LNG-IUS also contains progestogen hormone.

All hormonal contraception is category 4 for women with a current diagnosis of breast cancer. If a woman is diagnosed while taking a form of hormonal contraception this should be removed and an alternative form instituted. For women with a past history of breast cancer and no evidence of disease for the past five years, hormonal contraceptives are MEC category 3. This means that the risks generally outweigh the benefits in the setting of past breast cancer, however, in situations where alternative methods are not available or possible then they can be considered under careful clinical supervision. The available evidence suggests that use of the LNG-IUS in women taking tamoxifen after breast cancer does not increase recurrence [57].

For women with gynecological cancer, treatment usually signals the end of fertility. However, in rare situations where this is not the case, hormone-containing contraceptives can be used as they are known to lower the risk of both ovarian and endometrial cancer. It is important to note that this is only in the setting of primary prevention.

For women with a *BRCA* pathogenic variant, contraceptive decisions can be challenging as concerns may exist about the use of hormonal contraception in this cohort because of their higher risk of breast cancer. Current evidence, however, suggests that the breast cancer risk in this setting does not seem to be modified by hormonal contraceptives.

For women with other cancer diagnoses, there are unlikely to be concerns about the use of hormonal contraception, although little data exists in this area.

Case Resolution

CD's LNG-IUS is removed by her doctor due to her breast cancer diagnosis. She opts to rely on barrier methods of contraception during treatment. She returns to the office following completion of treatment. She has been started on tamoxifen as adjuvant endocrine therapy. Her menses have returned, and she is concerned about becoming pregnant. Following consultation, she opts for a copper-containing IUS (Cu-IUS).

She returns to the office several months later, complaining of heavy, irregular menstrual bleeding. She undergoes endometrial biopsy in view of her current tamoxifen use. The pathology result was benign. Following careful consultation with her treating oncologists and following counseling about the pros and cons, she has the Cu-IUS removed and a LNG-IUS reinserted. She returns for follow-up 12 weeks postinsertion of the LNG-IUS and her bleeding symptoms are controlled.

Take Home Points

- Contraceptive care is important for women with cancer and often overlooked.
- For many women, cancer treatment may make contraception unnecessary.
- Hormonal contraception is best avoided in women with a history of breast cancer but can be considered in certain clinical scenarios.
- The copper-containing IUS is the safest and most reliable form of contraception for women with a prior history of breast cancer.

References

1. Harlow S. D., Gass M., Hall J. E., et al. Executive summary of the Stages of Reproductive Aging Workshop + 10: Addressing the unfinished agenda of staging reproductive aging. *Menopause.* 2012;**19**(4):387–95.

2. Hickey M., Hunter M. S., Santoro N., Ussher J. Normalising menopause. *BMJ.* 2022;377:e069369.

3. "The 2022 Hormone Therapy Position Statement of The North American Menopause Society" Advisory Panel. The 2022 hormone therapy position statement of The North American Menopause Society. *Menopause.* 2022;**29**(7):767–94.

4. Lethaby A., Ayeleke R. O., Roberts H. Local oestrogen for vaginal atrophy in postmenopausal women. *Cochrane Database Syst Rev.* 2016; **31**(8):CD001500.

5. Haines C. J., Xing S. M., Park K. H., Holinka C. F., Ausmanas M. K. Prevalence of menopausal symptoms in different ethnic groups of Asian women and responsiveness to therapy with three doses of conjugated estrogens/medroxyprogesterone acetate: The Pan-Asia Menopause (PAM) study. *Maturitas.* 2005;**52**(3–4):264–76.

6. Anderson R. A., Cameron D., Clatot F., et al. Anti-Müllerian hormone as a marker of ovarian reserve and premature ovarian insufficiency in children and women with cancer: A systematic review. *Hum Reprod Update.* 2022;**28**(3):417–34.

7. Hickey M., Szabo R. A., Hunter M. S. Non-hormonal treatments for menopausal symptoms. *BMJ (Clinical research ed).* 2017;**23**(359):j5101.

8. Davis S. R., Baber R., Panay N., et al. Global consensus position statement on the use of

testosterone therapy for women. *J Clin Endocrinol Metab.* 2019;**104**(10):4660–6.

9. Sturgeon K. M., Deng L., Bluethmann S. M., et al. A population-based study of cardiovascular disease mortality risk in US cancer patients. *Eur Heart J.* 2019;**40**(48):3889–97.

10. Zhu D., Chung H. F., Dobson A. J., et al. Type of menopause, age of menopause and variations in the risk of incident cardiovascular disease: Pooled analysis of individual data from 10 international studies. *Hum Reprod.* 2020;**35**(8):1933–43.

11. Scarabin P. Y. Progestogens and venous thromboembolism in menopausal women: An updated oral versus transdermal estrogen meta-analysis. *Climacteric.* 2018;**21**(4):341–5.

12. Canonico M., Fournier A., Carcaillon L., et al. Postmenopausal hormone therapy and risk of idiopathic venous thromboembolism: Results from the E3 N cohort study. *Arterioscler Thromb Vasc Biol.* 2010;**30**(2):340–5.

13. Elkins G. R., Fisher W. I., Johnson A. K., Carpenter J. S., Keith T. Z. Clinical hypnosis in the treatment of postmenopausal hot flashes: A randomized controlled trial. *Menopause.* 2013;**20**(3):291–8.

14. Elkins G., Marcus J., Stearns V., et al. Randomized trial of a hypnosis intervention for treatment of hot flashes among breast cancer survivors. *J Clin Oncol.* 2008;**26**(31):5022–6.

15. Mann E., Smith M. J., Hellier J., et al. Cognitive behavioural treatment for women who have menopausal symptoms after breast cancer treatment (MENOS 1): A randomised controlled trial. *The Lancet Oncology.* 2012;**13**(3):309–18.

16. Green S. M., Donegan E., Frey B. N., et al. Cognitive behavior therapy for menopausal symptoms (CBT-Meno): A randomized controlled trial. *Menopause.* 2019;**26**(9):972–80.

17. Guthrie K. A., Larson J. C., Ensrud K. E., et al. Effects of pharmacologic and nonpharmacologic interventions on insomnia symptoms and self-reported sleep quality in women with hot flashes: A pooled analysis of individual participant data from four MsFLASH trials. *Sleep.* 2018 01;**41**(1).

18. Kauffman R. P. Telephone-based CBT reduced insomnia severity more than menopause education in menopausal women. *Ann Intern Med.* 2016;**165**(6): JC30.

19. Franzoi M. A., Agostinetto E., Perachino M., et al. Evidence-based approaches for the management of side-effects of adjuvant endocrine therapy in patients with breast cancer. *Lancet Oncol.* 2021;**22**(7):e303–13.

20. Pinkerton J. V., Abraham L., Bushmakin A. G., Cappelleri J. C., Komm B. S. Relationship between changes in vasomotor symptoms and changes in menopause-specific quality of life and sleep parameters. *Menopause (New York, NY).* 2016;**23**(10):1060–6.

21. Saadati N., Mohammadjafari R., Natanj S., Abedi P. The effect of gabapentin on intensity and duration of hot flashes in postmenopausal women: A randomized controlled trial. *Glob J Health Sci.* 2013;**5**(6):126–30.

22. Modi M., Dhillo W. S. Neurokinin 3 receptor antagonism: A novel treatment for menopausal hot flushes. *Neuroendocrinology.* 2019;**109**(3):242–8.

23. O'Meara E. S., Rossing M. A., Daling J. R., et al. Hormone replacement therapy after a diagnosis of breast cancer in relation to recurrence and mortality. *J Natl Cancer Inst.* 2001;**93**(10):754–62.

24. Ponzone R., Biglia N., Jacomuzzi M. E., et al. Vaginal oestrogen therapy after breast cancer: Is it safe? *Eur J Cancer.* 2005;**41**(17):2673–81.

25. Stuenkel C. A., Davis S. R., Gompel A., et al. Treatment of symptoms of the menopause: An Endocrine Society clinical practice guideline. *J Clin Endocrinol Metab.* 2015;**100**(11):3975–4011.

26. Dew J. E., Wren B. G., Eden J. A. A cohort study of topical vaginal estrogen therapy in women previously treated for breast cancer. *Climacteric.* 2003;**6**(1):45–52.

27. Le Ray I., Dell'Aniello S., Bonnetain F., Azoulay L., Suissa S. Local estrogen therapy and risk of breast cancer recurrence among hormone-treated patients: A nested case-control study. *Breast Cancer Res Treat.* 2012;**135**(2):603–9.

28. Melisko M. E., Goldman M. E., Hwang J., et al. Vaginal testosterone cream vs estradiol vaginal ring for vaginal dryness or decreased libido in women receiving aromatase inhibitors for early-stage breast cancer: A randomized clinical trial. *JAMA Oncol.* 2017;**3**(3):313–19.

29. Wills S., Ravipati A., Venuturumilli P., et al. Effects of vaginal estrogens on serum estradiol levels in postmenopausal breast cancer survivors and women at risk of breast cancer taking an aromatase inhibitor or a selective estrogen receptor modulator. *J Oncol Pract.* 2012;**8**(3):144–8.

30. Brennan A., Brennan D., Rees M., Hickey M. Management of menopausal symptoms and ovarian function preservation in women with gynecological cancer. *International Journal of Gynecologic Cancer* [Internet]. 2021;**31**(3). https://ijgc.bmj.com/content/31/3/352

31. Edwards D., Panay N. Treating vulvovaginal atrophy/genitourinary syndrome of menopause: How important is vaginal lubricant and moisturizer composition? *Climacteric.* 2016;**19**(2):151–61.

32. Mitchell C. M., Reed S. D., Diem S., et al. Efficacy of vaginal estradiol or vaginal moisturizer vs placebo for treating postmenopausal vulvovaginal symptoms: A randomized clinical trial. *JAMA Intern Med.* 2018;**178**(5):681–90.

33. Chan J. A., Meyerhardt J. A., Chan A. T., et al. Hormone replacement therapy and survival after colorectal cancer diagnosis. *J Clin Oncol.* 2006;**24**(36):5680–6.

34. Calle E. E., Miracle-McMahill H. L., Thun M. J., Heath C. W. Estrogen replacement therapy and risk of fatal colon cancer in a prospective cohort of postmenopausal women. *J Natl Cancer Inst.* 1995;**87**(7):517–23.

35. Mahase E. Colorectal cancer: Screening may need to change given rising incidence in under 50s. *BMJ.* 2019 May 17;365:l2249.

36. Tauchmanovà L., Selleri C., De Rosa G., et al. Estrogen-progestin therapy in women after stem cell transplant: Our experience and literature review. *Menopause.* 2007;**14**(2):320–30.

37. Holmberg L., Iversen O. E., Rudenstam C. M., et al. Increased risk of recurrence after hormone replacement therapy in breast cancer survivors. *J Natl Cancer Inst.* 2008;**100**(7):475–82.

38. von Schoultz E., Rutqvist L. E., Stockholm Breast Cancer Study Group. Menopausal hormone therapy after breast cancer: The Stockholm randomized trial. *J Natl Cancer Inst.* 2005;**97**(7):533–5.

39. Kenemans P., Bundred N. J., Foidart J. M., et al. Safety and efficacy of tibolone in breast-cancer patients with vasomotor symptoms: A double-blind, randomised, non-inferiority trial. *Lancet Oncol.* 2009;**10**(2):135–46.

40. Poggio F., Del Mastro L., Bruzzone M., et al. Safety of systemic hormone replacement therapy in breast cancer survivors: A systematic review and meta-analysis. *Breast Cancer Res Treat.* 2022;**191**(2):269–75.

41. Edey K. A., Rundle S., Hickey M. Hormone replacement therapy for women previously treated for endometrial cancer. *Cochrane Database Syst Rev.* 2018;5:CD008830.

42. Concin N., Matias-Guiu X., Vergote I., et al. ESGO/ESTRO/ESP guidelines for the management of patients with endometrial carcinoma. *International Journal of Gynecologic Cancer.* 2020;ijgc.

43. Pergialiotis V., Pitsouni E., Prodromidou A., et al. Hormone therapy for ovarian cancer survivors: Systematic review and meta-analysis. *Menopause.* 2016;**23**(3):335–42.

44. Li D., Ding C. Y., Qiu L. H. Postoperative hormone replacement therapy for epithelial ovarian cancer patients: A systematic review and meta-analysis. *Gynecol Oncol.* 2015;**139**(2):355–62.

45. MacKie R. M., Bray C. A. Hormone replacement therapy after surgery for stage 1 or 2 cutaneous melanoma. *Br J Cancer.* 2004;**90**(4):770–2.

46. Clague J., Reynolds P., Henderson K. D., et al. Menopausal hormone therapy and lung cancer-specific mortality following diagnosis: The California Teachers Study. *PLoS One.* 2014;**9**(7):e103735.

47. Katcoff H., Wenzlaff A. S., Schwartz A. G. Survival in women with NSCLC: The role of reproductive history and hormone use. *J Thorac Oncol.* 2014;**9**(3):355–61.

48. Ganti A. K., Sahmoun A. E., Panwalkar A. W., Tendulkar K. K., Potti A. Hormone replacement therapy is associated with decreased survival in women with lung cancer. *J Clin Oncol.* 2006;**24**(1):59–63.

49. Chlebowski R. T., Schwartz A. G., Wakelee H., et al. Oestrogen plus progestin and lung cancer in postmenopausal women (Women's Health Initiative trial): A post-hoc analysis of a randomised controlled trial. *Lancet.* 2009;**374**(9697):1243–51.

50. Kotsopoulos J., Gronwald J., Karlan B. Y., et al. Hormone replacement therapy after oophorectomy and breast cancer risk among BRCA1 mutation carriers. *JAMA Oncol.* 2018;**4**(8):1059–65.

51. Gordhandas S., Norquist B. M., Pennington K. P., et al. Hormone replacement therapy after risk reducing salpingo-oophorectomy in patients with BRCA1 or BRCA2 mutations: A systematic review of risks and benefits. *Gynecol Oncol.* 2019;**153**(1):192–200.

52. Siegel R. L., Miller K. D., Fuchs H. E., Jemal A. Cancer statistics, 2021. *CA: A Cancer Journal for Clinicians.* 2021;**71**(1):7–33.

53. Quinn M. M., Letourneau J. M., Rosen M. P. Contraception after cancer treatment: describing methods, counseling, and unintended pregnancy risk. *Contraception.* 2014;**89**(5):466–71.

54. Hadnott T. N., Stark S. S., Medica A., et al. Perceived infertility and contraceptive use in the female, reproductive-age cancer survivor. *Fertil Steril.* 2019;**111**(4):763–71.

55. Dominick S. A., McLean M. R., Whitcomb B. W., et al. Contraceptive practices among female cancer survivors of reproductive age. *Obstet Gynecol.* 2015;**126**(3):498–507.

56. World Health Organization. *Medical eligibility criteria for contraceptive use (MEC).* World Health Organization; 2015.

57. Romero S. A., Young K., Hickey M., Su H. I. Levonorgestrel intrauterine system for endometrial protection in women with breast cancer on adjuvant tamoxifen. *Cochrane Database Syst Rev.* 2020;12: CD007245.

Cervical Cancer Screening

Samantha H. Batman, Kathleen M. Schmeler,
and Mila P. Salcedo

Case Presentation

A 31-year-old woman is diagnosed with acute myeloid leukemia (AML). She is recommended by her oncologist to proceed with treatment involving both chemotherapy and an allogeneic hematopoietic stem cell transplant (SCT). Prior to her transplant, her oncologist refers her to gynecology for routine screening and to discuss fertility. She informs her gynecologist that she has never been vaccinated against human papillomavirus (HPV) and asks about the timing of vaccination. She has had regular cervical cancer screening and no history of abnormal cervical cytology. A pretransplant cervical cytology and HPV specimen are collected, which show atypical squamous cells of undetermined significance (ASCUS) and HPV-16 positive. She undergoes colposcopy which appears normal and no biopsies are taken. She then proceeds with her previously planned treatment for AML. Following her treatment, her oncologist wishes to discuss screening recommendations going forward as she will need to continue immunosuppressive medications. What would you recommend?

Epidemiology of Cervical Cancer

Incidence and Long-Term Prognosis

Though it is both preventable and curable, cervical cancer remains the fourth most common cause of cancer among women globally [1]. The morbidity and mortality associated with cervical cancer highlight great inequalities in care delivery worldwide, with nearly 90% of cervical cancer-related deaths occurring in low- and middle-income countries (LMICs) [1]. For those patients living in the highest-resource countries, the relative incidence of rate of cervical cancer is two to four times lower than those in LMICs [2].

These disparities in a preventable cancer ultimately led the World Health Organization (WHO) Director General to issue a global call to action to eliminate cervical cancer in May 2018 involving scaling up of prevention, screening, and treatment interventions [1]. In 2020, there were approximately 604,000 cases of cervical cancer and 342,000 related deaths [2]. Globally, the average age at diagnosis was 53 years and the average age at death from cervical cancer was 59 years [2]. The regions most affected include Southeast Asia, the Caribbean, sub-Saharan Africa, Latin America, Micronesia, and Melanesia [3].

Cervical cancer is a preventable disease, with a prolonged and treatable preinvasive phase prior to progression to invasive cancer. Furthermore, there are excellent tools for both prevention and screening, including the Papanicolaou (Pap) test (cervical cytology) and HPV testing. Cervical Intraepithelial Neoplasia (CIN) is a precancerous lesion of the cervical squamous epithelium and is a histologic diagnosis from tissue obtained at time of cervical biopsy. Mild dysplasia (CIN 1) frequently will spontaneously regress within six to 12 months [4]. The designation of CIN 2 is given to lesions in which cellular atypia affects two-thirds of the epithelial thickness. At this stage, the process is still reversible and approximately 40% of lesions will regress spontaneously without treatment [5]. However, 22% of CIN 2 will progress to CIN 3, defined as cellular atypia involving more than two-thirds of the epithelium, and 5% will progress to invasive cancer [5]. Although CIN 3 is considered a precursor to invasive cancer and treatment is recommended as approximately 15% of these cases will progress to invasive cancer, roughly one-third of these lesions may spontaneously regress [6].

Etiology and Risk Factors

It is well-established that the overwhelming majority of cervical cancer cases are caused by persistent infection with high-risk HPV [7]. HPV is a double-stranded DNA virus that infects epithelial cells and includes over 120 types, which can be either oncogenic or nononcogenic [8]. Nononcogenic types (such as types 6 and 11) do not integrate into the host cell genome and tend to be associated with genital warts and low-grade dysplasia. In contrast, oncogenic types integrate into the host cell genome and causes neoplastic changes that are associated with high-grade dysplasia and invasive cancer. HPV types 16 and 18, in particular, are associated with 70% of cervical cancer and 60% of high-grade dysplasia cases [9]. HPV infection does not persist in most women and the virus is cleared spontaneously and the dysplasia regresses. However, in a small percentage of women the infection persists and causes progression to dysplasia and cancer. Ultimately, HPV DNA is found in 80% of low-grade lesions and up to 77% of high-grade lesions [8].

HPV is the most common sexually transmitted infection, with an estimated average lifetime probability of acquiring HPV of more than 80% by age 45 if unvaccinated [10]. The initial infection with HPV is typically during adolescence or early adulthood, and approximately 80% of this group will clear the virus spontaneously within 18–24 months after infection [11]. For those that go on to have persistent infection, 3–5% develop preinvasive disease and less than 1% develop cervical cancer [12]. Persistent HPV infection is also associated with other cancer, including anal, vulvar, vaginal, penile, and oropharyngeal (head and neck) cancer.

Risk factors associated with the progression from CIN 3 to invasive cancer include history of smoking, long-term oral contraceptive use, multiparity, increased number of sexual partners, and immunosuppression from any cause [12]. With respect to tobacco use, cigarette smoking is associated with a 1.5 to 2.5-fold increased risk in developing cervical cancer [13]. The association between oral contraceptive use and cervical cancer is controversial, though it appears there is an increased risk in current users and that this risk declines after use is discontinued [14]. Number of sexual partners is a known risk factor for both dysplasia and invasive cancer, with an approximately threefold increased risk in women who have had six or more sexual partners. It is thought that this occurs due to the higher risk of HPV infection [14]. Lastly, it is well-established in the literature that there is an increased risk of both HPV infection and preinvasive/invasive disease in women with immunosuppression, such as those living with human immunodeficiency virus (HIV) and those with cancer [15]. In patients with a history of allogeneic stem cell transplantation, it has been confirmed that chronic graft-versus-host disease, particularly when vulvovaginal, is an independent risk factor for cervical dysplasia [16].

Primary Prevention and HPV Vaccination

HPV vaccination represents an opportunity for primary prevention of cervical cancer. There are currently three different prophylactic vaccines available commercially worldwide: Cervarix[TM] is a bivalent vaccine targeting HPV 16 and 18, Gardasil[TM] is a quadrivalent vaccine targeting HPV 16, 18, 6 and 11, and Gardasil-9[TM] is a nonavalent vaccine targeting the same HPV types as the quadrivalent vaccine in addition to types 31, 33, 45, 52, and 58 [17–19]. All three preparations have been shown to be extremely effective in the prevention of cervical dysplasia and cervical cancer in clinical trials, with efficacy rates ranging from 93–98% in women who were previously uninfected with HPV [20]. These vaccines also have a tolerable safety profile [17–19]. As of 2020, the nonvalent vaccine is the only one available in the United States.

The vaccines have been shown to be most effective when given prior to sexual debut and therefore prior to HPV exposure. As such, the Centers for Disease Control and Prevention (CDC) recommend vaccination against HPV to both boys and girls between the ages of 11 and 12 years, though it can be given as early as 9 years. Typically, two doses are recommended though certain populations are eligible for a three-dose schedule – namely, those who start the series after 15 years of age and those who are living with HIV or are immunocompromised [21]. For those who were not previously vaccinated and are between the ages of 13 to 26 years, catch-up vaccination should be offered [22]. In 2018, the US Food and Drug Administration (FDA) approved an extension for the Gardasil-9[TM] vaccine for persons up to the age of 45 years after discussion and shared decision-making with their providers [21].

HPV Vaccination in Cancer Survivors

Ideally, all eligible patients would receive the HPV vaccination prior to initiating treatment but there is rarely time to complete the series prior to starting therapy. The vaccine is not recommended during treatment due to limited efficacy associated with the patient's inability to mount an immune response. To date, there are no data on immunogenicity or safety regarding the HPV vaccine in the post-stem cell transplant population, however, there have been significant declines in HPV-related malignancies across multiple populations, including those with immunocompromised states. Thus, for patients between 9–45 years of age who may be immunosuppressed due to treatments related to malignancy, HPV vaccination may offer a means of primary prevention for HPV exposure and subsequent development of cervical dysplasia/invasive cancer as well as other HPV-related malignancies. The nonavalent HPV vaccine may be considered six months post-transplant and the full regimen (three doses at zero, two, and six months) is recommended. Preliminary data suggests that the immunologic response is robust and similar to immunocompetent women [23].

Importantly, the rate of HPV vaccination has remained low amongst pediatric cancer survivors, though this is a group that could potentially experience a longer period of benefit [24]. A study in Tennessee found female pediatric cancer survivors aged 9–17 years were less likely to both initiate and complete the HPV vaccine series compared with healthy age-matched controls (32.6% versus 34.3% initiation and 17.9% versus 20.0% completion), though this trend did not reach statistical significance [25]. As cancer survivors are potentially at increased risk for secondary malignancies, further efforts are needed to reach this population.

As vaccination does not provide protection against all known oncogenic HPV subtypes and has an unknown duration of protection, it is recommended that even women who have received the HPV vaccine undergo routine cervical cancer screening.

Cervical Cancer Screening

Screening tools for cervical cancer include cervical cytology (Pap testing), HPV testing, or a combination (also called "co-testing"). In many LMICs, these tests may not be readily available and therefore visual inspection with acetic acid (VIA) is used instead to identify precancerous cervical lesions. When used appropriate, screening is associated with a significantly decreased incidence and mortality from invasive cervical cancer.

Cervical Cytology

The conventional Pap test/cervical cytology is obtained by scraping cervical cells from the transformation zone via spatula and endocervical brush and smearing the cells on a glass slide for later review by a cytologist or pathologist. In recent years, some high-income countries including the US have moved to a liquid-based approach, with the sample placed in a liquid medium that can also be used for HPV DNA testing. Over the past 60–70 years, widespread screening with cervical cytology has reduced cervical cancer incidence by 50–70% in high-income countries despite its overall low sensitivity [26]. The screening success of cervical cytology has been due, in part, to the long preinvasive phase of the disease. In the United States, women who develop invasive cervical cancer are often those who have never been screened, were lost to follow up after an abnormal test, or have not had testing for many years [27].

HPV Testing

Multiple prior studies have demonstrate a higher sensitivity in HPV testing as compared to cervical cytology (96% versus 53%) in the detection of CIN 2 and CIN 3, while the specificity remains similar (91% versus 96%) [28–30]. Thus, co-testing with both cervical cytology and high-risk HPV testing is recommended and HPV testing is part of most screening algorithms in the United States.

There has been interest regarding the efficacy of primary HPV testing alone for cervical cancer screening. In their large randomized study, Ogilvie and colleagues looked at data from 19,009 women screened with HPV testing versus liquid-based cytology and demonstrated that negative HPV primary testing was associated with a significantly lower likelihood of CIN 3+ at 48 months than negative cytology [31]. Addition of HPV-based testing to routine screening has increased the negative predictive value of our screening methods, allowing the screening interval to be lengthened when co-testing is performed [30].

In considering timing and frequency of cervical cancer screening, it often helpful to categorize patients as either those with average risk or those with higher risk. Patients living with HIV, immunosuppression, or in-utero exposure to diethylstilbestrol (DES) are at an increased risk for developing cervical cancer and are therefore subject to different screening recommendations. In considering gynecologic care of the cancer patient and screening recommendations after cancer therapy, it is therefore helpful to consider whether the patient is in an immunosuppressed state (such as a patient who is on chronic immunosuppressants following SCT). Cervical cancer screening, to include both cytology and HPV testing, is also critical prior to any potential SCT or organ transplant and is considered a routine part of a pretransplant evaluation for those who have been sexually active, regardless of age [23].

Patients at Average Risk

Patients who are immunocompetent following cancer therapy and are HIV negative can be screened according to the guidelines for those at average risk.

The American Society of Colposcopy and Cervical Pathology (ASCCP) guidelines for screening patients at average risk are summarized below [32]:

- Screening is recommended for all persons with a cervix between the ages of 21 and 65
- Cervical cancer screening should begin at age 21, regardless of the age of onset of sexual activity
- Ages 21–29: screening via cervical cytology alone every 3 years is recommended
- Ages 30–65: co-testing with cervical cytology and HPV every 5 years (preferred) or cervical cytology alone every 3 years
- Age > 65: screening not recommended for those with a history of negative screening (defined as 3 consecutive negative cervical cytology or 2 consecutive negative HPV tests provided no history of CIN 2+ or cancer in the past 20 years)
- No screening recommended after hysterectomy with removal of the cervix for those without a history of CIN 2 +
- Screening does not differ based on HPV vaccination status

For asymptomatic, immunocompetent women, there is some discussion regarding optimal age to initiate screening and optimal screening modality, leading to variation in consensus guidelines from different expert organizations. For instance, the US Preventive Services Task Force (USPSTF) endorses the use of either cytology alone every 3 years, high-risk HPV testing alone every 5 years, or co-testing every 5 years in women aged 30–65 [33]. In a shift towards primary HPV testing, the American Cancer Society (ACS) recommends initiation of screening at age 25 with primary HPV testing every 5 years (preferred) but also considers cytology alone every 3 years (if HPV testing unavailable) or co-testing every 5 years acceptable [34].

Patients at Increased Risk

Patients who are immunosuppressed following cancer therapy or who are living with HIV should be screened according to the modified guidelines for those at higher risk.

Immunocompromised patients are those living with HIV, solid organ transplant, or allogeneic hematopoietic stem cell transplant, as well as those with systemic lupus erythematous, inflammatory bowel disease, or rheumatologic disease requiring ongoing immunosuppressant therapy. Although literature guiding screening in this population is limited, it is understood that these patients have a suppression of cell-mediated immunity and are therefore at risk for virally induced cancer. It is therefore recommended that immunosuppressed patients without HIV use the same guidelines recommended for persons living with HIV. Currently the recommendation is to begin screening within one year of first insertional sexual activity followed by annually for three years and then every three years (cytology alone) until the age of 30. After this period, screening should continue with either cytology alone or co-testing every three years throughout a patient's lifetime [35].

For stem cell transplant patients who subsequently develop a new diagnosis of genital graft-versus-host disease or chronic graft-versus-host disease, annual cervical cytology should be resumed until three consecutive normal results or a baseline co-test can be performed and, if normal, repeated at three-year intervals [36].

Questions remain as to whether cervical cytology abnormalities post-stem cell transplant reliably predict cervical cancer in the absence of HPV co-testing as abnormal cytology can occur transiently as a consequence of conditioning therapy (i.e. chemotherapy, radiation, or immunotherapy used prior to stem cell transplantation) [37]. Thus, in this population, it is important to use both screening modalities if available.

Another population considered at increased risk for the development of cervical cancer includes women who were previously treated for CIN 3 or cervical adenocarcinoma in situ (AIS). The risk for developing invasive cancer in this population is substantial for the first 10 years after treatment though continues to be elevated for up to 25 years after initial therapy. Thus, these women should continue to receive routine age-based screening for 20 years after completion of their initial post-treatment surveillance, which may extend beyond age 65 [38]. Given the risk of recurrent dysplasia or cancer at the vaginal cuff, they should also be considered for vaginal cytology testing after hysterectomy [38].

Treatment

In 2020, the ASCCP published updated consensus guidelines for the management of abnormal cervical cancer screening results. These recommendations align our understanding of the natural history of HPV and cervical carcinogenesis and are based on the principle that persistent HPV infection is necessary to develop dysplasia or invasive cancer. Both duration of HPV infection and HPV genotype are therefore important to understanding risk stratification and an individual's risk of developing CIN 3+ (CIN 3, AIS, or cancer)[35].

Of note, if primary HPV screening is being performed and the results are positive, the recommendation is to perform both reflex cytology if not already done and reflex HPV genotyping, ideally from the same specimen. If this is not feasible, it is acceptable to refer the patient for colposcopy [35].

Colposcopy

The traditional colposcope is a binocular microscope with a powerful light source used for closer examination of the cervix in women with an abnormal screening result. Prior to its use, acetic acid (3 to 5%) is applied to the cervix to enhance visualization of abnormal lesions [39]. A trained colposcopist can identify tissue patterns and lesions associated with cervical dysplasia and determine whether or not a biopsy is indicated.

Treatment of Cervical Intraepithelial Neoplasia

Per the updated ASCCP treatment guidelines (Table 7.1), observation is preferred for women with CIN 1 [35]. Treatment of CIN 2/3 is recommended given the higher risk of progression to invasive cancer. The choice of treatment depends heavily on availability of equipment and expertise of the providers and can include ablation (either cryotherapy or thermal ablation) or excision of the dysplastic area. Excisional procedures include loop electrosurgical excision procedure (LEEP), cold knife conization (CKC), and CO_2 laser conization. When used in properly selected patients, the success rate of these treatments is

Table 7.1 Summary of key ASCCP 2020 guideline changes [35]

Management Change	Notes
1. Recommendations are now based on risk	Recommendations are based on risk of CIN 3+ determined by a combination of current results and past history
2. Colposcopy can be deferred	In exchange for repeat HPV or co-testing at 1 year for patients with minor screening abnormalities
3. Expedited treatment is expanded	Now preferred for nonpregnant patients ≥ 25 years with HSIL cytology and HPV-16 positive or never/rarely screened patients with HPV-positive HSIL regardless of HPV genotype
4. Excision is preferred to ablation for CIN 2+ and AIS in the US	
5. Observation is preferred for CIN 1	
6. Continued surveillance recommended for at least 25 years after treatment of histologic HSIL, CIN 2+, or AIS	With HPV testing or co-testing at 3-year intervals for at least 25 years
7. Surveillance with cytology alone is acceptable only if testing with HPV or co-testing is not feasible	Cytology recommended at 6-month intervals when HPV testing/co-testing is recommended annually; cytology recommended annually when HPV/co-testing interval is 3 years

greater than 90% [40, 41]. In the United States, excision is preferred to ablative therapy for CIN 2+ (CIN 2, CIN 3, or cancer) and AIS [35]. The ASCCP guidelines should be referenced for specific treatment recommendations pertaining to specific clinical scenarios, as these are updated regularly. These guidelines are also published in a smartphone application for those who prefer to have a reference available on their phone.

For patients undergoing stem cell transplant, if the pretransplant screening is abnormal, treatment can be performed according to ASCCP guidelines depending on whether healing from biopsies or treatment can occur prior to transplantation. Given the risk of rapid progression of a high-grade cervical squamous intraepithelial lesion (HSIL) or cancer during immunodeficiency from transplant or while on immunosuppressants to prevent graft-versus-host disease, it is important to treat abnormalities pretransplant [23]. If there is not sufficient time for healing before transplant, treatment may be delayed until three to six months after transplant to allow for adequate recovery of platelets and white blood cell count [23].

For all immunocompromised patients, regardless of age, colposcopy should be performed for any patient with ASCUS/HPV-positive or worse results. If HPV testing cannot be performed in a patient with an ASCUS cytology, then repeat cytology is recommended in 6–12 months followed by colposcopy for an ASCUS or worse result. If the result of cytology is low-grade squamous intraepithelial lesion (LSIL) or worse, colposcopy is recommended regardless of HPV testing results [35].

Case Resolution

Six months after her allogeneic hematopoietic stem cell transplant, the 31-year-old patient with AML revisits her gynecologist. At that visit, she initiates the first of three doses of the 9-valent HPV vaccine with plans to receive the two remaining doses at two and six months from that visit. Her gynecologist informs her that, going forward, she should be screened with HPV and cytology co-testing yearly for the next three years and then every three years for her lifetime. She counsels the patient that should she develop graft-versus-host disease, her screening interval may need to be shortened.

Take Home Points

- HPV infection is necessary but not sufficient in the development of cervical dysplasia and cancer, and is associated with virtually all cases of cervical cancer.
- The majority of HPV infections will regress spontaneously, but persistent HPV infection is a risk factor for developing high-grade cervical dysplasia and cervical cancer.
- Immunosuppression is a risk factor that some cancer survivors may possess that increases the likelihood of progression to cervical cancer.
- Preventive vaccines are available to prevent HPV infection and the development of cervical cancer, and immunosuppressed patients are eligible for vaccination; the vaccine is most effective when given prior to sexual debut.
- Cervical cancer screening is performed via cervical cytology and/or HPV testing, and women can be categorized as being at average risk or at higher risk.
- Patients with immunosuppression are considered at higher risk and should be managed according to cervical cancer guidelines for people living with HIV.
- Colposcopy is used to evaluate women with abnormal screening results and the diagnosis of CIN 1, 2, or 3 is based on histologic review of a colposcopy-directed biopsy.
- For immunocompromised patients, colposcopy should be performed for any abnormal results of ASCUS/HPV-positive or worse.
- CIN 1 should be observed rather than treated as it will often regress spontaneously.
- CIN 2/3 should be treated either by ablative or excisional procedures, though excision (i.e. LEEP or cold knife conization) is preferred in higher-income countries.

References

1. World Health Organization. Cervical Cancer Elimination Initiative. www.who.int/initiatives/cervical-cancer-elimination-initiative#cms. Accessed 8 March 8, 2022.

2. Arbyn M., Weiderpass E., Bruni L., et al. Estimates of incidence and mortality of cervical cancer in 2018: A worldwide analysis. *Lancet Glob Heal.* 2020;**8**:e191–e203.

3. Bray F., Ferlay J., Soerjomataram I., et al. Global cancer statistics 2018: GLOBOCAN estimates of incidence and mortality worldwide for 36 cancer in 185 countries. *CA Cancer J Clin.* 2018;**68**:394–424.

4. Bansal N., Wright J. D., Cohen C. J., Herzog T. J. Natural history of established low grade cervical intraepithelial (CIN 1) lesions. *Anticancer Res.* 2008;**28**:1763–6.

5. Castle P. E., Schiffman M., Wheeler C. M., Solomon D. Evidence for frequent regression of cervical intraepithelial neoplasia-grade 2. *Obstet Gynecol.* 2009;**113**:18–25.

6. Ostör A. Natural history of cervical intraepithelial neoplasia: A critical review. *Int J Gynecol Pathol.* 1993;**12**:186–92.

7. Walboomers J., Jacobs M., Manos M., et al. Human papillomavirus is a necessary cause. *J Pathol.* 1999;**189**:12–19.

8. Wolf J. K., Ramirez P. T. The molecular biology of cervical cancer. *Cancer Invest.* 2001;**19**:621–9.

9. Bosch X., Harper D. Prevention strategies of cervical cancer in the HPV vaccine era. *Gynecol Oncol.* 2006;**103**:21–4.

10. Chesson H., Dunne E., Hariri S., Markowitz L. The estimated lifetime probability of acquiring human papillomavirus in the United States. *Sex Transm Dis.* 2014; **41**:660–4.

11. Moscicki A.-B. Management of adolescents with abnormal cytology and histology for OBGYN Clinics of North America. *Obs Gynecol Clin North Am.* 2008;**35**:633–43.

12. Schiffman M., Doorbar J., Wentzensen N., et al. Carcinogenic human papillomavirus infection. *Nat Rev Dis Prim.* 2016; https://doi.org/10.1038/nrdp.2016.86.

13. Lee Y. C. A., Hashibe M. Tobacco, alcohol, and cancer in low and high income countries. *Ann Glob Heal.* 2014;**80**:378–83.

14. Berrington De González A., Green J. Comparison of risk factors for invasive squamous cell carcinoma and adenocarcinoma of the cervix: Collaborative reanalysis of individual data on 8,097 women with squamous cell carcinoma and 1,374 women with adenocarcinoma from 12 epidemiological studies. *Int J Cancer.* 2007;**120**:885–91.

15. Ferenczy A., Coutlee F., Franco E., Hankins C. Human papillomavirus and HIV coinfection and the risk of neoplasias of the lower genital tract: A review of recent developments. *Can Med Assoc J.* 2003;**169**:431–4.

16. Wang Y., Brinch L., Jebsen P., Tanbo T., Kirschner R. A clinical study of cervical dysplasia in long-term survivors of allogeneic stem cell transplantation. *Biol Blood Marrow Transplant.* 2012;**18**:747–53.

17. The Future II Study Group. Quadrivalent vaccine against human pappilomavirus to prevent high-grade cervical lesions. *N Engl J Med.* 2006;**355**:11–20.

18. Paavonen J., Naud P., Salmerón J., et al. Efficacy of human papillomavirus (HPV)-16/18 AS04-adjuvanted vaccine against cervical infection and precancer caused by oncogenic HPV types (PATRICIA): Final analysis of a double-blind, randomised study in young women. *Lancet.* 2009;**374**:301–14.

19. Joura E. A., Giuliano A. R., Iversen O.-E., et al. A 9-valent HPV vaccine against infection and intraepithelial neoplasia in women. *N Engl J Med.* 2015;**372**:711–23.

20. Lei J., Ploner A., Elfström K. M., et al. HPV vaccination and the risk of invasive cervical cancer. *N Engl J Med.* 2020;**383**:1340–8.

21. HPV Vaccination Recommendations. In: Centers Dis. Control Prev. 2021. www.cdc.gov/vaccines/vpd/hpv/hcp/recommendations.html. Accessed April 8, 2022.

22. Meites E., Kempe A., Markowitz L. E. Use of a 2-dose schedule for human pappilomavirus vaccination: Updated recommendations of the Advisory Committee on Immunization Practices. *Morb Mortal Wkly Rep.* 2016;**65**:1405–8.

23. Murphy J., McKenna M., Abdelazim S., Battiwalla M., Stratton P. A practical guide to gynecologic and reproductive health in women undergoing hematopoietic stem cell transplant. *Biol Blood Marrow Transplant.* 2019;**25**:e331–e343.

24. Cherven B., Klosky J. L., Chen Y., et al. Sexual behaviors and human papillomavirus vaccine non-initiation among young adult cancer survivors. *J Cancer Surviv.* 2021;**15**:942–50.

25. Klosky J., Russell K., Canavera K., et al. Risk factors for non-initiation of the human papillomavirus (HPV) vaccine among adolescent survivors of childhood cancer. *Cancer Prev Res.* 2013;**6**:1101–10.

26. Wingo P. A., Cardinez C. J., Landis S. H., et al. Long-term trends in cancer mortality in the United States, 1930–1998. *Cancer.* 2003;**97**:3133–275.

27. Leyden W. A., Manos M. M., Geiger A. M., et al. Cervical cancer in women with comprehensive health care access: Attributable factors in the screening process. *J Natl Cancer Inst.* 2005;**97**:675–83.

28. Huh W. K., Ault K. A., Chelmow D., et al. Use of primary high-risk human papillomavirus testing for cervical cancer screening: Interim clinical guidance. *Gynecol Oncol.* 2015;**136**:178–82.

29. Monsonego J., Cox J. T., Behrens C., et al. Prevalence of high-risk human papilloma virus genotypes and associated risk of cervical precancerous lesions in a large U.S. screening population: Data from the ATHENA trial. *Gynecol Oncol.* 2015;**137**:47–54.

30. Cuzick J., Clavel C., Petry K. U., et al. Overview of the European and North American studies on HPV testing in primary cervical cancer screening. *Int J Cancer.* 2006;**119**:1095–101.

31. Ogilvie G. S., Van Niekerk D., Krajden M., et al. Effect of screening with primary cervical HPV testing vs cytology testing on high-grade cervical intraepithelial neoplasia at 48 months: The HPV FOCAL randomized clinical trial. *JAMA – J Am Med Assoc.* 2018;**320**:43–52.

32. Saslow D., Solomon D., Lawson H., et al American Cancer Society, American Society for Colposcopy and Cervical Pathology, and American Society for Clinical Pathology Screening Guidelines for the Prevention and Early Detection of Cervical Cancer. *CA Cancer J Clin.* 2012;**62**:147–72.

33. Curry S. J., Krist A. H., Owens D. K., et al Screening for cervical cancer us preventive services task force recommendation statement. *JAMA – J Am Med Assoc.* 2018;**320**:674–86.

34. Fontham E. T. H., Wolf A. M. D., Church T. R., et al Cervical cancer screening for individuals at average risk: 2020 guideline update from the American Cancer Society. *CA Cancer J Clin.* 2020;**70**:321–46.

35. Perkins R. B., Guido R. S., Castle P. E., et al. 2019 ASCCP risk-based management consensus guidelines for abnormal cervical cancer screening tests and cancer precursors. *J Low Genit Tract Dis.* 2020;**24**:102–31.

36. Moscicki A. B., Flowers L., Huchko M. J., et al. Guidelines for cervical cancer screening in immunosuppressed women without HIV infection. *J Low Genit Tract Dis.* 2019;**23**:87–101.

37. Chang H. A., Armenian S. H., Dellinger T. H. Secondary neoplasms of the female lower genital tract after hematopoietic cell transplantation. *JNCCN J Natl Compr Cancer Netw.* 2018;**16**:211–18.

38. Vegunta S., Files J. A., Wasson M. N. Screening women at high risk for cervical cancer: Special groups of women who require more frequent screening. *Mayo Clin Proc.* 2017;**92**:1272–7.

39. Hilal Z., Tempfer C. B., Burgard L., Rehman S., Rezniczek G. A. How long is too long? Application of acetic acid during colposcopy: A prospective study. *Am J Obstet Gynecol.* 2020;**223**(101):e1–101.e8

40. Massad L. S., Einstein M. H., Huh W. K., et al. 2012 Updated consensus guidelines for the management of abnormal cervical cancer screening tests and cancer precursors. *Obstet Gynecol.* 2013;**121**:829–46.

41. Martin-Hirsch P. P. L., Paraskevaidis E., Bryant A., Dickinson H. O. Surgery for cervical intraepithelial neoplasia. Cochrane Database Syst Rev. 2013. https://doi.org/10.1002/14651858.CD001318.pub3

Vulvar Lesions and Eruptions

Christina Kraus and Melissa Mauskar

Case Presentation

A 68-year-old patient presents to the clinic four weeks after receiving radiation of her vulva for cutaneous metastasis of lobular breast carcinoma to the vulva. She notes pain on her skin with edema, erythema, cutaneous erosions, and ulcerations (Figure 8.1). She is in significant pain and has been given oral antibiotics and oral antiviral medication without alleviation of symptoms. What are the next best steps?

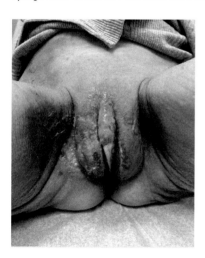

Figure 8.1 68-year-old patient with erythema, edema, desquamation, and erosions after radiation to her vulva

Morphologic Terminology

Macules – Flat lesions less than 1 cm in diameter

Patches – Flat lesions greater than 1 cm in diameter

Papules – Elevated lesions less than 1 cm in diameter

Plaques – Elevated lesions greater than 1 cm in diameter

Vesicle – Fluid-filled lesions less than 1 cm in diameter

Bullae – Fluid-filled lesions greater than 1 cm in diameter

Pustules – Vesicles that contain pus

Nodules – Firm papules or plaques that extend deeper into the dermis or subcutaneous tissue (i.e. cysts)

Petechia – Small punctate hemorrhage

Purpura – Larger hemorrhagic macules/patches or papules/plaques

Overview of Vulvar Skin and Mucosa

The vulvar skin and mucosa is made up of multiple types of epithelia including keratinized skin (hair-bearing labia majora and mons pubis), partially keratinized skin (medial labia majora, labia minora), and nonkeratinized mucous membranes (introitus, extending to vaginal mucosa) [1]. Due to the different types of epithelia and anatomic location, vulvar skin conditions can be challenging to diagnose and treat. For example, scale does not always appear in traditionally "scaly" conditions, (e.g., psoriasis or tinea) as the vulvar skin is damp, consists of folds, and is subject to friction [1]. While various common skin conditions can be present (e.g. psoriasis, atopic dermatitis), some conditions are more unique to vulvar skin (e.g. lichen sclerosus, erosive lichen planus). Additionally, in the oncology patient chemotherapy and/or immunotherapy, radiation, pelvic surgery or lymphatic dissection can predispose patients to developing a vulvar dermatosis or exacerbate a preexisting vulvar condition. Here, we will provide a framework for diagnosis based on morphology of individual lesions, focusing on those conditions most pertinent to the oncology patient.

Approach to General Vulvar Care

In general, "less is more" when it comes to vulvar care. Patients should be counseled that washing the vulva only once a day is sufficient and even mild soap should be avoided when the skin is irritated [2]. Tampons are preferred to pads, as pads can exacerbate wet conditions and cause an allergic or irritant contact dermatitis. White petrolatum ointment is a useful moisturizer and barrier. Zinc oxide ointment is also a useful barrier, which can be applied prior to urination for patients with open wounds or ulcers to prevent stinging and burning with urination.

Vaginal preparations can be cream- or ointment-based depending on the depth and number of lesions in this area. However, for almost all vulvar conditions where a topical medication is warranted, an ointment preparation is preferred over a cream, as creams are more likely to result in a burning sensation on the vulva. Steroid ointments are commonly utilized for inflammatory vulvar conditions and a list of commonly used steroids by potency can be a helpful resource when managing vulvar conditions (Table 8.1). While topical calcineurin inhibitors such as tacrolimus are useful adjuncts for various conditions, it is important to remind patients that application of tacrolimus can initially result in a burning sensation.

Vulvar Biopsy Considerations

Tissue biopsy plays a role in the diagnosis of vulvar conditions, both neoplastic (tumors) and inflammatory (dermatoses). For vulvar dermatoses that are not improving or are refractory to first-line therapy, a tissue biopsy should be considered. For example, a tissue biopsy may help differentiate lichen sclerosus from an allergic contact dermatitis or psoriasis. For lesions that are pigmented and appear clinically suspicious, tissue biopsy is important to differentiate vulvar melanosis/melanotic macules from atypical nevi or melanoma.

For inflammatory vulvar conditions it is important to remember that biopsies represent a "snapshot in time" of a complex and dynamic biologic process. When interpreting biopsy results, clinician must also take into consideration condition duration, use of immunosuppressive therapy, the possibility of more the one process, and the location and the quality of

Table 8.1 Examples of each class of topical steroids, all are ointment as vehicle. Ointments preferred for use on the vulvar skin

Potency	Generic	Brand
Ultra-High (Class I)	Augmented betamethasone dipropionate 0.05%	Diprolene
	Clobetasol propionate 0.05%	Clobex, Temovate
	Halobetasol propionate 0.05%	Ultravate
High (Class II)	Amcinonide 0.1%	Cyclocort
	Betamethasone dipropionate 0.05%	Diprolone
	Fluocinonide 0.05%	Lidex
Medium (Class III)	Betamethasone valerate 0.05%	Valisone
	Hydrocortisone valerate 0.2%	Westcort
	Triamcinolone acetonide 0.01%	Kenalog
Low (Class IV)	Aclometasone diproprionate 0.05%	Aclovate
	Desonide 0.05%	Desowen
	Hydrocortisone 1%	Cortaid

the sample [3]. Thus, histology must be considered in context with the clinical picture and not entirely relied upon for final diagnosis.

A shave biopsy is often sufficient to evaluate for an inflammatory condition such as lichen sclerosus or lichen planus. This can be performed by a procedure known as a "snip" biopsy (modified shave) for lesions where deeper biopsies are not required or challenging. Following lidocaine infiltration, a "snip" biopsy entails applying tension to the skin through use of a suture and snipping underneath the suture with curved iris scissors to free the skin sample.

For chemotherapy- and immunotherapy-related toxicities, there are often findings on skin biopsies that can serve as clues for a therapy-related adverse event. This may prompt the clinician to consider changing therapies depending on grade of toxicity. For infectious conditions, performing a biopsy for tissue culture may be warranted, particularly if the infection is not responding to standard therapy. Additionally, while largely outside the scope of the conditions we discuss here, biopsies can be performed for direct immunofluorescence (DIF) to evaluate for autoimmune blistering conditions that can affect the vulva including pemphigus and mucous membrane pemphigoid.

Infections

Folliculitis

Folliculitis is an inflammation of the hair follicle, which can affect any area of the body, but on the vulva affects only the hair-bearing vulvar skin, including labia majora, mons, and inner thighs. Clinical findings include acneiform appearing follicular-based red papules and pustules which may be few or diffuse. Diagnosis is usually based on patient history and physical exam. Folliculitis is generally treated with topical antibiotics (mupirocin), topical retinoids (tretinoin 0.05% cream), benzoyl peroxide wash (4% or 10% wash three times weekly), and/or oral antibiotics. Because staphylococcus aureus is the most common form of infectious folliculitis, options include treatment with an antistaphylococcal antibiotic such as topical mupirocin 3x/day for 5–7 days or topical clindamycin gel, lotion or solution twice daily for 7–10 days. Topical erythromycin is no longer first choice due to increasing erythromycin resistance. Resistant folliculitis may require oral antibiotics, such as dicloxacillin or cephalexin. If Methicillin-resistant Staphylococcus aureus is suspected, consideration of infectious disease consultation may be indicated.

In addition to bacterial folliculitis which includes staphylococcal, pseudomonal, and gram-negative folliculitis, there are other etiologies for folliculitis which are less commonly seen in this area and include viral and fungal causes. Pityrosporum folliculitis is less common in this area but can lead to a pruritic folliculitis and is usually treated with topical azoles such as ketoconazole cream or selenium sulfide washes. Candida albicans can rarely cause a fungal folliculitis and herpesvirus infections may target the hair follicle, which is more commonly seen with a varicella zoster virus infection than a herpes infection. For these other infectious etiologies, it is necessary to treat the underlying cause with antifungals like oral fluconazole for candida folliculitis and antivirals such as oral valacyclovir for herpes folliculitis.

While not an infectious etiology, Epidermal Growth Factor Receptors (EGFR) inhibitors, such as gefitinib and cetuximab, commonly cause folliculitis, which may involve the vulva. In such cases, oral antibiotics such as doxycycline or minocycline are usually first-line therapy, and are utilized for their anti-inflammatory effects instead of their antimicrobial properties. The previously mentioned topicals, such as benzyl peroxide wash and topical clindamycin can also be utilized in these cases as well as addition of topical triamcinolone cream 0.1% on trunk and body to target inflammation. The severity of EGFR inhibitor-induced folliculitis correlates with a better tumor response. Paclitaxel is another agent that often causes folliculitis as well as other cutaneous skin toxicities.

Abscesses and Furuncles

Bartholin's gland abscesses tend to be the most common abscesses that affect the vulva, but any area of the skin and hair follicles can be subject to infection, particularly in the immunosuppressed patient [4]. Shaving or waxing pubic hair can also increase the risk of infection in this area. The most common pathogens leading to an **abscess** are Staphylococcus aureus, streptococci, and normal skin flora. **Furuncles** are abscesses associated with hair follicles, while **carbuncles** are a continuous group of furuncles. Both furuncles and carbuncles may start as a small erythematous papule and/or pustule and progress in size, associated with fullness, pain, pressure, and tenderness. On exam, both tend to be fluctuant and have associated edema or induration. Gram stain and culture of purulent or serous contents should be performed. Empiric antibiotic coverage should be started with transition to a different antibiotic depending on organisms and sensitivities on culture. Treatment depends on the severity of the lesion(s), but if there is fluctuance, treatment consists of incision or drainage and may include systemic antibiotic therapy (examples include doxycycline 100 mg twice a day for seven days or cephalexin 500 mg 3 times a day for 10 days). Evaluation for a fluid collection a fluid collection can be performed by physical exam or ultrasound. If there is no local fluid collection to drain, patients are treated with systemic therapy, either oral or intravenous depending on severity. Local wound care including warm compresses and chlorhexidine washes (chlorhexidine applied to a gauze or a pad and allowed to come into contact with the area for a few minutes, prior to rinsing off) as well as topical antibiotics (such as mupirocin ointment) may also be utilized.

Angioinvasive Infections

In immunocompromised neutropenic patients, deep fungal infections should be considered in the differential of cutaneous infections, particularly in those that are refractory to antibacterial therapy. Angioinvasive fungal infections are caused by agents that invade blood vessel walls. While these can present as non-specific localized pink to purple papules, nodules, ulcers, eschars, or even red swollen plaques, they can also be vesicular, hemorrhagic, or necrotic in appearance due to tissue ischemia and necrosis. Fungal organisms include candidal (albicans, glabrata, tropicalis, parapsilosis, and krusei), aspergillus, mucor, rhizopus, and fusarium species. If there is any suspicion for an angioinvasive infection, blood cultures and biopsy with tissue culture should be performed and patients should be started on empiric therapy (usually lipid-based amphotericin b or posaconazole) to prevent morbidity and mortality [5].

Herpesvirus Infections

While herpes simplex virus (HSV) commonly affects the vulvovaginal area, patients who are immunosuppressed are at an increased risk of developing both HSV and varicella zoster virus (VZV) on the vulva. The primary lesions are vesicles or crusted papules with an erythematous base, often grouped in clusters. The VZV lesions (shingles), will be distributed along a dermatome. Treatment for both consists of oral acyclovir (typical dose) or valacyclovir (typical dose) with dosing dependent on type of infection. In the oncology population with recurrent outbreaks, suppressive therapy with daily dosing (Valtrex 500mg twice daily) should be considered with recurrent outbreaks.

Kaposi's sarcoma (KS) is a malignant neoplasm arising from endothelial cells that can occur on the vulva and is caused by human herpesvirus type 8 (HHV-8). The iatrogenic type of KS can arise from chronic systemic immunosuppression and should be considered in patients who present with a fixed purple to red nodule, plaque, or tumor. Skin biopsy is diagnostic, and treatment may consist of local or systemic therapies depending on severity of cutaneous disease and presence or absence of systemic involvement. Treatment modalities that have been utilized include: radiation therapy, systemic chemotherapy (gemcitabine, paclitaxel, bleomycin, vincristine, etoposide, among others), and intralesional chemotherapy (vincristine, vinblastine, or bleomycin directly injected into the KS lesion).

Candidal Infections

Vulvovaginal candidiasis (VVC) is common in patients on systemic and/or local immunosuppressants. There is also an increased risk of VVC with topical high-potency steroid application (to treat inflammatory vulvar dermatoses) or topical estrogen replacement therapy (to treat genitourinary syndrome of menopause). It is important to remember that vulvar involvement without vaginal involvement is common and patients may just have bright red erythematous macules, papules, or patches on the vulva (Figure 8.2) without vaginal discharge.

While candida can be invasive as discussed previously, angioinvasive candidal lesions have a different morphology than VVC. Potassium hydroxide (KOH) preparation, wet

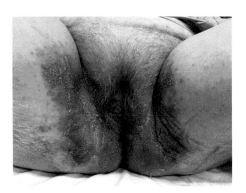

Figure 8.2 Vulvar candidiasis. There is erythema on the mons as well as the inguinal fold. Initially we were concerned for acute generalized exanthematous pustulosis (AGEP, a severe cutaneous adverse reaction to drug) but biopsy returned as candidiasis. Patient improved on topical zinc oxide paste and oral fluconazole 200 mg by mouth, for one dose

mount microscopy and cultures can be performed to evaluate for fungal elements. Additionally, as there may be differences between c. albicans and non-c. albicans infections, it is important to consider sending fungal cultures that identify the organism. For c. albicans infections, treatment usually consists of oral fluconazole 150 mg as a single dose or regimens of 1–3 day course, or topical agents such as clotrimazole 1% cream 5 g intravaginally for 7–14 days and miconazole 2–4% cream intravaginally for 3 days or miconazole 100–200 mg vaginal suppositories for 7 days. Candida glabrata, may be a part of normal vaginal flora but if it is present and thought to be symptomatic, it tends to be resistant to oral and topical azoles and often requires 17% flucytosine cream and/or 3% amphotericin B compounded in an ointment or gel base for 14 days or agents such as ibrexafungerp 300 mg every 12 hours for two doses or topical application of boric acid 600 mg intravaginally, which can be compounded or ordered online, nightly for 2–3 weeks.

Primary Inflammatory Dermatoses

Each of the following conditions can lead to vulvar architectural changes depending on the severity of the condition and the response of the disease to treatment.

Lichen Sclerosus

Lichen sclerosus (LS) is a chronic inflammatory dermatosis (Figure 8.3) that has a predilection for the anogenital area, with extragenital involvement reported in about 15% of patients [6]. While traditionally thought to affect only postmenopausal and pre-pubertal patients, recent studies have suggested increased prevalence in reproductive-age patients [7, 8]. Pruritus is a common presenting symptom, but patients may experience burning, irritation, pain, and dyspareunia. Clinically this may present with nonspecific erythema, whitening (hypopigmentation/depigmentation), and textural change. Patients may have fissures, erosions, or purpura/ecchymoses. Late-stage LS presents with chronic architectural changes (scarring) which include resorption of labia minora, fusion of clitoris to clitoral hood, and introital narrowing.

Diagnosis of LS is often clinical, and a biopsy is not required to initiate treatment. Tissue biopsy may be helpful in cases where the findings are not classic, response to appropriate therapy is minimal, or there is concern for a concomitant diagnosis. However, it is important to remember that LS may have nonspecific biopsy findings [8]. Treatment of LS consists

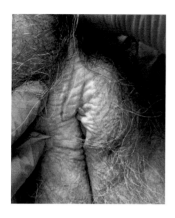

Figure 8.3 Severe hyperkeratotic lichen sclerosus. There is complete obliteration of anatomical structures

of a high-potency steroid ointment daily (clobetasol 0.05% ointment) while the disease is active for 8–12 weeks with decrease to maintenance therapy (twice to three times weekly) after active disease is controlled [6,9]. The amount of topical steroid to be applied to the entire vulva should be a lentil-size amount. Patients should be counseled to rub a thin layer into the affected skin. With the use of this limited amount of steroid and with tapering to maintenance dosing when disease is controlled, the risk of steroid atrophy on the vulvar skin and modified mucous membranes is very low.

There are various regimens for maintenance therapy including a high potency topical steroid (clobetasol 0.05% ointment) three times a week, a mid-potency topical steroid (triamcinolone 0.1% ointment) daily, or a calcineurin inhibitor (tacrolimus 0.1% ointment) daily [6]. Maintenance therapy is important even if patients are asymptomatic and disease is not active clinically, to prevent scarring and decrease the risk of squamous cell carcinoma (SCC) development [9]. Most cases of SCC develop in patients that are not on maintenance therapy, with SCC occurring in up to 5% of cases of uncontrolled vulvar LS. In severe or hypertrophic cases of LS, systemic agents or intralesional injections of steroids (triamcinolone 10 mg/cc) may be considered.

Clinically and histologically, LS may be confused with an allergic or irritant contact dermatitis (and contact dermatitis can exacerbate LS) so clinicians should obtain a thorough history of products used including topicals applied to the area, wipes, douches, and other products, particularly in patients who are not improving or recalcitrant to first-line therapy. Prior reports have noted onset of LS following radiation therapy and in the setting of pelvic malignancy; diagnosis of LS should be considered in patients with new onset vulvar pruritus following radiation. Patients with LS are more likely to have other autoimmune conditions including vitiligo and thyroid disease, so it is important to obtain a thorough history and physical exam for these patients.

Lichen Planus

Lichen planus (LP) is also a chronic immune-mediated inflammatory dermatosis that has a wide-range of cutaneous presentations, but when occurring on the vulva, the most common variant is erosive vulvovaginal LP (EVVLP) (Figure 8.4). Unlike LS, EVVLP often involves the vaginal mucosa and can involve the oral mucosa. Patients with EVVLP

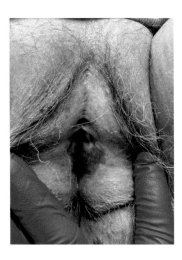

Figure 8.4 Erosive vulvovaginal lichen planus

are more likely to have lichen planus elsewhere on the skin and can have chronic nail changes as well as scalp itching/redness and hair loss due to a variant known as lichen planopilaris. Biopsy may be helpful for diagnosis but on the vulvar skin and mucosa, LP and LS can look similar histologically.

Treatment often requires systemic agents due to the severity of the erosive disease. Topical high-potency steroid ointments (clobetasol 0.05% ointment) are used for the vulva, along with hydrocortisone suppositories (Anusol[T] HC suppositories used for hemorrhoids, written for the vagina twice daily for two months then taper) if there is vaginal involvement [6]. These can also be kept in the refrigerator and cut in half if a lower dose is being utilized. We use once nightly for two months then maintenance of twice to three times weekly at night. Topical calcineurin inhibitors (such as tacrolimus 0.1% ointment) may also be utilized on the vulva and intravaginally. Dilators should be considered if vaginal introitus and/or vaginal mucosa is affected to maintain vaginal patency. Any underlying vulvovaginal estrogen deficiency should also be addressed, and patients may be treated as appropriate with topical estrogen regimens. Many patients require systemic agents for disease control, including methotrexate (usually dosed between 12.5–20 mg once weekly), mycophenolate mofetil (1000 mg twice a day, up to a maximum of 3 g per day), hydroxychloroquine, acitretin, tofacitinib, and other agents [10]. Due to the severity of this condition and the frequent need for multimodal therapies, we suggest combined gynecology and dermatology care for patients with vulvovaginal lichen planus.

Lichen Simplex Chronicus

We include lichen simplex chronicus (LSC) here because, while it is not considered a primary inflammatory dermatosis, it is a common mimicker of other conditions and can occur in the setting of any vulvar itchy rash, including LS. Vulvar LSC is intensely pruritic and patients often find relief with scratching initially. However, with constant rubbing and scratching, the skin becomes thicker (lichenified). Instead of bending, the skin is more prone to break, which often leads to pain and fissures over time. LSC usually occurs in the setting of an underlying inflammatory skin condition such as lichen sclerosus, allergic or irritant contact dermatitis, psoriasis, eczema, or an underlying infection. It can also occur in the setting of an underlying neuropathy. LSC presents as well-demarcated, lichenified, often hypopigmented or hyperpigmented plaques. It is often unilateral but can be bilateral. It may be accompanied by edema, or have overlying fissures, excoriations, or even erosions from constant scratching.

Treatment is focused on breaking the itch/scratch cycle and consists of short courses of a high-potency topical steroid (usually clobetasol 0.05% ointment daily for four to six weeks), oral antihistamines, and sometimes neuropathic agents (i.e. gabapentin, pregabalin, amitriptyline, etc.) to target itch. Depending on LSC severity, short courses of systemic steroids may be considered for acute relief. Patient should be counseled to stop using all products, avoid all wet wipes, and use only emollients or barrier cream such as white petrolatum or zinc oxide to the area. It is important to perform a thorough investigation of all the topical agents patients are using. Patients may not feel comfortable disclosing product use initially, so repeated questioning may be warranted. Frequently, a variety of topical agents are used to try to alleviate the itch associated with LSC. If patients cannot entirely discontinue wet wipes, we do recommend the Water Wipes brand if wet wipes are necessary.

Patients with LSC should also be evaluated for superinfection (fungal, bacterial, or viral) and should be treated as appropriate. Additionally, one should investigate for any underlying dermatosis that is contributing to LSC and this should be adequately treated. If a suspected case of LSC is not responding appropriately to first-line therapies or if the patient has atypical clinical findings, a biopsy is often warranted to rule out malignancies including SCC or extramammary Paget disease.

Treatment Side Effects

Genitourinary Syndrome of Menopause

Genitourinary syndrome of menopause (GSM), resulting from hypoestrogenic effects on the vulva and vagina, leads to symptoms of dryness, irritation, burning, urinary frequency, and dyspareunia [11]. While many postmenopausal women experience these symptoms, GSM is very common in women with malignancies, making this a significant survivorship issue. Surgery, radiation, endocrine therapies for breast and other cancer, and chemotherapy can predispose patients to develop menopausal symptoms earlier and at greater severity than the average age of menopause. It is important to note that LS spares the vagina but can have clinical findings similar to GSM including erythema, hypopigmentation, and architectural changes. Vulvar inflammatory disorders are usually multifactorial and addressing components of GSM in patient with vulvar LP or LS, can improve disease severity [12].

Nonhormonal therapies include vaginal moisturizers and lubricants. Hyaluronic acid containing moisturizers (Revaree® and Hyalogyn®) are effective moisturizers ordered online, while Replens® is an example of an over-the-counter FDA-approved vaginal moisturizer [13]. Moisturizers are used two to three times per week at night, when not sexually active. Vaginal lubricants are slippery products used to decrease friction during intercourse. Vaginal estrogen therapy can be administered locally in the form of a cream, ring, insert, or tablet [11]. Studies have shown local estrogen replacement is safe in most cancer survivors but is not first line therapy for breast cancer survivors receiving aromatase inhibitors but can be considered if non-hormonal treatments fail in collaboration with their medical oncologist [14–16]. In patients with a history of endometrial, ovarian, or cervical cancer who were prescribed topical estrogen for GSM, adverse outcomes including venous thromboembolism and recurrence, were infrequent [14].

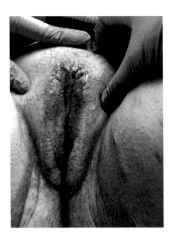

Figure 8.5 28-year-old patient that was treated for verruca for several months before lesions were diagnosed as acquired lymphatic anomalies (ALA). When you apply pressure to these lymphatic lesions, they will often become compressible. If in doubt, biopsy should be performed. This patient's lesions were biopsied to confirm clinical suspicion

Vulvar Lymphedema and Acquired Lymphatic Anomaly

Vulvar lymphedema and acquired lymphatic anomaly (ALA, previously known as lymphangioma circumscriptum) result as a late complication of anogenital or pelvic malignancies [17]. This is thought to occur due to obstruction or alteration of pelvic lymphatics, leading to edema and/or vesiculobullous lesions. Clinically, ALA can be mistaken for condyloma or herpes simplex virus based on morphology (Figure 8.5). Treatment is challenging for both vulvar lymphedema and ALA and involves regular compression, lymphatic massage, and addressing any underlying factors contributing to lymphatic disruption. For ALA, laser therapy and excision performed by dermatologic surgeons have been utilized with varying levels of efficacy [17].

Radiation Dermatitis

Radiation dermatitis is a common adverse effect of radiation therapy that can occur following initiation of radiation therapy or even decades later, with 95% of patients developing this condition following radiation [18]. Acute radiation dermatitis starts as erythema that progresses to eczema-like patches and plaques, blistering, desquamation, erosions or ulceration, and even necrosis. Chronic radiation dermatitis results in dry, atrophic skin, that often has increased telangiectasias and hypo- or hyper-pigmentation [19]. One study of patients with vulvar carcinoma found that age, radiotherapy dose, and pathological stage of disease, were associated with an increased risk of vulvar radiation dermatitis [20].

For acute radiation dermatitis, treatment consists of low- to mid-potency topical steroids (hydrocortisone 2.5% cream or triamcinolone 0.1% cream or ointment) [18]. If ulcers or open wounds are present, absorbent dressings and occlusive ointments (white petrolatum ointment) should be applied to the wounds. Vaseline-impregnated gauze (Xeroform^T) can also be helpful to cover the base of wounds. Hydrogel and hydrocolloid dressings as well as dressings containing silver (such as Mepilex Ag^T foam dressing) may be helpful in managing acute radiation dermatitis. Dressings such as Mepilex Ag can be purchased over the counter at most pharmacies and medical supply stores or online. Patients should be counseled to use only mild soap (avoid products with many additives including fragrance, some of the "unscented" products still contain a fragrance to cover up another scent) and water to cleanse the area. Clinicians should maintain a high index of suspicion for superinfection in open wounds, and culture and treat as appropriate.

Chronic radiation dermatitis is more challenging to treat and consists of modalities such as physical therapy and massage. Pentoxifylline 400 mg three times daily and hyperbaric oxygen therapy have been used with varying levels of success [21]. Pentoxifylline allows blood to be slightly less viscous and increases erythrocyte flexibility. For any chronic radiation-induced ulcers, treatment should focus on wound therapy and surgical intervention as skin flaps may be considered for radiation-induced ulcers where the underlying tissue lacks vascular supply [21].

Radiation Recall

Radiation recall is an acute inflammatory reaction that occurs at the site of previous radiation therapy following use of chemotherapy agents (i.e. cisplatin, 5-fluorouracil, etc) typically weeks to years following radiation. The skin findings can present as redness or ulceration/necrosis. Treatment is similar to that of radiation dermatitis depending on the morphology of the lesion: inflammatory lesions should be treated with mid potency topical steroids such as triamcinolone ointment 0.1%, while ulcers should be treated with appropriate wound care. Upon discontinuation of the inciting pharmacologic agent, the dermatitis will improve [22].

Vulvovaginal Graft-Versus-Host Disease

Genital chronic graft-versus-host-disease (cGVHD) is a complication of allogeneic hematopoietic stem cell transplantation (HSCT) and is likely underrecognized with early diagnosis and intervention critical to prevent sequalae [23]. Up to 60–70% of HSCT patients will experience chronic GVHD at some point. This can affect any area of the skin and mucosa and is treated with local or systemic therapies depending on extent and severity of skin/mucosa involvement. For example, mild oral or ocular involvement may be treated with topical steroids, but more severe symptoms require systemic therapy with steroids (prednisone) and other immunosuppressants including agents like oral tacrolimus. The most common presenting symptoms of vulvovaginal involvement are vaginal dryness, discharge, and vulvar pain. Early on, findings may include non-specific erythema or hypopigmentation. However, if untreated, this progresses to chronic architectural changes including introital narrowing and even complete vaginal closure. Genital cGVHD often spares the labia majora, involving the interlabial sulci, labia minora, peri-clitoral area, introitus, and vagina. Clinically, it can mimic LS or LP. Thus, genital cGVHD is often classified as LS- or LP-like, with a more sclerotic or erosive appearance, respectively. Vulvar cGVHD typically occurs prior to vaginal involvement [24]. Vaginal involvement includes erythematous growth like projections that cause narrowing of the vaginal vault.

Management focuses on topical immunosuppressive agents and estrogen therapies, similar to management of other inflammatory vulvar dermatoses that can progress to scarring. Initial treatment of the vulva should include a high-potency steroid (clobetasol 0.05% ointment) one to two times daily with assessment of response in 6-8 weeks and titrating steroid therapy as appropriate to control clinical symptoms and findings and prevent side effects. Topical tacrolimus 0.1% once to twice daily may be used as an adjunct maintenance therapy, however in acute cases this may burn significantly. Vaginal involvement is similar to that of erosive LP, with treatment recommendations including hydrocortisone suppositories (Annusol^T HC suppositories). Dilators should be utilized to maintain vaginal patency and vaginal estrogen deficiency should be treated with topical estrogens (creams or tablets preferable).

It is important to remember that allogeneic HSCT recipients are at higher risk of condylomas and cervical dysplasia, likely due to reactivation of human papillomavirus (HPV) in the setting of chronic immunosuppression (see Chapter 7) [25].

Toxic Erythema of Chemotherapy

Toxic Erythema of Chemotherapy (TEC) is a spectrum of skin reactions to chemotherapeutic agents (e.g. cytarabine, 5-fluorouracil, taxanes), which commonly involve the hands and feet or intertriginous areas (axillae, inguinal folds) including the vulva[26]. Lesions are most frequently red-purple patches, papules, and plaques but a toxic epidermal necrolysis (TEN)-like presentation has been described in the vulvar area with desquamation and skin sloughing [27]. TEC is not immune-mediated but occurs due to the toxic effects of anti-neoplastic agents on the skin and underlying sweat glands [26]. Biopsy is helpful in diagnosis as histology reveals changes in the eccrine glands and epidermis. Treatment is mostly supportive, consisting of emollients such as petroleum jelly and topical steroids, such as triamcinolone 0.1% ointment. However, more severe cases have been treated with oral steroids and intravenous immunoglobulin, among other agents [27].

Immune-Checkpoint Inhibitor Cutaneous Toxicities

Immune-checkpoint inhibitors (ICIs) have a wide-range of cutaneous toxicities but the following mucosal toxicities should be considered in patients with new vulvovaginal lesions on ICI therapy: aphthous ulcers, oral and genital lichen planus, mucous membrane pemphigoid, and lichen sclerosus [28, 29]. For blistering or ulcerative vulvovaginal conditions, biopsies for routine hematoxylin and eosin staining should be considered, along with direct immunofluorescence studies, to evaluate for an autoimmune blistering disorder (e.g. mucous membrane pemphigoid). Treatment of the cutaneous toxicities is that of standard treatment for each condition, with consideration of minimizing systemic steroids or other modalities that may alter response of malignancy to ICI-therapy. Ideally, topical steroids (triamcinolone 0.1% ointment) or locally injected steroids (triamcinolone 10 mg/cc) should be utilized. If not sufficient for disease control, systemic agents can be considered but it is important to avoid systemic agents that are more immunosuppressive in the setting of an underlying malignancy. If these reactions occur, consulting a dermatologist who is familiar with treating these conditions can be helpful.

Case Resolution

Over the next two months, this patient improved significantly (Figure 8.6). Initially, she was treated with zinc oxide 40% paste three times a day. After two weeks, when her pain had improved, vaseline-impregnated gauze (xeroform) was applied to the base of the wounds and the wounds re-epithelized.

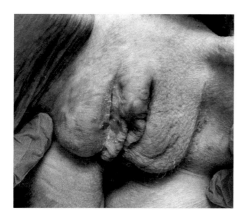

Figure 8.6 Improvement in radiation dermatitis with topical therapy

Take Home Points

- Chemotherapy, immunotherapy, radiation, pelvic surgery, or lymphatic dissection can predispose patients to developing a vulvar dermatosis or exacerbate a preexisting vulvar condition.
- Patients often overclean their genitals, causing more harm than good. Asking about washing techniques is very important. Less is better with nonscented soaps and gentle rinsing with water as opposed to using hard washcloths or scrubs.
- For almost all vulvar conditions where a topical medication is warranted, an ointment preparation is preferred over a cream.
- For vulvar rashes that are not improving or are refractory to first-line therapy, a tissue biopsy should be considered. Biopsies represent a "snapshot in time" and must be considered in the context of the clinical picture and not entirely relied upon for final diagnosis.
- Toxic erythema of chemotherapy (TEC) is very common in intertriginous areas such as the vulva. Treatment with one to two weeks of triamcinolone 0.1% ointment, followed by supportive care with emollients is helpful.
- Diagnosis of lichen sclerosus should be considered in patients with new onset vulvar pruritus following radiation.

References

1. Edwards L., Lynch P. J. *Genital Dermatology Atlas and Manual.* 3rd ed. Wolters Kluwer; 2018.

2. Mauskar M. M., Marathe K., Venkatesan A., Schlosser B. J., Edwards L. Vulvar diseases: Approach to the patient. *J Am Acad Dermatol.* 2020;82(6):1277–84. doi:https://doi.org/10.1016/j.jaad.2019.07.115

3. Shulman H. M., Cardona D. M., Greenson J. K., et al. NIH consensus development project on criteria for clinical trials in chronic graft-versus-host disease: II. The 2014 Pathology Working Group Report. *Biol Blood Marrow Transplant.* 2015;21(4):589–603. doi:https://doi.org/10.1016/j.bbmt.2014.12.031

4. Sally R., Shaw K. S., Pomeranz M. K. Benign "lumps and bumps" of the vulva: A review. *Int J Women's Dermatology.* 2021;7(4):383–90. doi:10.1016/j.ijwd.2021.04.007

5. Berger A. P., Ford B. A., Brown-Joel Z., et al. Angioinvasive fungal infections impacting the skin: Diagnosis, management, and complications. *J Am Acad Dermatol.* 2019;**80**(4):883–98.e2. doi: https://doi.org/10.1016/j.jaad.2018.04.058

6. Mauskar M. M., Marathe K., Venkatesan A., Schlosser B. J., Edwards L. Vulvar diseases: Conditions in adults and children. *J Am Acad Dermatol.* 2020;**82**(6):1287–98. doi:10.1016/j.jaad.2019.10.077

7. Krapf J. M., Smith A. B., Cigna S. T., Goldstein A. T. Presenting symptoms and diagnosis of vulvar lichen sclerosus in premenopausal women: A cross-sectional study. *J Low Genit Tract Dis.* 2022;**26**(3):271–5. doi:10.1097/LGT.0000000000000679

8. Kolitz E., Gammon L., Mauskar M. Vulvar lichen sclerosus in women of reproductive age. *Baylor Univ Med Cent Proc.* 2021;**34**(3):349–51. doi:10.1080/08998280.2021.1885093

9. Lee A., Bradford J., Fischer G. Long-term management of adult vulvar lichen sclerosus: A prospective cohort study of 507 women. *JAMA Dermatology.* 2015;**151**(10):1061–7. doi:10.1001/jamadermatol.2015.0643

10. Cooper S. M., Haefner H. K., Abrahams-Gessel S., Margesson L. J. Vulvovaginal lichen planus treatment: A survey of current practices. *Arch Dermatol.* 2008;**144**(11):1520–1. doi:10.1001/archderm.144.11.1520

11. Crean-Tate K. K., Faubion S. S., Pederson H. J., Vencill J. A., Batur P. Management of genitourinary syndrome of menopause in female cancer patients: A focus on vaginal hormonal therapy. *Am J Obstet Gynecol.* 2020;**222**(2):103–13. doi:10.1016/j.ajog.2019.08.043

12. Fischer G., Bradford J. Interactions between vulvovaginal disorders and urinary disorders: The case for an integrated view of the pelvis. *Int J Women's Dermatology.* 2021;7(5 Part A):600–05.

13. Bygdeman M., Swahn M. L. Replens versus dienoestrol cream in the symptomatic treatment of vaginal atrophy in postmenopausal women. *Maturitas.* 1996;**23**(3):259–63. doi:10.1016/0378-5122(95)00955-8

14. Chambers L. M., Herrmann A., Michener C. M., Ferrando C. A., Ricci S. Vaginal estrogen use for genitourinary symptoms in women with a history of uterine, cervical, or ovarian carcinoma. *Int J Gynecol Cancer.* 2020;**30**(4):515–24. doi:10.1136/ijgc-2019-001034

15. Simon J., Nachtigall L., Ulrich L. G., Eugster-Hausmann M., Gut R. Endometrial safety of ultra-low-dose estradiol vaginal tablets. *Obstet Gynecol.* 2010;**116**(4):876–83. doi:10.1097/AOG.0b013e3181f386bb

16. Lethaby A., Ayeleke R. O., Roberts H. Local oestrogen for vaginal atrophy in postmenopausal women. *Cochrane Database Syst Rev.* 2016;(8). doi:10.1002/14651858.CD001500.pub3

17. Luu Y. T., Kimmis B. D., Bodine J. S., Gloyeske N. C., Dai H. Malignancy-associated acquired vulvar lymphangioma circumscriptum: A clinicopathologic study of 71 cases. *J Cutan Pathol.* 2022;**49**(5):426–33. Doi:10.1111/cup.14181

18. Rosenthal A., Israilevich R., Moy R. Management of acute radiation dermatitis: A review of the literature and proposal for treatment algorithm. *J Am Acad Dermatol.* 2019;**81**(2):558–67. doi:10.1016/j.jaad.2019.02.047

19. Seité S., Bensadoun R.-J., Mazer J.-M. Prevention and treatment of acute and chronic radiodermatitis. *Breast cancer (Dove Med Press).* 2017;**9**:551–7. Doi:10.2147/BCTT.S149752

20. Teng X., Zhang X., Zhi X., et al. Risk factors of dermatitis during radiation for vulvar carcinoma. *Precis Med Sci.* 2022;**11**(3):106–10. doi:https://doi.org/10.1002/prm2.12077

21. Jia A. Y., Viswanathan A. N. Vaginal necrosis: A rare late toxicity after radiation therapy. *Gynecol Oncol.* 2021;**160**(2):602–9. doi:10.1016/j.ygyno.2020.11.025

22. Sweren E., Aravind P., Dembinski R., et al. Radiation recall dermatitis following letrozole administration in patient with

a remote history of radiation therapy. *NPJ Breast Cancer.* 2021;**7**(1):62. doi:10.1038/s41523-021-00271-3

23. Kornik R. I., Rustagi A. S. Vulvovaginal graft-versus-host disease. *Obstet Gynecol Clin North Am.* 2017;**44**(3):475–92. doi:10.1016/j.ogc.2017.05.007

24. Stratton P., Turner M. L., Childs R., et al. Vulvovaginal chronic graft-versus-host disease with allogeneic hematopoietic stem cell transplantation. *Obstet Gynecol.* 2007;**110**(5):1041–9. doi:10.1097/01.AOG.0000285998.75450.86

25. Grulich A. E., van Leeuwen M. T., Falster M. O., Vajdic C. M. Incidence of cancer in people with HIV/AIDS compared with immunosuppressed transplant recipients: a meta-analysis. *Lancet (London, England).* 2007;**370**(9581):59–67. doi:10.1016/S0140-6736(07)61050-2

26. Bolognia J. L., Cooper D. L., Glusac E. J. Toxic erythema of chemotherapy: A useful clinical term. *J Am Acad Dermatol.* 2008;**59**(3):524–9. Doi:10.1016/j.jaad.2008.05.018

27. Lu A., Endicott A., Tan S. Y., et al. Toxic epidermal necrolysis-like toxic erythema of chemotherapy: 2 illustrative cases. *JAAD case reports.* 2021;**15**:56–9. doi:10.1016/j.jdcr.2021.07.010

28. Fässler M., Rammlmair A., Feldmeyer L., et al. Mucous membrane pemphigoid and lichenoid reactions after immune checkpoint inhibitors: Common pathomechanisms. *J Eur Acad Dermatol Venereol.* 2020;**34**(2):e112–e115. Doi:10.1111/jdv.16036

29. Truong K., Jones-Caballero M., Chou S., et al. Lichen sclerosus and immune checkpoint inhibitors: A case and review of the literature. *Australas J Dermatol.* 2022;**64**(1):158–61. doi:10.1111/ajd.13941

Nonpregnant and False-Positive Causes of β-hCG Elevation

Timothy N. Dunn and Denise R. Nebgen

Case Presentation

A 38-year-old G2P2 Caucasian female with known metastatic adenocarcinoma of the gastro-esophageal junction presented with an elevated serum β-human chorionic gonadotropin (β-hCG). The patient previously received localized radiation followed by three different regimens of chemotherapy. Her recent hospitalization was complicated by pneumonia and an incidentally detected β-hCG of 293.3 milli-international units per milliliter (mIU/mL). The patient's previously regular menstrual cycles had stopped after her first round of chemotherapy, and she was using two forms of contraception including abstinence and partner vasectomy. What is your next step in the evaluation?

Epidemiology and Background

Introduction

For medical providers and patients alike, few clinical scenarios can incur as much surprise and concern as an unexpectedly positive β-hCG test upon hospital admission or prior to a surgical procedure. Although there are no universal guidelines mandating pregnancy testing prior to surgical intervention, discussing the possibility of pregnancy is imperative to determine if pregnancy testing is indicated. Screening pregnancy tests are often obtained prior to surgery or chemotherapy due to the concern for interrupting a developing pregnancy or exposing it to potentially teratogenic therapeutics [1, 2]. When these pregnancy tests return positive, the steps to either confirm pregnancy or explore etiologies if not pregnant can feel daunting. Requirements may include multiple additional tests, laboratory consultation, and oncological workup, which can cause delays in diagnosis or therapy for the patient.

There are multiple etiologies for a positive serum pregnancy test. The first and most likely explanation is pregnancy. If the clinical suspicion for pregnancy is low based on the patient's last menstrual period (LMP), age, or the type of contraception, other conditions such as kidney disease, pituitary hormonal changes, or laboratory error can cause positive β-hCG test results. Many malignancies, both gynecologic and nongynecologic, can cause positive β-hCG values. When malignancy is suspected, a more expanded oncological workup may be required to determine the cause.

We will review the underlying physiology of the HCG molecule, the basics of laboratory assessment of β-hCG, potential confounding laboratory etiologies, and benign and

Acknowledgements: The authors thank Rachel Hicklen in the Research Medical Library at The University of Texas MD Anderson Cancer Center for her assistance with the literature review.

malignant causes of positive tests to help guide clinicians in the care of patients with nonpregnant elevations of β-hCG.

The Human Chorionic Gonadotropin Molecule

The β-hCG assay or pregnancy test detects the presence of the β-hCG molecule. HCG is a heterodimeric glycoprotein that has five unique variants that share the same 145 amino acid β-subunit but differ based on changes in their final molecular structure. The five individual β-hCG variants and metabolites include heterodimeric hCG ("pregnancy" hCG), sulfated hCG, hyperglycosylated hCG, hCG free β-subunit, and hyperglycosylated hCG free β-subunit [3]. The first three variants of β-hCG are composed of both an alpha and beta-subunit, with the last two variants containing a β-subunit only [4]. The hCG molecule shares its amino acid composition of the α-subunit with thyroid-stimulating hormone (TSH), follicle-stimulating hormone (FSH), and luteinizing-hormone (LH) [5]. Circulating heterodimeric hCG has a long half-life of over 36 hours [6].

The five variants of hCG are produced by separate cells and have unique functions [4]. Heterodimeric hCG, or "pregnancy hCG," is produced by syncytiotrophoblasts of the placenta and promotes a large array of functions throughout pregnancy. Sulfated hCG is made by the pituitary during the menstrual cycle and potentially helps augment the ovulatory surge and corpus luteum production of progesterone. Hyperglycosylated hCG is produced by the placenta and cytotrophoblasts and promotes autocrine growth of cytotrophoblasts, implantation of the blastocyst neoplastic growth including choriocarcinoma, hydatidiform molar pregnancies, and germ cell tumors. Both hCG free β-subunit and hyperglycosylated hCG free β-subunit are produced by malignancies and cause cancer growth and invasion.

Heterodimeric or "pregnancy" hCG and sulfated hCG act on the dual LH/hCG receptor to exert their function. Hyperglycosylated hCG, hCG free β-subunit and hyperglycosylated hCG free β-subunit act by antagonizing transforming growth factor β (TGF- β) which in turn blocks cancer cell apoptosis leading to cancer growth and invasion. Commercially available assays can detect the pregnancy or heterodimeric form of hCG along with these variants. In this chapter, we will use "β-hCG" to refer to all forms of the hCG molecule [4]. Also, as β-hCG testing can be both qualitative and quantitative, we imply quantitative, serum β-hCG tests for this chapter.

Pregnancy Tests

The sensitivity of pregnancy tests has improved over time, with most urine pregnancy tests (UPTs) resulting positive at β-hCG values of 25 to 50 mIU/mL and serum testing detecting values as low as 1 mIU/mL [5, 7]. All commercial tests identify the β-hCG form present in pregnancy, but assay sensitivity varies across the numerous commercial hCG tests in their ability to detect other β-hCG isoforms. As these other β-hCG variants often occur in nonpregnant conditions, using the same commercial β-hCG test is important to avoid introducing test variation [4].

Assessing for Pregnancy

When a woman of reproductive age tests positive for β-hCG, the most likely cause is pregnancy. If an intrauterine gestational sac and a yolk sac or fetal pole is visualized with transvaginal sonography (TVS), the pregnancy is diagnosed as an intrauterine pregnancy [8]. If an extrauterine gestational sac and yolk sac or fetal pole is visualized, the patient is diagnosed with an ectopic pregnancy and requires surgical or medical management with a gynecologist. Heterotopic pregnancies, when an intrauterine and ectopic pregnancy occur simultaneously, can occur but are extremely rare [8].

In some clinical presentations of early pregnancy, TVS cannot give a definitive diagnosis at the time of a patient's positive pregnancy test, leaving clinicians with a "pregnancy of unknown location" (PUL). In these cases, serial β-hCG values and TVS can provide insight if the pregnancy is progressing as expected or if it is concerning for an abnormal or ectopic pregnancy [9]. Most normally progressing intrauterine pregnancies will show evidence of pregnancy on TVS if the serum β-hCG is over 3,500 mIU/mL, with this serum value referred to as the "discriminatory zone" [8]. If initial β-hCG values are below the discriminatory zone and TVS does not elucidate the pregnancy location, β-hCG trends over 48 hours become the cornerstone of monitoring. While the classic teaching for β-hCG trends in PUL cases is to expect intrauterine pregnancies to have a doubling in value over a 48-hour period, normal intrauterine pregnancies may have slower rates of rise of β-hCG than previously described. β-hCG increases of only 49% over 48 hours can occur in normally-progressing intrauterine pregnancies if the initial value was less than 1,500 mIU/mL, and normal pregnancies have also been seen in cases with increases of only 33% in β-hCG over 48 hours when starting values were over 3,000 mIU/mL [3, 8]. In the case of a pregnancy of unknown location, pregnancy location and subsequent management can often be determined with close follow-up and repeat imaging.

Laboratory Causes of β-hCG Elevation

The predominant laboratory cause of false-positive β-hCG results is heterophilic antibody-interference, which is sometimes referred to as "phantom HCG." Though modern testing approaches are designed to limit this interference, heterophilic antibodies remain an important etiology to consider, especially in populations at higher risk for these antibodies.

Heterophilic Antibodies

Urine and serum pregnancy tests are predominantly immunoassays [10]. β-hCG immuno-assays typically use mouse monoclonal antibodies against β-hCG as a "capture" antibody that is fixed to the assay plate. Patient sera or urine is added to this fixed phase, and then a second, or tracer, antibody against β-hCG is added. This second antibody is chemilumin-escent to then allow for quantification of the hormone levels in the sample [11].

Heterophilic antibodies are antibodies that interfere with immunoassays, often by cross-linking the antibodies used in the test. When this occurs, the assay reports a positive result even if there is no molecule of interest present [12]. The majority of heterophilic antibodies are from unknown exposures, and while patients with histories of working on animal farms, as animal laboratory technicians, or in veterin-ary care could be at higher risk, many cases of heterophilic antibodies are found in patients without known animal antibody exposure [12, 13]. For patients who have had prior treatments with mouse-derived antibodies, anti-mouse antibodies can develop and interfere with the immunoassay, particularly as the majority of antibodies used in commercial assays are mouse derived [12]. In 2000, Cole et al. reported a series of twelve women with positive β-hCG testing who underwent surgical intervention and/

or chemotherapy for presumed gestational trophoblastic disease (GTD), but after extensive laboratory investigation were all found to have false-positive β-hCG testing secondary to human heterophilic antibodies [14].

Assuming the initial serum value is above the sensitivity threshold for a urine pregnancy test (UPT), a UPT may be helpful to assess for the possibility of heterophilic antibodies. [12, 14]. The majority of heterophilic molecules are large and will not pass through the kidney's filtration barrier, producing a true negative UPT result (12–14). There are other laboratory approaches to evaluate for heterophilic antibodies, including serial dilutions, alternative immunoassays, or depleting antibodies where consultation with laboratory medicine could help provide guidance [12].

Two patient populations that have increased risk of heterophilic antibodies are patients with immunoglobulin A (IgA) deficiency and those with rheumatoid arthritis or serum rheumatoid factor. IgA-deficient patients may have more systemic exposure to antigens that were not removed by IgA at their mucosal surfaces, which could lead to increased serum production of heterophilic antibodies [11]. In one study, 30% of serum samples from patients with IgA deficiency caused false-positive serum pregnancy tests when evaluated [11]. Rheumatoid factors, since they are commonly immunoglobulin M heterophilic antibodies, can also cause false-positive pregnancy tests due to the ability of these antibodies to cross-link both phases of β-hCG tests. While rheumatoid factors are common and can be present in healthy individuals, they are at higher concentrations in patients with active rheumatologic disease [12].

Anti-β-hCG Antibody Formation

There is a report of antibody formation against β-hCG itself. The patient developed antibodies against the injectable form of β-hCG used in her fertility treatment [15]. Most patients using β-hCG injection therapies will not form these antibodies, making this etiology very unlikely to be encountered in clinical practice.

Non-neoplastic Causes of β-hCG Elevation

Non-neoplastic causes of serum β-hCG elevations include pituitary production, renal disease, familial HCG, and exogenous medications.

Pituitary Production of β-hCG

In normal physiologic states, both men and women produce a small amount of β-hCG from the pituitary gland. The secreted form is sulfated β-hCG, and in premenopausal women, it is nearly undetectable, averaging only 1.54 mIU/mL at the time of the LH surge [6]. In a woman of reproductive age, pituitary release of β-hCG is unlikely to cause a positive serum pregnancy test. However, as a woman progresses through the menopause transition and gonadotropin-releasing hormone (GnRH) activity increases due to decreased ovarian reserve, the pituitary will release higher levels of FSH, LH, and sulfated β-hCG. These β-hCG levels may increase sufficiently to cause positive pregnancy test results. Since 8% of menopausal women present with β-hCG levels > 5 mIU/mL, studies suggest expanding the normal serum β-hCG reference range for perimenopausal and post-menopausal women to allow levels up to 14.0 mIU/mL to be treated as negative given this pituitary β-hCG production [16, 17].

To assess if a positive β-hCG is related to pituitary production, measure FSH at the same time as the β-hCG test. Elevated FSH values would not be expected in pregnancy, indicating the β-hCG is likely pituitary in origin. An additional option is to prescribe estrogen for two to three weeks, often as an oral contraceptive pill (OCP) assuming no contraindications, to suppress GnRH and FSH levels [6]. If β-hCG levels fall in the presence of estrogen, this would confirm the diagnosis of pituitary β-hCG production [6].

End-Stage Renal Disease

While uncommon, women with chronic kidney disease (CKD) and end-stage renal disease (ESRD) have been found to have positive serum β-hCG values. In one series, 14.5% of premenopausal women aged 18–50 years on dialysis had positive serum β-hCG values, although many of these women had serum estradiol, FSH and anti-Müllerian hormone levels that were more consistent with menopausal values. The β-hCG values in postmenopausal women in this study were typically less than 25 mIU/mL [18]. Women on dialysis undergo menopause 4.5 years earlier than average and 14% are diagnosed with premature ovarian insufficiency. Therefore there is some debate as to whether the positive serum β-hCG result is due to renal dysfunction or due to pituitary production of β-hCG [18].

Familial β-hCG

Familial β-hCG is a benign, familial form of persistently positive β-hCG. The entity was described after evaluating several patients, both men and women, who had positive testing for β-hCG [19, 20]. Unfortunately, many of the index cases had significant interventions, such as chemotherapy and hysterectomy, prior to the correct diagnosis. The familial etiology was discovered after the patient's first-degree relatives also underwent testing, with all cases having a family member with persistently positive β-hCG testing [19]. Current estimates suggest this syndrome is as rare as 1 in 60,000 individuals [19]. Familial β-hCG is a diagnosis of exclusion, with the requirement for assessing for pregnancy, gestational trophoblastic disease, and nongestational trophoblastic disease prior to considering the diagnosis. In the setting of a reassuring gynecologic and oncologic workup, and the presence of similar β-hCG findings in a first-degree relative, the diagnosis would appear to be familial β-hCG.

Exogenous hCG injection

HCG is available in an injectable form, most often used in assisted-reproductive techniques (ART) (as a substitute for LH) and with testosterone-replacement regimens. HCG injections have been utilized for weight-loss assistance despite no rigorous scientific evidence to support this indication [3, 21]. In ART, HCG activates the LH receptor and is given to "trigger" ovulation for intrauterine insemination cycles. It is also commonly administered prior to oocyte retrieval during in vitro fertilization. As the half-life of HCG approaches 36 hours, patients can present several days after an oocyte retrieval or insemination and still have residual injected β-hCG present in their serum. With increasing utilization of fertility preservation procedures for women prior to chemotherapy or oncologic surgery, providers must be aware that serum β-hCG levels can remain detectable for up to two weeks after an oocyte retrieval depending on the dose used [22]. Through a careful review of the patient's history and medication use, one can easily determine if the etiology was HCG administration.

Neoplastic Causes of β-hCG Elevations

Clinicians must consider the role of neoplastic disease leading to elevations in β-hCG. While this commonly entails a gynecologic disorder, there are also nongynecologic malignancies documented in the medical literature that can cause positive β-hCG results.

Gestational Trophoblastic Disease and Gestational Trophoblastic Neoplasia

Gestational trophoblastic disease (GTD) and its associated disorders are the most common type of neoplastic hCG-related tumor. GTD can be classified as premalignant, including partial or complete hydatidiform moles, or malignant, when it is referred to as gestational trophoblastic neoplasia (GTN). GTN includes subtypes such as invasive mole, choriocarcinoma, placental-site trophoblastic tumor, and epithelioid trophoblastic tumors [23]. The diagnosis of GTN is typically made through serum β-hCG testing as opposed to requiring histologic identification, and GTN can arise even if the antecedent pregnancy was remote [23]. The World Health Organization (WHO) risk-scoring system notes that increased time since the index pregnancy confers higher risk than a more recent pregnancy. GTN cases typically occur after hydatidiform molar pregnancies but can also occur following term, preterm, miscarriage, and ectopic pregnancies [23]. As such, providers must consider GTD along with GTN in patients with persistently positive β-hCG testing [23].

Germ-Cell Tumors

Germ-cell tumors (GCT) can occur both within and outside of the gonad and comprise 1-2% of all ovarian malignancies. GCTs encompass a wide range of pathologies, including dysgerminomas and embryonal carcinoma, and often express tumor markers that can facilitate their identification [24]. β-hCG expression has been documented with nongestational choriocarcinoma, embryonal carcinoma and occasionally dysgerminomas. While the original prognosis for these malignancies was bleak, survival has improved dramatically with current chemotherapeutic regimens [24].

While GCTs are usually gonadal or ovarian in origin, there are cases in the literature of nongestational choriocarcinomas or extragonadal GCTs secreting β-hCG. Notable cases include primary esophageal choriocarcinoma, thoracic choriocarcinoma that mimicked primary lung carcinoma, postmenopausal choriocarcinoma, primary intracranial choriocarcinoma, and intracranial metastases of GTN (25–29). There are cases of intracranial GCTs that have induced precocious puberty across a wide range of β-hCG values [30, 31]. Although rare, in the setting of an elevated β-hCG result with a normal pelvic ultrasound, a GCT occurring outside of the gynecologic tract should be considered.

Nongynecologic Malignancies

There are multiple examples of nongynecologic malignancies producing β-hCG (Table 9.1). These have not been limited to a single organ system but rather show a wide degree of diversity. The dedifferentiated malignant tissue may acquire the ability to secrete β-hCG as a cell survival mechanism to escape regulation. Malignancies that produce β-hCG often secrete the free β-hCG molecule or hyperglycosylated free β-hCG as opposed to the heterodimeric form of β-hCG. As both free β-hCG variants antagonize TGF-β activity, this could allow increased malignant cell survival and invasion [4, 32]. β-hCG expression is

Table 9.1 Cases of nonpregnant or false-positive β-hCG elevations in malignancies

Malignancy type	Reported HCG ranges (mIU/mL)	References
Bone (Osteosarcoma)	25–1,008	(40–43, 63, 64)
Central Nervous System	8–2,747	[30, 31, 59, 60]
Colorectal	218	[33, 65]
Esophageal	190	[49, 51, 52]
Gallbladder	39–558	[50, 66]
Gastric	75–458	(67-69)
Gastro-Intestinal	17–1,317	[47, 48, 70]
Lung	54–11,286	(53, 55-58, 71)
Sarcoma	130–1,122	(44-46, 61)
Thyroid	48–2,800	[38, 39, 72]
Renal, Bladder, and Urothelial	1–469	[32, 34, 35, 73, 74]
Head and Neck	29–397	[36, 61, 62]
Ovarian mucinous adenocarcinoma	103–210	[75]
Cervical	50	[76]

associated with a worse prognosis in early-stage colorectal cancer, decreased survival in patients with renal cell carcinoma, worse prognosis in urothelial transitional cell carcinoma, and worse disease-specific survival in cases of oropharyngeal squamous cell carcinoma (33–36). β-hCG could correlate with disease progression or advanced-stage disease given its potential impact on malignant cell survival. Additional work is needed to determine if β-hCG can gauge cancer prognosis.

Ectopic β-hCG secretion is often described as a "paraneoplastic syndrome." In true paraneoplastic syndromes, autoantibodies, cytokine signaling, active peptides and hormones arise from tumor secretion or from the body's immune response against the malignant tissue to cause widespread symptoms [37]. While the cases presented in this chapter do secrete β-hCG, we recommend considering it as ectopic β-hCG production as opposed to a true paraneoplastic syndrome. The malignancies presented also can have variable β-hCG levels, so we caution providers from excluding a malignant pathology from the differential if the β-hCG values are not concordant with prior cases given the sparse data available.

Thyroid Malignancies

Papillary thyroid cancer (PTC) is the most common form of thyroid carcinoma, comprising 65–80% of cases, and has excellent survival rates [38]. Multiple subtypes of papillary thyroid cancer exist, including the more aggressive forms of cribiform-morular variant and columnar cell variant, with both having documented cases of β-hCG expression [38, 39]. A young woman with cribriform-morular papillary thyroid cancer was treated with thyroidectomy and radionucleotide iodine-ablation. She had recurrent disease and was also found to have a positive pregnancy test during a preoperative evaluation [39]. Pathology evaluation of her initial and subsequent tumor resections showed positive staining for β-hCG, consistent with tumor secretion of the β-hCG molecule [39]. Another patient with columnar-type papillary thyroid cancer had a positive β-hCG value arising from the tumor [38]. In patients with thyroid cancer, especially rare histologic subtypes, positive β-hCG values may reflect primary tumor activity as opposed to pregnancy or a gynecologic disorder.

Sarcoma

Osteosarcomas are a class of sarcomas that can produce β-hCG. A 26-year-old woman diagnosed with disseminated osteogenic sarcoma had a β-hCG level of 693 mIU/mL. She was treated with chemotherapy, and her β-hCG levels rose and fell in accordance with her tumor burden [40]. Harrold et al. reported a similar case of metastatic osteosarcoma with serum β-hCG levels reflecting tumor burden and response to therapy [41]. However, it appears that most cases of metastatic osteosarcoma do not cause positive serum β-hCG testing, despite some positivity on immunohistochemistry [42, 43].

Other sarcomas that have caused positive β-hCG results include dedifferentiated soft-tissue sarcomas, with one case of a postmenopausal woman with a preoperative β-hCG value of 1122 mIU/mL prior to excision of a posterior thigh lesion [44]. Her pathology was an unclassified pleomorphic sarcoma, but it showed strong positivity for β-hCG on immunohistochemistry. After resection and adjuvant radiotherapy, her β-hCG testing was negative [44]. Positive serum β-hCG values in the setting of dedifferentiated liposarcoma have also been described [45, 46].

Gastrointestinal Carcinomas

There are multiple reported cases of gastrointestinal carcinomas causing positive β-hCG values. An early series evaluated ectopic β-hCG secretion in gastrointestinal tumors and found 44.4% were positive for β-hCG, with elevated levels more commonly seen in patients with advanced disease [47]. Cases of gastric, metastatic duodenal, gallbladder, esophageal, and bile duct cancer have all been reported with positive β-hCG results (48–51). In one study, 29 esophageal carcinomas were assessed and β-hCG expression was seen in approximately 21% of tumors. These positive-staining regions tended to occur in regions of poor differentiation, high concentrations of pleiomorphic cells, and significant tissue invasion [52].

Pulmonary Lesions and Malignancy

Primary pulmonary lesions and pulmonary malignancies have shown ectopic β-hCG production. In one case, a 56-year-old woman was found to have an extremely elevated serum β-hCG in the setting of a large right-upper lobe mass. The mass was found to be a rare pulmonary pleomorphic carcinoma, which is an aggressive, poorly differentiated non-small cell lung carcinoma, with positive immunostaining for β-hCG that was driving the β-hCG secretion [53]. Two additional case reports of patients with non-small cell lung cancer also revealed positive serum β-hCG values, with one male patient demonstrating a β-hCG as high as 11,286 mIU/mL [54, 55]. Other pulmonary etiologies with secreted ectopic β-hCG are poorly differentiated lung adenocarcinoma and a solitary fibrous pleural tumor (56–58). While rare, tissue and serum β-hCG expression can be seen in pulmonary lesions.

Central Nervous System and Head-and-Neck

There are documented cases of central nervous system (CNS) malignancies producing β-hCG. One example was a primary CNS-germinoma causing β-hCG positivity, and a neuroblastoma that induced precocious puberty [59, 60].

In head-and-neck malignancies, one report detailed β-hCG positive findings in a patient with sinonasal terato-carcinosarcoma while another case reported positive β-hCG values in the setting of lingual squamous cell carcinoma [61, 62]. Lastly, in a case series of patients with oropharyngeal squamous cell cancer (OPSCC), the authors not only noted positive β-hCG values but that levels correlated with poor overall survival [36].

Evaluation of Elevated β-hCG (Figure 9.1 – Diagnostic Algorithm)

The differential for an elevated β-hCG, if not an obvious intrauterine pregnancy, is expansive. It includes ectopic pregnancy, heterophilic antibodies, pituitary β-hCG, exogenous hCG, end-stage renal disease, familial β-hCG syndrome, and gynecologic and non-gynecologic malignancies. We suggest the following evaluation when confronted with a patient with a potential false-positive or nonpregnant β-hCG value.

First, a thorough history and physical exam is required, remembering that the most common cause for a positive β-hCG in a reproductive-age woman is pregnancy. If pregnancy is excluded and the patient's serum β-hCG value is above the sensitivity threshold for UPTs (typically 20–25 mIU/m), collect a urine β-hCG. If the urine test is negative, heterophilic antibody interference is likely occurring where consultation with laboratory medicine may provide additional guidance as needed. If the urine β-hCG is positive, a detailed history should assess for possible medical causes of β-hCG elevations along with asking about medication use. If the patient used hCG injections within the last two weeks for ART, oocyte cryopreservation, weight loss, or other purposes, the result is likely due to residual medication. Lastly, if the patient has a history of renal disease on dialysis, low serum β-hCG values could be related to kidney dysfunction or increased pituitary secretion.

If the patient is perimenopausal or postmenopausal, consider checking FSH levels, for an elevated FSH suggests pituitary production of β-hCG. If the FSH value is inconclusive and time allows, consider giving the patient two to three weeks of oral estrogen to suppress pituitary function and recheck β-hCG. If the result has normalized, the test confirms pituitary production of β-hCG. If FSH is normal or suppressed or if β-hCG fails to normalize with estrogen suppression, further workup is indicated. TVS should then be ordered to assess for ovarian or adnexal masses or signs of GTD if it was not already performed.

If a pregnancy is visualized at any time in the algorithm, treatment should be provided as indicated. If any abnormalities are seen on the TVS, consider GCT, GTD, ectopic pregnancy, or PUL as the source. If the uterus and ovaries appear normal on TVS, consider a 48-hour trend of β-hCG for a possible PUL. If the patient has a known primary malignancy, consult with pathology to assess for tumor secretion of β-hCG by immunohistochemistry (IHC). If ultrasound and laboratory trends do not seem consistent with a gynecologic cause of the elevated β-hCG, consider more extensive imaging to assess for non-gynecologic malignancies. Lastly, if this assessment has not yet revealed a source of β-hCG, consider a broad oncologic workup and consider assessment for the rare etiology of familial hCG by familial testing.

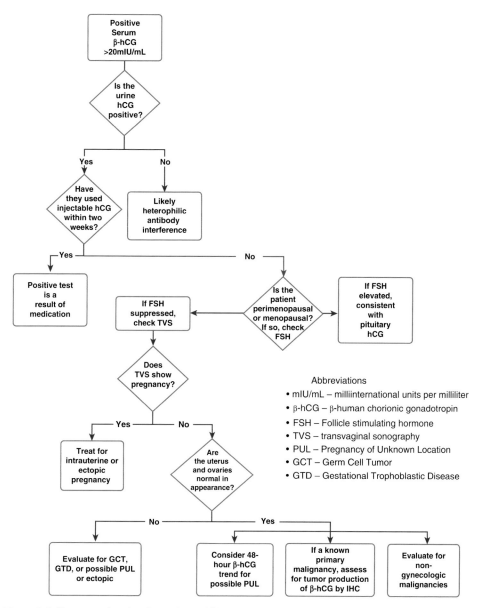

Figure 9.1 Diagnostic algorithm for an elevated β-hCG

We encourage all providers to think critically while working through this algorithm, as some steps may need to occur sooner than others based on clinical judgment in the management of the patient under their care. Through this evaluation, providers will likely be able to determine the cause of the patient's positive β-hCG, and with that knowledge, the clinician can then bring a measure of clarity to the challenges faced with a non-pregnant or false-positive elevation in β-hCG.

Case Resolution

The patient's UPT was positive, eliminating the concern for heterophilic antibody interference. TVS demonstrated no gestational sac or evidence of ectopic pregnancy, and normal appearing ovaries bilaterally. A CT of the chest, abdomen and pelvis was negative for any masses aside from her known malignancy. Repeat serial β-hCG at two-day intervals showed decreasing values from 293.3 mIU/mL to 195.5 mIU/mL and then to 162.6 mIU/mL. The patient was felt to have ectopic tumor-production of β-hCG and was cleared to resume chemotherapy. The patient received a total of four chemotherapy treatment regimens and an additional 12-day course of radiation therapy for curative intent. Despite these treatments, her cancer progressed with repeat β-hCG of 55,925 mIU/mL three months following the initial value with a further increase to a peak value of 136,054 mIU/mL one week later. No further values were drawn as they appeared to correspond with her cancer progression. Due to disease progression and considering the wishes of the patient and her family, she was transitioned to hospice care.

Take Home Points

- Positive serum testing for β-hCG can occur for reasons other than pregnancy.
- If the clinical suspicion for pregnancy is low based on the patient's LMP, age, and method of contraception, consider other conditions such as kidney disease, pituitary hormonal changes, laboratory error, or gynecologic and non-gynecologic malignancies.
- The classic teaching for β-hCG trends in pregnancies of undetermined location is to expect intrauterine pregnancies to have a doubling in the value over a 48-hour period. However, normal intrauterine pregnancies may exhibit slower rates of rise of β-hCG.
- When a false positive serum β-hCG is suspected, a negative urine pregnancy test may indicate assay interference from heterophilic antibodies.
- If the follicle stimulating hormone (FSH) is elevated at the time of a positive β-hCG, a pituitary etiology is suspected.
- If the patient has a known primary malignancy, consult with pathology to assess for tumor secretion of β-hCG by immunohistochemistry (IHC).
- If ultrasound and laboratory trends do not seem consistent with a gynecologic cause of the elevated β-hCG, consider more extensive imaging to assess for non-gynecologic malignancies.
- If a workup for pregnancy, laboratory error, pituitary hormonal production, or malignancy is negative, familial β-hCG syndrome should be considered.

References

1. Martin S. K., Cifu A. S. Routine preoperative laboratory tests for elective surgery. *JAMA*. 2017;**318**(6):567–8.

2. Anesthesiologists Committee on Quality Management and Departmental Administration. Pregnancy Testing Prior to Anesthesia and Surgery. 2021.

3. Herkert D., Meljen V., Muasher L., et al. Human chorionic gonadotropin: A review of the literature. *Obstet Gynecol Surv.* 2022;**77**(9):539–46.

4. Cole L. A. The hCG assay or pregnancy test. *Clin Chem Lab Med.* 2012;**50**(4):617–30.

5. Choi J., Smitz J. Luteinizing hormone and human chorionic gonadotropin: origins of

difference. *Mol Cell Endocrinol.* 2014;**383**(1–2):203–13.

6. Cole L. A. hCG, the wonder of today's science. *Reprod Biol Endocrinol.* 2012;**10**:24.

7. Harvey R. Human chorionic gonadotropin: biochemistry and measurement in pregnancy and disease. 2022.

8. ACOG Committee Opinion No. 191. Tubal ectopic pregnancy. *Obstet Gynecol.* 2018;**131**(2):e65–e77.

9. Carusi D. Pregnancy of unknown location: Evaluation and management. *Semin Perinatol.* 2019;**43**(2):95–100.

10. Chard T. Pregnancy tests: A review. *Hum Reprod.* 1992;**7**(5):701–10.

11. Knight A. K., Bingemann T., Cole L., Cunningham-Rundles C. Frequent false positive beta human chorionic gonadotropin tests in immunoglobulin A deficiency. *Clin Exp Immunol.* 2005;**141**(2):333–7.

12. Bolstad N., Warren D. J., Nustad K. Heterophilic antibody interference in immunometric assays. *Best Pract Res Clin Endocrinol Metab.* 2013;**27**(5):647–61.

13. ACOG Committee Opinion No. 278. Avoiding inappropriate clinical decisions based on false-positive human chorionic gonadotropin test results. *Obstet Gynecol.* 2002;**100**(5):1057–9.

14. Rotmensch S., Cole L. A. False diagnosis and needless therapy of presumed malignant disease in women with false-positive human chorionic gonadotropin concentrations. *The Lancet.* 2000;**355**(9205):712–15.

15. Heijboer A. C., Martens F., Mulder S. D., Schats R., Blankenstein M. A. Interference in human chorionic gonadotropin (hCG) analysis by macro-hCG. *Clin Chim Acta.* 2011;**412**(23–4):2349–50.

16. Snyder J. A., Haymond S., Parvin C. A., Gronowski A. M., Grenache D. G. Diagnostic considerations in the measurement of human chorionic gonadotropin in aging women. *Clin Chem.* 2005;**51**(10):1830–5.

17. Patel K. K., Qavi A. J., Hock K. G., Gronowski A. M. Establishing reference intervals for hCG in postmenopausal women. *Clinical Biochemistry.* 2017;**50**(4–5):234–7.

18. Haninger-Vacariu N., Herkner H., Lorenz M., et al. Exclusion of pregnancy in dialysis patients: Diagnostic performance of human chorionic gonadotropin. *BMC Nephrol.* 2020;**21**(1):70.

19. Cole L. A. Familial HCG syndrome. *J Reprod Immunol.* 2012;**93**(1):52–7.

20. Cole L. A., Butler S. Familial hCG syndrome: Production of variable, degraded or mutant forms of hCG. *J Reprod Med.* 2014;**59**(9–10):435–42.

21. Lijesen G. K., Theeuwen I., Assendelft W. J., Van Der Wal G . The effect of human chorionic gonadotropin (HCG) in the treatment of obesity by means of the Simeons therapy: A criteria-based meta-analysis. *Br J Clin Pharmacol.* 1995;**40**(3):237–43.

22. Damewood M. D., Shen W., Zacur H. A., Schlaff W. D., Rock J. A., Wallach E. E. Disappearance of exogenously administered human chorionic gonadotropin. *Fertility and Sterility.* 1989;**52**(3):398–400.

23. Horowitz N. S., Eskander R. N., Adelman M. R., Burke W. Epidemiology, diagnosis, and treatment of gestational trophoblastic disease: A Society of Gynecologic Oncology evidenced-based review and recommendation. *Gynecol Oncol.* 2021;**163**(3):605–13.

24. Pectasides D., Pectasides E., Kassanos D. Germ cell tumors of the ovary. *Cancer Treat Rev.* 2008;**34**(5):427–41.

25. Fujiwara Y., Okamoto K., Ninomiya I., Saito H., Yamaguchi T., Terai S, et al. Surgically resected primary esophageal choriocarcinoma accompanied with Barrett's adenocarcinoma: A case report. *Surg Case Rep.* 2020;**6**(1):227.

26. Gasparri R., Sedda G., Brambilla D., et al. When a differential diagnosis is fundamental: Choriocarcinoma mimicking lung carcinoma. *J Clin Med.* 2019;**8**(11).

27. Guo N., Yin R., Li Q., Song L., Wang D. Postmenopausal choriocarcinoma: A rare case report and review of the literature. *Menopause*. 2018;**25**(2):239–41.

28. Schrader E., Stephens A. J., Shroff S., Ahmad S., Holloway R. W. Widespread choriocarcinoma metastases from de-differentiated gastro-esophageal junction primary adenocarcinoma: A case report with literature review. *Gynecol Oncol Rep*. 2020;**31**:100513.

29. Xiao P., Guo T., Luo Y., Zhang M., Yin R. Real-world data of 14 cases of brain metastases from gestational trophoblastic neoplasia and a literature review. *Arch Gynecol Obstet*. 2022;**305**(4):929–35.

30. Chen H., Ni M., Xu Y., Zhong L. Y. Precocious puberty due to intracranial germ cell tumors: A case-control study. *Endocr Relat Cancer*. 2022;**29**(10):581–8.

31. Parra Villasmil M. G., Kim C., Sato M., Kanner L. A. Rapidly progressive precocious puberty with an elevated testosterone level in a 5-year-old boy with a beta-human chorionic gonadotropin-secreting intracranial germ cell tumor in the pineal gland. *AACE Clin Case Rep*. 2022;**8**(4):174–8.

32. Butler S. A., Ikram M. S., Mathieu S., Iles R. K. The increase in bladder carcinoma cell population induced by the free beta subunit of human chorionic gonadotrophin is a result of an anti-apoptosis effect and not cell proliferation. *Br J Cancer*. 2000;**82**(9):1553–6.

33. Li J., Yin M., Song W., et al. B subunit of human chorionic gonadotropin promotes tumor invasion and predicts poor prognosis of early-stage colorectal cancer. *Cell Physiol Biochem*. 2018;**45**(1):237–49.

34. Hotakainen K., Ljungberg B., Paju A., et al. The free beta-subunit of human chorionic gonadotropin as a prognostic factor in renal cell carcinoma. *Br J Cancer*. 2002;**86**(2):185–9.

35. Douglas J., Sharp A., Chau C., et al. Serum total hCGbeta level is an independent prognostic factor in transitional cell carcinoma of the urothelial tract. *Br J Cancer*. 2014;**110**(7):1759–66.

36. Sjoblom A., Carpen T., Stenman U. H., et al. The role of human chorionic gonadotropin beta (hCGbeta) in HPV-positive and HPV-negative oropharyngeal squamous cell carcinoma. *Cancer (Basel)*. 2022;**14**(12).

37. Pelosof L. C., Gerber D. E. Paraneoplastic syndromes: An approach to diagnosis and treatment. *Mayo Clin Proc*. 2010;**85**(9):838–54.

38. Gu H., Sui S., Cui X., et al. Thyroid carcinoma producing beta-human chorionic gonadotropin shows different clinical behavior. *Pathol Int*. 2018;**68**(4):207–13.

39. Alikhan M., Koshy A., Hyjek E., et al. Discrepant serum and urine beta-hCG results due to production of beta-hCG by a cribriform-morular variant of thyroid papillary carcinoma. *Clin Chim Acta*. 2015;**438**:181–5.

40. Glass R., Asirvatham J. R., Kahn L., Aziz M. Beta-human chorionic gonadotropin producing osteosarcoma of the sacrum in a 26-year-old woman: A case report and review of the literature. *Case Rep Pathol*. 2015;**2015**:897230.

41. Harrold E., McMahon E., McGing P., Higgins M. betahCG-secreting osteosarcoma. *BMJ Case Rep*. 2017;2017.

42. Lee A. F., Pawel B. R., Sullivan L. M. Significant immunohistochemical expression of human chorionic gonadotropin in high-grade osteosarcoma is rare, but may be associated with clinically elevated serum levels. *Pediatr Dev Pathol*. 2014;**17**(4):278–85.

43. Masrouha K. Z., Khattab R., Tawil A., et al. A preliminary investigation of Beta-hCG expression in patients with osteosarcoma. *J Bone Joint Surg Br*. 2012;**94**(3):419–24.

44. Blank A. T., Khalighi M., Randall R. L., Jones K. B. Don't cancel the surgery just yet! A case report of positive preoperative pregnancy test due to a soft tissue sarcoma production of ectopic beta human chorionic gonadotropin. *Rare Tumors*. 2018;**10**:2036361318789727.

45. Maryamchik E., Lyapichev K. A., Halliday B., Rosenberg A. E. Dedifferentiated liposarcoma with rhabdomyosarcomatous differentiation producing HCG: A case report of a diagnostic pitfall. *Int J Surg Pathol.* 2018;**26**(5):448–52.

46. Russell M. J., Flynt F. L., Harroff A. L., Fadare O. Dedifferentiated liposarcoma of the retroperitoneum with extensive leiomyosarcomatous differentiation and beta-human chorionic gonadotropin production. *Sarcoma.* 2008;**2008**:658090.

47. Birkenfeld S., Noiman G., Krispin M., Schwartz S., Zakut H. The incidence and significance of serum hCG and CEA in patients with gastrointestinal malignant tumors. *Eur J Surg Oncol.* 1989;**15**(2):103–8.

48. Kang S., Zaidi A. J., Shokouh-Amiri M., Wiley E., Venepalli N. K. A case report of paraneoplastic syndrome in beta-hCG-secreting duodenal adenocarcinoma. *J Gastrointest Oncol.* 2019;**10**(6):1151–6.

49. Kutty G., Gupta S., Yap J. E., McDunn S. Advanced esophageal carcinoma expressing beta-HCG: A case report. *American Journal of Gastroenterology.* 2013;**108**:S217–S8.

50. Leostic A., Tran P. L., Fagot H., Boukerrou M. Elevated human chorionic gonadotrophin without pregnancy: A case of gallbladder carcinoma. *J Gynecol Obstet Hum Reprod.* 2018;**47**(3):141–3.

51. Li D. M., Li S. S., Zhang Y. H., Zhang H. J., Gao D. L., Wang Y. X. Expression of human chorionic gonadotropin, CD44v6 and CD44v4/5 in esophageal squamous cell carcinoma. *World J Gastroenterol.* 2005;**11**(47):7401–4.

52. Trias I., Campo E., Benasco C., Palacín A., Cardesa A. Human chorionic gonadotropin in esophageal carcinomas: An immunohistochemical study. *Pathology – Research and Practice.* 1991;**187**(4):503–7.

53. Dinis de Sousa M., Barata M., Miranda A. R., et al. Beta-HCG secretion by a pulmonary pleomorphic carcinoma:

A case report. *Respir Med Case Rep.* 2021;**34**:101528.

54. Groza D., Duerr D., Schmid M., Boesch B. When cancer patients suddenly have a positive pregnancy test. *BMJ Case Rep.* 2017;2017.

55. Khattri S., Vivekanandarajah A., Varma S., Kong F. Secretion of beta-human chorionic gonadotropin by non-small cell lung cancer: A case report. *J Med Case Rep.* 2011;**5**:19.

56. Kugasia I. R., Alkayem M., Patel J. B. A rare case of beta-hCG production by a solitary fibrous tumor of the pleura. *Am J Case Rep.* 2014;**15**:518–22.

57. Peng J., Lv S., Liu L., Feng S., Xing N. Lung neoplasm mimicking as ectopic pregnancy due to paraneoplastic secretion of human chorionic gonadotropin:A case report and literature review. *Arch Gynecol Obstet.* 2021;**303**(3):607–14.

58. Wong Y. P., Tan G. C., Aziz S., Pongprakyun S., Ismail F. Beta-human chorionic gonadotropin-secreting lung adenocarcinoma. *Malays J Med Sci.* 2015;**22**(4):76–80.

59. Chou Y. C., Wu Y. Y., Hung S. P., et al. Treatment of primary central nervous system germinomas with short-course induction chemotherapy followed by low-dose radiotherapy without a tumor bed boost: Prognostic impact of human chorionic gonadotropin. *J Pediatr Hematol Oncol.* 2021;**43**(7):e907–e12.

60. Maeyama T., Ichikawa C., Okada Y., et al. Beta-human chorionic gonadotropin-producing neuroblastoma: An unrecognized cause of gonadotropin-independent precocious puberty. *Endocr J.* 2022;**69**(3):313–18.

61. Weinberg B. D., Newell K. L., Wang F. A case of a beta-human chorionic gonadotropin secreting sinonasal teratocarcinosarcoma. *J Neurol Surg Rep.* 2014;**75**(1):e103–7.

62. Wenneker E., Xu Y., Hernandez D. J. Two cases of beta-human chorionic gonadotropin-positive oral tongue cancer resulting in false-positive pregnancy tests.

Otolaryngol Head Neck Surg. 2022:1945998221095391.

63. Lawless M. E., Jour G., Hoch B. L., Rendi M. H. Beta-human chorionic gonadotropin expression in recurrent and metastatic giant cell tumors of bone: A potential mimicker of germ cell tumor. Int J Surg Pathol. 2014;22(7):617–22.

64. Morris C. D., Hameed M. R., Agaram N. P., Hwang S. Elevated beta-hCG associated with aggressive Osteoblastoma. Skeletal Radiol. 2017;46(9):1187–92.

65. Pokharel K., Gilbar P. J., Mansfield S. K., Nair L. M., So A. Elevated beta human chorionic gonadotropin in a non-pregnant female diagnosed with anal squamous cell carcinoma. J Oncol Pharm Pract. 2020;26(5):1266–9.

66. Michalski W., Poniatowska G. M., Jońska-Gmyrek J. G., et al. hCG-secreting malignancies: Diagnostic pitfalls. Oncology in Clinical Practice. 2020;15(6):331–5.

67. Ben Kridis W., Ben Hassena R., Charfi S., et al. Gastric signet-ring cell carcinoma with hypersecretion of β-Human chorionic gonadotropin and review of the literature. Experimental Oncology. 2018;40(2):144–8.

68. Brown J., Barrett-Campbell O., David Y., Luhrs C., McFarlane S. I. An unexpected pregnancy test result leading to the diagnosis of advanced gastric cancer. Am J Med Case Rep. 2019;7(7):148–50.

69. Kafka M., Woll E., Brunhuber T., et al. A presumed extragonadal germ cell tumor that turned out to be a gastric cancer: A case report. Transl Androl Urol. 2021;10(6):2528–33.

70. Daniel M., Das K. An atypical cause for a positive urine pregnancy test. Gastroenterology. 2022;162(6):e6–e7.

71. Fenichel P., Rouzier C., Butori C., et al. Extragestational betaHCG secretion due to an isolated lung epithelioid trophoblastic tumor: microsatellite genotyping of tumoral cells confirmed their placental origin and oriented specific chemotherapy. J Clin Endocrinol Metab. 2014;99(10):3515–20.

72. Becker N., Chernock R. D., Nussenbaum B., Lewis J. S., Jr. Prognostic significance of beta-human chorionic gonadotropin and PAX8 expression in anaplastic thyroid carcinoma. Thyroid. 2014;24(2):319–26.

73. Puco K., Bierner J., Muller S., et al. Abstract 481: Utility of hCG as a biomarker of treatment response in advanced urothelial cancer: A population based series at Akershus University Hospital, Norway. Cancer Research. 2021;81.

74. Gupta A. K., Charlton A., Prelog K., Kellie S. J. beta-HCG Elevation in Wilms Tumor: An Uncommon Presentation. Pediatr Blood Cancer. 2016;63(6):1105–6.

75. Goldstein J., Pandey P., Fleming N., Westin S., Piha-Paul S. A non-pregnant woman with elevated beta-HCG: A case of para-neoplastic syndrome in ovarian cancer. Gynecol Oncol Rep. 2016;17:49–52.

76. Mustafa A., Bozdağ Z., Tepe N. B., Ozcan H. C. An unexpected reason for elevated human chorionic gonadotropin in a young woman Cervical squamous carcinoma. Saudi Medical Journal. 2016;37(8):905–7.

Chapter 10

Cancer and Pregnancy

Jenifer Dinis Ballestas

Case Presentation

A 35-year-old G2P0010 at 34 weeks' gestation presents to a prenatal care visit complaining of a self-palpated, painless breast mass. On physical exam there is a 3 cm firm mass at 12 o'clock in the left breast. Patient was advised that she likely has pregnancy-related breast changes or fibrocystic breasts and the plan was for expectant management and re-examination postpartum. The patient subsequently had a vaginal delivery at 38 weeks' gestational age and then presented for a follow up examination four weeks postpartum. The mass was still painless and measured 3.5 cm. What is the best next step for this patient?

Introduction

Cancer during pregnancy is defined as a malignancy diagnosed either during gestation or within twelve months postpartum. Malignancies diagnosed during gestation pose a unique therapeutic challenge and a high level of suspicion is needed when evaluating women both during pregnancy and postpartum. Often there are delays in diagnosis as many symptoms are attributed to pregnancy.

There is a paucity of nationwide data regarding the incidence of cancer during pregnancy in the United States. Small regional studies from the 1990s estimate the incidence at 1:1000 pregnant women. Data from European registries report an incidence of approximately 1:2000 pregnant women and one year postpartum [1, 2].

Worldwide, the incidence of cancer during gestation has risen in the last few decades attributed partly to delayed conceptions and advanced maternal age (>35 years old at the time of delivery) [3]. In addition, treatment for cancer has continued to improve over the last several decades, resulting in longer life spans and a rising number of survivors who will then become pregnant and present for prenatal care. Other risks factors include obesity, smoking, and family history of malignancy.

A contemporary review in the United States demonstrated the most common type of cancer occurring during pregnancy are breast, followed by lymphoma, leukemia, and gynecologic cancer (cervix and ovary), whereas in northern Europe melanoma is the most common type, followed by breast and ovarian [1–3].

This chapter addresses care for women who are diagnosed with the most common malignancies during gestation and for survivors who become pregnant. Patients require a multidisciplinary team comprised of an oncologist, maternal fetal medicine specialist, mental health provider, and social worker.

Breast Cancer and Pregnancy

Epidemiology

Breast cancer is the malignancy most commonly diagnosed during pregnancy, affecting approximately 1 in every 3000 gestations with the majority diagnosed while breastfeeding or postpartum [4]. There is also a higher likelihood that breast cancer diagnosed during pregnancy will be estrogen and progesterone receptor negative, compared to women above age 40 or postmenopausal. HER 2 expression frequency is similar to that of non-pregnant women and invasive ductal carcinoma is the most common histological type [5].

Pregnant patients are more likely to have stage II breast cancer (60.1% versus 56.1%, p < 0.035), grade 3 tumors (74.0% versus 62.2%, p < 0.001), hormone receptor-negative tumors (48.4% versus 34.0%, p < 0.001) or triple-negative breast cancer (38.9% versus 26.9%, p < 0.001) compared to nonpregnant women. Outcome of women treated during pregnancy is similar to nonpregnant women.

Diagnosis and Workup

Signs and Symptoms

The most common presentation is a painless, palpable mass. During pregnancy, rising levels of estrogen and progesterone lead to changes in the breast such as proliferation and elongation of lobular-ductal units. Macroscopically this translates into enlargement of the breast and increased tissue nodularity [7]. This can make diagnosis challenging as palpation of new lesions may be more difficult, but also patients and clinicians may believe that a palpated mass during gestation is part of the physiological changes of pregnancy and thus tend to observe for longer before pursuing adequate imaging and biopsy.

Differential Diagnosis

It is important to remember that 80% of all breast lesions found during gestation will be benign, and the differential diagnosis shown in Table 10.1 should be considered when pursuing a workup for a breast mass [8, 9].

Physical Exam Findings

It is important to perform and document a breast exam during the first prenatal care visit, as well as any time the patient reports a mass or masses. The provider must ensure to examine all breast tissue, including the tail of Spence that may enlarge and reach the axilla and, in rare cases, may be the primary disease site. Nipple and areola should be examined for presence of skin retraction, color changes or nipple discharge. Superficial skin changes of *peau de orange* are an uncommon finding during gestation. Lastly, axillary, cervical, and supraclavicular regions should be palpated to detect lymphadenopathy.

Imaging Studies

All palpable masses require immediate evaluation, especially if present for >2 weeks [4, 10]. Pregnant and lactating patients should undergo workup in the same fashion as a nonpregnant patient. Observation leads to unnecessary delays in diagnosis which must be avoided as this contributes to pregnancy-associated cancer presenting in more advanced stages.

Table 10.1 Differential diagnosis of breast lesions during gestation

Lactating adenoma	Galactocele	Fibroadenoma	Other benign diagnosis	Other rare malignant diagnosis
• Most common etiology for a breast mass during pregnancy and lactation	• More common among lactating women • Can arise after duct blockages that occur with inflammation but on occasion occurs with other tumors that block the ducts	• Most common Lesion in nonpregnant women of reproductive age	• Fibrocystic changes • Lipoma • Hamartoma • Abscess	• Phylloides tumors • Sarcoma • Lymphoma • Leukemia

Several guidelines exist regarding breast imaging for pregnant and lactating women, as a large proportion of cases are diagnosed during the first year postpartum. Breast sonogram and mammogram are safe during pregnancy and lactation. The threshold radiation dose to cause fetal harm is 5 rads (50 mGy), with a two view mammogram resulting in only 0.001–0.1 mGy of fetal exposure [11]. During lactation interpretation of breast imaging may be more difficult, however this does not constitute a contraindication. Expressing milk immediately prior to the study by pumping or breastfeeding may improve visualization. In order to avoid delays in diagnosis, patients should not be counseled to stop breastfeeding or temporarily discontinue breastfeeding before performing a mammogram [4, 11, 12].

The use of magnetic resonance imaging (MRI) with gadolinium during pregnancy is not recommended due to concerns for fetal anomalies and some reports of increased risk of stillbirth. Due to increased vascularity of breasts during gestation, noncontrast MRI is of little use and thus is not recommended during pregnancy [11]. However, for patients who are breastfeeding, an MRI with gadolinium is safe. The total contrast dose the baby will receive through breastmilk is < 0.0004% of the maternal IV dose. Although the taste of the milk may change, the milk will be safe for feeding hence no need to "pump and dump" [9, 12]. Patients who have a high lifetime risk of developing breast cancer such as carriers of a pathogenic variant may have received screening contrast MRI before gestation. It is important for these women to have a discussion with their oncologist regarding screening strategies during pregnancy. According to their clinical situation, they may either forgo screening or obtain a mammogram during pregnancy.

Table 10.2 is a condensed summary of recommendations [10–13] regarding the use of diagnostic studies among pregnant and lactating women by the American College of Obstetricians and Gynecologists (ACOG), the Academy of Breastfeeding Medicine (ABM), the American College of Radiology (ACR), and the American Society of Breast Surgeons (ASBrS), with recommendations listed by patient's age:

Table 10.2 Diagnostic studies to be utilizing among pregnant and lactating women, stratified by age

Women under 30 years old	Women 30 to 39 years old	Women over 40 years old
A breast ultrasound should be the first diagnostic test. Mammogram is performed if there is a concerning finding on ultrasound or if the ultrasound does not find a mass that correlates with the finding on physical exam	Both mammogram and ultrasound should be obtained [*].	Both mammogram and ultrasound should be obtained

(*) It is acceptable to order an ultrasound as the first assessment for this age group, however, an early finding of breast cancer are microcalcifications, which can only be detected with a mammogram and can be present even without a palpable mass. Therefore, if an ultrasound is selected as the initial test (even with a normal result), a mammogram should still be obtained. This is crucial to help diagnose cancer in an earlier stage among pregnant and lactating women.

Diagnostic Tests

A core needle biopsy is preferred over fine needle aspiration during gestation as it decreases likelihood of indeterminate and/or false negative results [14]. The pathologist should be made aware of whether the patient is pregnant or breastfeeding.

Pregnant and breastfeeding women should be counseled that performing any breast procedure such as a biopsy carries a small risk (2.2%) of a milk fistula. To prevent fistula formation and to improve visualization of breast tissue during stereotactic biopsy, the lactating woman should empty her breasts shortly before and after biopsy via pumping or direct feeding [14, 15]. If a milk fistula does form, the breast should be emptied consistently to promote closure of the fistulous tract. If breastfeeding is stopped abruptly, this could increase risk of a fistula secondary to increased breast engorgement. Women should not be advised to interrupt breastfeeding in order to undergo a diagnostic biopsy, and these tests should be performed without delay at an experienced center.

Staging and Other Workup

Common sites of metastases are lungs, liver, and bone. A chest x-ray to exclude lung metastases can be obtained with low risk of fetal radiation exposure; only approximately 0.0005 to 0.01 mGy for a two-view study. If further evaluation is required, noncontrast chest MRI is recommended over chest CT. Chest CT can be safely performed as fetal exposure doses are also low (0.01–0.66 mGy), however a chest x-ray will usually suffice [11]. A liver ultrasound may be performed to rule out metastases. Alkaline phosphatase level is an unreliable marker as pregnancy induces a physiologic elevation. A bone scan may be performed postpartum in most cases, with MRI as a safer alternative during gestation. In select cases of symptomatic disease or advanced stages where an MRI was inconclusive, a bone scan can be performed if a low dose radiation protocol is available and with care to maintain hydration and frequent voiding. Brain MRI can be performed if indicated. A sentinel lymph node biopsy is acceptable during gestation using tecnethium-99, which is injected in the tumor site. As it remains locally without systemic exposure, risks to the fetus are minimal and lymph node mapping has high accuracy [16, 17]. If the patient declines tecnethium-99, injection with methylene blue is an alternative. Isosulfan blue is usually avoided due to a 1% risk of anaphylaxis [16, 17].

Treatment

Termination

Termination of pregnancy is not routinely recommended with a desired pregnancy as young women treated with chemotherapy during gestation have comparable survival to their nonpregnant counterparts [6]. Patients with advanced or metastatic disease diagnosed in the first trimester (up to 14 weeks of gestation) may elect to terminate the pregnancy in order to expedite neoadjuvant therapy and radiation.

Radiation

Radiation is deferred until postpartum to avoid fetal exposure [4, 6, 18–20]. The more advanced the gestation, the closer the fetus is to the chest and thus the higher risk. Among women who are candidates for lumpectomy and radiotherapy, surgery is performed during gestation and radiotherapy is administered postpartum.

Chemotherapy and Neoadjuvant Agents

Anthracycline-based chemotherapy regimens are the most widely used, consisting of doxorubicin with cyclophosphamide (AC) with or without 5-fluorouracil (FAC). In Europe epirubicin has been increasingly used in place of doxorubicin. Chemotherapy administered after 14 weeks is not associated with an increases risk of anomalies. Methotrexate is a well-known teratogen and it is best avoided during pregnancy [4, 6, 18–20].

Herceptin is contraindicated during gestation due to increased risk of oligohydramnios and fetal pulmonary hypoplasia. Tamoxifen and raloxifene are also contraindicated due to increased risk of miscarriage and multiple anomalies, including ambiguous genitalia. All of these agents may be initiated postpartum [19–23].

Surgery

Surgery is safe during any trimester of pregnancy. Either a lumpectomy or mastectomy can be performed. After 20 weeks the gravid uterus may be large enough to compress the inferior vena cava while laying supine which can lead to decreased venous return and hypotension, thus the patient should be positioned in the operating room using a left tilt.

Before viability, fetal heart tones need to be documented via doppler before and after surgery. After viability (23 weeks), a nonstress test should be performed before and after surgery, and ideally intraoperative fetal monitoring should be utilized [24]. If intraoperative monitoring reveals fetal distress an emergency cesarean can be performed; thus it is important to make preparations such as performing the surgery in a center with an appropriate obstetric and neonatal team.

When undergoing surgery during pregnancy there is always a risk of an emergency cesarean. Procedures that don't involve entry into the abdominal cavity are typically low risk as long as the patient remains hemodynamically stable.

If a mastectomy is performed, a tissue expander can be placed during the same procedure. Reconstruction is preferably delayed until the postpartum period to decreased maternal and fetal risks from surgery and to obtain a better aesthetic result, particularly if only unilateral mastectomy was performed, as the contralateral breast will undergo size changes postpartum.

Deferral of Treatment:

Women presenting with early-stage breast cancer during gestation, particularly during the third trimester, may choose to defer treatment until after delivery. It is important to stress that treatment should always be offered.

Obstetric Management of the Pregnant Patient with Breast Cancer

Maternal Risks

There is an increased risk of miscarriage if chemotherapy is administered during the first trimester, thus initiation is typically delayed until after week 14. This delay does not adversely impact the mother's expected survival or morbidity. All pregnant patients with cancer, regardless of type, have increased risk of severe maternal morbidity such as anemia requiring transfusion, pulmonary embolism, hysterectomy, and mechanical ventilation [25].

Risks for the Fetus

Risk of fetal anomalies is not increased if chemotherapy is avoided during the first trimester and radiation is delayed until postpartum. There is an increased risk of preterm birth (before 37 weeks) and the subsequent neonatal morbidity among those born preterm. There is an increased risk of low birth weight, however this is typically determined by gestational age at delivery.

There is a theoretical risk of fetal anemia induced by chemotherapy during pregnancy, however fetal middle cerebral artery (MDA) doppler monitoring for fetal anemia is often normal during gestation. If emergency delivery is performed less than three to four weeks after the last chemotherapy treatment, there can be increased risk of neonatal leukopenia and anemia [26, 27]. There are no adverse developmental outcomes reported among children exposed to chemotherapy in utero [28].

Antenatal Testing

Women receiving chemotherapy should have a baseline echocardiogram, as well as baseline renal and hepatic function testing. A growth ultrasound is recommended every three to four weeks, typically the day prior to each chemotherapy session. Consideration may be given to adding MCA doppler assessment for fetal anemia at this time. After 32 weeks, weekly antenatal testing is indicated. The placenta should be sent to pathology after delivery. Consider referral to a clinical psychologist specialized in oncologic patients at least once at the onset of care.

Delivery Route and Timing

Vaginal delivery is preferred, with cesarean reserved for usual obstetric indications. Ideal timing of delivery is at term (37 weeks) to improve fetal outcomes, however occasionally late preterm delivery (35 to 36 weeks) may be suggested according to chemotherapy timing. Three to four weeks should be allowed to pass between the last chemotherapy and delivery to allow for fetal and maternal cell counts to recover and decrease likelihood of maternal complications such as infection. Thus, the last round of chemotherapy is typically administered at 34–35 weeks [5, 6, 18, 24, 27].

Breastfeeding

Breastfeeding during chemotherapy is discouraged. Although only a small amount of the maternal dose is present in breastmilk, there is still a concern for cytotoxicity for the newborn [18, 20]. If radiation is performed postpartum, breastfeeding is not recommended.

Pregnancy Among Survivors of Breast Cancer

Pregnancy does not affect the likelihood of recurrence. For *BRCA* mutation carriers, abortion does not improve disease-free survival after cancer and continuation of pregnancy does not worsen disease-free survival [29].

For patients with advanced stage disease, pregnancy may limit treatment options and thus worsen prognosis. Based on that concern, avoidance of pregnancy is recommended. Survivors previously treated for early-stage disease are typically counseled to wait two years after completion of treatment to conceive. Most recurrences will occur within the first two years after treatment completion and pregnancy may render treatment more challenging.

Fertility declines after maternal age 30 and even more so after chemotherapy. Consideration may be given to allow women with favorable prognosis to conceive earlier than two years from treatment completion. A recent large cohort study with over 7500 Canadian women indicated that pregnancy occurring 6 months or more after a breast cancer diagnosis did not incur additional risk for recurrence, suggesting a reduced interval to conception may be considered for select patients [30]. Preconception consultation with a maternal fetal medicine specialist is recommended.

If methotrexate is utilized, conception must be delayed three to six months to avoid teratogenicity. Tamoxifen or trastuzumab should be stopped for approximately three months before attempting conception and can be restarted postpartum. Prior to stopping these medications a patient should be evaluated by her oncologist to discuss her personal recurrence risk.

If a patient has a unilateral tissue expander, reconstruction is completed after pregnancy for best cosmesis. For patients undergoing autologous tissue reconstruction, as long as the flap has healed there is no contraindication to vaginal delivery, even for flaps involving part of the abdominal wall [20, 31].

The rate of fetal anomalies among cancer survivors is similar to that of the general population. If the patient has a genetic pathogenic variant, her child may inherit this mutation; many of which are autosomal dominant. In vitro fertilization with preimplantation genetic screening allows selection of an embryo that does not carry the mutation of interest.

Anthracyclines confer risk of cardiotoxicity. A maternal echocardiogram to assess cardiac function is indicated prior to pregnancy. Other recommended tests are EKG, renal, and hepatic function testing.

An ultrasound may be performed at 32 weeks to screen for fetal growth restriction but this is optional. There is no indication for weekly antenatal testing unless other obstetrical or medical complications arise.

Vaginal delivery is preferred; cesarean is reserved for obstetric indications. There is no indication for a preterm birth or early term (37 week) delivery as long as there are no other obstetrical complications.

If a patient underwent a unilateral mastectomy, she can attempt to breastfeed with her remaining breast although formula supplementation may be necessary. Some women report inadequate milk supply with one breast which can cause distress and lead to shorter duration of breastfeeding. Breastfeeding is also possible from a breast treated with lumpectomy and radiation, although milk production will be lower from that side [32, 33]. The most common reason for survivors to not breastfeed is receiving instructions from their doctors discouraging them. These patients require a multidisciplinary strategy to successfully breastfeed if they desire, which includes early and frequent access to certified lactation consultants, access to breast pump equipment (a hospital grade pump if possible) and extensive support from family, friends, and their physicians.

Cervical Cancer and Pregnancy

Epidemiology

Although cervical cancer is the fourth most common cancer among nonpregnant women of reproductive age, it is relatively rare during gestation with an approximate incidence of 3.6 per 100,000 live births [1]. The majority of cases are actually detected within the first year postpartum. When diagnosed during gestation, it is typically in the second trimester (reported median at 18 weeks) [2].

Fortunately, most patients are at an early stage at diagnosis (commonly IB1), histologic grade 1 or 2, squamous, and without lymphovascular invasion [2]. Perhaps this cancer is found more frequently in early stages because the Pap smear is part of routine prenatal care evaluation.

FIGO staging for cervical cancer was amended in 2021 with two key differences to the FIGO staging 2009 versions (inclusion of stages IB3 and IIIC). Tumor size has been further stratified as IB1 ≤2 cm, IB2 >2–≤4 cm, and IB3 >4 cm (previously referred to as bulky IB2). Lymph node involvement confers poor prognosis, which is now acknowledged as stage IIIC1(pelvic) and IIIC2 (para-aortic) [35]. Most of the existing cohort studies refer to the FIGO 2009 or 2018 classification, but acknowledge presence of lymph nodes and tumors > 4 cm as poor prognosis. For the purpose of this section we will consider early disease stages I to IB2 and advanced disease IB3 to IV.

Cervical cancer is one of the most challenging cancer to treat during pregnancy. Among patients with early-stage disease (stages I through IB2), survival is comparable to nonpregnant women. Some women presenting after 22 weeks are candidates to delay treatment until postpartum [35].

Diagnosis and Workup

Signs and Symptoms

Most women are asymptomatic (over 70%), as early-stage disease is more common and can only be diagnosed by histopathology. When symptoms are present, the most common symptom is vaginal bleeding (which can be postcoital) and increased vaginal discharge (usually watery, blood-tinged). Advanced stages may be associated with a pelvic mass found on exam, pelvic pain, flank or lower extremity pain [36]. All symptoms can be attributed to normal changes in pregnancy which explains why many cases are discovered postpartum. To avoid delays in diagnosis, any complaints of vaginal bleeding or discharge during pregnancy should be evaluated by a speculum exam and a Pap smear as indicated. Cytobrush use in pregnancy is safe.

Differential Diagnosis

Includes other benign etiologies for vaginal bleeding and discharge such as vaginal infections (i.e. trichomoniasis), cervical ectropion or polyps, obstetrical causes such as vasa previa, placenta previa, abruption, threatened abortion, and precancerous lesions or cervical intraepithelial neoplasia (CIN).

Physical Exam

For any suspicious lesions on speculum examination, a Pap smear and colposcopy are indicated. If there is a mass, then evaluation will also include a biopsy. Evaluation of abnormal Pap smears during pregnancy is as follows in Table 10.3 [37].

The use of acetic acid during colposcopy is safe during pregnancy, but endocervical curettage is contraindicated. If there are any suspicious lesions a punch biopsy can be performed. A common complication after biopsies is bleeding, as the cervix becomes more friable and vascular during gestation. The bleeding can be arrested with topical agents in the office (Monsels or silver nitrate), vaginal packing or, very rarely, suture ligation in the OR. For the following biopsy results see below management as shown in Table 10.4.

Table 10.3 Evaluation of abnormal cytology in pregnancy

Pap smear result	ASCUS HPV negative	ASCUS HPV positive and LSIL	HSIL or higher
Treatment plan	No colposcopy, follow age indicated screening	If under 25 years old may repeat pap and HPV testing in a year, over 25 years old can opt for colposcopy immediately or 4-6 weeks postpartum	Immediate colposcopy

Table 10.4 Evaluation of abnormal cervical biopsy in pregnancy

Colposcopy result	CIN 1	CIN 2 or CIN 3	Carcinoma in situ
Treatment plan	Repeat colposcopy at 6 weeks postpartum if initial procedure was adequate and there was no concern for malignancy on exam	If there is a high suspicion of invasive disease based on patient's history, an excision with LEEP or CKC can be performed, however the ASCCP recommends repeating colposcopy at 12–24 week intervals during gestation and repeat biopsy if lesion appearance is worsening [37]. A consultation with a gynecologic oncologist may be appropriate for these patients.	Refer to gynecologic oncologist; likely will need excision to rule out invasive disease.

CIN: Cervical intraepithelial neoplasia
LEEP: Loop electrosurgical excision procedure
CKC: Cold knife cone

Loop electrosurgical excision procedure (LEEP) and cold knife cone (CKC) should be reserved to rule out invasive malignancy in highly suspicious cases. Frequently CIN lesions are stable or regress after pregnancy, with CIN 1 being more likely to regress than CIN 2–3. The likelihood of developing invasive carcinoma during gestation is low [38]. LEEP and CKC have a modestly increased risk of pregnancy loss (particularly if performed in the first trimester), bleeding, infection, preterm labor and delivery. Complications are reduced if the procedures are performed at 14–20 weeks gestational age [36, 39].

Staging and Other Workup

Chest xray via a two-view study with abdominal shielding is safe for the fetus [11]. Abdominopelvic MRI may be performed in lieu of intravenous pyelogram and barium enema. Ultrasound can also be utilized to assess urinary tract patency; however MRI is preferred. If cystoscopy is needed, it may be performed. Lymphadenectomy can dictate recommendations for treatment during pregnancy, therefore when indicated and feasible it should be performed. The gynecologic oncologist may complete lymphadenectomy via laparotomy or laparoscopy. When the gravid uterus has reached 20 weeks (plus or minus 2 weeks) the size impedes adequate visualization and the procedure cannot be performed. Feasibility is also dependent on surgeon experience. For those women presenting with a gestational age too advanced for lymphadenectomy, treatment recommendations will be based on histopathological and clinical staging with plans to complete this procedure postpartum [34, 35].

Treatment

Choice of treatment will depend on stage, gestational age at the time of diagnosis, patient's desire to continue the pregnancy and/or retain future fertility.

Termination of Pregnancy

This is an option if the patient does not wish to continue the pregnancy and is under the legal gestational age cut-off according to local regulations. Termination of pregnancy is not routinely offered to women with early-stage disease as it does not improve outcome.

For women with advanced stage disease, immediate start of chemoradiation is recommended to improve survival. If the patient elects chemoradiation, due to deleterious effects of radiation on the fetus, expedited termination of pregnancy is then recommended, especially if the patient is <18–20 weeks per FIGO guidelines (up to 22 weeks as recommended by the European Society of Gynecological Oncology) [34, 35].

A patient with advanced disease may decline termination, in which case chemotherapy is started, radiotherapy is omitted, and she should be counseled regarding paucity of data describing outcomes and the theoretical risk of decreased survival due to delay or omission of treatment.

Radiation

Pelvic radiation has deleterious consequences for the fetus and effects vary by gestational age of exposure and dose. The typical threshold dose for deleterious effects is 5 rads (0.05 Gy). A dose of 100 rads (1 Gy) is considered extremely high exposure and will most likely result in demise of a pregnancy, particularly prior to 14 weeks gestation. Exposure to >2 Gy at 8–15 weeks gestation is associated with fetal growth restriction and microcephaly. Severe intellectual disability has been reported with exposures as low as 0.6 Gy. Exposures of >2.5 Gy at 15–25 weeks increase risk of fetal growth restriction and severe intellectual disability. Malformations are typically only seen with exposures above >2 Gy during the first trimester, however doses as low as 0.05 Gy may induce pregnancy loss [11, 35].

The total treatment radiation dose suggested by FIGO is 80–90 Gy. Administering this high of a dose will most likely result in embryonic or fetal demise [35]. Patients must be aware of the possibility of severe impairment in the unlikely event that the fetus does survive treatment. Patients should be counseled that after embryonic or fetal demise there may be complications such as spontaneous passage of products of conception, hemorrhage, disseminated intravascular coagulation (DIC) and infection. To avoid these potential complications, uterine dilation and evacuation (D&E) before therapy should be offered, particularly for those receiving treatment after the first trimester.

Chemotherapy

The most commonly used chemotherapy drug in pregnancy is cisplatin. When possible, it is employed as single agent therapy to decrease fetal exposure to multiple chemotherapeutic agents. Other combinations of cisplatin, carboplatin, paclitaxel or ifosfamide have also been reported in pregnancy. If indicated, chemotherapy is started after 14 weeks to avoid teratogenicity [34, 41, 42].

Surgery

CKC and LEEP have approximately a 5–15% risk of bleeding, premature rupture of membranes, preterm birth, pregnancy loss and, rarely, infection [39]. Trachelectomy (abdominal and vaginal) has a higher hemorrhage risk and pregnancy loss rate of 33% [40], hence only CKC and LEEP are recommended during pregnancy. For women with positive margins that require re-excision, simple trachelectomy is preferred over abdominal and vaginal radical trachelectomy due to higher risk of pregnancy loss and hemorrhage. Risks are reduced if procedures are completed between 14–20 weeks. At the time of CKC or trachelectomy a cervical cerclage may be placed at the discretion of the surgeon. Particularly if the remaining cervical length is short, cerclage may decrease chances of preterm birth.

Hysterectomy with lymph node dissection may be performed simultaneously with a cesarean (cesarean-hysterectomy) or at six to eight weeks postpartum (postpartum hysterectomy) when the uterus has involuted thus facilitating visualization of the surgical field.

If the patient chooses termination of pregnancy and will require a hysterectomy (gravid hysterectomy), management depends on gestational age. During the first trimester and early second trimester, a hysterectomy can be performed with the fetus in situ. After mid second trimester, the uterus may be evacuated by hysterotomy during the surgery. Fetal intracardiac potassium chloride (KCL) injection may be administered pre-operatively. Gravid hysterectomy and cesarean hysterectomy have increased hemorrhage and transfusion rates compared to postpartum surgery [34–36, 41, 43].

Delay of Treatment Until Postpartum

Recommended only for early-stage disease, diagnosed during the third trimester when delivery could be feasible. Any patient at any stage may opt to decline treatment [34, 35, 41]. Table 10.5 summarizes treatment alternatives per stage. Each patient will need a tailored plan with her care team.

Obstetric Management of the Pregnant Patient with Cervical Cancer

Risks for the Mother

All pregnant patients with cancer, regardless of type, have an increased risk of severe maternal morbidity such as need for transfusion, pulmonary embolism, hysterectomy, and mechanical ventilation [25]. For patients with advanced disease that choose to delay treatment or omit radiation, there may be decreased survival in theory but there is a paucity of data among this population. Risks of hysterectomy should be discussed (hemorrhage, transfusion, infection, damage to surrounding organs).

Table 10.5 Treatment options, mode and timing of delivery for cervical cancer diagnosed during pregnancy, stratified by stage

Stage	Gestational age at presentation (weeks)	Possible treatment	Mode of delivery	Timing of delivery
IA1	<20–22	CKC, ST or D	SVD if negative margins and desiring fertility**, otherwise	- 37 weeks, - Consider 39 weeks if negative margins on excision
	>20–22	CKC, ST or D	CD with PP-Hyst, CD with ST postpartum or C-hyst are more appropriate	
IA2 – IB1	<20–22	CKC, ST or D	SVD if negative margins, otherwise	- 37 weeks, up to 39 weeks if negative margins on excision.
	>20–22	Chemo or D	CD with PP-Hyst or C-hyst are more appropriate	- As early as 34–35 weeks if D was chosen
IB2*	<20–22	Chemo after 14 weeks	CD with PP-Hyst or C-hyst	- 37 weeks - As early as 34–35 weeks if D was chosen
	>20–22	Chemo or D		
IB3 and above	<20–22	TOP with usual treatment, if patient declines: Chemo after 14 weeks	If pregnancy continued, CD with PP-Hyst or C-hysterectomy	- 34–35 weeks
	>20–22	TOP with usual treatment, if patient declines: Chemo or D		

(*) On a case by case basis, some women staged as IIA may be eligible for this management

(**) If lymphovascular invasion is found, a cesarean may be recommended

CKC: cold knife cone. ST: simple trachelectomy. D: delay treatment until postpartum, CD: cesarean delivery. PP-hyst: Postpartum hysterectomy at 6–8 weeks after delivery. C-hyst: cesarean hysterectomy. TOP: termination of pregnancy, it is an option for every patient at any stage.

Fetal Risks

Women who have a LEEP or CKC while pregnant may be at increased risk of pregnancy loss or preterm birth. There is risk of fetal demise or severe impairment if radiotherapy is administered, and in these cases, termination is recommended before radiotherapy (see above).

If chemotherapy is administered after 14 weeks gestational age, the risks of anomalies is not increased from baseline. There is increased risk of low birth weight and neonatal morbidity which is predominantly determined by gestational age at delivery.

There is potential risk of fetal anemia induced by chemotherapy during pregnancy, however MCA doppler monitoring for fetal anemia is typically normal during gestation. If emergency delivery is performed less than three to four weeks after the last chemotherapy treatment, there can be increased risk of neonatal neutropenia [26, 27]. There are no reported adverse developmental outcomes among children exposed to chemotherapy during pregnancy [28].

Antenatal Testing

If a patient has undergone cervical surgery resulting in decreased cervical length, there may be increased risk of preterm birth [44]. LEEP procedures typically retain a greater portion of the cervix than CKC, which in turn is less aggressive than trachelectomy. For this reason, some providers place a cerclage at the time of trachelectomy, in an attempt to decrease likelihood of preterm birth.

At this time the Society for Maternal Fetal Medicine acknowledges that there is insufficient evidence to recommend cervical length screening solely for history of LEEP or CKC. However, a provider may opt for universal cervical length screening for all pregnant patients in an effort to prevent preterm birth [44, 45]. Under this premise, if the patient has a singleton gestation and has not had a previous preterm birth, a transvaginal cervical length may be performed at the time of the anatomy scan (18–20 weeks). If cervical length is less than 2.5 cm, vaginal progesterone may be initiated; if cervical length is shorter than 1.0 cm, the patient may benefit from cerclage placement. If a cerclage has been placed after CKC or trachelectomy, transvaginal ultrasound for cervical length screening is not indicated.

Baseline renal and hepatic function testing should be performed. Ultrasound for viability and growth should be performed every three to four weeks prior to chemotherapy administration. Consideration can be given to adding MCA doppler monitoring to screen for fetal anemia. After 32 weeks, weekly antenatal testing is initiated. The placenta should be sent to pathology after delivery.

Serial colposcopic examinations during pregnancy should be undertaken as recommended by their treating gynecologic oncologist. If the patient has delayed treatment until postpartum, serial pelvic exams should be documented upon discretion of gynecologic oncologist and maternal fetal medicine specialists. Follow up MRI is recommended to rule out disease progression. Consider referral to a clinical psychologist specialized in oncologic patients at least once at the onset of care.

Delivery Route and Timing

See Table 10.5 for recommended mode of delivery and gestational age at delivery per stage.

For women receiving chemotherapy, three weeks should be allowed to pass between the last treatment and delivery. The final round of chemotherapy is typically administered at

34–35 weeks if a term delivery is planned, however delivery timing or date of last treatment may need to be adjusted according to patient's clinical scenario.

For early-stage disease such as IA1 or IA2, vaginal delivery may be possible even if treatment has been delayed to the postpartum period. For women undergoing cesarean, a classical incision is recommended to avoid incising close to the cervix which could increase the likelihood of bleeding and tumor spread [35, 41, 45]. There are case reports of women who delivered vaginally with subsequent episiotomy site recurrences of cervical cancer 12 weeks to 5 years after initial diagnosis. The majority of these women were stage IB1 or higher [46]. Although episiotomy is not routinely performed at the time of delivery, on occasion there can be large vaginal tears that require repair or an episiotomy may be needed. Hence vaginal delivery is considered on a case-by-case basis and typically reserved for stage IA. Notably, vertical transmission of cervical cancer to fetal lungs has been reported among two women who delivered vaginally but had advanced stage disease [47].

Breastfeeding

Breastfeeding is encouraged only among women who are not receiving chemotherapy postpartum.

Pregnancy Among Survivors of Cervical Cancer

Pregnancy does not increase risk of recurrence. Cerclage erosion and cervical stenosis sometimes occur after fertility sparing procedures and should be evaluated by physical examination.

Patients are typically advised to wait 6–12 months after cervical surgery before attempting to conceive. There is evidence that the cervix can heal and increase in length 3–12 months after an excision, particularly after LEEP and CKC. Awaiting more time after the surgery may allow for more cervical regeneration and decrease the likelihood of preterm birth. For women with a short residual cervical length, a cerclage may be the only treatment available to decrease risk of preterm birth. There are no randomized trials to address timing of delivery after cervical surgery, however there is evidence that conceiving earlier than three months may lead to preterm birth, especially if the remaining cervix is short. Delaying conception at least for 3–6 months decreases chances of a preterm birth [48, 49]. Preconception consultation with a maternal fetal medicine specialist is recommended.

There are no reported cases of pregnancy after radiation for cervical cancer. The high radiation doses alter uterine vascularity and viability of the endometrial layer. Surrogacy is the best option for these patients desiring future childbearing [50].

There is an increased risk of preterm birth and pregnancy loss among survivors with fertility sparing surgery. Procedure type and subsequent birth rates are summarized in Table 10.6, based on a systematic review of over 2000 patients, of which majority had cerclages placed at the time of fertility sparing surgery [51].

In addition to routine prenatal testing, the prior chemotherapeutic agents utilized should be noted in the patient's record. Baseline liver function testing is recommended. If a patient does not have a cerclage in place then cervical length may be evaluated with transvaginal ultrasound at the time of the anatomy scan (18–20 weeks) [43]. An ultrasound can be performed at 32 weeks to screen for fetal growth restriction, but this is optional.

Table 10.6 Live birth and preterm birth rates among fertility sparing treatments for cervical cancer

Procedure Tyle	Subsequent live birth rate (%)	Preterm birth rate (%)
Simple trachelectomy and cold knife cone	74	15
Vaginal radical trachelectomy	67	39
Radical trachelectomy via laparotomy	68	57
Radical trachelectomy via minimally invasive surgery	78	50
Chemotherapy in addition to radiation, cold knife cone or simple trachelectomy	76	15

There is no indication for weekly antenatal testing unless other obstetrical or medical complications arise. Lastly, surveillance Pap smear and colposcopy as indicated by gynecologic oncologist should be continued during gestation.

If the patient has an abdominal or a vaginal Shirodkar cerclage, cesarean delivery is indicated at 39 weeks or earlier if other complications arise. If cerclage is not present and there is no evidence of local recurrence, vaginal delivery may be feasible. Breastfeeding is encouraged.

Lymphoma

Epidemiology

The incidence of lymphoma during pregnancy is 1:6,000 live births, with Hodgkin's lymphoma (HL) more common than non-Hodgkin's lymphoma (NHL). The incidence of NHL is increasing, which is associated with advanced maternal age (> 35 years) at delivery [1, 52].

The most common histological subtypes are classic, nodular sclerosis for HL (93%) and diffuse large B-cell for NHL (50%). Most women present with early-stage disease (Ann Arbor I and II) and are more commonly diagnosed during the second trimester of gestation. Patients with HL are often nulliparous and present without B symptoms, while those with NHL are typically multiparous and do exhibit B symptoms (fever, night sweats and weight loss). Women diagnosed during pregnancy have similar survival rates than their non-pregnant counterparts for both HL and NHL [52, 53].

As with other malignancies, some of the symptoms of lymphoma resemble common innocuous pregnancy complaints, thus diagnosis requires a high level of suspicion.

Diagnosis and Workup

Signs and Symptoms

Common symptoms are fatigue, night sweats, weight loss, shortness of breath, persistent cough, nausea and vomiting, appetite changes, abdominal discomfort, constipation and pruritus. Routine prenatal screening complete blood count (CBC) may reveal anemia, leukocytosis, neutrophilia, and thrombocytopenia.

Physical Exam Findings

Cervical, supraclavicular, and axillary lymphadenopathy is a common finding. Mediastinal lymphadenopathy in a patient with HL may manifest as cough [54]. Women with Burkitt's NHL frequently have extranodal involvement and during pregnancy there is an increase of breast, ovarian, and uterine involvement which may present with breast or ovarian masses.

Staging and Other Workup

Blood testing may include CBC, liver function testing, and creatinine. Erythrocyte sedimentation rate (ESR) has limited use as it is physiologically increased in pregnancy. Lactate dehydrogenase (LDH) does not physiologically increase in pregnancy however some obstetric conditions such as preeclampsia may be associated with an increase. Pregnant women are routinely tested for HIV as part of prenatal care upon the first visit [54].

A chest x ray can be performed with abdominal shielding (up to 0.01 mGy exposure). A CT scan of the chest is also safe during gestation (up to 0.66 mGy), however the preferred imaging modality during pregnancy is non contrast MRI of chest, abdomen and pelvis [11]. If required, bone marrow biopsy can be performed to complete staging. Excisional or core needle biopsy with local anesthesia is safe during pregnancy. PET scans are postponed until after delivery even among patients with aggressive NHL subtypes, to reduce fetal exposure to radiation and 18F-FDG which is fetotoxic [55].

Treatment

Termination of Pregnancy

For patients diagnosed in the first trimester or early second trimester who have aggressive NHL types, advanced stage or symptomatic high disease burden, termination of pregnancy should be offered. Radiation therapy is the cornerstone of treatment outside of pregnancy and it is usually avoided during gestation. A woman can opt to terminate a pregnancy in order to receive treatment including radiotherapy at any gestational age, as long as it is within the gestational age criteria established by local regulations. Otherwise, termination is not expected to improve outcomes [52–57].

Radiation

Radiation is traditionally avoided during pregnancy. While there have been some reports of women receiving radiotherapy while pregnant, this is carefully considered on a case-by case basis. If the uterine fundus has not grown above the pubic symphysis, the target lesions are above the diaphragm and/or there is no response to chemotherapy, radiation may be undertaken. As the uterine fundus grows towards the sternum after week 12, radiation will result in increasing levels of fetal exposure. Depending on the dose and gestational age at treatment, radiation exposure can result in pregnancy loss, anomalies, fetal growth restriction, severe mental disability and increase in risk of childhood cancer. Radiation treatment with the associated fetal risks typically preclude consideration [52–59].

Chemotherapy and Immunotherapy

For HL patients the standard regimen is ABVD (doxorubicin, bleomycin, vinblastine, and dacarbazone). NHL patients are typically treated with either CHOP or R-CHOP (Rituximab-cyclophosphamide, doxorubicin, vincristine, and prednisone). Etoposide may be added to CHOP or R-CHOP regimens. Chemotherapeutic regimen may vary for some NHL subtypes.

Chemotherapy is typically initiated after week 14 of gestation to avoid risks of malformations. Women with aggressive subtypes that require immediate therapy in the first trimester and opt to continue their pregnancy can be treated with vinblastine and steroids (HL) or steroids alone (NHL). Standard regimen therapy can then be initiated in the second trimester, instead of delaying treatment [52–59].

Rituximab administration has been associated with neonatal B-cell depletion and cases of neonatal infection. Lymphocyte depletion is more likely if administered in the late third trimester or if the baby is delivered prematurely soon after treatment. There is no known increased risk of malformation with Rituximab even among women receiving in the first trimester for other indications such as those with autoimmune disorders [60, 61].

Surgery

There is no role for surgical treatment.

Delay of Treatment Until Postpartum

Patients that are asymptomatic with low disease burden may opt to delay therapy until delivery regardless of gestational age. They should be kept under close observation and be offered treatment if they become symptomatic or disease is noted to progress. For patients with early-stage disease and wish to delay treatment, survival outcomes are similar to that of non-pregnant women [53, 57]. Treatment can be considered as follows (Table 10.7) for each type of lymphoma and pregnancy, according to trimester of pregnancy when diagnosis was made.

Obstetric Management of Pregnant Patients with Lymphoma

Maternal Risks

All pregnant patients with cancer, regardless of type, have increased risk of severe maternal morbidity such as need for transfusion, pulmonary embolism, hysterectomy, and mechanical ventilation [25]. Patients receiving steroids for extended periods are at risk for diabetes and/or hypertension however, an increased incidence of diabetes has not been reported. There are inconsistent reports of increased risk of preeclampsia [62, 63].

Fetal Risks

Preterm delivery and small for gestational age (SGA) are the most common fetal risks. Approximate rates of each for HL are 41% and 18% and for NHL 51% and 38%. SGA is more common among those receiving chemotherapy. Use of vinblastine and steroids in the first trimester appears to be safe [53, 57]. Neurodevelopmental outcome for children of women who receive chemotherapy is expected to be normal [28].

Antenatal Testing

If receiving chemotherapy, baseline liver function testing, baseline EKG, and maternal echocardiogram should be performed. Ultrasound is indicated every three to four weeks prior to each chemotherapy session to document fetal viability and growth. Consideration may be given to adding MCA doppler monitoring to screen for fetal anemia. After 32 weeks

Table 10.7 Treatment options for lymphoma in pregnancy, stratified by trimester

First Trimester	Second Trimester	Third Trimester
- Asymptomatic and low disease burden: Can delay treatment until postpartum while undergoing close observation or plan to start chemotherapy in the second trimester. For women with HL can also consider a bridge to the second trimester with steroids or vinblastine. - Advanced/aggressive disease, women desiring usual treatment with radiation: Can offer termination of pregnancy and usual treatment with chemoradiation.	- Asymptomatic and low disease burden: Can delay treatment until postpartum while undergoing close observation or start chemotherapy - Advanced/aggressive disease, women desiring usual treatment with radiation: Termination of pregnancy and usual treatment as non-pregnant women can be offered to those who present at a gestational age that is under the cut off for local regulations, otherwise can start chemotherapy	- Asymptomatic and low disease burden: Can delay treatment until postpartum while undergoing close observation or start chemotherapy, especially if diagnosed early in the third trimester. For women diagnosed close to term, delivery with postpartum treatment may be preferred - Advanced/aggressive disease: start chemotherapy. Can consider delivery if diagnosed close to term and/or immediate need for radiation.

gestational age, weekly antenatal testing is initiated. The placenta should be sent to pathology after delivery. Consider referral to a clinical psychologist specialized in oncologic patients at least once at the onset of care.

Delivery Route and Timing

Vaginal delivery is preferred; cesarean is reserved for usual obstetric indications. Recommended gestational age at delivery is term (37 weeks) if the patient does not go into spontaneous labor or there is no other indication for delivery [52–57].

For women receiving chemotherapy, three weeks should be allowed to pass from the last treatment to delivery for recovery of maternal immunity. The final round of chemotherapy is typically given at 34–35 weeks gestational age if a term delivery is planned, but delivery timing or date of last chemotherapy may need to be adjusted according to patient's progression.

Breastfeeding

Breastfeeding is not encouraged among women who are receiving chemotherapy postpartum.

Pregnancy Among Survivors of Lymphoma

If there are secondary effects from treatment such as cardiomyopathy and pulmonary fibrosis, risks of maternal morbidity are increased. Pregnancy may exacerbate symptoms of congestive heart failure, which can be life threatening if baseline left ventricular ejection fraction is poor.

Pregnancy itself does not increase risk of relapse [64]. The majority of the recurrences have been noted within two years of diagnosis and/or treatment. Recommendation has been to wait two years before attempting conception in order to promptly treat a potential relapse.

The largest cohort study to date among pregnant lymphoma survivors included 449 Swedish women, of which 144 conceived. There were 47 reported relapses and only one was diagnosed during pregnancy. Most relapses occurred within two to three years after remission. A patient may need to consider her chances of spontaneous conception and her initial cancer staging before deciding how long to delay childbearing [65]. Preconception consultation with a maternal fetal medicine specialist is recommended.

The rates of fetal anomalies, preterm birth, and fetal growth restriction are not increased [66]. In addition to routine prenatal testing, the chemotherapeutic agents utilized should be noted in the patient's record. Baseline renal and hepatic testing should be obtained, as well as a baseline maternal EKG and echocardiogram to exclude underlying conduction anomalies or cardiomyopathy. This is particularly important among childhood survivors that are now contemplating pregnancy and have received mediastinal radiation and/or anthracycline therapy. Baseline thyroid stimulating hormone (TSH) and free thyroxine (FT4) should also be obtained during the first visit. An ultrasound may be performed at 32 weeks to screen for fetal growth restriction, but this is optional. There is no indication for weekly antenatal testing unless other obstetrical or medical complications arise.

Finally, mothers treated with radiation are at risk of secondary malignancies including breast cancer and melanoma. A mammogram can be performed while pregnant. It is important to ensure continued care with appropriate oncologic surveillance during gestation.

There is no indication for a preterm birth or early term delivery if there are no other obstetrical complications. Vaginal delivery is preferred, cesarean reserved for usual obstetric indications.

After chest wall radiation there may be decreased milk production, however this concern should not be an impediment to breastfeeding. Survivors should be encouraged to breastfeed. Among a cohort of 94 lymphoma survivors, there was a 61% breastfeeding success rate [67]. To facilitate success, these patients need extensive support such as encouragement from their oncologist and maternal fetal medicine specialists, ample social support at home and antenatal and postnatal lactation consults; the latter a factor that significantly increases the chances of success.

Leukemia and Pregnancy

Epidemiology

The incidence of leukemia in pregnancy is estimated to be 1 in 75,000 to 100,000 pregnancies. Among women of reproductive age acute leukemias are more frequent than chronic types [67].

The most common acute leukemia is myeloid (AML); promyelocytic (APL) and lymphoblastic (ALL) are less common. Unlike other cancer, acute leukemias usually require immediate treatment upon diagnosis to avoid severe maternal morbidity and mortality. Thus, termination of pregnancy is usually recommended if diagnosis is made during the first trimester. Chronic myeloid Leukemia (CML) is more common than chronic lymphocytic leukemia (CLL), but chronic types are less common in reproductive aged women [67, 68]. With prompt treatment likelihood of remission is high, but likelihood of relapse may be greater than for other malignancies associated with pregnancy.

Diagnosis and Workup

Signs and Symptoms

Patients may be asymptomatic and the disease may be apparent only during routine CBC performed during prenatal care. Neutropenia in the setting of fever or infection should be suspicious. A common symptom is fatigue, which can also be normal during gestation. Some patients present with gingival enlargement or bleeding. Advanced cases may present with DIC, hemorrhage (AML) or thrombotic events (APL, CML). Other symptoms include anorexia, weight loss, cough, and bone pain [70].

Physical Exam Findings

Suspicion for a hematologic malignancy should be heightened if petechiae, ecchymosis, lymphadenopathy or hepato-splenomegaly are detected in combination with hematological anomalies.

Staging and Other Workup

Peripheral blood smear, flow cytometry, and molecular analysis can suffice for diagnosis in some cases. Bone marrow biopsy can safely be performed as indicated [69].

Patients may require a retinal evaluation (if retinal hemorrhage is suspected), dental care, or a lumbar puncture, all of which can be performed during pregnancy. If lumbar puncture is recommended, a provider with experience performing punctures in pregnant women may be required, as with advancing uterine size the procedure can become more challenging due to patient's positioning.

A spine MRI can be performed if the patient reports severe bone pain or lower extremity neurological symptoms such as paresthesia or weakness. A baseline echocardiogram is needed before onset of most chemotherapeutic regimens.

Treatment

Termination of Pregnancy

For women diagnosed during the first trimester with acute leukemia and/or blast crisis, a delay in treatment is not advisable. Termination of pregnancy followed by immediate initiation of treatment is recommended. Chemotherapy during the first trimester leads to multiple fetal anomalies and increases risk of spontaneous miscarriage. There is an inherent risk of hemorrhage during miscarriage, which could be life threatening. If the patient is already anemic or has had a hemorrhage upon diagnosis, blood products or one round of chemotherapy may be necessary to improve blood count prior to surgical abortion [68–72].

Radiation

Although nonpregnant women with ALL may receive radiotherapy, this treatment is not an option during gestation due to fetal toxicity.

Chemotherapy

Table 10.8 summarizes different regimens used according to type of Leukemia [68–72].

Surgery

There is no surgical treatment for this cancer during gestation. Stem cell transplantation is performed postpartum if needed.

Delay of Treatment Until Postpartum

This option is only available to select patients diagnosed late in the third trimester without life threatening symptoms. Delays in treatment can increase maternal morbidity and mortality and are not routinely recommended [68–72].

In summary, during the first trimester, termination of pregnancy followed by standard treatment should be offered to women with acute leukemia or with CML-blast crisis. Others with chronic leukemia may be able to utilize leukapheresis to bridge to the second trimester. In the second and third trimester chemotherapy can be initiated safely. There are rare instances of women diagnosed close to term who have delayed treatment until after delivery in the absence of other complications. With ALL, termination of pregnancy may be advised even after first trimester (up to week 20), due to a more aggressive nature of disease and need to initiate agents like methotrexate sooner for maternal health benefit [68–72]. These complex therapeutic decisions require input from a multidisciplinary team.

When thrombotic events are a concern, lovenox and heparin can be used during any trimester in prophylactic or therapeutic dosage. Oral anticoagulant use is not recommended during gestation, warfarin is a known teratogen but it can be used safely postpartum. Regarding direct oral anticoagulants such as rivaroxaban and apixaban, recent data suggests

Table 10.8 Treatment options for leukemia diagnosed during pregnancy

Type of Leukemia	Treatment during pregnancy
AML	Cytarabine and an anthracycline (most commonly, daunorubicin or idarubicin) and occasionally with etoposide.
APL	All-trans retinoic acid (ATRA) with cytarabine and daunorubicin or idarubicin. Retinoic acid is a known teratogen when used in the first trimester but can be used after this time.
ALL	Due to low incidence during pregnancy, there is little consensus on the most appropriate regimen.
	Regimens typically include cytarabine, anthracyclines, cyclophosphamide, vincristine, prednisone and can be combined with L-asparaginase.
	The use of methotrexate is not recommended in pregnancy due to teratogenicity, although there have been some reports of use after the first trimester with reassuring fetal outcomes. Irrespective of trimester, this antimetabolite may have deleterious effects for the fetus and thus it is best to avoid if possible
CML	Leukapheresis is the mainstay of treatment during gestation. For patients in whom leukapheresis is not an option, interferon alpha and hydroxyurea may be administered after the first trimester.
	Tyrosine-kinase inhibitors are first line therapy outside of pregnancy; however they are known to be teratogenic if used during the first trimester. If a woman conceives while on tyrosine-kinase inhibitors, they should be discontinued. There are some reports of successful use during the second trimester, but it is also possible to restart the medication postpartum and obtain remission again, therefore tyrosine-kinase inhibitors are not routinely used during gestation.
CLL	There is a paucity of data due to a very low incidence during gestation, but regimens include leukapheresis, chlorambucil, and rituximab.

that teratogenicity risk may not be as high as previously thought [75] but at this time they are not recommended for pregnant or breastfeeding women.

Obstetric Management of the Pregnant Patient with Leukemia

Maternal Risks

Patients are at significant risk for infection, sepsis, hemorrhage and DIC, and is dependent on blood counts and response to treatment [71]. All pregnant patients with cancer, regardless of type, have increased risk of severe maternal morbidity such as need for transfusion, pulmonary embolism, hysterectomy, and mechanical ventilation [25].

As many as 92% of patients have been reported to achieve remission with treatment during pregnancy, however recurrence rates are approximately 30% [69, 71]. Most cases recur in the first two years, but late recurrences beyond five years have been reported [76].

Fetal Risks

There is increased risk of miscarriage, stillbirth, fetal growth restriction, and premature birth, and these risks are independent of chemotherapeutic treatment. Transient neonatal cardiomyopathy has been reported with second trimester exposure to idarubicin and ATRA, and the pediatric team should be aware of neonate's fetal exposure. If there is an emergency preterm birth shortly after chemotherapy administration, the neonate can exhibit transient myelosuppression [77–79].

Antenatal Testing

Baseline renal and hepatic function testing are recommended as well as baseline EKG and echocardiogram. Ultrasound should be performed every three to four weeks, prior to chemotherapy to document fetal viability or growth. Consideration can be given to adding MCA doppler monitoring to screen for fetal anemia, as fetal anemia has been detected [26]. After 32 weeks gestational age, weekly antenatal testing is initiated. The placenta should be sent to pathology after delivery. Consider referral to a clinical psychologist specialized in oncologic patients at least once at the onset of care.

Delivery Route and Timing

Vaginal delivery is preferred, with cesarean reserved for usual obstetric indications. If the patient's blood count is stable and there is a good response to treatment, delivery can be performed at term. Otherwise, preterm delivery may be planned. For patients who deteriorate or those who would like to defer therapy until postpartum, delivery can be facilitated as early as 32–34 weeks. Three weeks is recommended to pass after chemotherapy administration before delivery to decrease likelihood of hemorrhage and infection. The final round of chemotherapy is typically given at 34–35 weeks gestational age if a term delivery is planned. However, delivery timing or date of last chemotherapy may need to be adjusted according to patient status.

Breastfeeding

Breastfeeding is usually not recommended due to the need for chemotherapy postpartum.

Pregnancy Among Survivors of Leukemia

According to a recent cohort study including over 4000 childhood survivors that conceived, history of stem cell transplantation was associated with severe maternal morbidity such as hemorrhage, ICU admission, and sepsis, but there was not an increase in the incidence of preeclampsia, gestational diabetes, or cesarean delivery [77]. If there is preexisting cardiomyopathy or renal impairment, then maternal morbidity is further increased.

CML survivors on tyrosine kinase inhibitors such as imatinib/Gleevec and dasatinib should be counseled to stop these medications before conception. Although tyrosine kinase inhibitors do not cross the placenta, first trimester embryonic exposure has been associated with skeletal, renal, and respiratory anomalies and omphalocele. There are reports of patients restarting this medication in the second trimester, however current recommendations are to delay restart of all tyrosine kinases until postpartum [73]. For those who relapse during pregnancy, interferon-alpha and hydroxyurea may be used after the first trimester.

Pregnancy itself does not increase risk of cancer relapse. The majority of the recurrences have been noted within two years of diagnosis and/or treatment completion. Hence, expert recommendation has been to delay conception for two years in order to avoid a relapse during pregnancy. There are no adequate studies to challenge the recommendation to delay conception. In addition, most cases of ALL occur during childhood, hence patients will usually present with pregnancy decades after treatment. Preconception consultation with a maternal fetal medicine specialist is recommended.

The rate of anomalies is that of the expected general population. History of alkylating agents and stem cell transplantation has been associated with increased risk of preterm birth [79].

Total body irradiation (TBI) may be performed prior to stem cell transplantation. TBI reduces myometrial and endometrial thickness, and impairs uterine vascularity resulting in decreased uterine blood flow and ovarian reserve [80]. All TBI recipients are at risk for infertility; risk is higher with high TBI doses (>800 cGy) and younger age at therapy [80–82]. Among survivors that received TBI, only 22% of teenager survivors report regular menses, 45% have iatrogenic premature ovarian insufficiency [83] and the pregnancy rate is approximately 22% (with 7.5% of those women reporting use of assisted reproductive techniques) [84]. There is an increased risk of preterm birth, low birth weight and miscarriage[80, 83, 84]. Placental abnormalities such as placenta accreta have been reported after TBI among survivors of myelodysplastic syndrome, CML, HL, and also after pelvic radiation for Wilms tumor and anal cancer [85–87].

A preconception ultrasound can be performed to assess uterus size, although this does not reliably predict fertility or pregnancy outcome. Careful examination of the placenta should be performed during fetal anatomy scan.

Previous chemotherapeutic agents should be recorded. Baseline renal and hepatic function testing should be obtained. An ultrasound can be performed at 32 weeks to screen for fetal growth restriction but this is optional. There is no indication for weekly antenatal testing unless other obstetrical or medical complications arise. Baseline EKG and maternal echocardiogram should be performed as most treatment regimens for leukemia include cardiotoxic medications.

There is no indication for a preterm birth or early term delivery as long as there are no other obstetrical complications. Vaginal delivery is preferred, cesarean reserved for usual obstetric indications. Breastfeeding is encouraged. Survivors that have a history of cranial radiation may have decreased milk production due to hypopituitarism, and support from a lactation consultant should be provided [80].

Additional Considerations

Pregnancy After Remote History of Anthracycline Use

Anthracycline based chemotherapeutic agents (e.g. Daunorubicin, doxorubicin, epirubicin. idarubicin, mitoxantrone, calrubicin) are utilized for various malignancies. Each agent has a different threshold cumulative dose, but typically with doses that exceed 250 mg/m2, there is increased risk of cardiotoxicity [89]. Cardiac damage is progressive, and symptoms may not present for months or years following treatment. The physiologic changes of pregnancy may unmask underlying heart failure.

Anthracycline related cardiomyopathy is a diagnosis of exclusion, defined as a decrease in left ventricular ejection fraction of at least 10% from baseline. Factors that increase risk are younger age at cancer diagnosis, longer time from cancer treatment to pregnancy and higher cumulative dose [89, 90]. Cardiotoxicity may be exacerbated by additional treatment such as radiation to the chest, trastuzumab, cyclophosphamide, protein kinase inhibitors, and tyrosine kinase inhibitors.

Patients with cancer related cardiac dysfunction have a 47.4-fold higher odds of experiencing left ventricular dysfunction and heart failure during pregnancy [91]. Cardiovascular disease remains a leading cause of maternal death in the United States. It is imperative to perform routine echocardiograms among survivors that received anthracyclines, particularly those treated during childhood. For those considering pregnancy, an echocardiogram within twelve months prior to conception is recommended, even if they are well-appearing and asymptomatic. If an echocardiogram was not performed prior to conception, then one should be obtained at time of presentation to prenatal care.

If cardiac dysfunction is confirmed then the patient should be assessed by a cardiologist regularly and assigned a modified WHO pregnancy risk classification, to determine pregnancy monitoring and delivery strategy [92].

Counseling Women Who Desire to Breastfeed Despite Receiving Chemotherapy Postpartum

Some women will elect to "pump and dump" their milk while they are receiving chemotherapy in an effort to establish and maintain their milk supply. Once chemotherapy is completed and the metabolites are no longer present in the breast milk, they will then initiate breastfeeding. The specific window of time required for drug clearance from the breast milk varies by drug and can be days to months [93]. A lactation consultation should be arranged for all women receiving chemotherapy postpartum to advise regarding drug clearance timeframe, milk suppression strategies, and/or to provide education on breast pumping and latching of the baby after prolonged bottle feeding.

Case Resolution

For the 35-year-old woman complaining of a breast mass the next step in management is bilateral mammogram without delay, complemented with a breast ultrasound. Breast biopsy should be performed without delay if indicated, regardless of patient's pregnancy or breastfeeding status. This patient eventually underwent mammogram and stereotactic biopsy that confirmed a ductal carcinoma.

Take Home Points

- Expedite diagnostic testing; do not delay solely because of pregnancy or postpartum state. Delays in diagnosis can lead to more advanced stages of disease.
- Breast sonogram and mammogram are safe during pregnancy and lactation.
- Most patients who are treated for cancer during pregnancy have similar outcomes to non-pregnant patients and thus termination of pregnancy is not routinely recommended. However, patients with aggressive or advanced disease who present early in gestation can consider termination.
- Radiotherapy is generally avoided during gestation.
- Chemotherapy can be safely started after the first trimester (14 weeks) with some modifications to avoid highly fetotoxic drugs.
- Offspring of women that received chemotherapy while pregnant have normal neurodevelopmental outcomes.
- Iatrogenic premature delivery must be avoided whenever possible, as gestational age at delivery is the main determinant of neonatal outcomes. Term deliveries (37 weeks) are preferred.
- Vaginal delivery is the preferred route of delivery, with exceptions for some patients with cervical cancer for whom a cesarean delivery may be recommended.
- Cancer survivors considering pregnancy should be screened for baseline renal, hepatic, and cardiac function. Echocardiogram should be ordered if the patient received anthracyclines.
- Women with history radiation to the chest, including left sided radiation for breast cancer, should be screened for delayed cardiac toxicity with EKG and echocardiogram.
- Consistent communication between oncology and maternal fetal medicine is imperative during pregnancy.

References

1. Smith L. H., Danielsen B., Allen M. E., Cress R. Cancer associated with obstetric delivery: results of linkage with the California cancer registry. *American journal of obstetrics and gynecology.* 2003;**189**(4):1128–35.

2. Stensheim H., Møller B., Van Dijk T., Fosså S. D. Cause-specific survival for women diagnosed with cancer during pregnancy or lactation: a registry-based cohort study. *Journal of Clinical Oncology.* 2009;**27**(1):45–51.

3. Eibye S., Kjær S. K., Mellemkjær L. Incidence of pregnancy-associated cancer in Denmark, 1977–2006. *Obstetrics & Gynecology.* 2013;**122**(3):608–17.

4. Boere I., Lok C., Poortmans P., et al. Breast cancer during pregnancy: epidemiology, phenotypes, presentation during pregnancy and therapeutic modalities. *Best Pract Res Clin Obstet Gynaecol.* 2022;**82**:46–59.

5. Navrozoglou I., Vrekoussis T., Kontostolis E., et al. Breast cancer during pregnancy: A mini-review. *European Journal of Surgical Oncology (EJSO).* 2008;**34**(8):837–43.

6. Amant F., Nekljudova V., Maggen C., et al. Outcome of breast cancer patients treated with chemotherapy during pregnancy compared with non-pregnant controls. *European Journal of Cancer.* 2022;**170**:54–63.

7. Alex A., Bhandary E., McGuire K. P. *Anatomy and Physiology of the Breast during Pregnancy and Lactation.* Diseases of the Breast during Pregnancy and Lactation. 2020;**1252**:3–7.

8. Vashi R., Hooley R., Butler R., Geisel J., Philpotts L. Breast imaging of the pregnant and lactating patient: Physiologic changes and common benign entities. *American Journal of Roentgenology*. 2013;**200**(2):329–36.

9. Mitchell K. B., Johnson H. M., Eglash A. Academy of Breastfeeding Medicine. *ABM Clinical Protocol# 30: breast masses, breast complaints, and diagnostic breast imaging in the lactating woman. Breastfeeding Medicine*. 2019;**14**(4):208–14.

10. American College of Obstetricians and Gynecologists Practice Bulletin No. 164 Summary. Diagnosis and management of benign breast disorders. *Obstet Gynecol*. 2016 Jun;**127**(6):1181–3.

11. ACOG Committee Opinion No. 273. Guidelines for diagnostic imaging during pregnancy and lactation. *Obstet Gynecol*. 2017;**130**(4):e210–e216.

12. Slanetz P. J., Moy L., Baron P., et al. ACR Appropriateness Criteria® breast imaging of pregnant and lactating women. *Journal of the American College of Radiology*. 2018;**15**(11):S263–75.

13. American Society of Breast Surgeons. Position Statement on Screening Mammography. 2018. www.breastsur geons.org/docs/statements/Position-State ment-on-Screening-Mammography.pdf

14. Collins J. C., Liao S., Wile A. G. Surgical management of breast masses in pregnant women. *The Journal of Reproductive Medicine*. 1995;**40**(11):785–8.

15. Johnson H. M., Mitchell K. B. Low incidence of milk fistula with continued breastfeeding following radiologic and surgical interventions on the lactating breast. *Breast Disease*. 2021;**40**(3):183–9.

16. Keleher A., Wendt III R., Delpassand E., Stachowiak A. M., Kuerer H. M. The safety of lymphatic mapping in pregnant breast cancer patients using Tc-99 m sulfur colloid. *The Breast Journal*. 2004;**10**(6):492–5.

17. Han S. N., Amant F., Cardonick E. H., et al. Axillary staging for breast cancer during pregnancy: Feasibility and safety of sentinel lymph node biopsy. *Breast Cancer Research and Treatment*. 2018;**168**(2):551–7.

18. Wolters V., Heimovaara J., Maggen C., et al. Management of pregnancy in women with cancer. *International Journal of Gynecologic Cancer*. 2021;**31**(3):314–22.

19. Loibl S., Han S. N., von Minckwitz G., et al. Treatment of breast cancer during pregnancy: an observational study. *The Lancet Oncology*. 2012;**13**(9):887–96.

20. Shah N. M., Scott D. M., Kandagatla P., et al. Young women with breast cancer: Fertility preservation options and management of pregnancy-associated breast cancer. *Annals of Surgical Oncology*. 2019;**26**(5):1214–24.

21. Reprotox. Herceptin. 2022. www.reprotox .org/member/agents/25182/printSummary

22. Reprotox. Tamoxifen. 2022. www.reprotox .org/member/agents/17850

23. Schuurman T. N., Witteveen P. O., Van Der Wall E., et al. Tamoxifen and pregnancy: An absolute contraindication?. *Breast Cancer Research and Treatment*. 2019;**175**(1):17–25.

24. Keyser C. E., Staat M. B., Fausett C. M., Shields L. C. Pregnancy-associated breast cancer. *Reviews in Obstetrics and Gynecology*. 2012;**5**(2):94–9.

25. Matsuo K., Klar M., Youssefzadeh A. C., et al. Assessment of severe maternal morbidity and mortality in pregnancies complicated by cancer in the US. *JAMA Oncology*. 2022;**8**(8):1213–16.

26. Nowik C. M., Gerrie A. S., Wong J. Conservative management of presumed fetal anemia secondary to maternal chemotherapy for acute myeloid leukemia. *American Journal of Perinatology Reports*. 2021;**11**(04):e137–41.

27. La Nasa M., Gaughan J., Cardonick E. Incidence of neonatal neutropenia and leukopenia after in utero exposure to chemotherapy for maternal cancer. *American Journal of Clinical Oncology*. 2019;**42**(4):351–4.

28. Cardonick E. H., Gringlas M. B., Hunter K., Greenspan J. Development of children born to mothers with cancer during pregnancy: Comparing in utero chemotherapy-exposed children with

nonexposed controls. *American Journal of Obstetrics and Gynecology.* 2015;**212**(5):658–e1.

29. Lambertini M., Ameye L., Hamy A. S., et al. Pregnancy after breast cancer in patients with germline BRCA mutations. *Journal of Clinical Oncology.* 2020;**38**(26):3012–23.

30. Iqbal J., Amir E., Rochon P. A., et al. Association of the timing of pregnancy with survival in women with breast cancer. *JAMA Oncology.* 2017;**3**(5):659–65.

31. Alipour S., Omranipour R., editors. *Diseases of the Breast during Pregnancy and Lactation.* Springer; 2020.

32. Azim Jr H. A., Bellettini G., Liptrott S. J., et al. Breastfeeding in breast cancer survivors: Pattern, behaviour and effect on breast cancer outcome. *The Breast.* 2010;**19**(6):527–31.

33. Bhurosy T., Niu Z., Heckman C. J. Breastfeeding is possible: A systematic review on the feasibility and challenges of breastfeeding among breast cancer survivors of reproductive age. *Annals of Surgical Oncology.* 2021;**28**(7):3723–35.

34. Halaska M. J., Uzan C., Han S. N., et al. Characteristics of patients with cervical cancer during pregnancy: A multicenter matched cohort study. An initiative from the International Network on Cancer, Infertility and Pregnancy. *International Journal of Gynecologic Cancer.* 2019;**29**(4).

35. Bhatla N., Aoki D., Sharma D. N., Sankaranarayanan R. Cancer of the cervix uteri: 2021 update. *International Journal of Gynecology & Obstetrics.* 2021;**155**:28–44.

36. Beharee N., Shi Z., Wu D., Wang J. Diagnosis and treatment of cervical cancer in pregnant women. *Cancer Medicine.* 2019;**8**(12):5425–30.

37. Perkins R. B., Guido R. S., Castle P. E., et al. Erratum: 2019 ASCCP risk-based management consensus guidelines for abnormal cervical cancer screening tests and cancer precursors. *Journal of Lower Genital Tract Disease.* 2021;**25**(4):330–1.

38. Mailath-Pokorny M., Schwameis R., Grimm C., Reinthaller A., Polterauer S. Natural history of cervical intraepithelial neoplasia in pregnancy: Postpartum histo-pathologic outcome and review of the literature. *BMC Pregnancy and Childbirth.* 2016;**16**(1):1–6.

39. Robinson W. R., Webb S., Tirpack J., Degefu S., O'Quinn A. G. Management of cervical intraepithelial neoplasia during pregnancy with LOOP excision. *Gynecologic Oncology.* 1997;**64**(1):153–5.

40. Han S. N., Mhallem Gziri M., Van Calsteren K., Amant F. Cervical cancer in pregnant women: treat, wait or interrupt? Assessment of current clinical guidelines, innovations and controversies. *Therapeutic Advances in Medical Oncology.* 2013;**5**(4):211–19.

41. European Society of Gynaecological Oncology. Cervical cancer chapter. https://eacademy.esgo.org/pdfviewer/web/viewer.html?file=https%3A//eacademy.esgo.org/util/document_library%3Fdc_id%3D3351%26g_id%3D41%26vxc%3D/esgo/document_library%3Fdc_id%3D3351

42. Ilancheran A. Neoadjuvant chemotherapy in cervical cancer in pregnancy. *Best Practice & Research Clinical Obstetrics & Gynaecology.* 2016;33:102–7.

43. Bigelow C. A., Horowitz N. S., Goodman A., et al. Management and outcome of cervical cancer diagnosed in pregnancy. *American Journal of Obstetrics and Gynecology.* 2017;**216**(3):276–e1.

44. American College of Obstetricians and Gynecologists. Prediction and prevention of spontaneous preterm birth: ACOG Practice Bulletin, Number 234. *Obstetrics and Gynecology.* 2021;**138**(2):e65–90.

45. McIntosh J., Feltovich H., Berghella V., Manuck T. The role of routine cervical length screening in selected high-and low-risk women for preterm birth prevention. *American Journal of Obstetrics and Gynecology.* 2016;**215**(3):B2–7.

46. Cliby W. A., Dodson M. K., Podratz K. C. Cervical cancer complicated by pregnancy: episiotomy site recurrences following vaginal delivery. *Obstetrics and Gynecology.* 1994;**84**(2):179–82.

47. Arakawa A., Ichikawa H., Kubo T., et al. Vaginal transmission of cancer from

mothers with cervical cancer to infants. *New England Journal of Medicine.* 2021;**384**(1):42–50.

48. Paraskevaidis E., Bilirakis E., Koliopoulos G., et al. Cervical regeneration after diathermy excision of cervical intraepithelial neoplasia as assessed by transvaginal sonography. *European Journal of Obstetrics & Gynecology and Reproductive Biology.* 2002;**102**(1):88–91.

49. Himes K. P., Simhan H. N. Time from cervical conization to pregnancy and preterm birth. *Obstetrics & Gynecology.* 2007;**109**(2):314–19.

50. Baucom A., Herzog T., Jackson A., Wahab S. A., Billingsley C. A case of placenta previa with increta with a history of pelvic radiation. *Gynecologic Oncology Reports.* 2021;37:100800.

51. Bentivegna E., Maulard A., Pautier P., et al. Fertility results and pregnancy outcomes after conservative treatment of cervical cancer: A systematic review of the literature. *Fertility and Sterility.* 2016;**106**(5):1195–211.

52. Pinnix C. C., Osborne E. M., Chihara D., et al. Maternal and fetal outcomes after therapy for Hodgkin or non-Hodgkin lymphoma diagnosed during pregnancy. *JAMA oncology.* 2016;**2**(8):1065–9.

53. Maggen C., Dierickx D., Cardonick E., et al. Maternal and neonatal outcomes in 80 patients diagnosed with non-Hodgkin lymphoma during pregnancy: Results from the International Network of Cancer, Infertility and Pregnancy. *British Journal of Haematology.* 2021;**193**(1):52–62.

54. Shah M. R., Brandt J. S., David K. A., Evens A. M. Lymphoma occurring during pregnancy: Current diagnostic and therapeutic approaches. *Current Oncology Reports.* 2020;**22**(11):1–3.

55. Kritharis A., Walsh E. P., Evens A. M. Managing lymphoma during pregnancy. In Azim H. A. (ed.), *Managing Cancer During Pregnancy* (pp. 159–73). Springer; 2016.

56. Pinnix C. C., Andraos T. Y., Milgrom S., Fanale M. A. The management of lymphoma in the setting of pregnancy. *Current Hematologic Malignancy Reports.* 2017;**12**(3):251–6.

57. Maggen C., Dierickx D., Lugtenburg P., et al. Obstetric and maternal outcomes in patients diagnosed with Hodgkin lymphoma during pregnancy: A multicentre, retrospective, cohort study. *The Lancet Haematology.* 2019;**6**(11): e551–61.

58. Kal H. B., Struikmans H. Radiotherapy during pregnancy: Fact and fiction. *The Lancet Oncology.* 2005;**6**(5):328–33.

59. Woo S. Y., Fuller L. M., Cundiff J. H., et al. Radiotherapy during pregnancy for clinical stages IA–IIA Hodgkin's disease. *International Journal of Radiation Oncology* Biology* Physics.* 1992;**23**(2):407–12.

60. Das G., Damotte V., Gelfand J. M., et al. Rituximab before and during pregnancy: a systematic review, and a case series in MS and NMOSD. *Neurology-Neuroimmunology Neuroinflammation.* 2018;**5**(3):e453.

61. Reprotox. Rituximab 2022. www.reprotox .org/member/agents/28797

62. Anand S. T., Ryckman K. K., Baer R. J., et al. Hypertensive disorders of pregnancy among women with a history of leukemia or lymphoma. *Pregnancy Hypertension.* 2022;29:101–7.

63. Evens A. M., Advani R., Press O. W., et al. Lymphoma occurring during pregnancy: antenatal therapy, complications, and maternal survival in a multicenter analysis. *Journal of Clinical Oncology.* 2013;**31**(32):4132–9.

64. Gaudio F., Nardelli C., Masciandaro P., et al. Pregnancy rate and outcome of pregnancies in long-term survivors of Hodgkin's lymphoma. *Annals of Hematology.* 2019;**98**(8):1947–52.

65. Weibull C. E., Eloranta S., Smedby K. E., et al. Pregnancy and the risk of relapse in patients diagnosed with Hodgkin lymphoma. *J Clin Oncol.* 2016;**34**:337–44.

66. Shliakhtsitsava K., Romero S. A., Dewald S. R., Su H. I. Pregnancy and child health outcomes in pediatric and young

adult leukemia and lymphoma survivors: A systematic review. *Leukemia & Lymphoma.* 2018;**59**(2):381–97.

67. McCullough L., Ng A., Najita J., et al. Breastfeeding in survivors of Hodgkin lymphoma treated with chest radiotherapy. *Cancer.* 2010;**116**(20):4866–71.

68. Fracchiolla N. S., Sciumè M., Dambrosi F., et al. Acute myeloid leukemia and pregnancy: Clinical experience from a single center and a review of the literature. *BMC Cancer.* 2017;**17**(1):1–8.

69. Milojkovic D., Apperley J. F. How I treat leukemia during pregnancy. *Blood, The Journal of the American Society of Hematology.* 2014;**123**(7):974–84.

70. Vandenbriele C., Dierickx D., Amant F., Delforge M. The treatment of hematologic malignancies in pregnancy. *Facts, Views & Vision in ObGyn.* 2010;**2**(2):74–87.

71. Chelghoum Y., Vey N., Raffoux E., et al. Acute leukemia during pregnancy: A report on 37 patients and a review of the literature. *Cancer.* 2005;**104**(1):110–17.

72. Brenner B., Avivi I., Lishner M. Haematological cancer in pregnancy. *The Lancet.* 2012;**379**(9815):580–7.

73. Cortes J., O'Brien S., Ault P., et al. Pregnancy outcomes among patients with chronic myeloid leukemia treated with dasatinib. *Blood.* 2008;**112**(11):3230.

74. Reprotox. Imatinib. 2022. www.reprotox .org/member/agents/25202

75. Beyer-Westendorf J., Tittl L., Bistervels I., et al. Safety of direct oral anticoagulant exposure during pregnancy: A retrospective cohort study. *The Lancet Haematology.* 2020;**7**(12):e884–91.

76. Aldoss I., Pillai R., Yang D., et al. Late and very late relapsed acute lymphoblastic leukemia: Clinical and molecular features, and treatment outcomes. *Blood Cancer Journal.* 2021;**11**(7):1–4.

77. Zgardau A., Ray J. G., Baxter N. N., et al. Obstetrical and perinatal outcomes in female survivors of childhood and adolescent cancer: A population-based cohort study. *JNCI: Journal of the National Cancer Institute.* 2022;**114**(4):553–64.

78. Siu B. L., Alonzo M. R., Vargo T. A., Fenrich A. L. Transient dilated cardiomyopathy in a newborn exposed to idarubicin and all-trans-retinoic acid (ATRA) early in the second trimester of pregnancy. *International Journal of Gynecologic Cancer.* 2002;**12**(4):399–402.

79. Anand S. T., Chrischilles E. A., Baer R. J., et al. The risk of preterm birth among women with a history of leukemia or lymphoma. *The Journal of Maternal-Fetal & Neonatal Medicine.* 2021;**8**:1–9.

80. Teh W. T., Stern C., Chander S., Hickey M. The Impact of Uterine Radiation on Subsequent Fertility and Pregnancy Outcomes. *BioMed research international.* 2014;**2014**:482968.

81. Loren A. W., Chow E., Jacobsohn D. A., et al. Pregnancy after hematopoietic cell transplantation: A report from the late effects working committee of the Center for International Blood and Marrow Transplant Research (CIBMTR). *Biology of Blood and Marrow Transplantation.* 2011;**17**(2):157–66.

82. Balas N., Hageman L., Wu J., et al. Conditioning intensity and probability of live birth after blood or marrow transplantation, a BMTSS report. *Blood Advances.* 2022;**6**(8):2471–9.

83. Chiodi S., Spinelli S., Bruzzi P., et al. Menstrual patterns, fertility and main pregnancy outcomes after allogeneic haematopoietic stem cell transplantation. *Journal of Obstetrics and Gynaecology.* 2016;**36**(6):783–8.

84. Gerstl B., Sullivan E., Koch J., et al. Reproductive outcomes following a stem cell transplant for a haematological malignancy in female cancer survivors: A systematic review and meta-analysis. *Supportive Care in Cancer.* 2019;**27**:4451–60.

85. Sasagasako N., Tani H., Chigusa Y., et al. Placenta Accreta in a woman with childhood uterine irradiation: A case report and literature review. *Case Reports in Obstetrics and Gynecology.* 2019;**2019**:2452975.

86. Bowman Z. S., Simons M., Sok C., Draper M. L. Cervical insufficiency and

placenta accreta after prior pelvic radiation. *Journal of Obstetrics and Gynaecology.* 2014;**34**(8):735.

87. Baucom A., Herzog T., Jackson A., Wahab S. A., Billingsley C. A case of placenta previa with increta with a history of pelvic radiation. *Gynecologic Oncology Reports.* 2021;37:100800.

88. Ogg S. W., Hudson M. M., Randolph M. E., Klosky J. L. Protective effects of breastfeeding for mothers surviving childhood cancer. *Journal of Cancer Survivorship.* 2011;**5**(2):175–81.

89. Bansal N., Hazim C. F., Badillo S., et al. Maternal cardiovascular outcomes of pregnancy in childhood, adolescent, and young adult cancer survivors. *Journal of Cardiovascular Development and Disease.* 2022;**9**(11):373.

90. Thompson K. A. Pregnancy and cardiomyopathy after anthracyclines in childhood. *Frontiers in Cardiovascular Medicine.* 2018;5:14.

91. Nolan M., Oikonomou E. K., Silversides C. K., et al. Impact of cancer therapy-related cardiac dysfunction on risk of heart failure in pregnancy. *Cardio Oncology.* 2020;**2**(2):153–62.

92. American College of Obstetricians and Gynecologists Practice Bulletin No. 212. Pregnancy and heart disease. *Obstet Gynecol.* 2019 May;**133**(5): e320–56.

93. Drugs and Lactation Database (LactMed®) [Internet]. Bethesda (MD): National Institute of Child Health and Human Development; 2006. www.ncbi.nlm.nih .gov/books/NBK500576/

Survivorship Care of Gynecologic Cancer

Ana C. Nelson and Therese B. Bevers

Case Presentation

Ms. Smith is a 60-year-old female with a history of right breast ductal carcinoma in situ (DCIS), estrogen receptor/progesterone receptor (ER/PR) positive diagnosed at age 50, treated with segmental mastectomy, radiation, and tamoxifen for 5 years. She then developed stage 1 endometrial adenocarcinoma at the age of 55, treated with hysterectomy and bilateral salpingo-oophorectomy. She complains of hot flashes, night sweats, and dyspareunia. She is currently not exercising. Screening mammogram was benign. Bone density testing revealed osteopenia and vitamin D level was low (28 ng/ml). She smokes one pack of cigarettes a day for the past 20 years. Body mass index (BMI) is 40. Physical exam was unremarkable, except for evidence of vaginal atrophy. What are your recommendations for care?

Epidemiology

More women are surviving gynecologic cancer secondary to advances in cancer screening, diagnosis, and treatment. From 2012 to 2018, the 5-year survival rates for cervical, endometrial, and ovarian cancer were 66.7%, 81.3%, and 49.7%, respectively [1, 2, 3]. The overall 5-year survival for breast cancer was 90.6% from 2011 to 2017 [4], achieving a rate of 99% for women treated for localized invasive breast cancer [5]. Furthermore, the 5-year survival rate for women treated for ductal carcinoma in situ (DCIS) with ipsilateral mastectomy is 95.6% and survival with breast conserving therapy and radiation is 94.8% [6]. Cancer patients are typically followed by their oncologist for a period of time after diagnosis that varies by the specific cancer site. This chapter will discuss the care of women with female cancer after five years of diagnosis – typically referred to as survivorship care.

Survivorship Care

Survivorship care typically starts at the five-year point and may be provided by the primary care team or general gynecology. The four domains of survivorship care include: surveillance, monitoring for late effects, risk reduction and early detection, and psychological functioning (Table 11.1) [7].

Surveillance and Monitoring for Late Effects

Patients with a history of cancer are seen annually to assess for disease recurrence. The clinician should review the patient's allergies, medications, past medical history, surgical history, family history of cancer, psychosocial history, and perform a focused physical exam, depending on the cancer specific site. Routine blood work is not typically performed for

Ana C. Nelson, Therese B. Bevers, MD

Table 11.1 Core domains of survivorship care

Surveillance

- Detection of cancer recurrence

Monitoring for Late Effects

- Maintenance and observation of vital organ function

Risk Reduction and Early Detection

- Lifestyle changes to reduce cancer risk and screening to detect a second cancer early

Psychosocial Function

- Support services to maintain healthy relationships and restore life

female cancer survivors, although tumor markers, such as CA-125, βhCG, and CEA, will be obtained for some cancer types. Imaging with chest x-ray, computed tomography, or magnetic resonance imaging is not recommended for asymptomatic patients. Patients are encouraged to visit their primary care providers or internist on an annual basis for a general physical exam and routine blood work, and other specific testing such as cardiac screening after anthracycline exposure.

The treatment of gynecologic cancer includes a combination of surgery, radiation, and/ or chemotherapy. Breast cancer treatment will include possible use of endocrine therapy with tamoxifen or aromatase inhibitors, such as anastrozole, exemestane, or letrozole. While late effects are spelled out in site specific chapters, it is important to note late conditions for survivorship patients of female cancer, such as bone health and sexual function.

There are various survivorship algorithms in clinical use. Listed below are our institutional algorithms for managing the survivorship care of cervical, endometrial, ovarian, and breast cancer patients.

Cervical Cancer Survivorship

Patients with a history of cervical cancer with no evidence of disease (NED) are transitioned to survivorship care at five years post-treatment (Figure 11.1). Cervical cancer survivors are seen annually for history and physical exams, including pap tests and pelvic exams. These patients should also start annual screening mammogram with a clinical breast exam (CBE) at the age of 40 and colonoscopy for colon cancer screening at the age of 45. Bone and sexual health are also assessed at every clinic visit [8].

Endometrial Cancer Survivorship

Patients with a history of endometrial cancer with NED are transitioned to survivorship care at three to five years post-treatment depending on whether they are considered low- or high-risk survivors (Figure 11.2). Low-risk survivors are those that presented with early-stage disease and were treated with surgery alone. High-risk survivors are defined as those who received surgery plus chemotherapy or radiation therapy. These patients are seen annually for history and physical with a pelvic exam. In addition, patients with a history of endometrial cancer whose pathology revealed adenosarcoma and/or high-grade serous subtypes

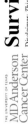
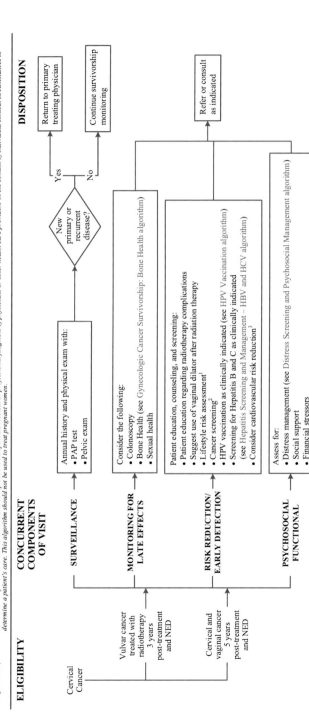

Figure 11.1 Cervical cancer survivorship algorithm. 2021. The University of Texas MD Anderson Cancer Center [8]

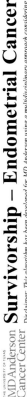

MD Anderson Cancer Center
THE UNIVERSITY OF TEXAS
Making Cancer History®

Survivorship – Endometrial Cancer

Disclaimer: This algorithm has been developed for MD Anderson using a multidisciplinary approach considering circumstances particular to MD Anderson's specific patient population, services and structure, and clinical information. This is not intended to replace the independent medical or professional judgment of physicians or other health care providers in the context of individual clinical circumstances to determine a patient's care. This algorithm should not be used to treat pregnant women.

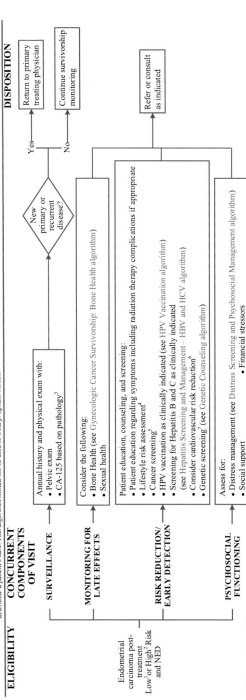

ELIGIBILITY	CONCURRENT COMPONENTS OF VISIT		DISPOSITION

ELIGIBILITY

Endometrial carcinoma post-treatment Low[1] or High[2] Risk and NED

SURVEILLANCE

Annual history and physical exam with:
- Pelvic exam
- CA-125 based on pathology[3]

MONITORING FOR LATE EFFECTS

Consider the following:
- Bone Health (see Gynecologic Cancer Survivorship: Bone Health algorithm)
- Sexual health

RISK REDUCTION/ EARLY DETECTION

Patient education, counseling, and screening:
- Patient education regarding symptoms including radiation therapy complications if appropriate
- Lifestyle risk assessment[4]
- Cancer screening[5]
- HPV vaccination as clinically indicated (see HPV Vaccination algorithm)
- Screening for Hepatitis B and C as clinically indicated (see Hepatitis Screening and Management – HBV and HCV algorithm)
- Consider cardiovascular risk reduction[6]
- Genetic screening[7] (see Genetic Counseling algorithm)

PSYCHOSOCIAL FUNCTIONING

Assess for:
- Distress management (see Distress Screening and Psychosocial Management algorithm)
- Social support
- Financial stressors

New primary or recurrent disease?

Yes → Return to primary treating physician

No → Continue survivorship monitoring

Refer or consult as indicated

NED = no evidence of disease

[1] Low risk endometrial cancer is defined as any patient who did not receive chemotherapy or radiotherapy as adjuvant treatment after their initial surgery. Survivorship begins 3 years post-treatment and NED.
[2] High risk defined as patients who received chemotherapy or radiotherapy as adjuvant treatment after their surgery. Survivorship begins 5 years post-treatment and NED.
[3] • Uterine carcinosarcoma – CA-125 annually
• High grade, serous types – CA-125 annually, if previously elevated
[4] See Physical Activity, Nutrition, and Tobacco Cessation algorithms; ongoing reassessment of lifestyle risks should be a part of routine clinical practice
[5] Includes breast, cervical (if appropriate), colorectal, liver, lung, pancreatic, and skin cancer screening
[6] Consider use of Vanderbilt's ABCDE's approach to cardiovascular health
[7] Consider genetic counseling if there has been a significant family history change since the last genetic consult, or if the patient has not previously had genetic counseling and has Lynch Syndrome risk factors. Lynch Syndrome risk factors: personal history of colon or rectal cancer; immediate family (first degree relatives such as parent, child, or sibling) with colorectal or endometrial cancer; immediate or extended family (first, second or third degree relatives including parent, child, sibling, aunt, uncle, nieces, nephews, grandparents, and first cousins) diagnosed before age 50 with colon, rectal or uterine cancer; any relatives tested positive for a Lynch Syndrome mutation (EPCAM, MLH1, MSH2, MSH6, PMS2 genes).

Department of Clinical Effectiveness V8
Approved by the Executive Committee of the Medical Staff on 05/18/2021

Copyright 2021 The University of Texas MD Anderson Cancer Center

Figure 11.2 Endometrial cancer survivorship algorithm. 2021. The University of Texas MD Anderson Cancer Center [9]

should undergo annual CA-125 testing if previously elevated [9]. These patients should also start annual screening mammogram with a CBE at the age of 40 and colonoscopy for colon cancer screening at the age of 45. Bone and sexual health are also assessed at every clinic visit [9].

Ovarian Cancer Survivorship

Patients with a history of ovarian cancer with NED are transitioned to survivorship care at five years post-treatment (Figure 11.3). These patients are seen in clinic on an annual basis for history and physical exams including pelvic examination. Annual assessment of CA-125 is performed for all types of ovarian cancer. Patients with a history of ovarian choriocarcinoma and gestational trophoblastic disease should obtain annual βhCG assessments; patients with a history of ovarian mucinous cancer should obtain annual CEA testing [10]. These patients should also start annual screening mammogram with a clinical breast exam at the age of 40 and colonoscopy for colon cancer screening at the age of 45. Bone and sexual health are also assessed at every clinic visit [10].

Breast Cancer Survivorship

Women with a history of noninvasive breast cancer with NED are transitioned to survivorship care at 6–24 months from date of diagnosis (Figure 11.4). These patients are seen for a history and physical exam to include a clinical breast exam every 6 to 12 months and annual mammogram [11]. Women with a history of invasive breast cancer who are NED are transitioned to survivorship care three to five years from the date of diagnosis (Figure 11.5). Annual history and physical exam with CBE and annual mammogram are recommended. In the first five years after diagnosis, these patients should obtain an annual diagnostic mammogram, but after five years of diagnosis, annual screening mammogram is acceptable [12]. It is preferred that the mammograms are with tomosynthesis.

Premenopausal patients with estrogen receptor (ER) positive breast cancer are typically treated with tamoxifen for five years. Postmenopausal patients with ER positive breast cancer are typically treated with an aromatase inhibitor (AI), such as anastrozole, exemestane, letrozole, or tamoxifen for 5–10 years. It is important to assess compliance and toxicity of these medications. Selective estrogen receptor modulators (SERMs) and AIs are associated with hot flashes, night sweats, vaginal dryness, and joint pain. Tamoxifen has an increased risk of uterine cancer if the patient is postmenopausal, so patients should be monitored for any abnormal vaginal bleeding. If abnormal vaginal bleeding occurs, a transvaginal ultrasound and an endometrial biopsy are recommended. Aromatase inhibitors confer an increased risk of osteopenia and osteoporosis, so bone density screening every one year is indicated.

Bone Health

Bone loss is a frequent late treatment effect for female cancer survivors. Some studies have found that 46.9% and 13.6% of women treated for gynecologic cancer were diagnosed with osteopenia and osteoporosis, respectively [13]. Other studies have found that 66% of the breast cancer survivors were diagnosed with osteoporosis [14].

Health care providers should recommend 1,000–1,200 mg daily consumption of calcium (divided am and pm) and 800–1,000 IU of vitamin D, engagement in weight bearing

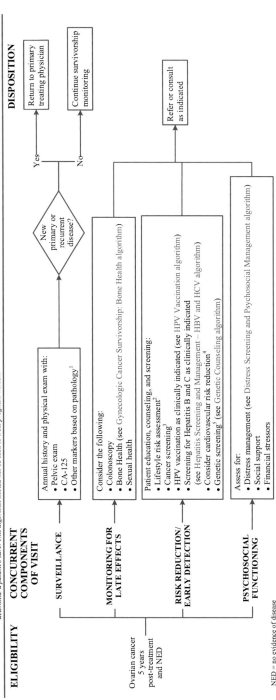

Figure 11.3 Ovarian cancer survivorship algorithm. 2021. The University of Texas MD Anderson Cancer Center [10]

THE UNIVERSITY OF TEXAS
MD Anderson Cancer Center
Making Cancer History®

Survivorship – Noninvasive Breast Cancer

Disclaimer: This algorithm has been developed for MD Anderson using a multidisciplinary approach considering circumstances particular to MD Anderson's specific patient population, services and structure, and clinical information. This is not intended to replace the independent medical or professional judgment of physicians or other health care providers in the context of individual clinical circumstances to determine a patient's care. This algorithm should not be used to treat pregnant women.

Note: Mammograms may continue as long as the patient has a 10-year life expectancy and no co-morbidities that would limit the diagnostic evaluation or treatment of any identified problem.

| ELIGIBILITY | CONCURRENT COMPONENTS OF VISIT | | DISPOSITION |

ELIGIBILITY

Female or male with noninvasive breast cancer, 6-24 months from date of diagnosis and NED

CONCURRENT COMPONENTS OF VISIT

SURVEILLANCE
- History and physical with clinical breast exam annually
- Imaging recommendations:
  - Routine imaging of the chest wall or reconstructed breast following mastectomy is not indicated
  - Diagnostic mammography[2,3] with or without tomosynthesis annually for patients who had breast conservation therapy for the first 5 years, followed by screening mammography thereafter
- Assess for compliance with hormone therapy and assess for toxicities if appropriate

MONITORING FOR LATE EFFECTS

Consider the following based on risk factors:
- Bone health[5] (see Breast Cancer Survivorship: Bone Health algorithm)
- Sexual health/fertility
- Gynecologic assessment if on tamoxifen
- Patient education regarding symptoms including radiation therapy complications if appropriate

RISK REDUCTION/ EARLY DETECTION

See Page 2

PSYCHOSOCIAL FUNCTIONING

DISPOSITION

Suspect new primary or biopsy-proven recurrence?

Yes → See evaluation for recurrence in Breast Cancer – Invasive Stage I-III algorithm

No → Continue survivorship monitoring

Refer or consult as indicated

NED = no evidence of disease
USPSTF = United States Preventive Services Task Force

[1] Completion of all treatment with the exception of hormonal agents
[2] Diagnostic mammography for up to 5 years post diagnosis then screening mammography thereafter
[3] Consider additional MRI breast with and without contrast annually for patients with germline mutations (see Appendix A in the Breast Cancer Screening algorithm for type of mutation and recommended screening interval) or diagnosis prior to age 50 years and have dense breasts[4]. Alternating mammography and MRI breast every 6 months is suggested if feasible.
Note: Additional imaging can be considered as delineated in the recommendation from the American College of Radiology (ACR) and the American Cancer Society (ACS). Note that the data supporting these guidelines are outdated (as per our internal analysis) and additional imaging is not recommended by the National Comprehensive Cancer Network (NCCN) survivorship guidelines.
[4] Dense breast is defined as heterogeneously dense or extremely dense
[5] All postmenopausal women (especially those on aromatase inhibitors) and premenopausal women on ovarian suppression

Department of Clinical Effectiveness V10
Approved by the Executive Committee of the Medical Staff on 03/21/2023

Figure 11.4 Noninvasive breast cancer survivorship algorithm. 2023. The University of Texas MD Anderson Cancer Center [11]

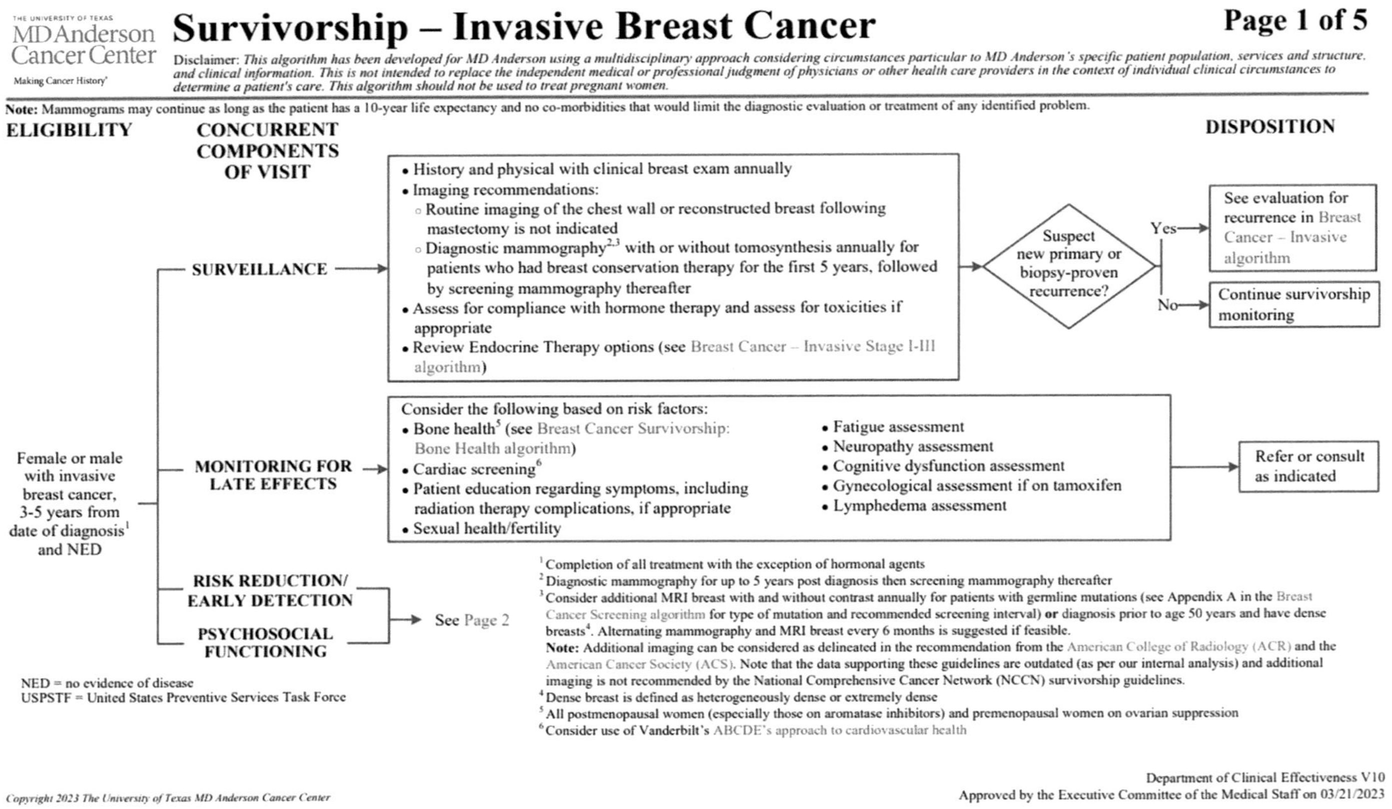

Figure 11.5 Invasive breast cancer survivorship algorithm. 2023. The University of Texas MD Anderson Cancer Center [12]

exercise three to five times a week (exercise on your feet, such as walking, jogging, tennis), muscle strengthening exercises at least two times a week, limiting alcohol consumption to one drink or less per day, limiting caffeine intake, and avoidance of tobacco. Bone mineral density (BMD), vitamin D level (25-OH Vit D), and evaluation for low impact fractures are recommended for women with risk factors including age above 50 years, postmenopausal status and/or other risk factors, such as low body weight, family history of hip fracture, rheumatoid arthritis, prior fracture, high risk medical conditions, or history of prior steroid use of three months or longer (Figure 11.6) [15].

Women with a normal BMD (T score ≥ -1.0) and vitamin D level (OH Vit D ≥ 30 ng/dl) should repeat the bone density testing in two years. Women with osteopenia (T score between -1.0 and -2.5) should continue with universal recommendations, repeat the BMD in two years, and consider medical therapy. Women with osteoporosis or a low impact fracture should be referred to a bone specialist to discuss benefits and risks of medical therapy, such as bisphosphonates, denosumab, and raloxifene. Women with low vitamin D level should start ergocalciferol weekly (50,000 IU) for 8–12 weeks, to maintain a vitamin D level at 30–50 ng/dl (Figure 11.6) [15].

Sexual Function

Some studies have found that about 60% of gynecologic cancer survivors experience sexual dysfunction [16]; therefore, sexual function should be assessed during the survivorship annual visit. For patients who indicate a concern and would like to discuss their sexual health, health care providers should conduct a history and physical, review their prior treatment, assess for signs and symptoms of estrogen deprivation, and review conditions and medications that may affect sexual function [17].

Many survivors of gynecologic cancer will experience vasomotor symptoms including hot flashes and night sweats. This is common among breast cancer survivors taking endocrine therapy, such as tamoxifen and aromatase inhibitors, and gynecological cancer survivors following bilateral oophorectomy. Hormone therapy (HT) with estrogen and progestogen is contraindicated for survivors of hormone-mediated cancer, such as breast cancer, low grade serous ovarian cancer, advanced endometrial cancer, and desmoid tumors, but may be considered for other survivors of gynecological cancer. Custom-compounded bioidentical hormone therapy is not recommended as they are not appropriately regulated by the Food and Drug Administration (FDA). Non-hormonal pharmacologic treatments with selective serotonin uptake inhibitors (SSRIs), gabapentin, and clonidine may be initiated as needed (see Chapter 6). Other nonpharmacological options include acupuncture, physical activity, lifestyle modifications, and integrative therapies of yoga and hypnosis [17].

Endocrine therapy for breast cancer can cause vaginal dryness leading to painful vaginal intercourse. Vaginal stenosis and dryness are common late effects of radiation therapy to the pelvis. Patients are encouraged to use vaginal dilators before and after their radiation treatment. Some patients benefit from pelvic floor physical therapy. Patients with a history of cervical cancer can use local estrogens, such as vaginal rings, suppositories, and creams, but these therapies should not be used for patients with a history of breast cancer or estrogen-receptor positive tumors. For those patients, nonhormonal vaginal moisturizers, vaginal gels, and hyaluronic acid containing moisturizers are options. Patients are also encouraged to use lubricants during sexual activity [17].

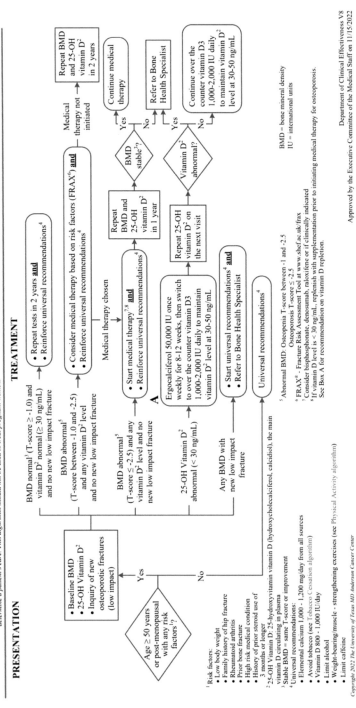

Figure 11.6 Survivorship – gynecologic cancer: Bone health algorithm. [2022]. The University of Texas MD Anderson Cancer Center [15]

Cancer survivors might also experience a low or lack of sexual desire, libido, orgasm, or altered intimacy. Other patients can experience global symptoms of distress, anxiety, or depression that affects their sexual function. Referral to a mental health counselor, psychologist, psychiatrist, sexual health specialist, or gynecologist who specializes in these treatments may be indicated [18].

Risk Reduction and Early Detection

Patients with a history of cancer are at a higher risk for other types of cancer. Early detection or screening are interventions to detect a cancer at an early stage, whereas risk-reduction strategies are interventions to decrease the risk of additional cancer.

Lifestyle Assessment

The physical activity level assessment can be performed by qualified clinical personnel and starts by identifying the current physical activity (PA) frequency, intensity, type, and duration. The American College of Sports Medicine (ACSM) guidelines for patients not undergoing cancer treatment includes weekly activity of at least 150 minutes of moderate-intensity activity, or 75 minutes of vigorous-intensity activity, or equivalent combination, plus two or more weekly sessions of strength training that includes major muscle groups [19]. For patients who are meeting the ACSM guidelines, clinicians should provide positive reinforcement and encourage maintenance of the current activity level. For patients who are not meeting the ACSM guidelines, but are interested in starting or increasing PA, clinicians should assess for conditions that require medical clearance, and then refer the patient to an exercise physiology technologist (EPT) or a community exercise program. For patients who are not meeting the ACSM PA guidelines and are not interested in starting or increasing PA, clinicians should conduct motivational interviewing (MI), for example open questions, affirmation, reflective listening, and summary reflections, to encourage physical activity and limit sedentary behaviors to reduce the risk of subsequent cancer and other chronic diseases [19].

The nutrition assessment includes the patient's body mass index (BMI), which is categorized as follows: underweight (BMI less than 18.5 kg/m2), normal weight (BMI 18.5–24.9 kg/m2), overweight (BMI 25–29.9 kg/m2), and obese (BMI greater than or equal to 30 kg/m2). Patients should be counseled that it is important to maintain a normal body weight throughout their lifetime to reduce the risk of additional cancer, such as breast, pancreatic, colorectal, liver, endometrial, and ovarian. The American Institute for Cancer Research (AICR) guidelines recommend individuals engage in regular physical activity, and eat a diet high in whole grains, vegetables, fruits, and beans. It is also highly recommended for people to limit consumption of sugary foods and drinks (less than 10% of daily calories), red meats (12–18 ounces or less per week), alcohol (no more than 1 drink a day for women), and avoid processed meats and foods [20].

Clinicians should assess the nonmedical and medical barriers to healthy eating, such as gastrointestinal dysmotility, swallowing problems, bowel dysfunction, poor dental health, oropharyngeal changes, digestive enzyme insufficiency, and gastrointestinal tract reconstruction or anastomoses. A referral to a registered dietician (RD) is indicated for patients with the following: diabetes, gastrointestinal, thyroid, renal or liver disease, malnutrition, or concerns about medications and supplements. Overweight and obese patients, who are interested and clinically appropriate for diet or weight changes, should be referred to a diet and exercise counseling program and RD as clinically indicated [20].

Tobacco use assessment should be performed at every clinic visit. Patients who have never smoked more than 100 cigarettes in their lifetime should be applauded and encouraged to remain tobacco-free. Former smokers, who have not smoked or used tobacco within the last 12 months, are to be congratulated for quitting tobacco use and encouraged to remain tobacco-free. Current smokers should be counseled regarding the importance of tobacco cessation, which can improve survivorship by as much as 30–40%. Current smokers who are ready to make a change should be referred to a tobacco treatment program, which will include a combination of behavioral therapy and pharmacotherapy. Health care providers should also inquire survivors about the use of other tobacco products, such as electronic cigarettes and smokeless tobacco [21].

First line pharmacologic interventions are varenicline and bupropion [21]. Varenicline dosage is titrated up in the first week (Days 1 to 3: 0.5 mg once a day; Days 4 to 7: 0.5 mg two times a day; Days 8 to end of treatment: 1 mg two times a day). The most common side effects of varenicline are insomnia, nausea, and abnormal dreams. Varenicline is contraindicated in patients with a previous known history of serious hypersensitivity reactions or skin reactions to Chantix. Patients should stop taking varenicline and contact their health care provider if they experience agitation, depressed mood, or changes in behavior, or develop suicidal ideation or behavior. Bupropion dosage is started at 150 mg once a day and increased to twice a day after 3 days with at least 8 hours between dosages. The most common side effects of bupropion are restlessness, agitation, tremor, ataxia, gait disturbance, vertigo, and dizziness. Bupropion is contraindicated with seizure disorders or disorders that increase the risk of seizures.

Second line therapy is nicotine replacement therapy (NRT), such as lozenges or gum. For current smokers who are not ready to make a change, clinicians should use motivational interviewing about smoking cessation, which includes reviewing the risks of smoking and benefits of quitting, providing education resources, assessing barriers and concerns of patients, and recommending a reduction of total cigarettes smoked per day using medications or NRT [21].

Cancer Screening

Breast cancer screening with annual screening mammogram and CBE should be performed for all gynecologic cancer survivors who are ≥ 40 years old. Supplemental breast cancer screening with annual breast magnetic resonance imaging (MRI) should be offered for women at risk of breast cancer related to family history of breast cancer, pathogenic mutation with *BRCA1* and *BRCA2*, or have a history of atypical ductal hyperplasia (ADH), atypical lobular hyperplasia (ALH), or lobular carcinoma in situ (LCIS) [22].

Cervical cancer screening should start for breast cancer survivors who are ≥ 21 years old. Women who are 21 to 29 years old should undergo a screening Pap test every 3 years, without human papilloma virus (HPV) testing. Women who are 30 to 65 years old should obtain co-testing with Pap and HPV test every 5 years (preferred), or primary HPV testing with reflex cytology every 5 years (preferred), or Pap test with reflex HPV test every 3 years, or Pap test alone every 3 years. Women older than age 65 and have had at least 3 consecutive negative Pap tests or 2 consecutive negative Pap and HPV tests within the past 10 years, and no history of cervical dysplasia or cancer, may discontinue cervical cancer screening [23].

Colon cancer screening for average risk patients, such as those without a history of adenomas, inflammatory bowel disease, or family history of colorectal cancer, should start at the age of 45. Colonoscopy is the preferred method for colorectal cancer screening. Other options for colorectal cancer screening are computed tomographic colonography, fecal immunochemical test, or multifocal stool DNA test. Patients with an increased risk of colon cancer secondary to a family history of colon cancer should start colorectal cancer screening at 40 years old or 10 years before the youngest colorectal cancer case in the family. The need for follow-up colorectal cancer screening will be dependent on the initial findings [24].

Lung cancer screening with a low-dose computed tomography (LDCT) should be offered for patients who are 50 to 80 years old, have at least a 20-year pack history of tobacco use, are current smokers or have quit tobacco within the past 15 years, do not have symptoms concerning for lung cancer, and are willing to undergo treatment if diagnosed with lung cancer [25].

HPV Vaccination

Human papilloma virus (HPV) is associated with an increased risk of cervical, penile, vulvar, vaginal, anal, and oropharyngeal cancer, so it is important to incorporate HPV vaccination into survivorship care. HPV vaccination is strongly recommended for all males and females from the age of 9 to 26 years old. The Advisory Committee on Immunization Practices (ACIP) recommends that the HPV vaccine series should be completed by the age of 11 to 12 years old and strongly recommends that the two- vaccine series be completed before age 15 (administered at 0 and 6–12 months). Patients from ages 15 to 26 years require a three-shot series (9vHPV-Gardasil administered at 0, 2, and 6 months) [26]. This three-dose vaccine series may also be considered for males and females between 27 to 45 years after a discussion with the clinician about the vaccine benefits and limitations in this age group. Patients should be counseled about the decreased effectiveness of the vaccine for those who have been sexually active and may have already been infected with one or more types of HPV in the vaccine.

Screening for Hepatitis B and C

The CDC recommends the following patients to be screened for hepatitis B [27]:

- people born in countries with prevalence of hepatitis B virus (HBV) infection >2%
- people born in the United States that were not vaccinated as infants whose parents were born in regions with a high rate of HBV infection
- men who have sex with men
- people who inject drugs
- people with HIV
- people with household and sexual contacts of people with HBV infection
- people requiring immunosuppressive therapy
- people with end-stage renal disease
- blood and tissue donors
- people with elevated alanine aminotransferase levels
- pregnant people
- infants born to people with HBV infection

The CDC also recommends screening for hepatitis C in all patients ≥ 18 years old and patients with risk factors, such as intravenous (IV) drug users [28].

Cardiovascular Risk Reduction

Survivorship patients should be evaluated for their risk of heart disease. The ABCDE approach is an effective method to assess cardiovascular health and prevent heart disease (Table 11.2) [29]. Patients who received chemotherapy with anthracycline or radiation to the chest have increased risk of developing heart disease, so they should be assessed for symptoms of shortness of breath, dyspnea on exertion and chest pain. Female cancer survivors should be encouraged to establish with a community primary care provider who can perform this assessment.

Table 11.2 ABCDEs of cardiovascular wellness in cancer survivors. 2020. NCCN.

A	•	Awareness of the risk factors and symptoms of heart disease
	•	Assessment of being at risk for or having heart disease
	•	Aspirin used as needed
B	•	Blood pressure management
C	•	Cholesterol management
	•	Cigarette and tobacco cessation [quit smoking]
D	•	Diet and weight management
	•	Doses of anthracyclines, radiation to the heart, or both
	•	Diabetes prevention and treatment
E	•	Exercise
	•	Echocardiogram, Electrocardiogram, or both, as needed

Genetic Screening

Genetic counseling is recommended for many patients with a history of female cancer. The genetic counselor will assess the patient's relevant personal and family history, cancer risk, and testing guidelines.

Patients with a history of **endometrial cancer** should be referred to genetic counseling in the following circumstances [29]:

- There is a significant change in family history since the last genetic consult
- They have not received previous genetic counseling
- Risk factors for Lynch syndrome exist, such as a personal history of colon or rectal cancer or immediate family with colorectal or endometrial cancer
- An immediate or extended family was diagnosed with colon, rectal, or uterine cancer before the age of 50
- Any relative tested positive for a Lynch syndrome pathogenic variant (*EPCAM*, *MLH1*, *MSH2*, *MSH6*, *PMS2* genes)

Patients with a history of **ovarian cancer** should be referred to genetic counseling in the following circumstances [29]:

- There is a significant family history change since the last genetic consult
- They have not received previous genetic testing for *BRCA1* and *BRCA2* or associated genes
- Histology of high grade non-mucinous epithelial ovarian cancer

Patients with a personal history of **breast cancer** should be referred to genetic counseling in the following circumstances [29]:

- Breast cancer diagnosis ≤ 50 years of age
- Triple negative breast cancer diagnosed at age ≤ 60 years
- Multiple breast cancers when first breast cancer was diagnosed at age ≤ 65 years
- Breast cancer diagnosed at any age with one or more:
  - Personal history of ovarian or pancreatic cancer
  - Family history of ovarian cancer
  - Family history of breast cancer diagnosed at age ≤ 50 years
  - Family history of male breast cancer
  - Family history of ≥ 2 relatives diagnosed with breast cancer at any age
  - Family history of metastatic prostate or high-grade prostate cancer
  - Family history of pancreatic cancer
  - Family history of cancer and/or dermatological manifestations suggestive of Cowden syndrome, such as thyroid cancer or endometrial cancer
  - Family history of cancer suggestive of Li-Fraumeni syndrome, such as sarcoma, adrenocortical cancer, brain tumors
  - Ashkenazi Jewish ancestry
  - Any member of the family with a known pathogenic variant (PV)
  - Metastatic breast cancer patient with *BRCA1/2* PV detected on tumor testing in the absence of a germline PV
  - An affected patient with a first- or second-degree relative meeting any of the above criteria

Vaccinations

Patients who are age ≥ 19 years should follow the latest adult immunization schedule from the Center of Disease and Prevention (CDC) guidelines (Figure 11.7) [30].

Psychosocial Functioning

Distress Management

About 25% of cancer survivors have persistent psychological distress after treatment [32]. Survivorship patients should undergo screening for distress at every clinical encounter by asking them to score their distress on a 0 to 10 scale with 10 being extreme distress. If patients score greater than 6 on distress, they should be referred to a social worker to complete a psychosocial assessment and receive appropriate interventions. The clinician should also address physical symptoms during the visit and provide a referral to the appropriate provider or ancillary service [33]:

(1) Psychiatry will provide assessment and management of cancer-related behavioral symptoms as well as neuropsychiatric side effects of cancer and its treatment. Priority is given to the management of anxiety, depression, and delirium. The treatment involves psychotherapy, medication, or both, which will be coordinated with care provided by a mental health counselor.

Table 1 Recommended Adult Immunization Schedule by Age Group, United States, 2023

Vaccine	19–26 years	27–49 years	50–64 years	≥65 years
COVID-19	2- or 3- dose primary series and booster (See Notes)			
Influenza inactivated (IIV4) or Influenza recombinant (RIV4) or	1 dose annually			
Influenza live, attenuated (LAIV4)	1 dose annually			
Tetanus, diphtheria, pertussis (Tdap or Td)	1 dose Tdap each pregnancy; 1 dose Td/Tdap for wound management (see notes) 1 dose Tdap, then Td or Tdap booster every 10 years			
Measles, mumps, rubella (MMR)	1 or 2 doses depending on indication (if born in 1957 or later)			For healthcare personnel, see notes
Varicella (VAR)	2 doses (if born in 1980 or later)		2 doses	
Zoster recombinant (RZV)	2 doses for immunocompromising conditions (see notes)		2 doses	
Human papillomavirus (HPV)	2 or 3 doses depending on age at initial vaccination or condition	27 through 45 years		
Pneumococcal (PCV15, PCV20, PPSV23)		1 dose PCV15 followed by PPSV23 OR 1 dose PCV20 (see notes)		See Notes See Notes
Hepatitis A (HepA)	2, 3, or 4 doses depending on vaccine			
Hepatitis B (HepB)	2, 3, or 4 doses depending on vaccine or condition			
Meningococcal A, C, W, Y (MenACWY)	1 or 2 doses depending on indication, see notes for booster recommendations			
Meningococcal B (MenB)	19 through 23 years	2 or 3 doses depending on vaccine and indication, see notes for booster recommendations		
Haemophilus influenzae type b (Hib)	1 or 3 doses depending on indication			

Recommended vaccination for adults who meet age requirement, lack documentation of vaccination, or lack evidence of past infection

Recommended vaccination for adults with an additional risk factor or another indication

Recommended vaccination based on shared clinical decision-making

No recommendation/ Not applicable

Figure 11.7 Recommended adult immunization schedule for adults. 2023. CDC available at: www.cdc.gov/vaccines/schedules/hcp/imz/adult.html

(2) Internal medicine will provide evaluation of patients experiencing fatigue-related to the cancer treatment. The internal medicine provider will assess multiple symptoms, such as depression, anxiety, sleep dysfunction, and pain, obtain a history, perform a physical examination, and review laboratory and diagnostic testing. The etiology of fatigue is often multifactorial and may need several recommendations. Exercise is the main treatment in cancer-related fatigue. Other interventions may include stimulants, behavioral modification therapy, and treatment of medical and mood disorders.

(3) Integrative medicine takes a global approach to wellness, incorporating Western and Eastern medicine, and it is practiced by physicians, advanced practice providers, and therapists. Integrative medicine provides a variety of group and individual clinical services to help patients to improve their physical, psycho-spiritual, and social health. Integrative medicine services can be individualized, such as nutrition, exercise, oncology massage, acupuncture, music therapy, and psychological consultation. Integrative services can also be group clinical programs, such as meditation, yoga, cooking classes, support groups, and education forums.

(4) Neuropsychology services provided by neurologists provide cognitive assessment and interventions for adults who experience symptoms or complaints involving memory and other thinking skills, or changes in behaviors, such as changes in concentration, organization, and reasoning.

(5) Onco-fertility services provided by reproductive endocrinologists assist with fertility after cancer treatment and exploration of other options for family building, such as donor eggs and embryos, child adoption, use of a gestational carrier, and referral to psychological and financial support services.

(6) Pain management should be available for patients who experience pain related to cancer treatment. The optimum pain control is achieved by formulating an individualized plan of care based on the patient's needs using a combination of pain management strategies such as nonpharmacologic methods, pharmacotherapy, nerve blocks, and vertebroplasty.

(7) Rehabilitation services provide patients with client-centered physical and occupational therapy. The patient and the therapist work together to identify strategies to compensate for the cognitive or physical impairment. The therapist also provides specific programs for management of lymphedema, fatigue, and chemo-brain.

(8) Sleep lab services are provided by pulmonologists to evaluate and manage cancer survivors experiencing symptoms of sleep deprivation and fatigue from their cancer treatment.

Body Image

Body image changes are common among breast cancer survivors who underwent partial or total mastectomies. Some women may have undergone several breast reconstruction surgeries without achieving the desired outcome, resulting in frustration and depression. Others may experience fear of being intimate with their partners and may benefit from referral to body image counselor who can help them to overcome their fears. Breast cancer survivors should also be offered prescriptions for postmastectomy bras and breast prosthesis. Most insurance plans will provide financial coverage for bras and prothesis with a prescription.

Financial Stressors

Financial stressors in cancer survivors are related to cancer treatment being one of the most expensive health care treatments in the United States, which uses a combination of surgery, radiation, chemotherapy, and more recent costly biologic therapies, combined with patients' inability to works because of the cancer diagnosis [34]. Even those with health insurance often do not have the entire cost of their treatment covered by the insurance and will incur substantial debt. Following completion of treatment, patients may be unable to return to work or to perform the same type of work. These patients may benefit from a referral to social work to help the patient access community services and navigate disability and/or social security programs.

Social Support

Many cancer survivors rely on their families and friends after cancer treatment, but not all patients have an effective support system. It is important to assess a patient's support system at every encounter. This will help to identify patients who might benefit from additional support services. Social workers provide counseling to patients and their families and help to connect patients with local and online support groups, special services, and programs in the community. In addition, social workers can provide patients with information about advance directives and advanced care planning [29].

Case Study Questions

Question 1: How can Ms. Smith decrease her risk of cancer recurrence or development of another cancer?
Question 2: How can Ms. Smith decrease her vaginal pain during intercourse?
Question 3: How can Ms. Smith improve her vasomotor symptoms?
Question 4: How can Ms. Smith improve her bone health?

Case Resolution

Question 1: The risk of cancer recurrence or development of another cancer is decreased by lifestyle modifications. Patients who have a diagnosis of overweight or obesity are encouraged to lose weight. They can be referred to weight loss programs that can focus on dietary modifications and engagement in regular physical activity. Patients are also encouraged to stop smoking. They can be referred to tobacco treatments programs.

Question 2: Vaginal pain during intercourse can be improved by using vaginal moisturizers regularly and vaginal lubricant during intercourse. Women with hormone-mediated cancer are instructed not to use oral estrogen therapy.

Question 3: Vasomotor symptoms can be decreased with weight loss, and regular physical exercise. Some patients might benefit from a nonhormonal therapy such as an SSRI. Women with history of hormone-mediated cancer should not take oral estrogen therapy.

Question 4: Patients with osteopenia should have Calcium 1,000–1,200 mg daily and 800–1,000 IU Vitamin D3 daily. The calcium should preferably come from their diet. Vitamin D level should be between 30–50 ng/dl. If the Vitamin D level is low, patient will need to be prescribed Vitamin D 50,000 IU weekly for 8 weeks, then Vitamin D3 800–1,000 IU daily. They should have weight bearing activity 5 days a week, and lift weights 2 days a week. Patients with osteopenia should also stop smoking. The bone density testing should be repeated in two years.

Take Home Points

- Survivorship care involves surveillance for recurrence of disease, monitoring for late effects of treatment, reducing the risk and early detection of other cancer, and assessment of psychosocial function.
- Patients are transitioned to survivorship when the cancer treatment is completed, and they have no evidence of disease.
- Survivorship care of patients with a history of cervical, endometrial, ovarian, noninvasive, and invasive breast cancer has some overlap, but demonstrate key differences based on the cancer specific site.
- Bone and sexual health should be assessed at every clinical visit.
- Risk reduction and early detection involves lifestyle assessment and recommendations, cancer screening, genetic screening, immunizations, and cardiovascular risk reduction.
- Psychosocial assessment includes evaluation of emotional distress, altered body image, financial toxicity, and degree of social support.

References

1. National Cancer Institute/Surveillance, Epidemiology, and End Results Program. Cancer Stat Facts: Cervical Cancer (NCI/SEER) (August 10, 2022). https://seer.cancer.gov/statfacts/html/cervix.html

2. National Cancer Institute/Surveillance, Epidemiology, and End Results Program (NCI/SEER) (August 10, 2022). Cancer Stat Facts: Uterine Cancer. https://seer.cancer.gov/statfacts/html/corp.html

3. National Cancer Institute/Surveillance, Epidemiology, and End Results Program (NCI/SEER) (August 10, 2022). Cancer Stat Facts: Ovarian Cancer. https://seer.cancer.gov/statfacts/html/ovary.html

4. National Cancer Institute/Surveillance, Epidemiology, and End Results Program (NCI/SEER) (August 10, 2022). Cancer Stat Facts: Female Breast Cancer. https://seer.cancer.gov/statfacts/html/breast.html

5. American Cancer Society (August 10, 2022). Survival Rates for Breast Cancer. www.cancer.org/cancer/breast-cancer/understanding-a-breast-cancer-diagnosis/breast-cancer-survival-rates.html

6. Brian L., McLaughlin V., Trentham-Dietz A. Disease-free survival by treatment after DCIS diagnosis in population-based cohort study. *Breast Cancer Research Treatment.* 2013;**14**(1):145–54.

7. Rodriguez M. A. and Lewis-Patterson P. Defining Cancer Survivorship. *In Handbook of Cancer Survivorship Care.* Springer Publishing Company, 2019. pp. 3–9.

8. UT MD Anderson Cancer Center (2021). Survivorship – Cervical Cancer. www.mdanderson.org/content/dam/mdanderson/documents/for-physicians/algorithms/survivorship/survivorship-cervical-web-algorithm.pdf

9. UT MD Anderson Cancer Center (2021). Survivorship – Endometrial Cancer. www.mdanderson.org/content/dam/mdanderson/documents/for-physicians/algorithms/survivorship/survivorship-endometrial-web-algorithm.pdf

10. UT MD Anderson Cancer Center (2021). Survivorship – Ovarian Cancer. www.mdanderson.org/content/dam/mdanderson/documents/for-physicians/algorithms/survivorship/survivorship-ovarian-web-algorithm.pdf

11. UT MD Anderson Cancer Center (2023). Survivorship – Noninvasive Breast Cancer. www.mdanderson.org/content/dam/mdanderson/documents/for-physicians/algorithms/survivorship/survivorship-breast-noninvasive-web-algorithm.p

12. UT MD Anderson Cancer Center (2023). Survivorship – Invasive Breast Cancer. www.mdanderson.org/content/dam/mdanderson/documents/for-physicians/algorithms/survivorship/survivorship-breast-invasive-web-algorithm.pdf

13. Lee J. E, Park C. Y., Lee E., Ji Y. I. Effect of gynecological cancer and its treatment on bone mineral density and the risk of osteoporosis and osteoporotic fracture. *Obstetrics & Gynecology Science.* 2020;**63**(4):470–9.

14. Ramin C, May B. J., Robden R. et al. Evaluation of osteopenia and osteoporosis in younger breast cancer survivors compared with cancer-free women: a prospective cohort study. *Breast Cancer Research.* 2018;**20**: article 132.

15. UT MD Anderson Cancer Center (2022). Survivorship – Gynecology Cancer: Bone Health. www.mdanderson.org/content/dam/mdanderson/documents/for-physicians/algorithms/survivorship/survivorship-gyn-bone-health-web-algorithm.pdf

16. Lin H., Fu H., Wu C., Tasai, et al. Evaluation of sexual dysfunction in gynecologic cancer survivors using DSM-5 diagnostic criteria. *BMC Women's Health.* 2022;**22**:Article number 1.

17. NCCN [2022]. NCCN Guidelines Version 1. (2022). Survivorship: Sexual Function. www.nccn.org/

18. NCCN [2022]. NCCN Guidelines Version 1. (2022). Survivorship: Hormone-Related. Symptoms. www.nccn.org/

19. UT MD Anderson Cancer Center (2021). Physical Activity – Adult. www.mdanderson.org/content/dam/mdanderson/documents/for-physicians/algorithms/screening/risk-reduction-physical-activity-web-algorithm.pdf

20. UT MD Anderson Cancer Center (2021). Nutrition – Adult. www.mdanderson.org/content/dam/mdanderson/documents/for-physicians/algorithms/screening/risk-reduction-nutrition-web-algorithm.pdf

21. UT MD Anderson Cancer Center (2021). Tobacco Cessation. www.mdanderson.org/content/dam/mdanderson/documents/for-physicians/algorithms/screening/risk-reduction-tobacco-cessation-web-algorithm.pdf

22. UT MD Anderson Cancer Center (2020). Breast Cancer Screening. www.mdanderson.org/content/dam/mdanderson/documents/for-physicians/algorithms/screening/screening-breast-web-algorithm.pdf

23. UT MD Anderson Cancer Center (2021). Cervical Cancer Screening. www.mdanderson.org/content/dam/mdanderson/documents/for-physicians/algorithms/screening/screening-cervical-web-algorithm.pdf

24. UT MD Anderson Cancer Center (2021). Colorectal Cancer Screening. www.mdanderson.org/content/dam/mdanderson/documents/for-physicians/algorithms/screening/screening-colorectal-web-algorithm.pdf

25. UT MD Anderson Cancer Center (2021). Lung Cancer Screening. www.mdanderson.org/content/dam/mdanderson/documents/for-physicians/algorithms/screening/screening-lung-web-algorithm.pdf

26. UT MD Anderson Cancer Center (2020). Human Papillomavirus [HPV] Vaccination for Prevention of HPV – Related Cancer. www.mdanderson.org/content/dam/mdanderson/documents/for-physicians/algorithms/screening/risk-reduction-hpv-vaccination-web-algorithm.pdf

27. CDC (2021). Hepatitis b questions and answers for health professionals. www.cdc.gov/hepatitis/hbv/hbvfaq.htm#b4

28. CDC (2021). Screen all patients for hepatitis C. www.cdc.gov/hepatitis/hcv/index.htm

29. NCCN (2020). Guidelines for Patients. Survivorship Care for Cancer-Related Late and Long-Term Effects. www.nccn.org/patients/guidelines/content/PDF/survivorship-crl-patient.pdf

30. MD Anderson Cancer Center (2021). Genetic Counseling. www.mdanderson.org/content/dam/mdanderson/documents/for-physicians/algorithms/clinical-management/clin-management-genetic-counseling-web-algorithm.pdf

31. CDC (2022). Adult Immunization Schedule. Recommendations for Ages 19 Years or Older, United States. www.cdc.gov/vaccines/schedules/downloads/adult/adult-combined-schedule-bw.pdf

32. National Institute of Health (2022). Meeting Cancer Survivors' Psychosocial Health Needs: A Conversation with Dr. Patricia Ganz. www.cancer.gov/news-events/cancer-currents-blog/2022/psychosocial-cancer-survivors-patricia-ganz

33. UT MD Anderson Cancer Center (2020). Distress Screening and Psychosocial Management of Adult Cancer Patients. www.mdanderson.org/content/dam/mdanderson/documents/for-physicians/algorithms/clinical-management/clin-management-distress-web-algorithm.pdf

34. National Cancer Institute (September 9, 2022). Financial Toxicity and Cancer Treatment. www.cancer.gov/about-cancer/managing-care/track-care-costs/financial-toxicity-hp-pdq#

Anal and Colorectal Cancer

Emma B. Holliday, Van K. Morris, and Craig Messick

Case Presentation

A 40-year-old, premenopausal woman was diagnosed with a clinical stage T3N1a squamous cell carcinoma of the anal canal. The primary anal cancer measured 5.5 cm in length and abutted but did not invade the posterior wall of the vagina on initial staging MRI (Figure 12.1a). She was treated with definitive chemoradiation therapy, including 58 Gray (Gy) radiation to the primary tumor and 47 Gy to the pelvis and inguinal lymph node basins in 29 daily fractions over 6 weeks (Figure 12.1b). Due to pain and mucositis, she was not able to initiate vaginal dilator use immediately after completion of treatment. By three months post definitive chemoradiation, she had a complete clinical response to therapy and was without evidence of disease. At her three-month follow-up visit, she reported not having had a menstrual period since prior to chemoradiation. She reported hot flashes, vaginal dryness, and dyspareunia. On pelvic exam she had a thin adhesion in the upper vagina, just before the level of the cervix. She was given a graduated set of vaginal dilators and lidocaine jelly with instructions on their use. She was without evidence of cancer. What would be your next recommendation?

Epidemiology

In 2022, there were an estimated 106,180 new cases of colon cancer, 44,850 cases of rectal cancer, and 9,440 cases of anal cancer [1]. Of those, women comprise approximately two-thirds of anal cancer diagnoses, one-third of rectal cancer diagnoses and one-half of colon cancer diagnoses. While overall rates of colorectal cancer have declined significantly in recent decades, rates in younger adults have increased with projections that by 2030, 10.9% of colon cancer and 22.9% of rectal cancer will be diagnosed in adults aged <50 years [2]. Rates of anal cancer have also increased, particularly in younger people [3]. Risk factors for colorectal cancer include hereditary syndromes such as Lynch syndrome and hereditary polyposis syndromes that are associated with mutations in genes such as *MLH1*, *MSH2*, *MSH6*, and *PMS2* for Lynch syndrome and *APC*, *MUTYH*, *SMAD4*, *BMPR1Am*, *PTEN*, and *POLE* for the hereditary polyposis syndromes. Hereditary factors are thought to be responsible for approximately 10% of colorectal cancer diagnoses after age 50 and 18% of colorectal cancer diagnoses before age 50. Inflammatory bowel disease also increases the risk of colorectal cancer. Dietary and lifestyle factors that have been associated with increased risk of colorectal cancer include consumption of red and/or processed meats as well as sugar and refined grains. Factors associated with decreased risk of colorectal cancer

(a)

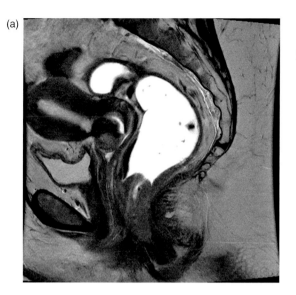

Figure 12.1a A sagittal image from the initial staging MRI for a woman with T3N1a squamous cell carcinoma of the anal canal. The tumor abuts but does not invade the posterior vagina.

(b)

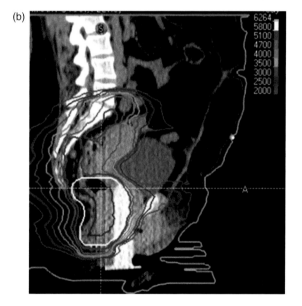

Figure 12.1b A sagittal image from the radiation treatment plan from her definitive treatment. A vaginal dilator was used daily during treatment to displace the anterior vaginal wall from the high radiation dose region.

include aspirin or non-steroidal anti-inflammatory drug (NSAID) use, calcium, vitamin D and folate use, and regular physical exercise [4]. In contrast, over 90% of anal cancer are associated with human papilloma virus (HPV). Other risk factors include smoking, immune suppression, or chronic inflammation from anal/perianal wounds [5]. Despite increasing incidence, fortunately, long-term survival in these populations is increasing, with five-year overall survival rates of 76% and 78% for colorectal and anal cancer, respectively [6, 7].

Presentation, Evaluation, and Treatment of Colorectal and Anal Cancer

Many colorectal and some anal cancer are diagnosed on screening colonoscopy. The age at which current guidelines recommend starting colorectal cancer screening is 45 years unless higher than average risk. Early detection and improved multidisciplinary treatment have been shown to contribute to improvements in outcomes [8]. Typical presenting symptoms of colorectal cancer include rectal bleeding and iron deficiency anemia [9]. Anal cancer, however, typically presents with anal pain and symptoms similar to hemorrhoidal irritation [5].

The diagnostic evaluation of rectal bleeding, unexplained iron deficiency anemia and/or anorectal pain should begin with a colonoscopy. This will allow for visualization of abnormalities in the lower gastrointestinal tract and biopsy of any suspicious masses or lesions. Staging workup differs somewhat based on the location of the confirmed cancer. Computed tomography scan is typically sufficient to stage colon cancer, whereas magnetic resonance imaging of the pelvis if vital to determine stage and extent of rectal cancer. Positron emission tomography is usually added for the work up of anal cancer [10–12]. Staging based on the American Joint Committee on Cancer Tumor-Node-Metastasis (TNM) classification is shown in Tables 12.1 and 12.2 for colorectal and anal cancer, respectively. Multidisciplinary evaluation is vital, particularly for rectal and anal cancer.

Colon cancer is treated primarily with surgical resection. Chemotherapy is given post-operatively for patients with high risk T3, T4, and/or node positive disease [10]. Rectal cancer is also treated primarily with total mesorectal excision (TME) surgery for T1, T2, but preoperative radiation and chemotherapy are given for T3, T4, and/or node positive disease [11]. Anal cancer, on the other hand, is primarily treated with definitive chemoradiation. Surgical resection consisting of an abdominoperineal resection (APR) with permanent colostomy is reserved for patients who have residual or recurrent disease after chemoradiation [12]. Salvage surgery (APR) results posttreatment in roughly 15–20% of all treated anal squamous cell carcinomas. The surgery requires partial removal of the sigmoid colon, complete removal of the mesorectum (TME) to include all draining lymph nodes, entire rectum and anus, including a wide skin resection to ensure completeness of the resection. Upon completion of the operation, the patient must have a permanent colostomy as there is no continence mechanism after the anus (sphincter muscles) have been removed. Additionally, in females with anteriorly located cancer of the anal canal, often the post-treatment scar or residual cancer infiltrates the posterior vaginal wall. This is very challenging for clinicians to distinguish, necessitating a partial (posterior) vaginal wall resection to ensure the adequacy of oncologic resection and obtain negative margins for disease. These patients are often reconstructed by a plastic surgery team and as part of the reconstruction to fill the void of resection in the pelvis, they will recreate the posterior wall of the vagina using a rotational abdominal wall (muscle, fat, and skin) flap.

Gynecologic problems after treatment of colorectal and anal cancer will differ in nature and severity depending on which modalities are used for treatment. Chemotherapy, pelvic surgery and pelvic radiation therapy can all lead to gynecologic problems for patients with colorectal and anal cancer. Of the three major modalities, pelvic radiation therapy is the most detrimental to gynecologic health. Patients with anal and rectal cancer are often treated with radiation fields that extend all the way down to the pelvic floor and include at least the posterior wall of the vagina. Cumulative dose to the vagina typically ranges from

Table 12.1 American Joint Committee on Cancer Tumor-Node-Metastasis (TNM) classification for Colorectal Cancer, 8th edition

T		N		M		Stage	
Tx	Primary tumor cannot be assessed	Nx	Regional lymph nodes cannot be assessed			0	TisN0M0
T0	No evidence of primary tumor	N0	No regional lymph node metastases			I	T1-2N0M0
Tis	Carcinoma in situ, intramucosal adenocarcinoma	N1a	1 regional lymph node is positive			IIA	T3N0M0
T1	Tumor invades submucosa	N1b	2–3 regional lymph nodes are positive			IIB	T4aN0M0
T2	Tumor invades muscularis propria	N1c	No regional lymph nodes are positive, but there are tumor deposits in subserosa, mesentery, or nonperitonealized pericolic or perirectal tissues without regional nodal metastases			IIC	T4bN0M0
T3	Tumor invades through the muscularis propria into pericolonic tissue	N2a	4–6 regional lymph nodes are positive			IIIA	T1-2N1M0 T1N2a
T4a	Tumor penetrates to the surface of the visceral peritoneum	N2b	7+ regional lymph nodes are positive			IIIB	T3-4aN1M0 T2-3N2aM0 T1-2N2bM0
T4b	Tumor invades and/or is adherent to other organs or structures					IIIC	T4aN2aM0 T3-T4aN2bM0 T4bN1-2M0
				M0	No distant metastases	IVA	M1a
				M1a	Metastasis confirmed in one organ/site without peritoneal metastases	IVB	M1b
				M1b	Metastasis confirmed in 2+ organs/sites without peritoneal metastases	IVC	M1c
				M1c	Metastases to the peritoneal surface alone or with other site of metastasis		

Table 12.2 American Joint Committee on Cancer Tumor-Node-Metastasis (TNM) Classification for Anal Cancer, 8th edition

Tx	Primary tumor cannot be assessed	Nx	Regional lymph nodes cannot be assessed	0	TisN0M0
T0	No evidence of primary tumor	N0	No regional lymph node metastases	I	T1N0M0
Tis	Carcinoma in situ, intramucosal squamous cell carcinoma	N1a	Positive lymph node in the inguinal, perirectal or internal iliac nodal basins	II	T2-3N0M0
T1	Tumor $\leq$2cm	N1b	Positive lymph node in the external iliac nodal basin	IIIA	T1-2N1M0 T4N0M0
T2	Tumor >2cm=/<5cm	N1c	Positive lymph nodes in the external iliac as well as inguinal, perirectal and/or internal iliac nodal basins.	IIIB	T4N1M0
T3	Tumor >5cm				
T4	Tumor invades other organs such as bladder, prostate or vagina	M0	No distant metastases	IV	Any M1
		M1	Metastasis to other parts of the body.		

(a)

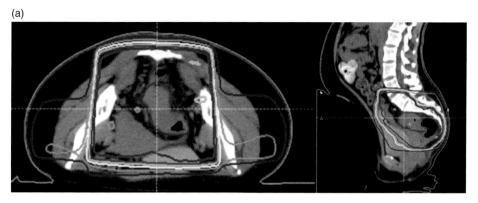

Figure 12.2a Radiation plan for a premenopausal women receiving preoperative chemoradiation for stage III rectal cancer. Note the proximity of the uterus to both the primary tumor (dark red) as well as positive lymph nodes (light red)

(b)

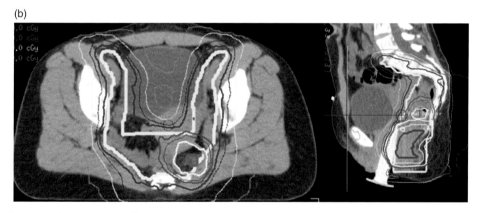

Figure 12.2b Radiation plan for a perimenopausal woman receiving definitive chemoradiation for stage III anal cancer. Note the proximity of the uterus to the elective nodal basins and involved lymph nodes

the equivalent of 45–58 Gy in 25 to 30 daily fractions. The ovaries and uterus are typically in the radiation fields for patients treated for anal (Figure 12.2a) and rectal (Figure 12.2b) cancer and receive approximately the equivalent of 45 Gy in 25 daily fractions. Gynecologic problems from pelvic radiation can be divided into acute and late toxicities related to the vagina, ovaries, and uterus. While most gynecologic toxicity is attributable, at least in part, to pelvic radiation, partial or total surgical removal of the vaginal wall, uterus and/or ovaries can lead to gynecologic concerns. Chemotherapy for colorectal and anal cancer can also contribute to treatment-induced ovarian insufficiency failure as well.

Gynecologic Problems after Pelvic Radiation

Radiation is not often used in the treatment of colon cancer but is given in the preoperative setting for patients with locally advanced rectal cancer and in the definitive setting for patients with nonmetastatic anal cancer. The typical dose is 45–54 Gy delivered in 1.8–2 Gy fractions over the course of 5–6 weeks. For rectal cancer, radiation targets the tumor in the rectum as well as the adjacent draining nodal basins to include those along the internal iliac vessels, obturator vessels, presacral space and mesorectum. For anal cancer, the draining nodal basin volume also includes the external iliac vessels and inguinal regions. Concurrent chemotherapy is typically given as a radiosensitizer [11, 12].

Vaginal Toxicity

Acute radiation-related vaginal mucosal toxicity typically starts around the second week of a 5–6 week course of pelvic radiation therapy when erythema and edema develop secondary to capillary dilation and intercellular edema. By the third or fourth week of radiation, the erythema evolves to confluent vaginal mucositis as the submucosal edema progresses to cause lifting and sloughing of the epithelium and thinning of the mucosal lining. The peak in acute vaginal toxicity is typically 1–2 weeks after the completion of radiation [13]. Biopsy is neither recommended nor necessary to confirm acute radiation toxicity, but histologic changes in the vaginal mucosa after radiation include lymphocytic infiltration of the epithelium, vascular congestion, endothelial swelling, submucosal hemorrhage, and hyalinization within the lamina propria [14].

Late vaginal toxicity typically appears months or years after the completion of pelvic radiation therapy and commonly include vaginal bleeding, vaginal dryness, and vaginal stenosis [15]. Rarely, vaginal fistula or necrosis can occur, although these toxicities typically require doses to the vagina higher than are typically prescribed in the treatment of rectal or anal cancer [16]. Vaginal stenosis is particularly common after definitive chemoradiation for anal cancer. One older study of patients receiving chemoradiation for anal cancer reported 78.5% of women reported any degree of vaginal stenosis, and 37.1% reported grade 3 stenosis, as defined as significant vaginal narrowing and/or shortening and dryness that interfere with use of tampons, causes dyspareunia or severe discomfort during intercourse, pain with dilator use, and interferes with physical examination (Table 12.3) [17]. Three studies of patients receiving pelvic radiation for rectal cancer reported reduced vaginal dimension in 29–35% of patients [18–20]. Vaginal stenosis is a major contributor to the high rates of dyspareunia reported by 35–60% of women after pelvic radiation for anal or rectal cancer [21–23]. Chronic vaginal dryness postradiation is another contributing factor to painful intercourse, and 41–83% of women report this chronic toxicity as well [18–20, 24]. Female sexual dysfunction is undoubtedly a multifactorial issue. Increasingly, studies are including validated patient reported outcome instruments to describe and quantify female sexual dysfunction after cancer treatment. One study of women treated with chemoradiation for anal cancer used the Female Sexual Function Index (FSFI) which includes domains for sexual interest, arousal, lubrication, orgasm, satisfaction, and pain. This study found 80% of women had FSFI scores compatible with sexual dysfunction at least two years after completion of chemoradiation [25].

Table 12.3 Grades of vaginal stenosis

Grade	Description
Grade 0	Normal sexual function, dilator compliance without pain, no vaginal dryness, and normal pelvic examinations.
Grade 1	Asymptomatic mild vaginal shortening/narrowing or dryness not interfering with sexual function, dilator use, or physical examination.
Grade 2	Symptomatic vaginal narrowing and/or shortening and dryness that did not significantly affect sexual function, dilator use, or the pelvic examination.
Grade 3	Significant vaginal narrowing and/or shortening and dryness that interfere with use of tampons, causes dyspareunia or severe discomfort during intercourse, pain with dilator use, and interferes with physical examination.

Adapted by Mirabeau-Beale et al. [17] based on the National Cancer Institute Common Terminology Criteria for Adverse Events version 4 scoring system.

Ovarian and Uterine Toxicity

Although the median age at diagnosis for colorectal and anal cancer is 60–70 years, premenopausal women can experience additional ovarian and uterine toxicities from treatment. Oocytes and granulosa cells are extremely sensitive to radiation damage even at low doses. Sterilization is predicted in 5% of women who receive 2–3 Gy to the ovaries and in 50% of women who receive 6–12 Gy. Within the ovarian stroma, radiation can lead to late tissue atrophy and fibrosis, which can contribute to endocrine dysfunction [26]. One study of premenopausal women who received standard doses of 45–50 Gy for rectal cancer reported 90% of patients developed premature menopause [27].

Additionally, pelvic radiation can thin the uterine lining such that implantation cannot successfully occur and cause myometrial fibrosis such that the uterus itself is not able to accommodate the normal growth of a pregnancy to term [28]. It can be difficult to separate out the effects of ovarian versus uterine damage on fertility and pregnancy outcomes, but one study of 74 women who underwent orthotopic ovarian transplantation prior to cancer therapy reported 21 pregnancies with four miscarriages. None of the patients in this cohort who received pelvic radiation became pregnant despite resuming normal menstrual cycles after transplantation; the reason for this was thought to be radiation-induced uterine fibrosis [29]. Another study of women who underwent in vitro fertilization with donor oocytes after cancer treatment reported 9% of embryo transfers were cancelled due to insufficient endometrial thickness. This also suggests direct impact of cancer therapies on the uterus itself. Unfortunately, detailed information about cumulative radiation doses and the specific radiation fields was not provided in this study [30].

Gynecologic Problems after Colorectal Surgery

Surgery can cause or contribute to gynecologic issues for women undergoing treatment for colorectal or anal cancer. Gynecologic toxicity of surgical intervention is directly related to the location and extent of the operation. For colon cancer, the oncologic operation includes mucosal margins that are at least 5 cm proximal and distal to the tumor as well as removal of at least twelve pericolic lymph nodes and removal of the mesentery to the origin of the named primary feeding vessel [31]. Colectomy will not typically result in gynecologic problems given the location of the operative field outside the pelvis. For rectal cancer, low risk, early-stage tumors are increasingly managed with transanal excision or transanal minimally invasive surgery due to decreased acute toxicity and better long-term bowel function [32]. For stage 1a rectal cancer without high-risk features (lymphovascular invasion, perineural invasion, signet ring pathology, poorly differentiated) transanal excision is appropriate, but for stage 1b rectal cancer or other stage 1a tumors with high-risk features, the standard of care is a TME or tumor specific mesorectal excision (TsME), with either a low anterior resection (LAR) or abdominal perineal resection (APR). Mid to high rectal tumors can also be removed with a LAR. LAR involves mobilizing the rectosigmoid colon and rectum and removing the structure *en block* down to the pelvic floor or 5 cm below the tumor. The reconstruction includes a mid to low rectal anastomosis. If pelvic radiation has been delivered prior to LAR, a temporary diverting ileostomy is required to allow the anastomosis to heal [33]. Low rectal tumors require an APR to obtain an adequate distal margin. An APR involves removing the entire rectum, anal canal, and anus followed by creation of a permanent end-colostomy from the sigmoid or descending colon and either the anus is closed using the remaining half of the anal canal (if an intersphincteric APR is performed or the perineum is closed with a myocutaneous flap) [33]. Anal cancer are treated with definitive chemoradiation but may require an APR for salvage surgery in the event of persistent or recurrent disease after chemoradiation.

For rectal or anal cancer operations in the pelvis where the tumor is near the posterior vagina, posterior vaginectomy may be performed along with total mesorectal excision surgery. This procedure can result in vaginal foreshortening which can contribute to dyspareunia. Additionally, patients whose surgery requires a permanent ostomy have higher rates of sexual inactivity and decreased sexual interest [20].

For colorectal cancer involving or metastatic to the ovaries or uterus, surgical removal is required and will lead to immediate and permanent loss of function. Acute ovarian insufficiency can also occur during or shortly after pelvic radiation and/or chemotherapy, and this can lead to infertility as well as the endocrine dysfunction of premature menopause [34]. Surgical removal of the uterus necessitates the use of a gestational surrogate if pregnancy is desired in the future.

Gynecologic Problems after Chemotherapy

The primary chemotherapy agents used in the treatment of colorectal cancer include 5-fluorouracil and oxaliplatin. Irinotecan is increasingly used in the metastatic setting and/or for young patients with high risk locally advanced disease. The primary chemotherapy agents used in the treatment of anal cancer include mitomycin c and 5-fluorouracil or cisplatin and 5-fluorouracil [10–12].

These agents have the potential to cause damage to the oocytes and granulosa cells of the ovaries. The mechanism of action for this damage depends on the specific chemotherapy agent. 5-fluorouracil is an antimetabolite that works by inhibiting DNA replication; it is thought to carry a low risk for infertility because it is not thought to cause DNA damage to human follicles. Cisplatin and oxaliplatin covalently bind to DNA and form intra- and interstrand cross links leading to DNA breakage during replication. Platinum-based compounds are thought to carry an intermediate risk to fertility, though specific toxicity has not been shown in human primordial follicles [35]. In one study on premenopausal women treated with FOLFOX (5-fluorouracil, leucovorin, and oxaliplatin) for colorectal cancer, 16% of patients experienced persistent amenorrhea more than one-year post treatment. That risk increased to 24% for women over the age of 40 at the time of treatment [36].

Patients who receive chemotherapy without pelvic radiation also have some risk of uterine dysfunction after treatment. Studies have shown women who have received chemotherapy have lower pregnancy rates, even when using donor oocytes [30]. Cancer survivors also have higher rates of spontaneous miscarriage following pregnancy resulting from oocyte donation embryo transfer [37]. Studies like these suggest there may be some degree of myometrial atrophy, damage to uterine vasculature and depletion of the endometrial stem cell niche [28].

Screening for Gynecologic Problems after Colorectal and Anal Cancer Treatment

Ideally, women should be seen by a gynecologist prior to starting treatment for colorectal or anal cancer, particularly if their treatment will include pelvic radiation. The care team should ensure that women are up to date on age-appropriate cervical cancer screening prior to starting treatment, discuss hormone therapy if necessary following treatment, and discuss vaginal dilator therapy after treatment. Radiation can induce cytologic changes evident on Papanicolaou (Pap) staining including cytoplasmic vacuolation, nuclear and cellular enlargement, multinucleation and inflammatory exudate for 6–12 months posttreatment, necessitating Pap smear before treatment when possible [38].

Premenopausal women who have not completed childbearing should also consult with a fertility/oncofertility specialist prior to treatment to discuss options for oocyte or embryo cryopreservation, and/or ovarian transplantation [39].

Prevention and Treatment of Gynecologic Problems During Survivorship

When possible, proactive strategies for toxicity risk reduction during the treatment planning phase are much more effective than treatment of side effects once they occur.

Prevention and Treatment of Vaginal Toxicity

In the treatment planning stage, the radiation oncologist can first attempt to limit dose to the vulva and vagina when planning radiation treatments to minimize early inflammation and late fibrosis. One dosimetric study showed reduced chronic dyspareunia when the percentage of the total vaginal volume receiving 20 Gy or more was kept to less than 35% [40]. Another dosimetric analysis showed that the mean vaginal doses for patients undergoing radiation for anal and rectal cancer were 50 Gy and 36.8 Gy, respectively. Patients who experienced posttreatment stenosis had a mean vaginal dose of 45.9 Gy while patients who did not experience posttreatment stenosis had a mean vaginal dose of 38.4 Gy, however patients began to experience vaginal stenosis at a mean dose of 25 Gy [41]. Minimizing vaginal and vulvar radiation dose is sometimes impossible, however, as the tumor target volume is typically near the posterior wall of the vagina for anal and low rectal tumors.

During treatment, the radiation oncologist can minimize radiation dose to the anterior vaginal wall and anterior half of the introitus by placing a dilator in the vaginal canal during each daily radiation treatment. This is performed at some institutions for patients undergoing treatment for anal and low rectal cancer to physically displace the anterior vagina and minimize the risk of circumferential fibrosis and stenosis. One study showed daily dilator use resulted in 5.5 Gy average dose reduction to the anterior vaginal wall compared with no daily dilator use [42]. A prospective phase II study investigating the benefit of daily vaginal dilators during radiation for anal cancer is currently underway [43].

After treatment, patients should also receive thorough teaching in vaginal dilator use from the radiation oncologist, gynecologist, or both, starting approximately four to six weeks after completion of pelvic radiation to reduce the risk of vaginal stenosis [44]. Although recommendations vary, most recommend vaginal dilator use at least three times per week, 5–10 minutes each session for at least one year after pelvic RT, although there may be benefit in continuing dilator use longer as stenosis can be seen as far out as 5 years from radiation therapy [45]. Vaginal intercourse may be utilized in lieu of dilator therapy to maintain patency.

For patients who develop vaginal stenosis, dryness, and/or dyspareunia, there are therapeutic interventions that can help. The NCCN survivorship guidelines recommend topical estrogens as the first-line posttreatment therapy for dyspareunia or vaginal pain after pelvic radiation for colorectal or anal cancer [46]. Psychotherapeutic interventions and pelvic floor exercises have also had modest effects [47]. Hyperbaric oxygen treatment or surgical neovagina reconstruction are also potential options but are supported by lower level evidence [48].

Prevention and Treatment of Ovarian Toxicity

Pretreatment evaluation is critical for premenopausal women in order to discuss potential options for fertility preservation and ovarian endocrine preservation. From the radiation planning standpoint, there is not much that can be done to prevent ovarian toxicity. The location, mobility and exquisite radiosensitivity of ovaries within the pelvis make it impossible to shield them from radiation doses that will likely lead to premature ovarian insufficiency. Therefore, gamete cryopreservation is considered first-line therapy for fertility preservation. It will often result in at least a two-week delay in initiation of chemotherapy and/or radiation, so swift referral is crucial. Another option for preservation of both the fertility and endocrine function of the ovary is ovarian transposition or oophoropexy. This involves laparoscopic surgery to mobilize both or at least one ovary to the abdominal sidewall above the pelvic brim. Transposition minimizes the radiation dose to the ovaries but does not eliminate it completely. Studies suggest internal scatter results in approximately 8–15% of the prescription dose still reaching the ovaries [49]. However, some studies report up to a 70–88% success rate of ovarian preservation following ovarian transposition [50].

Prevention and Treatment of Uterine Toxicity

Similar to the anatomic challenges of shielding the ovaries from damaging radiation, the uterus is in close proximity to the tumor for patients with anal and colorectal cancer. There have been case reports presented where advanced radiation techniques such as proton therapy are used to reduce uterine dose and increase the chances of successful pregnancy following treatment. There are also reports of surgical uterine transposition and fixation to the upper abdomen before radiation treatment with relocation back to the pelvis upon completion of radiation [51]. Both approaches are considered experimental, as robust data concerning subsequent pregnancy outcomes don't exist.

For women who have received pelvic radiation for anal or rectal cancer, the best outcomes for those desiring children posttreatment are to utilize cryopreserved oocytes or embryos prior to cancer therapy and subsequently utilize a gestational carrier.

Case Resolution

The patient was referred to gynecology and prescribed topical estrogen therapy, encouraged and counseled on vaginal dilator therapy, and adhesions were manually lysed by the gynecologist in office. She was also referred to a certified pelvic floor physical therapist with a treatment plan of three visits weekly for six weeks. Manual therapy with a graduated set of vaginal dilators as well as biofeedback were employed. Her dyspareunia improved and she was able to resume vaginal intercourse with the use of water-based lubricants.

Take Home Points

- Lower gastrointestinal cancer, particularly colorectal cancer, is on the rise in premenopausal women.
- Radiation, chemotherapy, and surgery can have toxicities that lead to permanent vaginal, ovarian, and uterine dysfunction.
- Pretreatment referral to reproductive endocrinology and gynecology for discussion of fertility preservation and hormone therapy is key for premenopausal women.
- Topical vaginal estrogens and vaginal dilator therapy can improve pain and sexual dysfunction associated with vaginal stenosis.

References

1. Siegel R. L., Miller K. D., Fuchs H. E., Jemal A. Cancer statistics, 2022. *CA Cancer J Clin.* 2022;**72**(1):7–33.

2. Bailey C. E., Hu C. Y., You Y. N., et al. Increasing disparities in the age-related incidences of colon and rectal cancer in the United States, 1975–2010. *JAMA Surg.* 2015;**150**(1):17–22.

3. Nelson V. M., Benson A. B. Epidemiology of anal canal cancer. *Surg Oncol Clin N Am.* 2017;**26**(1):9–15.

4. Stoffel E. M., Murphy C. C. Epidemiology and mechanisms of the increasing incidence of colon and rectal cancer in young adults. *Gastroenterology.* 2020;**158**(2):341–53.

5. Eng C., Ciombor K. K., Cho M., et al. Anal cancer: Emerging standards in a rare disease. *J Clin Oncol Off J Am Soc Clin Oncol.* 2022;**40**(24):2774–88.

6. Sauer R., Liersch T., Merkel S., et al. Preoperative versus postoperative chemoradiotherapy for locally advanced rectal cancer: Results of the German CAO/ARO/AIO-94 randomized phase III trial after a median follow-up of 11 years. *J Clin Oncol Off J Am Soc Clin Oncol.* 2012;**30**(16):1926–33.

7. Gunderson L. L., Winter K. A., Ajani J. A., et al. Long-term update of US GI intergroup RTOG 98-11 phase III trial for anal carcinoma: Survival, relapse, and colostomy failure with concurrent chemoradiation involving fluorouracil/mitomycin versus fluorouracil/cisplatin. *J Clin Oncol Off J Am Soc Clin Oncol.* 2012;**30**(35):4344–51.

8. Bretthauer M., Løberg M., Wieszczy P., et al. Effect of colonoscopy screening on risks of colorectal cancer and related death. *N Engl J Med.* 2022;**387**(17):1547–56.

9. Rex D. K., Boland C. R., Dominitz J. A., et al. Colorectal cancer screening: Recommendations for physicians and patients from the U.S. Multi-Society Task Force on Colorectal Cancer. *Am J Gastroenterol.* 2017;**112**(7):1016–30.

10. NCCN Guidelines: Colon Cancer v2.2022 [Internet]. [cited November 21, 2022]. www.nccn.org/professionals/physician_gls/pdf/colon.pdf

11. NCCN Clinical Practice Guidelines in Oncology: Rectal Cancer v1.2022 [Internet]. National Comprehensive Cancer Network. 2022. www.nccn.org/professionals/physician_gls/pdf/rectal.pdf

12. National Comprehensive Cancer Network. NCCN Guidelines Version 2. 2020 Anal Carcinoma [Internet]. [cited February 5, 2021]. www.nccn.org/professionals/physician_gls/pdf/anal.pdf

13. Hall E., Giaccia A. *Radiobiology for the Radiologist.* 7th ed. Philadelphia, PA: Lippincott, Williams & Watkins; 2011.

14. Abitbol M. M., Davenport J. H. The irradiated vagina. *Obstet Gynecol.* 1974;**44**(2):249–56.

15. Delanian S., Lefaix J. L. Current management for late normal tissue injury: Radiation-induced fibrosis and necrosis. *Semin Radiat Oncol.* 2007;**17**(2):99–107.

16. Kaidar-Person O., Abdah-Bortnyak R., Amit A., et al. Tolerance of the vaginal vault to high-dose rate brachytherapy and concomitant chemo-pelvic irradiation: Long-term perspective. *Rep Pract Oncol Radiother J Gt Cancer Cent Poznan Pol Soc Radiat Oncol.* 2014;**19**(1):56–61.

17. Mirabeau-Beale K., Hong T. S., Niemierko A., et al. Clinical and treatment factors associated with vaginal stenosis after definitive chemoradiation for anal canal cancer. *Pract Radiat Oncol.* 2015;**5**(3):e113-8.

18. Bregendahl S., Emmertsen K. J., Lindegaard J. C., Laurberg S. Urinary and sexual dysfunction in women after resection with and without preoperative radiotherapy for rectal cancer: A population-based cross-sectional study.

Colorectal Dis Off J Assoc Coloproctology G B Irel. 2015;**17**(1):26–37.

19. Bruheim K., Tveit K. M., Skovlund E., et al. Sexual function in females after radiotherapy for rectal cancer. *Acta Oncol Stockh Swed.* 2010;**49**(6):826–32.

20. Thyø A., Elfeki H., Laurberg S., Emmertsen K. J. Female sexual problems after treatment for colorectal cancer: A population-based study. *Colorectal Dis Off J Assoc Coloproctology G B Irel.* 2019;**21**(10):1130–9.

21. Provencher S., Oehler C., Lavertu S., et al. Quality of life and tumor control after short split-course chemoradiation for anal canal carcinoma. *Radiat Oncol Lond Engl.* 2010;**5**:41.

22. Fakhrian K., Sauer T., Dinkel A., et al. Chronic adverse events and quality of life after radiochemotherapy in anal cancer patients. A single institution experience and review of the literature. *Strahlenther Onkol Organ Dtsch Rontgengesellschaft Al.* 2013;**189**(6):486–94.

23. Sunesen K. G., Nørgaard M., Lundby L., et al. Long-term anorectal, urinary and sexual dysfunction causing distress after radiotherapy for anal cancer: A Danish multicentre cross-sectional questionnaire study. *Colorectal Dis Off J Assoc Coloproctology G B Irel.* 2015;**17**(11):O230–239.

24. Koerber S. A., Seither B., Slynko A., et al. Chemoradiation in female patients with anal cancer: Patient-reported outcome of acute and chronic side effects. *Tumori J.* 2019;**105**(2):174–80.

25. Corrigan K. L., Rooney M. K., De B., et al. Patient-reported sexual function in long-term survivors of anal cancer treated with definitive intensity modulated radiation therapy and concurrent chemotherapy. *Pract Radiat Oncol.* 2022;**12**(5):e397–405.

26. Wallace W. H. B., Thomson A. B., Kelsey T. W. The radiosensitivity of the human oocyte. *Hum Reprod Oxf Engl.* 2003;**18**(1):117–21.

27. Schüring A. N., Fehm T., Behringer K., et al. Practical recommendations for fertility preservation in women by the FertiPROTEKT network. Part I:

Indications for fertility preservation. *Arch Gynecol Obstet.* 2018;**297**(1):241–55.

28. Griffiths M. J., Winship A. L., Hutt K. J. Do cancer therapies damage the uterus and compromise fertility? *Hum Reprod Update.* 2020;**26**(2):161–73.

29. Van der Ven H., Liebenthron J., Beckmann M., et al. Ninety-five orthotopic transplantations in 74 women of ovarian tissue after cytotoxic treatment in a fertility preservation network: Tissue activity, pregnancy and delivery rates. *Hum Reprod Oxf Engl.* 2016;**31**(9):2031–41.

30. Muñoz E., Fernandez I., Martinez M., et al. Oocyte donation outcome after oncological treatment in cancer survivors. *Fertil Steril.* 2015;**103**(1):205–13.

31. Vogel J. D., Felder S. I., Bhama A. R., et al. The American Society of Colon and Rectal Surgeons Clinical Practice Guidelines for the Management of Colon Cancer. *Dis Colon Rectum.* 2022;**65**(2):148–77.

32. Kidane B., Chadi S. A., Kanters S., Colquhoun P. H., Ott M. C. Local resection compared with radical resection in the treatment of T1N0M0 rectal adenocarcinoma: a systematic review and meta-analysis. *Dis Colon Rectum.* 2015;**58** (1):122–40.

33. Rajput A., Bullard Dunn K. Surgical management of rectal cancer. *Semin Oncol.* 2007;**34**(3):241–9.

34. Kim S., Kim S. W., Han S. J. et al. Molecular mechanism and prevention strategy of chemotherapy- and radiotherapy-induced ovarian damage. *Int J Mol Sci.* 2021;**22** (14):7484.

35. Bedoschi G., Navarro P. A., Oktay K. Chemotherapy-induced damage to ovary: Mechanisms and clinical impact. *Future Oncol Lond Engl.* 2016;**12**(20):2333–44.

36. Cercek A., Siegel C. L., Capanu M., Reidy-Lagunes D., Saltz L. B. Incidence of chemotherapy-induced amenorrhea in premenopausal women treated with adjuvant FOLFOX for colorectal cancer. *Clin Colorectal Cancer.* 2013;**12**(3):163–7.

37. Sauer M. V., Paulson R. J., Ary B. A., Lobo R. A. Three hundred cycles of oocyte donation at the University of Southern California: Assessing the effect of age and infertility diagnosis on pregnancy and implantation rates. *J Assist Reprod Genet.* 1994;**11**(2):92–6.

38. Gupta S., Gupta Y. N., Sanyal B. Radiation changes in vaginal and cervical cytology in carcinoma of the cervix uteri. *J Surg Oncol.* 1982;**19**(2):71–3.

39. Shandley L. M., McKenzie L. J. Recent advances in fertility preservation and counseling for reproductive-aged women with colorectal cancer: A systematic review. *Dis Colon Rectum.* 2019;**62**(6):762–71.

40. Koerber S. A., Seither B., Slynko A., et al. Chemoradiation in female patients with anal cancer: Patient-reported outcome of acute and chronic side effects. *Tumori.* 2019;**105**(2):174–80.

41. Son C. H., Law E., Oh J. H., et al. Dosimetric predictors of radiation-induced vaginal stenosis after pelvic radiation therapy for rectal and anal cancer. *Int J Radiat Oncol Biol Phys.* 2015;**92**(3):548–54.

42. Briere T. M., Crane C. H., Beddar S., et al. Reproducibility and genital sparing with a vaginal dilator used for female anal cancer patients. *Radiother Oncol J Eur Soc Ther Radiol Oncol.* 2012;**104**(2):161–6.

43. Arians N., Häfner M., Krisam J., et al. Intrafractional vaginal dilation in anal cancer patients undergoing pelvic radiotherapy (DILANA): A prospective, randomized, 2-armed phase-II-trial. *BMC Cancer.* 2020;**20**(1):52.

44. Miles T., Johnson N. Vaginal dilator therapy for women receiving pelvic radiotherapy. *Cochrane Database Syst Rev.* 2010;9:CD007291.

45. Stahl J. M., Qian J. M., Tien C. J., et al. Extended duration of dilator use beyond 1 year may reduce vaginal stenosis after intravaginal high-dose-rate brachytherapy. *Support Care Cancer Off J Multinatl Assoc Support Care Cancer.* 2019;**27**(4):1425–33.

46. NCCN. NCCN Clinical Practice Guidelines: Survivorship Guidelines [Internet]. National Comprehensive

Cancer Network. [cited July 17, 2020]. www.nccn.org/professionals/physician_gls/default.aspx#survivorship

47. Candy B., Jones L., Vickerstaff V., Tookman A., King M. Interventions for sexual dysfunction following treatments for cancer in women. *Cochrane Database Syst Rev.* 2016;2:CD005540.

48. Denton A. S., Maher E. J. Interventions for the physical aspects of sexual dysfunction in women following pelvic radiotherapy. *Cochrane Database Syst Rev.* 2003;2003(1): CD003750.

49. Wo J. Y., Viswanathan A. N. Impact of radiotherapy on fertility, pregnancy, and neonatal outcomes in female cancer patients. *Int J Radiat Oncol Biol Phys.* 2009;**73**(5):1304–12.

50. Bisharah M., Tulandi T. Laparoscopic preservation of ovarian function: An underused procedure. *Am J Obstet Gynecol.* 2003;**188**(2):367–70.

51. Ribeiro R., Rebolho J. C., Tsumanuma F. K., et al. Uterine transposition: Technique and a case report. *Fertil Steril.* 2017;**108** (2):320–324.e1.

Chapter 13

Bladder Cancer

Valentina Grajales, Suzanne Lange and Kelly K. Bree

Case Presentation

A 70-year-old female presents to her PCP with recurrent urinary tract infections and hematuria. The patient initially presented with urgency, frequency, and gross hematuria. She was treated empirically with a course of antibiotics with some improvement in symptoms. She was also referred to Gynecology for concern of uterine bleeding. A month later she experienced recurrence of symptoms, and she was again treated with antibiotics but this time a urine culture was obtained. Urine culture was negative for infection; thus, she was referred to Urology for further work-up. Of note, the patient has a 20-pack year smoking history but quit 10 years ago.

Epidemiology

It is estimated that in 2023, a total of 82,290 new cases of bladder cancer will be diagnosed in the USA. Of these, 19,870 will occur in females with 4,500 expected female bladder cancer-related deaths [1]. Bladder cancer is the 11th most common cancer in women with a median age at diagnosis of 73 years [1, 2]. Survival is highly associated with stage, with a 5-year relative survival of 69.6% for localized disease and a dismal 5% for distant disease. Although males have a fourfold higher incidence of bladder cancer, female sex portends a worse prognosis [2–4]. The primary risk factor for development of bladder cancer is tobacco smoking, accounting for approximately 50% of cases [5]. Additional risk factors include: occupational exposures (i.e. paint, dyes, metals, petroleum), environmental exposures (i.e. arsenic), genetic mutations, race, prior pelvic radiation therapy, inflammatory inducing conditions (chronic indwelling urinary catheters and recurrent urinary tract infection) and Schistosoma haematobium infections [3], [5–7].

Presentation and Evaluation

Bladder cancer is often asymptomatic and may present with painless gross hematuria, microscopic hematuria or as an incidental bladder lesion on pelvic imaging [8]. Bladder cancer risk in patients with gross and microscopic hematuria is approximately 13.2% and 3.1%, respectively [4]. **Female patients often experience delays in diagnosis as hematuria can be presumed to be secondary to urinary infections or uterine bleeding, which may result in presentation with more advanced disease** [4, 8]. When symptomatic, patients may have associated irritative voiding symptoms such as dysuria, urgency, and frequency without the presence of a urinary infection [6]. In patients with bulky tumors or advanced cancer, obstructive voiding symptoms or flank pain due to hydroureteronephrosis may be present. The differential diagnosis for hematuria in females includes infection, inflammation, urolithiasis, malignancy (renal cancer, urothelial cancer, urethral cancer or invasion of other cancer into the urinary system), and gynecological sources of bleeding [4].

The diagnostic evaluation of gross hematuria includes visual evaluation of the bladder and urethra with cystourethroscopy and upper urinary tract imaging (cross sectional imaging with an urographic phase preferred, i.e. CT Urogram) [4]. Microscopic hematuria (defined as ≥3 RBC/HPF on microscopic evaluation; microscopic hematuria is NOT the presence of trace/moderate/large blood on urine dipstick alone) evaluation is now risk stratified based upon the degree of hematuria, age, smoking history and other risk factors (Figure 13.1) [4]. Urinary cytology or other urinary markers in the diagnostic setting are reserved for patients with gross hematuria or persistent microscopic hematuria, negative work-up and symptoms suggestive of carcinoma in situ (CIS) [4].

Fortunately, most patients (85%) will present with localized disease [2], however, about one quarter of these patients will have muscle invasion at diagnosis [3]. Treatment is dependent on cancer stage and grade at presentation. Bladder cancer staging is based on the American Joint Committee on Cancer (AJCC) Tumor-Node-Metastases (TNM) classi-fication (Table 13.1). Tumor grade is defined by the World Health Organization (WHO)/ International Society of Urological Pathology (ISUP) 2004 grading system, which designates tumors as low or high-grade and is an important prognostic factor in both recurrence and progression [6].

Among patients with nonmuscle invasive bladder cancer (NMIBC) (pTa, pTis, pT1), treatment will vary depending on risk of recurrence and/or progression. The American Urological Association (AUA) classifies patients into low, intermediate and high-risk categories with risk-stratified surveillance and treatment schedules [6]. Management of NMIBC is burdensome generally requiring multiple courses of adjuvant intravesical ther-apy, frequent cystoscopy +/- urine cytology and cross-sectional imaging studies [6, 7]. Despite this, survival outcomes are favorable in NMIBC. Approximately 30–40% of patients with low-risk NMIBC will recur at five years but with very low rates of progression or

Table 13.1 Staging of primary tumors (T) in bladder cancer

TX	Primary tumor cannot be assessed
Ta	Noninvasive papillary carcinoma
Tis	Carcinoma in situ (CIS)
T1	Tumor invades lamina propria
T2	Tumor invades muscularis propria
T2a	Tumor invades superficial muscularis propria (inner half)
T2b	Tumor invades deep muscularis propria (outer half)
T3	Tumor invades perivesical tissue/fat
T3a	Tumor invades perivesical tissue/fat microscopically
T3b	Tumor invades perivesical tissue fat macroscopically (extravesical mass)
T4	Tumor invades prostate, uterus, vagina, pelvic wall, or abdominal wall
T4a	Tumor invades adjacent organs (uterus, ovaries, prostate stoma)
T4b	Tumor invades pelvic wall and/or abdominal wall

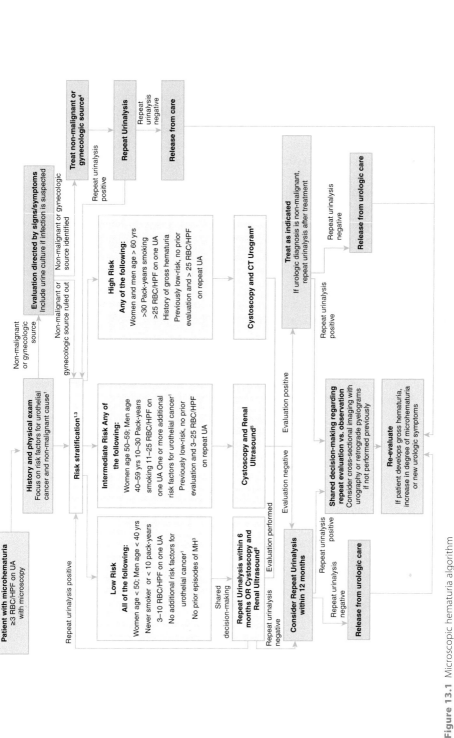

Figure 13.1 Microscopic hematuria algorithm

cancer-specific mortality [6]. Conversely, high-risk tumors (e.g. High-grade T1 or CIS) have high rates of recurrence (60–70% at 5 years), as well as 5-year progression to MIBC rates as high as 40% [9].

In patients with localized NMIBC, surgery with transurethral resection (TUR) +/- perioperative intravesical chemotherapy instillation is the gold standard treatment [6]. A bimanual exam is also performed at the time of TUR to better assess clinical staging. Following NMIBC diagnosis, adjuvant intravesical treatment options include the immuno-therapy agent Bacillus Calmette-Guerin (BCG) and chemotherapy agents such as mitomy-cin, gemcitabine, docetaxel and valrubicin. In addition, systemic immunotherapy with pembrolizumab has been approved by the FDA for patients with BCG-unresponsive, high-risk NMIBC with carcinoma in situ who are ineligible for or have elected to forgo cystectomy.

If patients present with or progress to MIBC, treatment options and prognosis differ from NMIBC. In patients with localized MIBC, radical cystectomy with urinary diversion +/- platinum-based neoadjuvant chemotherapy is the gold standard treatment [7]. Neoadjuvant chemotherapy (chemotherapy administered prior to surgery) with Methotrexate, Vinblastine, Doxorubicin, and Cisplatin (MVAC) has been shown to improve overall survival [10]. Since then, additional chemotherapeutic regimens including dose dense MVAC and gemcitabine and cisplatin have also been shown to improve survival outcomes [11, 12]. In females, radical cystectomy historically involves removing the bladder, urethra, uterus, fallopian tubes, ovaries, and part of the anterior vagina, in addition to a bilateral pelvic lymph node dissection [7, 8]. More recently, the AUA and the European Association of Urology (EAU) guidelines include consideration and discussion of reproductive organ sparing surgery in female patients who have organ confined disease [6, 13].

Trimodal therapy with transurethral resection, radio-sensitizing chemotherapy, and radiation represents another treatment option for highly selected patients with MIBC who prefer bladder preservation. Currently, there are no randomized trials comparing radical cystectomy and trimodal therapy [7].

At the time of radical cystectomy, concomitant urinary diversion is also performed. When selecting the type of urinary diversion to perform, one must take into consideration the patient's lifestyle, preference, medical history, and surgeon's experience. There are several reconstruction types including ileal conduit, orthotopic neobladder, or a continent cutaneous diversion [8]. The most common urinary diversion is the ileal conduit (Figure 13.2) with approximately 80% of patients undergoing this diversion as it involves shorter operation times, surgeon familiarity, and potentially reduced rates of post-operative complications [8]. Metabolic derangements associated with urinary diversions depend on the segment of bowel used, for example hyperchloremic metabolic acidosis and vitamin B12 deficiency can be seen with ileum segment diversions. Despite advancements in surgical technique and enhanced recovery pathways, radical cystectomy with urinary diversion has high morbidity and mortality rates. Nearly two-thirds of patients have a postoperative complication and approximately one-fourth are readmitted to the hospital after a radical cystectomy [8]. Perioperative mortality rate ranges from 1.5–2%.

Adjuvant therapies for patients with high-risk features after cystectomy such as locally advanced or node positive disease have been evaluated. These include cisplatin-based chemotherapy (if not given in the neoadjuvant setting), check-point inhibitors, and radi-ation. Data in this setting are not as robust as in the neoadjuvant setting, however, studies suggest that adjuvant systemic therapy may delay recurrences and improve overall survival

Ileal Conduit with Stoma

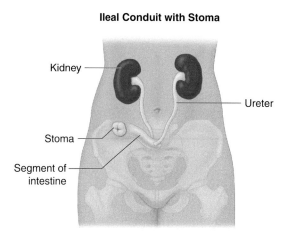

Figure 13.2 Ileal conduit urinary diversion, reproduced with permission from National Institute of Diabetes and Digestive and Kidney Diseases, National Institutes of Health

(albeit there are no robust randomized studies confirming definitive survival benefit) [14, 15].

In patients with metastatic disease, platinum-based chemotherapy is the mainstay of treatment. For those platinum-ineligible patients or those who fail platinum-based chemotherapy, alternative chemotherapy regimens, immunotherapy, or enrollment in clinical trials can be considered [12]. The most common sites of metastases include lymph nodes, lung, bone, and liver.

Special Considerations

Females are affected by multiple malignancies involved in the urologic system, including the kidney, ureters, bladder, and urethra; however, bladder cancer imparts a unique burden of disease and treatment effects for females as compared to males.

Gender-Based Disparities

While the incidence of bladder cancer is lower in females than males, when females are diagnosed with bladder cancer it is more often diagnosed at a higher stage [16–18]. The majority of data supporting inferior outcomes in women comes from the MIBC literature; however, differences appear to be present in NMIBC and metastatic settings as well [18]. Differences in presentation between sexes has been attributed to multiple etiologies. Anatomically, women have thinner bladders and embryologically close association of the trigone to the vagina without a robust fascial plane [18]. This close association of the bladder is thought to lead to higher risk for local invasion as compared to men, as they often have thickened bladders with age due to BPH and more robust fascial planes (i.e. Denonvillier's fascia) [19]. Another possible explanation for the disparity in outcomes between sexes involves differences in sex steroid hormone receptor-mediated signals that may lead to more aggressive cancer in females [16, 17, 19]. Genetic causes (e.g. X-chromosome associated, sex-specific degradation of carcinogens, etc.) are also being studied [16–19]. Lastly, population-level studies suggest that differences in outcomes for females compared to males may be due to disparities of care [16–18]. Females experience delayed diagnosis, likely due to lower rates of referral to urology and less frequent receipt of diagnostic imaging and/or cystourethroscopy [20]. These disparities may be secondary to attribution of lower urinary tract symptoms and gross hematuria to recurrent urinary tract infections or vaginal/uterine bleeding.

Role of Gynecologic Organ Sparing

Significant work is being performed to improve outcomes and the care for women who need radical cystectomy. As previously discussed, historically, radical cystectomy has included hysterectomy, anterior vaginectomy, and bilateral salpingo-oophorectomy. Recent studies have been performed evaluating pathology specimens from extirpative surgery and resultant long-term outcomes [21, 22]. A single institution, retrospective study of 186 women undergoing radical cystectomy found gynecological organ involvement in 5.7% of patients, with the vagina being the most common site of involvement, followed by the uterus. The vast majority of females had direct invasion of their bladder cancer rather than metastatic spread to these sites [21]. In females who had not had prior bilateral salpingo-oophorectomy, they did not identify any fallopian tube or ovarian involvement. A multi-institutional study of females who underwent anterior exenteration for high stage (≥pT3a) tumors found rare involvement of the ovaries [22]. When comparing vaginal involvement versus uterine or ovarian involvement, cancer specific survival was better for those with only vaginal involvement [22]. Taken together, these studies highlight the low risk of gynecologic organ involvement at the time of radical cystectomy, and thus the opportunity for gynecologic organ sparing in appropriately selected patients.

Ovarian Preservation

There is limited evidence supporting complete anterior pelvic exenteration (removal of all gynecologic organs) and growing evidence supporting possible detrimental physiologic and psychosocial impacts of complete gynecologic organ removal. Removal of the ovaries was previously thought to decrease risk for primary ovarian malignancy and eliminate risk of metastatic disease; however, increasing evidence now supports the notion that "ovarian" malignancies actually arise from the fallopian tubes [23, 24]. In lieu of bilateral oophorectomy at time of hysterectomy, some professional gynecological societies have expressed support of opportunistic salpingectomy in patients with normal risk at time of hysterectomy to decrease the risk of ovarian cancer – this procedure adds minimal surgical risk and simultaneously preserves ovarian function [25, 26]. One large, population-based study demonstrated significantly decreased incidence of serous and epithelial ovarian cancer among those who underwent opportunistic salpingectomy, as compared to those who had hysterectomy without salpingectomy or tubal ligation alone [25].

Ovarian removal can affect women of all ages. Despite the rarity of MIBC in pre-menopausal women with interest in fertility preservation, it can occur. Removal of the ovaries (and other gynecologic organs) would have direct impacts on fertility, especially if egg or embryo preservation are not feasible pre-operatively. Anecdotally, complete preservation of fertility is possible; however, relatively no research or reporting has been completed relating to surgical factors affecting fertility outcomes in this population [27]. Concerns also exist over the impact of chemotherapy on fertility. However, Solheim et al. demonstrated promising results of successful maternity in those who have received cisplatin-based therapy, which is commonly used in this urologic population [28].

In addition to the undisputed impacts on fertility, additional risks associated with surgically induced menopause include cardiovascular disease and cognitive impairment, as well as deleterious effects on sexual function [29]. Additionally, post-oophorectomy estrogen deficiency may lead to osteoporosis and increased risk of hip fracture [30, 31], as well as urinary symptoms related to vaginal atrophy (genitourinary syndrome of menopause) [32]. While there previously was believed to be minimal utility in ovarian preservation in postmenopausal women, new research suggests ovarian testosterone production impacts libido and sexual function – calling into question the potential impact of oophorectomy even in the postmenopausal patient population [31]. Considering these factors, discussion of potential risks versus benefits of ovarian removal is imperative with women of all ages.

With increasing data in support of ovarian preservation, and limited data in support of routine removal, mounting research suggests that the majority of women may benefit from ovary-sparing cystectomy [31–34]. Implementation of these practices may take time. A 2017 survey of urologic oncologists found that many providers were not aware of the benefits of salpingectomy and possible risks of oopoherectomy [35]. Fortunately, principles of gynecologic organ preservation are beginning to become incorporated into professional guidelines and hopefully will become more widely utilized for those with organ-confined disease [9].

Vaginal Preservation

Additional gynecological organs to spare at the time of radical cystectomy include the vagina and pelvic nerves [31, 33, 34]. Traditionally the anterior vagina is removed, and the remaining tissue is closed in a tubular or clamshell fashion, either narrowing or shortening the vagina, respectively. These reconstructed vaginal canals can lead to sexual dysfunction, dyspareunia, and prolapse. Data suggest that in women with nonbulky, non-trigonal, or nonbladder neck tumors vaginal-sparing procedures are likely safe [33]. Additionally, preservation of the vagina and pelvic floor may decrease risk of complications such as neobladder-vaginal fistula, bowel evisceration, and urinary retention (or "hyper-continence") [36].

Reported rates of vaginal complications vary and are likely underreported. However, a study utilizing Medicare claims data reported an overall vaginal complication rate of more than 20% [37]. Vaginal cuff dehiscence was the most frequent complication (10%) with a median time to occurrence of 25 days [37]. Data on cuff dehiscence are also quite limited in the gynecologic literature and are primarily comprised of case reports, however, a recent literature review noted that minimally invasive approaches to hysterectomy may be associated with higher risk of dehiscense [38]. In addition to cuff dehiscence, prolapse also represents another important, yet likely underreported, complication following cystectomy. A recent literature review identified only five studies discussing rates of prolapse following cystectomy [36]. There was significant heterogenicity among these limited studies with only one study using a validated instrument to assess subjective symptoms. Despite these gaps in the literature, the review noted prolapse rates of 0–23% following cystectomy [36]. In order to improve these outcomes, more research is paramount to understand the true incidence and risk factors associated with vaginal complications, as well as which surgical techniques minimize these complications. Assessment of baseline sexual function, physical exam with evaluation of preexisting vaginal atrophy and pelvic organ prolapse, and discussion of potential postoperative vaginal-related complications should become standard for clinicians performing radical cystectomy in females.

Neurovascular Preservation

Neurovascular preservation can be performed by carefully preserving the tissue lateral to the vagina during dissection, and potentially sparing the distal urethra in selected patients, which may facilitate preserved sexual function [31, 33, 34]. There is extensive men's health research evaluating the optimal technique for preservation of the neurovascular bundles during radical prostatectomy in hopes of retaining sexual function. Ideally, with ongoing research, similar practices can become standard of care when performing female radical cystectomy.

Survivorship Following Bladder Cancer Surgery

Aside from oncologic outcomes and technical improvements in surgery, improvements are necessary in understanding functional outcomes and quality of life following this major extirpative surgery. Patients may suffer from generalized negative effects on physical and social functioning, in addition to chronic physical and emotional side effects from treatment [39]. Utilization of Patient Reported Outcomes surveys is an important method to assess both the baseline and ongoing patient experience of cancer diagnosis and treatment [34]. One focus of functional and patient-reported outcomes is improving sexual function [40]. Postoperatively, or if a patient has received pelvic radiation, patients may have significant vaginal discomfort or dysfunction, which could benefit from interventions like lubricants, vaginal estrogen, or vaginal dilation [41]. Many patients would benefit from assistance of the gynecologist, pelvic floor physical therapists and/or sexual health therapists in management of these post-operative issues.

In addition to sexual symptoms, treatment of bladder cancer can have emotional and psychological impacts including decreased self-esteem and body image [34, 42]. Generally, bladder cancer has been found to be associated with increased anxiety, stress, and depression [32]. A recent cross-sectional survey of near 1,800 individuals, across bladder cancer stages and treatments, found reduced quality of life in multiple facets of physical and psychological function including decreased mobility, sexual dysfunction, and changes to body image [43]. The authors noted that health-related quality of life overall, aside from anxiety and depression, are worse than other pelvic malignancies like prostate or colorectal cancer [43]. Worse outcomes were generally associated with increased age and comorbidities. However, anxiety and depression were noted to be highest in younger age groups, who were also more concerned about the financial toxicities associated with management of their cancer. This study highlights the psychologic stress associated with a cancer diagnosis across all cancer types, while emphasizing that bladder cancer patients in particular have reduced quality of life, even when compared to patients with other common pelvic malignancies. Support in regards to physical therapy, access to mental health providers, and social work intervention is imperative.

Barriers in Delivery of Care to Women with Bladder Cancer

For various reasons, patients and providers find it difficult to discuss treatment options associated with the management of bladder cancer. A 2018 survey of urologic oncologist assessing pre-operative counseling prior to radical cystectomy found a wide variety of practices in assessment of baseline sexual dysfunction and counseling regarding perioperative and post-operative expectations [44]. Notably, almost 40% did not routinely discuss potential for pelvic organ preservation with sexually active females. Inadequate counseling was attributed to numerous barriers including advanced patient age, inadequate time during clinic visit and uncertainty of baseline sexual function. Difficulty with communication regarding sexual function is not limited to urology and is prevalent among multiple other cancer types [45, 46]. However, urologists are poised to lead the charge in improving understanding of women's sexual function and improved education of healthcare professionals [40].

Case Resolution

After referral to urology, the patient underwent clinic cystoscopy which demonstrated a large papillary bladder mass on the anterior bladder wall. She was then taken to the operating room, where exam under anesthesia and transurethral resection of this bladder mass was performed which revealed localized MIBC with lymphovascular invasion. Staging imaging was negative for any metastatic disease or involvement of the upper tracts (kidneys or ureters). The patient was referred to medical oncology and received neoadjuvant chemotherapy prior to undergoing radical cystectomy with ileal conduit urinary diversion. Prior to her surgery she had a pelvic exam that did not reveal any pelvic organ prolapse. The patient was single and not currently sexually active but stated that she may be interested in sexual activity in the future. Given the location of her tumor, a gynecologic organ sparing radical cystectomy was able to be completed. Postoperatively, the patient did experience change to self-esteem as she began dating with a new ileal conduit. Referrals to mental health providers and online support groups were helpful as the patient began to navigate her new life following cystectomy.

Take Home Points

- Female patients with microscopic or gross hematuria in the absence of other etiologies (i.e. active urinary tract infection, vaginal bleeding) should be referred to urology for evaluation.
- Hematuria is often attributed to other causes in females, leading to delays in diagnosis which may result in presentation with more advanced disease.
- While males are more likely to be diagnosed with bladder cancer, when females are diagnosed, they are more often diagnosed with later stage disease.
- Treatment of bladder cancer is largely dependent on stage and grade. Patients with non-muscle invasive bladder cancer can often be managed with transurethral resection +/- adjuvant intravesical therapy, while those with muscle-invasive disease often require radical cystectomy +/- neoadjuvant chemotherapy.
- Historically, radical cystectomy in the female has also included anterior pelvic exenteration with removal of the uterus, ovaries and anterior vagina. However, mounting research suggests that gynecologic organ preservation is likely safe in many patients.
- Radical cystectomy is associated with multiple gynecologic-specific complications including vaginal cuff dehiscence, pelvic organ prolapse, dyspareunia, iatrogenic menopause, and vaginal fistula.
- Ongoing research is needed to better understand the patient-related risk factors and surgical techniques associated with improved outcomes in female patients undergoing radical cystectomy.

- The treatment of bladder cancer, especially muscle invasive bladder cancer, has significant impacts on psychological, physical and sexual health. Open discussions with healthcare providers about the effect of bladder cancer diagnosis and treatment are paramount, as is referral to specialists as needed.

References

1. Siegel R. L., Miller K. D., Wagle N. S., Jemal A. Cancer statistics, 2023. *CA Cancer J Clin.* 2023;**73**:17–48.

2. SEER Cancer Stat Facts: Bladder Cancer. https://seer.cancer.gov/statfacts/html/urinb.html. Published 2022.

3. Burger M., Catto J. W., Dalbagni G., et al. Epidemiology and risk factors of urothelial bladder cancer. *Eur Urol.* 2013;**63**(2):234–41.

4. Barocas D. A., Boorjian S. A., Alvarez R. D., et al. Microhematuria: AUA/SUFU Guideline. *J Urol.* 2020;**204**(4):778–86.

5. Lobo N., Afferi L., Moschini M, et al. Epidemiology, screening, and prevention of bladder cancer. *Eur Urol Oncol.* 2022; **5**(6):628–39.

6. Chang S. S., Boorjian S. A., Chou R., et al. Diagnosis and treatment of non-muscle invasive bladder cancer: AUA/SUO guideline. *J Urol.* 2016;**196**(4):1021–9.

7. Chang S. S., Bochner B. H., Chou R., et al. Treatment of non-metastatic muscle-invasive bladder cancer: AUA/ASCO/ASTRO/SUO guideline. *J Urol.* 2017;**198**(3):552–9.

8. Lenis A. T., Lec P. M., Chamie K., Mshs M. D. Bladder cancer: A review. *JAMA.* 2020;**324**(19):1980–91.

9. Babjuk M., Burger M., Capoun O., et al. European Association of Urology Guidelines on Non-muscle-invasive Bladder Cancer (Ta, T1, and Carcinoma in Situ). *Eur Urol.* 2022;**81**(1):75–94.

10. Grossman H. B., Natale R. B., Tangen C. M., et al. Neoadjuvant chemotherapy plus cystectomy compared with cystectomy alone for locally advanced bladder cancer. *N Engl J Med.* 2003;**349**(9):859–66.

11. von der Maase H., Hansen S. W., Roberts J. T., et al. Gemcitabine and cisplatin versus methotrexate, vinblastine, doxorubicin, and cisplatin in advanced or metastatic bladder cancer: Results of a large, randomized, multinational, multicenter, phase III study. *J Clin Oncol.* 2000;**18**(17):3068–77.

12. Flaig T. W., Spiess P. E., Abern M., et al. NCCN Guidelines(R) Insights: Bladder Cancer, Version 2.2022. *J Natl Compr Canc Netw.* 2022;**20**(8):866–78.

13. Witjes J. A., Bruins H. M., Cathomas R., et al. European Association of Urology Guidelines on muscle-invasive and metastatic bladder cancer: Summary of the 2020 Guidelines. *Eur Urol.* 2021;**79**(1):82–104.

14. Millikan R., Dinney C., Swanson D., et al. Integrated therapy for locally advanced bladder cancer: Final report of a randomized trial of cystectomy plus adjuvant M-VAC versus cystectomy with both preoperative and postoperative M-VAC. *J Clin Oncol.* 2001;**19**(20):4005–13.

15. Leow J. J., Martin-Doyle W., Rajagopal P. S., et al. Adjuvant chemotherapy for invasive bladder cancer: A 2013 updated systematic review and meta-analysis of randomized trials. *Eur Urol.* 2014;**66**(1):42–54.

16. Dobruch J., Daneshmand S., Fisch M., et al. Gender and bladder cancer: A collaborative review of etiology, biology, and outcomes. *Eur Urol.* 2016;**69**(2):300–10.

17. Gul Z. G., Liaw C. W., Mehrazin R. Gender differences in incidence, diagnosis, treatments, and outcomes in clinically localized bladder and renal cancer. *Urology.* 2021;**151**:176–81.

18. Mun D. H., Kimura S., Shariat S. F., Abufaraj M. The impact of gender on oncologic outcomes of bladder cancer. *Curr Opin Urol.* 2019;**29**(3):279–85.

19. Moorthy H. K., Prabhu G. G. L., Venugopal P. Clinical and therapeutic implications of sex steroid hormone receptor status in urothelial bladder cancer. *Indian J Urol.* 2020;**36**(3):171–8.

20. Ngo B., Perera M., Papa N., Bolton D., Sengupta S. Factors affecting the timeliness and adequacy of haematuria assessment in bladder cancer: A systematic review. *BJU Int.* 2017;**119** Suppl 5:10–18.

21. Bree K. K., Hensley P. J., Westerman M. E., et al. Contemporary rates of gynecologic organ involvement in females with muscle invasive bladder cancer: A retrospective review of women undergoing radical cystectomy following neoadjuvant chemotherapy. *J Urol.* 2021;**206**(3):577–85.

22. Avulova S., Benidir T., Cheville J. C., et al. Prevalence, predictors, and oncologic outcomes of pelvic organ involvement in women undergoing radical cystectomy. *Arch Pathol Lab Med.* 2023;**147**(2):202–7.

23. Erickson B. K., Conner M. G., Landen C. N., Jr. The role of the fallopian tube in the origin of ovarian cancer. *Am J Obstet Gynecol.* 2013;**209**(5):409–14.

24. Karnezis A. N., Cho K. R., Gilks C. B., Pearce C. L., Huntsman D. G. The disparate origins of ovarian cancer: Pathogenesis and prevention strategies. *Nat Rev Cancer.* 2017;**17**(1):65–74.

25. Hanley G. E., Pearce C. L., Talhouk A., et al. Outcomes from opportunistic salpingectomy for ovarian cancer prevention. *JAMA Netw Open.* 2022;**5**(2): e2147343.

26. ACOG Committee Opinion No. 774. Opportunistic salpingectomy as a strategy for epithelial ovarian cancer prevention. *Obstet Gynecol.* 2019;**133**(4):e279–e284.

27. Fukushima H., Nakanishi Y., Kataoka M., Tobisu K. I., Koga F. Clinically node-positive micropapillary bladder cancer in a young female desiring to spare functional bladder and fertility. *Int Cancer Conf J.* 2020;**9**(3):151–4.

28. Solheim O., Trope C. G., Rokkones E., et al. Fertility and gonadal function after adjuvant therapy in women diagnosed with a malignant ovarian germ cell tumor (MOGCT) during the "cisplatin era". *Gynecol Oncol.* 2015;**136**(2):224–9.

29. Adelman M. R., Sharp H. T. Ovarian conservation vs removal at the time of benign hysterectomy. *Am J Obstet Gynecol.* 2018;**218**(3):269–79.

30. Liedberg F., Jancke G., Sorenby A., Kannisto P. Should we refrain from performing oophorectomy in conjunction with radical cystectomy for bladder cancer? *Eur Urol.* 2017;**71**(6):851–3.

31. Escott M., Avulova S., Bree K. K., Westerman M. E. Radical cystectomy and women's sexual health: Can we do better? *Curr Opin Urol.* 2022;**32**(5):545–53.

32. Vencill J. A., Kacel E. L., Avulova S., Ehlers S. L. Barriers to sexual recovery in women with urologic cancer. *Urol Oncol.* 2022;**40**(8):372–8.

33. Avulova S., Chang S. S. Role and indications of organ-sparing "radical" cystectomy: The importance of careful patient selection and counseling. *Urol Clin North Am.* 2018;**45**(2):199–214.

34. Tyson M. D., 2nd, Barocas D. A. Quality of life after radical cystectomy. *Urol Clin North Am.* 2018;**45**(2):249–56.

35. Sussman R. D., Han C. J., Marchalik D., et al. To oophorectomy or not to oophorectomy: Practice patterns among urologists treating bladder cancer. *Urol Oncol.* 2018;**36**(3):90 e1–90.

36. Richter L. A., Egan J., Alagha E. C., Handa V. L. Vaginal complications after radical cystectomy for bladder cancer: A systematic review. *Urology.* 2021;**156**: e20–e29.

37. Richter L. A., Osazuwa-Peters O. L., Routh J. C., Handa V. L. Vaginal complications after cystectomy: Results from a medicare sample. *J Urol.* 2022;**207**(4):789–96.

38. Cronin B., Sung V. W., Matteson K. A. Vaginal cuff dehiscence: Risk factors and

management. *Am J Obstet Gynecol.* 2012;**206**(4):284–8.

39. Mohamed N. E., Pisipati S., Lee C. T., et al. Unmet informational and supportive care needs of patients following cystectomy for bladder cancer based on age, sex, and treatment choices. *Urol Oncol.* 2016;**34**(12): e7–531.

40. Avulova S., Wittmann D. Optimizing women's sexual function and sexual experience after radical cystectomy. *Urology.* 2021;**151**:138–44.

41. Arthur S. S., Dorfman C. S., Massa L. A., Shelby R. A. Managing female sexual dysfunction. *Urol Oncol.* 2022;**40**(8):359–65.

42. Hedgepeth R. C., Gilbert S. M., He C., Lee C. T., Wood D. P., Jr. Body image and bladder cancer specific quality of life in patients with ileal conduit and neobladder urinary diversions. *Urology.* 2010;**76**(3):671–5.

43. Catto J. W. F., Downing A., Mason S., et al. Quality of life after bladder cancer: A cross-sectional survey of patient-reported outcomes. *Eur Urol.* 2021;**79**(5):621–32.

44. Gupta N., Kucirka L. M., Semerjian A., et al. Comparing provider-led sexual health counseling of male and female patients undergoing radical cystectomy. *J Sex Med.* 2020;**17**(5):949–56.

45. Reese J. B., Bober S. L., Daly M. B. Talking about women's sexual health after cancer: Why is it so hard to move the needle? *Cancer.* 2017;**123**(24):4757–63.

46. Reese J. B., Sorice K., Beach M. C, et al. Patient-provider communication about sexual concerns in cancer: A systematic review. *J Cancer Surviv.* 2017;**11**(2):175–88.

Breast Cancer

Giancarlo Moscol, Melissa Mitchell, and Rosa F. Hwang

Introduction

Case Presentation

BW is a 48-year-old premenopausal female with no significant past medical history presenting to clinic after self-palpating a right breast mass three weeks ago while showering. She has not had a prior screening mammogram. The mass is increasing in size, is hard and nontender. She also reports new right axillary fullness. Family history is significant for metastatic breast cancer in her paternal aunt (deceased at age 50) and father was diagnosed with metastatic prostate cancer four years ago at age 76.

Diagnostic mammogram demonstrates a 3 x 4 cm mass located at 3 o'clock 4 cm from nipple. Breast sonogram shows increased vascularity associated with the mass and two suspicious level I axillary lymph nodes. Biopsy reveals invasive ductal carcinoma, grade 3, with evidence of lympho-vascular invasion. Axillary lymph node biopsy is positive for metastatic disease. Tumor profile is negative for estrogen receptor, negative for progesterone receptor, and negative for human epidermal growth factor receptor-2 (HER2) with Ki-67=75%. What are the next steps?

Epidemiology

Breast cancer is the most common cancer diagnosed among women in the United States, excluding skin cancer. It is the second leading cause of cancer death among women overall, but the leading cause of cancer death among Black and Hispanic women. Approximately 287,850 new cases of invasive breast cancer and 51,400 cases of ductal carcinoma in situ (DCIS) were diagnosed in women in the United States in 2022 with 43,250 deaths reported [1].

The incidence of breast cancer has been increasing among women in the United States for the past 50 years. In 1975, the lifetime risk of breast cancer in women was 9.09% or 1 in 11. In 2022 this lifetime risk had increased to 12.9% or 1 in 8 women [2]. Interestingly, in less developed regions, the lifetime cumulative breast cancer risk is significantly lower than in developed countries (3.3%). These differences in incidence are related to risk factor exposure as well as availability of early detection methods.

Although the etiology of breast cancer remains largely unknown, several risk factors have been identified. Risk factors can be classified as non-modifiable (age, race, density of

Acknowledgements: The authors thank Debasish Tripathy, MD, Chair Breast Medical Oncology at The University of Texas MD Anderson Cancer Center for his council.

breast tissue, presence of germline mutations and positive family history) and modifiable (elevated body mass index (BMI), low exercise and activity levels, diet, alcohol consumption, radiation exposure, use of HT, parity, and history of breastfeeding among others). There is a clear association between breast cancer and estrogen exposure. Use of HT (particularly estrogen plus progesterone) leads to higher stimulation of cellular proliferation, increased mutation rates and higher rates of breast cancer as demonstrated in the Women's Health Initiative Hormone Trials [3].

Screening

Screening and diagnostic mammograms facilitate early diagnosis and prompt surgical intervention, which improves morbidity, decreases mortality, and helps save lives. As with other cancer screenings, their use may also lead to overdiagnosis of low risk or preinvasive conditions that may not improve mortality. Various guidelines differ regarding when to initiate screening. Most recently, the United States Preventative Services Task Force (USPSTF) (2023) updated their screening recommendations to include screening mammograms for all women every other year starting at age 40 [4]. Supplemental screening with breast ultrasound may be considered for women with dense fibroglandular tissue that obscures a potential breast cancer and decreases mammogram effectiveness [5]. Additional research is needed to understand the benefits and harms of screening women older than age 75, and we recommend extending screening mammograms for those with overall good general health, limited number of comorbidities and with at least 10 years of life expectancy.

Risk assessment tools provide a better way to assess lifetime risk of breast cancer and guide when to initiate screening mammograms. These models incorporate multiple clinical variables (age, ethnicity, previous biopsies, parity, age at menarche and previous family members with breast cancer) to estimate a woman's risk of developing breast cancer in the next five years and during her lifetime. These tools are not indicated for women with a known pathogenic variant (PV) (*BRCA1/2, PTEN, PALB2*) or with a previous diagnosis of ductal carcinoma in situ (DCIS) or lobular carcinoma in situ (LCIS). We recommend using the Breast Cancer Risk Assessment Tool available online (bcrisktool.cancer.gov) to help predict the five -year and lifetime risk for breast cancer for women. The average lifetime risk for developing breast cancer is calculated at 12.4%. For women with slightly elevated risk (between 12% and 20% lifetime risk) annual screening mammograms should begin at age 40 (with no role for breast MRI), while for those with a lifetime risk >20%, screening mammograms alternating with breast MRIs 6 months apart are recommended beginning at age 40.

Pathology

Benign breast lesions can be incidentally found as part of the workup for abnormal mammogram findings including microcalcifications. They are usually asymptomatic and include proliferative lesions with and without atypia. There are two subtypes of particular interest: atypical ductal hyperplasia (ADH) and atypical lobular hyperplasia (ALH). These lesions are managed more as indicators of subsequent malignancy risk rather than precursor lesions that may evolve into invasive breast cancer. The presence of ADH or ALH on previous biopsy increases the lifetime risk of breast cancer and is incorporated in the Breast Cancer Risk Assessment Tool.

Table 14.1 Breast lesions: Continuum from benign to invasive breast cancer

Benign lesions with associated risk of invasive disease:	Atypical lobular hyperplasia, Atypical ductal hyperplasia
Preinvasive lesions:	Ductal carcinoma in situ (DCIS), Lobular carcinoma in situ
Invasive disease:	Invasive ductal carcinoma, Invasive lobular carcinoma

Malignant breast lesions or carcinomas of the breast are broadly divided into two major categories:

- Noninvasive carcinomas (malignant cells are confined by the basement membrane). Two subtypes are identified based on histology: ductal carcinoma in situ (DCIS) and lobular carcinoma in situ (LCIS). These lesions are considered preinvasive and are staged as stage 0.
- Invasive carcinomas (malignant invasion through the basement membrane and possible spread to the lympho-vascular space, possible distant metastases). The two most common subtypes include invasive ductal carcinoma (accounting for 75% of all newly diagnosed breast cancer) and invasive lobular carcinoma (approximately 15% of all newly diagnosed cases). Other less frequent subtypes include mucinous, tubular or papillary and comprise the remaining 10% of new cases.

There is a continuum of lesions that can be identified as precursors for invasive breast cancer (Table 14.1).

Biomarkers

Estrogen receptors (ER) and progesterone receptors (PR) play a critical role in breast development, differentiation, and tumorigenesis. The majority (68%) of newly diagnosed breast cancer are ER/PR positive [6]. These receptors can be targeted in the neoadjuvant (before surgery) and adjuvant (after surgery) setting with use of hormone blockers such as selective estrogen receptor modulators [(SERMs), tamoxifen] in premenopausal women as well as aromatase inhibitors [(AIs) anastrozole, letrozole or exemestane] in postmenopausal females. ER and PR expression is detected using immunohistochemical staining (IHC), with positive considered as >10% expression, low positive as 1–10% expression, and negative <1% expression.

HER2 is a member of the tyrosine kinase growth factor receptor family. HER2 positivity indicates worse biological behavior, high clinical aggressiveness and leads to uncontrolled tumor growth in breast cancer. Testing for HER2 can be performed using two different modalities: IHC (assessing the amount of protein expression in the breast cancer cell membrane) and FISH (fluorescence in situ hybridization) that evaluates the number of copies of the HER2 gene in the nucleus of the cancer cell. HER2 expression by IHC staining is graded into three levels: IHC negative (0 and 1+), IHC equivocal (2+), and IHC positive (3+). Equivocal (2+) IHC should prompt ordering a reflex confirmatory FISH test.

Ki-67 is a marker of cellular proliferation in breast cancer. A high Ki-67 index generally correlates with high tumor grade and more aggressive disease, as is the case for HER2 positive and triple negative breast cancer. Breast carcinomas with a high Ki-67 index (>20%) usually respond well to chemotherapy.

PD-L1 (programmed death ligand-1) is a protein expressed on the surface of some cancer cells. When expressed, it inactivates T-lymphocytes and suppresses the immune response against breast cancer proliferation. It is measured with IHC, and reported using the combined positive score (CPS) system. A CPS >10% predicts response to immunotherapy (with an agent called pembrolizumab) for patients with metastatic triple negative breast cancer in their first line of therapy (see later section on management of triple negative breast cancer) [7, 8].

Workup and Staging

Initial diagnostic workup for a breast mass should include physical examination with special attention to location of the mass, extension to skin and attachment to posterior chest wall, changes in skin density, nipple retraction, and palpation of axillary and supraclavicular lymph nodes. Diagnostic mammogram allows the diagnosis of soft tissue masses with associated microcalcifications and spiculations, while breast ultrasound (US) can differentiate other features associated with malignancy including hypoechogenicity, internal calcifications, shadowing and irregular or indistinct margins. Breast US also helps characterize any suspicious lymph nodes (axillary, supraclavicular or internal mammary) that should be targeted for biopsy.

Staging for newly diagnosed breast cancer follows the 8th American Joint Committee on Cancer (AJCC) TNM system (Table 14.2). The most recent edition differentiates between anatomic and prognostic staging, recognizing that tumor grade, hormone and HER2 receptor status refine prognosis [9]. The use of the prefix "c" indicates clinical staging (physical exam and imaging), "p" indicates pathological assessment, "y" indicates post therapy (systemic or radiation), and "r" indicates recurrent disease.

Staging scans including CT chest/abdomen/pelvis and bone scan are recommended to rule out distant metastatic disease for patients with breast masses bigger than 5 cm or with multiple biopsy positive enlarged or matted axillary lymph nodes. Additionally, they should be considered for patients with symptoms concerning for distant metastatic disease (localized bone pain, elevated alkaline phosphatase, abnormal liver function tests, abdominal or pelvic masses on physical exam). As endorsed by NCCN guidelines, routine systemic staging is not indicated for early localized cancer patients in the absence of systemic symptoms [10].

Treatment for Breast Cancer

The management of breast cancer is multidisciplinary, including breast surgical oncology (to discuss surgical modalities: segmental mastectomy versus mastectomy, role of sentinel lymph node biopsy and axillary management for more advanced cases), radiation oncology (to discuss the use of adjuvant radiotherapy to reduce the risk of local recurrence) and medical oncology (to identify modifiable risk factors, administer endocrine therapy and/or chemotherapy for patients with high risk features to prevent recurrence and progression into metastatic disease).

Surgical Management of Breast Cancer

The surgical options for patients with breast cancer have expanded considerably in the past few decades. As a result, the decision-making process has become more complicated and

Table 14.2 TNM staging categories of breast cancer [11]

Category	Definitions
Tis	In situ (ductal not lobular), should specify separately if Paget's disease
T1	≤ 2 cm (invasive component)
T1mic	≤ 1 mm
T1a	> 1 mm and ≤ 5 mm
T1b	> 5 mm and ≤ 10 mm
T1 c	> 10 mm and ≤ 2 cm
T2	> 2 cm and ≤ 5 cm
T3	> 5 cm
T4	Any size with extension to chest wall/skin as described below
T4a	Extension to chest wall with adherence (does not pertain to pectoralis muscle involvement)
T4b	Extension to skin with ulceration, satellitosis, edema and/or redness (not meeting T4d criteria)
T4 c	Both T4a and T4b apply
T4d	Inflammatory breast cancer (peau d'orange edema and erythema involving more than 1/3 of the breast with clinically rapid onset)
cN0	No palpable or imaging-apparent adenopathy
cN1a	Ipsilateral mobile axillary level I or II nodes
cN2a	Fixed or matted axillary nodes
cN2b	No axillary node, but ipsilateral internal mammary (IM) nodes present
cN3a	Ipsilateral infraclavicular (axillary level 3) node(s)
cN3b	Ipsilateral and internal mammary and axillary nodes
cN3 c	Ipsilateral supraclavicular node
pN0	Histologically negative axillary nodes
pN0[i+] / pN0[mol+]	Isolated tumor cells only, ≤ 0.2 mm / molecularly + (by RT-PCR*)
pN1	Involvement of 1 to 3 axillary nodes (> 0.2 mm)
pN1mic	Micrometastases only to axillary nodes (> 0.2 mm and ≤ 2 mm)
pN1a	Involvement of 1-3 axillary nodes, at least one > 2 mm
pN1b	Involvement of IM node > 0.2 mm
pN1 c	Both pN1a and pN1b apply
pN2	Refers to either pN2a or pN2b
pN2a	Involvement of 4-9 nodes, at least one > 2 mm
pN2b	Involvement of IM node(s),withnegativeaxillary nodes on pathologic review
pN3	Refers to either pN3a, pN3b or pN3 c

Table 14.2 (cont.)

Category	Definitions
pN3a	Involvement of 10+ nodes, at least one > 2 mm, or infraclavicular (axillary level 3) node(s)
pN3b	pN1a or pN2a with cN2b or pN2a with pN1b
pN3 c	Involvement of ipsilateral supraclavicular node(s)
For all pN categories, suffix (sn) used if regional node metastasis identified only by sentinel node, or suffix (f) if by fine needle aspirate or core biopsy	
cM0	No tissue-based, clinical or radiographic distant metastases (beyond breast and ipsilateral regional nodes). Imaging not required.
cM0[i+]	cM0, but circulating or bone marrow tumor cells or tissue deposits ≤ 0.2 mm
cM1	Distant metastases noted by physical exam or imaging
pM1	Histologically demonstrated distant metastases > 0.2 mm

IM= internal mammary; RT-PCR=reverse transcriptase polymerase chain reaction, T=tumor, c=clinical, p=pathological, N=nodes, M=metastasis

should be carefully considered in a multidisciplinary fashion with medical oncology, radiation oncology, plastic/reconstructive surgery (when appropriate) as well as the patient's preferences.

Surgery for the primary breast tumor (or "local treatment") includes breast-conserving surgery (BCS, or lumpectomy) and mastectomy. With lumpectomy surgery, adjuvant radiation therapy (RT) to the remaining ipsilateral breast is typically recommended for complete breast-conserving therapy (BCT) which provides equivalent disease-free and overall survival compared to total mastectomy [12, 13]. Recent studies suggest that BCT may even confer improved overall- and disease specific survival compared to mastectomy in early-stage breast cancer with very low rates of local/regional recurrence of 4.6% at 5 years [14–17]. In general, patients who are appropriate candidates for BCS should have a favorable breast-to-tumor ratio, which is subjectively determined by the breast surgeon and relies on accurate breast imaging, and the patient should be willing and able to undergo adjuvant RT. The conventional eligibility criteria for BCS have broadened with the advent of oncoplastic reconstruction techniques to include patients with tumors that are relatively large, multicentric or located in unfavorable locations (e.g.-medial quadrants) [18, 19]. Broadly, oncoplastic reconstruction techniques combine cancer treatment surgery with cosmetic surgery to reconstruct the breast following lumpectomy surgery. These techniques include mobilizing breast tissue surrounding a lumpectomy cavity to fill the cavity to avoid a contour deformity, excising skin to avoid any dimpling and repositioning the nipple to avoid or correct deviation or ptosis of the nipple-areolar complex.

Although many more women are now eligible for BCS due to the improved response seen with modern neoadjuvant systemic therapy and the increasing use of oncoplastic reconstruction, there remain a few relative contraindications to BCS for whom total mastectomy would be indicated. These include patients who have inflammatory breast cancer, those with large volume disease for whom oncoplastic reconstruction is not available or adequate, or patients with contraindications to RT such as a prior history of chest RT or scleroderma. In addition, women with pathogenic germline mutations that confer an increased risk of breast cancer, such as *BRCA1/2* mutations, may elect to undergo prophylactic mastectomies (PM) to decrease their risk of breast cancer. In a large prospective, multicenter study of 2482 women with *BRCA1* or *BRCA2* mutations, none of the women who underwent PM developed breast cancer, compared to 7% of those who did not undergo PM surgery [20].

For those women who are interested in reconstruction after mastectomy, the cosmetic outcome is improved with immediate reconstruction compared to delayed reconstruction. In the setting of immediate reconstruction, the breast surgeon will perform either skin-sparing or nipple- and skin-sparing mastectomy in order to preserve the skin envelope with or without the nipple [21, 22]. Reconstruction after mastectomy can be with either breast implants or autologous tissue or occasionally implants combined with autologous tissue for additional volume when needed. Autologous flap reconstruction is performed most often using donor tissue from the lower abdomen or latissimus dorsi muscle from the back. Other potential donor sites include tissue from the inner thigh or buttock [23]. Reconstruction is be performed in a staged fashion (also called "delayed-immediate") with initial placement of a temporary tissue expander (TE) after skin- or nipple-sparing mastectomy, followed by definitive reconstruction with either implant or autologous tissue at a later date. This approach is often used for patients with locally advanced breast cancer who may need postmastectomy radiation in order to avoid radiating the final reconstructed breast. Staged reconstruction with TEs is also used when the mastectomy skin needs to be stretched (expanded) to create additional space when a larger final breast size is desired. Many women will opt to forego reconstruction after mastectomy in order to have a faster recovery or avoid placement of a foreign body with surveys showing good satisfaction scores [24].

Surgical Management of Lymph Nodes

The goals of surgical evaluation of regional lymph nodes for patients with breast cancer are to provide information that will help guide treatment decisions and to help determine prognosis, but it is not performed primarily for a therapeutic purpose. This section will focus on management of the lymph nodes in the axilla which are more likely to be involved with breast cancer compared to other nodal basins such as the internal mammary or supraclavicular nodes. During the initial workup for a patient with newly diagnosed breast cancer, physical exam of the axilla and other regional nodal basins and possibly imaging with ultrasound should be performed to evaluate for lymph node involvement. Any clinically suspicious nodes should be biopsied to assess for metastasis.

For patients with clinically node-negative disease, sentinel lymph node biopsy (SLNB) is performed to remove the first few lymph nodes in the axilla to which a breast cancer is likely to spread. SLNB accurately stages the axilla with multiple large series reporting 95-100% accuracy in predicting the status of axillary nodes [25]. However, SLNB has less morbidity than axillary lymph node dissection (ALND) which removes more lymph nodes and is associated with significantly higher risk of neuropathy, shoulder dysfunction and lymphedema [26, 27]. Patients with early-stage breast cancer with negative SLNs do not need to have ALND as demonstrated in the NSABP B-32 trial that enrolled 5611 patients with no significant differences in regional control, overall survival (92.9% versus 91.6%) or disease free survival (75.1% versus 76.1%) between the groups [28]. For patients with one to two metastatic SLNs, ALND can be safely omitted if they undergo BCS with whole-breast radiation [29, 30].

Axillary lymph node dissection (ALND) removes nodes in levels I and II of the axilla, which are located inferior/lateral to the pectoralis minor (level I) and posterior to the pectoralis minor and inferior to the axillary vein (level II). Dissection of level III of the axilla (infraclavicular) is usually reserved for patients with locally advanced disease involving that nodal basin. Typically, ALND is performed for patients with clinically node positive nodes at initial presentation. However, if the patient receives neoadjuvant systemic treatment and has a good response, they may be eligible for targeted axillary dissection which is a more limited procedure to remove only the biopsy-confirmed positive node along with SLNs [31]. ALND is also performed for clinically node-negative breast cancer patients who have a positive SLN but do not meet the criteria for the ACOSOG-Z0011 trial. This would include patients with three or more positive SLNs, those who are not candidates for whole breast irradiation, have large tumors >5 cm or the presence of extranodal extension, although radiation to the nodal basins may be appropriate instead of ALND. Finally, for patients with clinically node-positive disease who undergo neoadjuvant therapy and have residual positive nodes on targeted axillary dissection, the standard of care is to perform completion ALND although clinical trials are in progress to determine whether axillary radiation is as effective as ALND. As the algorithms for management of axillary nodes continue to evolve, it is critical for surgeons to work closely with colleagues in medical oncology, radiation oncology and the patient to determine the best approach individually tailored for each patient.

Radiotherapy for Breast Cancer

Radiation Therapy for Early-Stage Breast Cancer

Radiation plays a role in curative treatment for most breast cancer patients undergoing partial mastectomy (also known as segmental mastectomy or lumpectomy). Mastectomy does not completely reduce the risk of local recurrence, even in early-stage breast cancer, as a small amount of breast tissue remains between the pectoralis muscle and skin, even with a total mastectomy. Thus, large randomized studies comparing mastectomy to lumpectomy and whole breast radiotherapy show no difference in local control, distant disease or metastases with breast conserving treatment, consisting of lumpectomy and radiation, as compared to mastectomy [32]. Recent retrospective studies in the modern era suggest that lumpectomy and radiation may even have improved outcomes over mastectomy in patients matched for clinical tumor and patient characteristics [33, 34]. This observation has been especially notable for hormone positive patients; it has also been consistently noted in hormone negative breast cancer, which has been theorized to be related to immune stimulation from radiation exposure [35, 36]. Based on equivalency in oncologic outcomes across multiple studies, options of breast conservation or mastectomy should be routinely offered to all patients who are surgical candidates, regardless of age or tumor subtype. However, diffuse disease throughout the breast or unfavorable ratio of tumor size to breast size that would lead to poor cosmetic outcomes, despite oncoplastic rearrangement, may still require mastectomy. Prior radiation, such as for mediastinal lymphoma, or connective tissue disorders, such as scleroderma or active lupus, are also contraindications for radiation therapy, and thus breast conserving treatment.

Lumpectomy is routinely followed by radiation, as meta-analyses show it reduces recurrence at 10 years from 35% to 19.2% and reduces the 15-year risk of breast cancer death from 25.2 to 21.4% [37]. However, there is a subset of patients for whom lumpectomy alone is an acceptable option. Two large studies of lumpectomy alone versus lumpectomy with radiation have now been published for hormone positive pT1N0 patients > 65 years old [38] or >70 years old [39]. These studies both show a reduction from 10% to 2% in 10-year local recurrence for patients treated with adjuvant radiation as compared to lumpectomy alone. However, as recurrences are still rare and usually salvaged with repeat surgery and radiation, there was no survival advantage noted. As such, omission of radiation should be an option for patients over 65 with small, node negative, hormone positive, and Her-2 negative tumors. Patients with favorable DCIS, low grade, measuring less than 2.5 cm in size, excised with more than 3 mm clear margins, also have a low risk of recurrence, approximately 1% per year [40]. The RTOG 9804 randomized study of radiation therapy verses omission after lumpectomy for this subset of DCIS patients also suggested minimal reduction in recurrence, supporting omission as a reasonable option for these patients [41]. Ongoing large cooperative group studies will help determine whether omission will be an option for younger patients with hormone positive and/or Her-2 positive T1N0 breast cancer, including the DEBRA trial (ClinicalTrials.gov number, NCT04852887) and HERO (NCT05705401). Outside of trials, all patients under 65 with invasive cancer, patients with tumors greater than 3 cm, Her-2 positive patients, and all triple negative breast cancer patients are recommended for radiation therapy.

For whole breast radiation, high energy photons are directed at the breast using tangent fields designed using CT modeling to pass through the breast tissue and minimize exposure to heart and lung. Radiation causes DNA damage to tumor cells as well as normal tissue. Giving a small dose daily allows for normal tissue to repair, but confers irreparable damage to the tumor tissue. By administering multiple sessions over the course of several weeks, there is an additive preferential damage to tumor tissue. Historically, patients received conventional doses of radiation, consisting of 1.8 to 2.0 Gy per fraction, given 5 days a week, for 5–7 weeks of therapy, for total tumor bed doses of ~60 Gy. Hypofractionation is the term used when treatment is given over a shorter time by using less fractions to get to an equivalent effective radiation dose. When treatment is given over a shorter time by using less fractions to get to an equivalent effective radiation dose, this is termed hypofractionation. Studies comparing conventional fractionation with moderate hypofractionation, using 2.6 to 2.7 Gy per fraction for 3–4 weeks of therapy, for total tumor bed doses of ~ 50 Gy, showed similar results with regards to oncologic outcomes of local control and survival [42, 43]. These studies also showed reduced acute toxicity to the skin and improved cosmesis, making hypofractionation standard of care for early-stage node negative breast cancer [44]. Early results were recently published from randomized trials on ultrahypofractionated radiation, treating patients with 5.2 Gy per fraction for just one week, with a total dose of 26 Gy [45]. At five years of follow-up, oncologic outcomes were equivalent and cosmesis was similar, although critics caution routine use of this regimen until longer follow-up is available [46].

In extremely low risk patients, accelerated partial breast irradiation (APBI) therapy is an acceptable treatment option. There are several dosing options for partial breast radiation, which generally delivers 26–38.5 Gy to the tumor bed with a margin. This spares a portion of the normal breast and treatment is delivered over only five days. Randomized studies comparing partial breast radiation to whole breast radiation have shown similar rates of local control and survival, however, initial studies of APBI used doses and fields that impaired cosmesis [47, 48]. More recent studies using modern techniques to spare normal tissue have shown improved cosmesis as compared to whole breast treatment and equivalent oncologic control for low risk patients [49, 50]. Guidelines for the use of APBI have been published by the ASTRO task force, with the most suitable patients over 50 years of age with T1N0 hormone positive tumors excised with widely negative margins [51].

Radiation Therapy for Locally Advanced Breast Cancer

In patients with positive lymph nodes or tumors greater than 5 cm in size, comprehensive radiation may be recommended to the breast and lymph nodes. Recently published MA.20 and EORTC 22922 trials show improved oncologic outcomes with nodal treatment, as compared to breast radiation alone [52, 53]. Decisions to treat the whole breast alone or to include the axilla, supraclavicular, infraclavicular and internal mammary nodes are based on extent of axillary surgery as well as the presence and number of high-risk features. High-risk features include young age, large primary tumor size, medial tumor location, presence of multiple positive nodes, lymphovascular invasion, high grade disease, and ER negative disease. Current studies are assessing the role of genomic assays to predict potential benefit of nodal radiation in low risk patients, such as Tailor RT, which is enrolling ER+ patients with node positive disease or T3N0 tumors (NCT03488693).

Patients undergoing mastectomy with low risk T1-2N0 disease do not require post-mastectomy radiation therapy, but as with breast-conserving patients, tumor size greater than 5 cm or presence of positive nodes may warrant comprehensive radiation treatment. In a meta-analysis of mastectomy alone versus mastectomy with radiation therapy, local recurrence risk was reduced from 26% to 8.1% with radiation, while breast cancer specific mortality was reduced from 66.4% to 58.3% with postmastectomy radiation [54]. The aforementioned high-risk features are utilized to guide radiation decisions in these patients. Patients requiring radiation who had sentinel node biopsy alone may be considered for omission of axillary dissection, as long as the radiation oncologist plans to intentionally target the level I and II axilla. However, in hormone positive and node positive patients with no adverse features, axillary dissection is recommended if radiation is not anticipated [55].

The radiation recommendations above are based on pathologic findings from upfront surgical treatment. However, many patients are recommended for neoadjuvant chemotherapy, including most Her-2 positive or triple negative patients with tumors more than 2 cm in size or positive nodes, as well as young node positive patients with hormone positive tumors. In patients undergoing surgery after systemic therapy, radiation recommendations are routinely based on clinical stage, regardless of the response to the systemic therapy. Any patient with cT3N0 disease or a biopsy proven node prior to systemic therapy should routinely receive radiation therapy while awaiting the results of the NSABP B51 trial, which randomized mastectomy patients with a pathologic complete treatment response to observation vs postmastectomy radiation therapy and breast conserving patients to whole breast radiation +/- regional nodal radiation (NCT01872975). Any patient with a positive node following systemic therapy, regardless of surgical type or clinical stage, should receive comprehensive radiation therapy to include treatment of all the nodal basins and the breast or chest wall.

Patients requiring comprehensive radiation are typically treated with conventional radiation, using 1.8–2.0 Gy per fraction over 25–30 fractions, for a total dose of ~60 Gy. Initial hypofractionation studies were performed primarily in patients receiving whole breast radiotherapy and there was concern for greater long term toxicity to critical structures, such as the brachial plexus [42, 43]. However, trials of hypofractionation in patients undergoing comprehensive radiation to include the nodes are well underway and starting to report outcomes. Early reports suggest reduced toxicity with hypofractionation, especially with regards to acute symptoms of fatigue and skin reaction [56]. Early results suggest a possible reduction in lymphedema and equivalent local control.

Radiation Toxicity and Developing Technology

Acute side effects of radiotherapy include mild fatigue, skin erythema, pruritus, and breast or chest wall edema or tenderness. These usually resolve following radiation. Patients receiving comprehensive radiation therapy may also experience mild esophagitis, transient thyroid inflammation, decreased range of motion or ipsilateral extremity lymphedema. Long term, patients may see a change in the shape, size, or color of the breast. Injury to underlying tissue, such as the heart or lung, are rare, with very low incidence of pneumonitis or heart disease, especially with modern planning techniques. Secondary malignancies, rib fractures, and brachial plexopathy are also rare.

It has been estimated that one breast cancer death is avoided for every four breast cancer local recurrences prevented with radiation [57]. While radiation can reduce the risk of local recurrence in breast cancer patients, which often translates into a survival advantage, it is not without risk. Survival gains are countered by increased risk of heart disease, pulmonary disease, contralateral breast cancer, and lung cancer, especially in patients treated in prior eras. Newer technology may improve survival gains by reducing risk of long-term radiation-related morbidity.

A case-control study of major coronary events in over 2000 patients treated between 1958 and 2001 showed a linear correlation between radiation dose to the heart and risk of cardiac sequelae [58]. Heart doses were seen to decrease over time during this period. With modern radiation treatment, great attention is placed on reducing dose to the heart. With 3D conformal radiation, the angle for the path of beam is optimized to exclude or minimize cardiac radiation exposure. In patients with challenging anatomy, chest motion during a deep inspiratory breath hold can move the target tissue anteriorly, away from the heart, while diaphragmatic breathing pulls the heart downwards in the thoracic cavity, also away from the radiation field. Current recommendations for limiting heart dose place risk far below what was observed in the aforementioned study.

Other new technology to improve the safety of radiation treatment includes surface guidance, which employs 3D cameras to monitor the surface of the patient, in order to ensure correct positioning of the patient before and during treatment [59]. This technique can help to monitor accurate deep inspiration breath hold for patients, as well as eliminate the need for external markings or tattoos for breast cancer patients. Volumetric modulated arc therapy allows for delivery of radiation in a continuous arc around the patient, with constant computer generated modulation of the beam to deliver radiation to target tissue. This minimizes the dose to organs at risk, leading to a more conformal dose of radiation to the patient. Proton therapy is also gaining popularity in breast cancer treatment [60]. Unlike photons, which pass all the way through the body, the depth of proton radiation can be controlled with modification of beam energy, which can also allow radiation to be delivered conformally with exceptional sparing of the normal tissues. However, the treatment is sensitive to set-up errors, patient motion, and changes in tissue volume during treatment, such as seroma formation or resolution. The ongoing RADCOMP trial comparing proton radiation to photon treatment is powered to detect a reduction in cardiac toxicity with the use of proton treatment (NCT01766297).

Systemic Therapy for Breast Cancer

Systemic therapy for breast cancer includes the use of antihormonal therapies, chemotherapy, immunotherapy, targeted agents, antibodies and antibody drug conjugates. The goal of systemic therapy is to eliminate occult metastases and reduce the risk of local and distant recurrence. Different factors such as the size of the breast tumor, number of lymph nodes involved, tumor grade, menopausal status and genomic risk help understand the aggressiveness of the disease, risk of recurrence and overall benefit from systemic chemotherapy and/or endocrine therapy. Depending on the timing, treatment can be given before (neoadjuvant) or after surgery (adjuvant). Neoadjuvant chemotherapy is given with intent to shrink the tumor size in order to facilitate improved rates of breast conservation surgery, achieve negative margins and to serve as an in-vivo sensitivity test. Adjuvant chemotherapy is given after surgical resection to reduce the risk of local and distant recurrence and increase overall survival.

Genomic testing refers to the evaluation of certain genes in the breast cancer cell associated with high risk of recurrence, aggressiveness and sensitivity to chemotherapy. Genomic testing is usually recommended for ER positive tumors after surgical resection. There are multiple platforms available to perform this testing, but we recommend using the Oncotype Dx Recurrence Score (RS). Oncotype Dx score has been validated in multiple randomized prospective studies [61] and is both prognostic for risk of recurrence (identifies patients with a high risk breast cancer independent of tumor size) as well as predictive for benefit of chemotherapy (patients with scores >25 benefit from use of adjuvant chemotherapy to reduce their risk of recurrence). We recommend checking OncotypeDx score on postmenopausal patients with ER+ breast cancer measuring between 5 mm–50 mm and up to 3 positive axillary lymph nodes (LN). For premenopausal women, this test should only be offered if the breast cancer measures between 5 mm–50 mm but with no evidence of LN involvement by cancer. Premenopausal women with evidence of positive LNs benefit from the use of chemotherapy. Women with high genomic score (>25) have a higher risk of distant recurrence and benefit from the use of adjuvant chemotherapy.

The choice of therapy depends on staging of the tumor, tumor profile (presence of estrogen, progesterone and HER2 receptors) and patient factors (age, past medical history, comorbidities). We will discuss the different treatment options available for patients in the following three categories: estrogen receptor (ER) positive HER2 negative breast cancer, triple negative breast cancer, and HER2 positive breast cancer.

ER Positive HER2 Negative Breast Cancer

Neoadjuvant Therapies for ER+ HER2- Breast Cancer

The use of neoadjuvant chemotherapy (NACT) should be restricted to patients with locally advanced and high-risk ER+ HER2- breast cancer. This includes any premenopausal patient with a breast mass larger than 5 cm or with any evidence of metastatic disease to axillary lymph nodes. For postmenopausal women, we recommend NACT for patients presenting with masses larger than 5 cm or if there is initial evidence of 4 or more positive axillary LN with metastatic disease, based on results from the Rxponder trial [62].

Current regimens incorporate use of anthracycline and cyclophosphamide (in a dose dense fashion, if tolerated, for 4 cycles with use of growth factors) followed by weekly paclitaxel for 12 weeks. The use of anthracyclines with cyclophosphamide showed lower risk of recurrence and also a 4.2% reduction in 10-year breast cancer mortality (versus non-anthracycline regimens) [63]. Dose dense cycles are given every 14 days (instead of the historical every-three-week schedule) and are associated with a reduction in the risk of recurrence and breast cancer mortality. The more frequent administration also increases the rate of myelosuppression, neutropenia, and infectious complications. The use of colony stimulating growth factors (pegfilgrastim) is recommended to prevent infectious complications and treatment delays.

For high risk patients that are considered poor anthracycline candidates (elderly age, Eastern Cooperative Oncology Group (ECOG) performance score greater than 2, multiple cardiac comorbidities) and without evidence of lymph node involvement, using an anthracycline-free regimen (such as docetaxel and cyclophosphamide every three weeks for four to six cycles with use of growth factor) has shown to be noninferior to anthracycline based regimens and has better tolerability [64].

There is limited data about the efficacy and use of neoadjuvant endocrine therapy (NET). In premenopausal females, use of NET produced significantly lower response rates vs chemotherapy (44% versus 75%) [65]. In postmenopausal women, use of NET had similar rates of response as neoadjuvant chemotherapy with lower toxicity, but the long-term benefits in term of risk of relapse and overall survival remain largely unknown [66]. We only recommend NET for elderly and frail postmenopausal women that due to comorbidities may not be considered ideal candidates for upfront surgery. The ideal duration of therapy is unknown; we recommend it not to exceed six months in the neoadjuvant setting (followed by at least five years of adjuvant therapy), with close monitoring of the breast response using breast ultrasound at three and six months.

Adjuvant Chemotherapy for ER+ HER2- Breast Cancer

Based on the final pathology after surgery, the use of adjuvant chemotherapy is warranted if the size of the primary breast tumor is bigger than 5 cm, or if there are more than three lymph nodes with metastatic disease. For patients that do not meet this criteria, we recommend using genomic testing like OncotypeDx to help guide adjuvant recommendations (see section on Systemic Therapy for Breast Cancer).

The choice of adjuvant chemotherapy depends on patient's age, comorbidities, ECOG performance status, and past medical history. The standard of care recommendation is a regimen of dose dense anthracycline and cyclophosphamide for 4 cycles (with growth factor support) followed by weekly paclitaxel for 12 weeks. This combination provides the best balance between efficacy, reduction in the risk of recurrence and reduction in 10-year breast cancer mortality. For elderly or frail patients, or those with a large primary but no lymph node involvement, an anthracycline sparing regimen is a reasonable approach (see section on neoadjuvant therapies for ER + HER2-breast cancer).

Adjuvant Endocrine Therapy (ET) for ER+ HER2- Breast Cancer

Patients with ER+/PR+ breast cancer benefit from various antihormonal agents.

Based on menopausal status, OncotypeDx genomic recurrence score (RS) and risk of recurrence, the following options can be considered:

- Premenopausal women with low risk of recurrence (pT1-2, N0 disease, grade 1–2, genomic recurrence score <25): Use of adjuvant endocrine therapy (ET) with tamoxifen daily for at least 5 years is recommended. Tamoxifen is a selective estrogen receptor modulator (SERM) that binds to the estrogen receptor and inhibits estrogen effects. Five years of adjuvant tamoxifen reduces the risk of recurrence by 39% and reduces the risk of breast cancer mortality by 30% at 15 years [67]. Some of the toxicity associated with use of tamoxifen includes vasomotor symptoms (hot flushes, night sweats), increased risk of venous thrombosis and thromboembolic events, risk of endometrial cancer and cataract formation.

- Premenopausal women with high risk of recurrence (age <35years, primary tumor >5 cm, lymph node positive disease, genomic recurrence score >25): given high-risk features, these patients will require use of chemotherapy (either in the neoadjuvant or adjuvant setting). Upon completion of chemotherapy and radiation, we recommend ET with combination of suppression of ovarian function (SOF) using a monthly gonadotropin releasing hormone agonist such as goserelin, leuprolide or triptorelin, and an aromatase inhibitor (anastrozole, letrozole or exemestane). Other means to achieve SOF such as prophylactic oophorectomy or bilateral ovarian irradiation may be considered. This combination approach using SOF and an aromatase inhibitor is superior than single agent tamoxifen as published in the SOFT (Suppression of Ovarian Function Trial) [68] and TEXT (Tamoxifen and Exemestane Trial) trials, with lower risk of recurrence and a trend to decreasing breast cancer related mortality [69]. When SOF is considered for high-risk patients, extending ET duration to 10 years further decreases the risk of relapse.

  Recognizing the increased risk of relapse in these patients, newer agents have recently been approved to be used in the adjuvant setting in combination with endocrine therapy and suppression of ovarian function. The CDK4-6 inhibitor abemaciclib used for two years in combination with endocrine blockers reduces the risk of recurrence in high-risk patients. Its use is indicated for patients at high risk of recurrence, defined as having 4 or more positive axillary lymph nodes (LN) or 1–3 positive axillary LN and either tumor grade 3 or tumor >5 cm [70].

- Postmenopausal women with low risk of recurrence (low grade, tumor size <5 cm, genomic recurrence score <25): Adjuvant ET with an aromatase inhibitor for a duration of 5 years is the preferred option. Toxicity associated with the use of aromatase inhibitors includes vasomotor symptoms (hot flushes, night sweats), decreased libido, vaginal dryness, and increased risk of osteopenia and osteoporosis.

Duration of Adjuvant Endocrine Therapy

The minimum duration of adjuvant ET is five years. Unfortunately, the risk of distant recurrence for ER+ breast cancer remains high for up to 20 years following five years of ET [71]. In the ATLAS trial, extending adjuvant tamoxifen to 10 years reduced the risk of breast cancer recurrence and lowered breast cancer specific mortality, as well as overall mortality, compared to only 5 years of adjuvant tamoxifen [72]. Based on this, for women with high-risk features extending ET to complete 10 years is recommended. If the pre/peri-menopausal patient started endocrine therapy with tamoxifen and reached menopause, it is reasonable to offer five additional years of an aromatase inhibitor to maximize endocrine blockage.

Metastatic ER+ HER2- Breast Cancer (mBC)

The goal in metastatic disease is to help patients live longer (improve overall survival (OS)) without exposing the patient to excessive toxicity. The management is centered on the use of sequential hormone blockers which delay the need for chemotherapy. Also, the use of next generation sequencing of the metastatic tumor helps identify different actionable mutations for which newer therapies are becoming quickly available (for example alpelisib for PI3KCA mutation, elacestrant for ESR1 mutation).

Development of CDK4-6 inhibitors (palbociclib, ribociclib, and abemaciclib) has drastically changed the first line therapy for metastatic breast cancer and these are the preferred first line therapy option in combination with a hormone blocker. These molecules hit pause in the cell-cycle at phase G1, inhibiting progression into S phase (where DNA replication occurs) and inducing cancer cell arrest. The choice of hormone blocker depends on previous exposure to adjuvant endocrine therapy. For patients with de novo metastatic breast cancer, any aromatase inhibitor (letrozole, anastrozole or exemestane) may be combined with any CDK 4-6 inhibitors. For patients with recurrent metastatic disease and previously exposed to an aromatase inhibitor in the adjuvant setting, fulvestrant is the preferred hormone blocker.

The choice of CDK 4-6 inhibitor is user specific. Clinical data is more robust for the use of ribociclib or abemaciclib (with evidence of delay in the risk of progression as well as reduction in the risk of death), while palbociclib appears to have a better toxicity profile.

Subsequent lines of treatment take into consideration previous therapies, existing toxicities, and goals of care. For patients with ESR1 mutation, elacestrant appears to be more effective than fulvestrant in delaying disease progression in second line therapy. Phosphatidylinositol 3-kinase catalytic subunit alpha (PI3KCA) mutations occur in 35% of patients progressing into second line therapy and have a worse prognosis [73]. Alpelisib is a PI3KCA inhibitor that helps delay the risk of progression in second line patients post CDK inhibitors (Bylieve trial), but is associated with a high risk of rash, diarrhea, and hyperglycemia, limiting its use [73].

Everolimus and exemestane can be considered for third line treatment in patients that remain endocrine sensitive. Otherwise, for endocrine refractory patients, single agent chemotherapy (paclitaxel versus capecitabine) is preferred.

Antibody drug conjugates (ADC) are a new treatment modality that combine the precision of monoclonal antibodies with powerful chemotherapy agents. First, the ADC recognizes the specific antigen expressed in the breast cancer cell membrane (i.e. HER2, Trop2, HER3 among others). Then, the ADC is internalized. Once inside the cell, it releases the chemotherapy (also known as payload) to destroy the cancer cell while sparing normal cells that do not express the antigen. Current examples of this technology include ADC against HER2 (trastuzumab deruxtecan) [74] and against Trop2 (Sacituzumab govitecan) [75] (see Table 14.3).

Table 14.3 Common breast cancer treatments and newer agents

Drug	Mechanism of Action	Indication	Toxicity
Doxorubicin	Inhibits DNA and RNA synthesis by obstructing DNA base pairs	High risk ER+ breast cancer (neoadjuvant, adjuvant) TNBC (neoadjuvant, adjuvant)	Cytopenias, mucositis, cardiomyopathy
Cyclophosphamide	Alkylating agent, cross links DNA and prevents DNA synthesis	Similar to doxorubicin	Bone marrow suppression, cystitis, liver toxicity, cytopenias
Paclitaxel	Taxane, stabilizes microtubules interfering in mitosis and inhibits cell replication	High risk ER+ breast cancer (neoadjuvant, adjuvant) TNBC (neoadjuvant, adjuvant) Metastatic breast cancer (ER+, TNBC)	Cytopenias, neuropathy, nausea, vomiting, diarrhea, alopecia
Capecitabine	Prodrug metabolized to fluorouracil (active chemotherapy). Interferes with DNA and RNA synthesis	TNBC (adjuvant setting in patients with evidence of residual disease post NACT) Metastatic breast cancer (ER+, TNBC)	Hand-foot syndrome, nausea, vomiting, diarrhea, fatigue.
Trastuzumab	Antibody against HER2-2	Neoadjuvant treatment for HER2+ (in combination with docetaxel, carboplatin, pertuzumab) Adjuvant treatment for early-stage HER2+ (in combination with weekly paclitaxel) Metastatic HER2+ breast cancer (first line in combination with pertuzumab and docetaxel)	Diarrhea, cardiomyopathy
Pertuzumab	Antibody against HER2-4	Neoadjuvant treatment for HER2+ (in combination with docetaxel, carboplatin, trastuzumab). Metastatic HER2+ breast cancer (first line in combination with trastuzumab and docetaxel)	Diarrhea, cardiomyopathy, fatigue

Drug	Mechanism	Indication	Side effects
Ado-trastuzumab emtansine (T-DM1)	ADC against HER2 (payload DM1 is a microtubule inhibitor that inhibit mitosis and induce cell cycle arrest)	Adjuvant HER2+ therapy (in patients with residual disease post trastuzumab/pertuzumab) HER2+ metastatic breast cancer: can be used in 2nd line and beyond	Hepatotoxicity (increased transaminases), neuropathy, fatigue.
Sacituzumab govitecan	ADC against Trop-2 (payload SN-38 is a topoisomerase inhibitor that interrupts replication of DNA)	2nd line agent for metastatic TNBC In ER+ metastatic breast cancer: after endocrine resistance and progression on 1 line of chemotherapy.	Nausea, vomiting, diarrhea, cytopenias.
Trastuzumab deruxtecan	ADC against HER2 (payload deruxtecan is a topoisomerase inhibitor that induces DNA damage and cell death)	2nd line HER2+ metastatic breast cancer HER2 low metastatic breast cancer (either ER + or ER-) after at least one previous line of therapy.	Cytopenias, cardiomyopathy, nausea, vomiting, diarrhea, risk of interstitial lung disease and pulmonary fibrosis.
Tucatinib	Tyrosine kinase inhibitor against intracellular HER2 domain	2nd line HER2+ metastatic breast cancer in combination with trastuzumab and capecitabine (high BBB penetration is especially useful in patients with progression limited to the CNS)	Hand foot syndrome, rash, diarrhea, hepatotoxicity.

ADC=antibody drug conjugate, BBB=blood brain barrier, CNS=central nervous system, ER=estrogen receptor, HER2= Human epidermal receptor-2, NACT= neoadjuvant chemotherapy, TNBC=triple negative breast cancer.

Triple Negative Breast Cancer (TNBC)

Neoadjuvant chemotherapy for localized TNBC

Triple negative breast cancer is an aggressive subtype with no approved targeted agents. Neoadjuvant chemotherapy (NACT) is the preferred modality because it achieves a faster onset of response, with better local control while reducing the risk of distant relapse. It also helps downstage tumor size prior to surgery, helps eliminate micrometastasis and shows a biologic proof of chemotherapy sensitivity. Among the most used regimens, dose dense Doxorubicin and Cytoxan (ddAC) given every 2 weeks for 4 cycles (with use of prophylactic growth factors) followed by weekly paclitaxel for 12 weeks is considered the standard of care for early localized TNBC.

For TNBC patients with high-risk features (tumor>2 cm, positive LN), adding immuno-therapy (pembrolizumab) to NACT helps increase rates of complete cancer cell elimination (also called pathological complete response or pCR) and decreases the risk of early relapse. Higher toxicity rates are expected with this approach, with overlap between chemotherapy and immunotherapy induced adverse events [76].

For germline mutated *BRCA1/2* patients with evidence of residual disease post-NACT, the use of the poly(ADP-ribose) polymerase (PARP) inhibitor olaparib in the adjuvant setting is the preferred option, and may be added to adjuvant pembrolizumab to further reduce the risk of relapse [77].

Advanced Metastatic TNBC

Initial biopsy for evaluation of the distant metastasis is highly recommended. This includes immunohistochemistry (testing for PD-L1 and HER2 low expression) and use of next generation sequencing to discover other genomic alterations (*BRCA1/2* germline and somatic mutations, *AKT, PI3KCA,* mismatch repair deficiencies among others).

The choice for first line treatment depends on the expression of PD-L1 protein in the cell surface. If PD-L1 expression is higher than 10%, the combination of immunotherapy (pembrolizumab) with chemotherapy (paclitaxel, nab-paclitaxel, or carboplatin/gemcita-bine) produces higher responses, delays the progression of metastatic disease and allows the patients to live longer [78]. If the tumor shows low level of PD-L1 expression (<10%), single agent chemotherapy (either weekly paclitaxel or capecitabine) is a reasonable option. The final agent decision should also take into consideration the patient's comorbidities, past medical history, previous treatments, and goals of care.

Second line treatment options vary based on the presence of *BRCA* germline muta-tions. For *BRCA* mutated patients, PARP inhibitors (olaparib, talazoparib) are the pre-ferred agents. If the patient is *BRCA* wildtype, the antibody drug conjugate sacituzumab govitecan (SG, directed against the Trop-2 receptor in breast cancer cells) helps delay the rate of progression and allows patients to live longer versus use of chemotherapy. Diarrhea and neutropenia are most commonly seen with SG and require use of growth factors and anti-motility agents (to slow down peristalsis in GI tract and decrease diarrhea) [79].

Newer targets are being incorporated in the management of metastatic TNBC. Up to 35% of TNBC patients can be categorized as having HER2-low expression (HER2 IHC=1+ or 2+ with FISH negative). An exploratory analysis from the Destiny-Breast04 trial showed that using the ADC trastuzumab deruxtecan greatly delayed the risk of progression and improved survival versus chemotherapy in this subset of patients [80].

HER2 Positive Breast Cancer

As described previously, HER2 is a member of the tyrosine kinase growth factor receptor family. HER2 positivity indicates worse biological behavior, high clinical aggressiveness and leads to uncontrolled tumor growth in breast cancer. Treatment for this cancer subtype combines chemotherapy, monoclonal antibodies against HER2 receptor, antibody drug conjugates, small molecule inhibitors of the HER2 intracellular receptor among other mechanisms (Table 14.3).

Early Localized HER2+ Breast Cancer

For tumors smaller than 3 cm and without LN involvement, upfront resection and adjuvant trastuzumab/paclitaxel for 12 weeks followed by trastuzumab to complete one year allows a reduction in toxicity while significantly reducing the risk of relapse. The most recent 10-year update for the APT trial shows 96% of patients did not experience distant recurrence following this sequence [81].

For tumors larger than 3 cm or with positive LN involvement, neoadjuvant chemotherapy combining two chemotherapy agents (docetaxel and carboplatin) with two anti-HER2 antibodies (Herceptin and Perjeta) given every three weeks for six cycles showed superior rates of pathological complete response (pCR is the absence of cancer cells in surgical specimen) in the Tryphaena trial [82]. Based on final pathology, for patients with evidence of residual disease, switching to adjuvant trastuzumab emtansine (T-DM1) for 14 cycles every 3 weeks further reduces the risk of recurrence versus continuation of adjuvant trastuzumab. If pCR is achieved, continuation of adjuvant trastuzumab and pertuzumab to complete one year of therapy is the preferred option [83].

Metastatic HER2+ Breast Cancer

The preferred frontline therapy in the metastatic setting includes a combination of one chemotherapy agent (docetaxel) with two anti-HER2 antibodies (trastuzumab and pertuzumab) given every three weeks (Cleopatra trial) [84]. The chemotherapy backbone docetaxel can be discontinued after six to eight cycles (assuming no evidence of progression) to prevent worsening compounding toxicity. This allows the patient to be switched to a chemo-free "maintenance" with significantly lower toxicity but continuing with close monitoring for cardiac toxicity.

Upon progression, the antibody drug conjugate (ADC) trastuzumab deruxtecan is the preferred second line option based on the Destiny-Breast03 trial [85]. The use of this new ADC produced better rates of response and more than quadrupled the duration of treatment on these patients (versus previous standard of care ado-trastuzumab emtansine), allowing them to live longer. As with any new agents, special toxicities of interest are arising. Interstitial lung disease is a new life-threatening toxicity that has been described with trastuzumab deruxtecan and warrants close surveillance and monitoring. Patients may present with new onset shortness of breath, dry cough, progressive difficulty breathing and dyspnea or incidental findings of ground glass opacities in surveillance CT scans. Prompt initiation of steroids and pulmonary referral has helped prevent more fatalities while on treatment.

Up to 50% of HER2-positive metastatic breast cancer patients may develop brain metastases during their illness. Usual regimens including chemotherapy and antibodies (like trastuzumab or pertuzumab) do not cross the blood-brain barrier and therefore have limited clinical benefit with intracranial disease. Recently, the development of newer oral small molecule tyrosine kinase inhibitors like tucatinib has allowed for greater central nervous system penetration and better local disease control. Tucatinib is used in combination with trastuzumab and capecitabine in patients with metastatic HER2+ breast cancer with multiple untreated brain metastases that opt not to receive whole brain radiation due to risk of worsening cumulative neurotoxicity. This combination achieved better rates of intracranial response, delayed the rate of progression among patients with brain metastasis, allowing them to live longer [86].

Inflammatory Breast Cancer (IBC)

IBC is not a histologic subtype but rather an aggressive clinical presentation of a rare breast cancer. It affects between 0.5% to 2% of all newly diagnosed breast cancer patients and presents with diffuse skin erythema and edema (also called peau d'orange) due to dermal lymphatic infiltration of tumor cells. As compared with locally advanced breast cancer, IBC is diagnosed at an earlier age (a median of 59 versus 66 years of age) and has higher incidence in Black Americans compared with White Americans [87].

A mass is not always present on the initial clinical presentation, and sometimes these patients may be treated for cellulitis or abscess without clinical improvement. Usually patients are afebrile and demonstrate progressive swelling and redness over a short period of time. If there has been no improvement after a short course of antibiotics (a week or less), biopsy is indicated to determine the diagnosis.

The initial diagnostic workup includes ultrasound guided biopsy of the underlying mass (if present) and at least two skin punch biopsies to document the extension of dermo-lymphatic invasion. However, pathologic confirmation of skin involvement is not required for diagnosis, as diagnosis is based on rapid development of erythema and peau d'orange encompassing 1/3 or more of the breast. As with any other subtype, tumor profiling should include testing for estrogen, progesterone and HER2 receptor status. Confirmation of IBC is staged as T4d as per AJCC 8th edition. After diagnosis, we recommend completion of staging scans (CT chest, abdomen, and pelvis) as well as bone scan. If the patient also complains of altered vision, persistent headaches or paresthesias/numbness over face and head, completion of staging with brain MRI is recommended [88].

Given the aggressiveness of this subtype, we recommend prompt initiation of neoadjuvant chemotherapy with an anthracycline and taxane based regimen (with addition of anti-HER2 antibodies as appropriate). Neoadjuvant chemotherapy is given to reduce tumor burden, facilitate surgical resection, and decrease risk of local and distant recurrence. Comprehensive radiation always follows surgery, regardless of response to neoadjuvant therapy. Based on pathologic response and tumor profile, adjuvant treatment recommendations should follow the same principles previously discussed for management of non-IBC breast cancer.

Hereditary Breast Cancer

BRCA1 and BRCA2 genes play a crucial role in maintaining genomic integrity by repairing double-strand DNA breaks via homologous recombination pathways. A PV in BRCA1 and

BRCA2 subsequently causes accumulation of additional deleterious genetic mutations, leading to cancer development [89]. Approximately 5 to 10% of breast cancer are associated with germline alterations in *BRCA1* and *BRCA2*. The prevalence of *BRCA1/2* PVs vary widely based on geographic region, age and ethnicity. A *BRCA1* PV is associated with a 55–72% lifetime risk of breast cancer, while a BRCA2 PV is associated with a 45%–69% lifetime risk of breast cancer [90]. Other genetic PVs associated with an increased incidence of breast cancer include *PALB2, PTEN*, and *CHEK2*.

Women with germline *BRCA1/2* mutations should start self-breast exams beginning at age 18 to facilitate awareness of morphologic changes. Clinical breast examination performed every 6 to 12 months should begin at age 25. High risk screening using breast MRI is also recommended by age 25, while screening mammograms with tomosynthesis can start at age 30, or earlier depending on the earliest age of breast cancer in the family. Breast MRI allows for better sensitivity and identification of underlying masses compared to mammogram, especially in patients with dense breast tissue or where underlying fibrosis may obscure other masses. When the patient qualifies for both imaging modalities, we recommend performing them 6 months apart [7]. This recommendation can also be extended to carriers of other PVs (*PTEN, CHEK2*), untested women with a first-degree relative with a *BRCA* PV or to women with a 20% or higher lifetime risk of breast cancer (see Breast Cancer Risk Assessment Tool under the section entitled Screening above).

Prophylactic mastectomy is indicated for *BRCA1* and *BRCA2* PV carriers and is supported by National Comprehensive Cancer Network (NCCN) guidelines. Multiple prospective and retrospective studies show that prophylactic bilateral mastectomy decreases the incidence of breast cancer by 90% or more in at risk patients [91, 92]. Skin-sparing mastectomy with preservation of the nipple-areola complex offers superior cosmetic results, with low recurrence risk. The role of risk reducing bilateral salpingo-oophorectomy is discussed under Chapter 3.

The use of hormone therapy (HT) in *BRCA* carriers who have undergone risk reducing salpingo-oophorectomies is acceptable in women who have had prophylactic mastectomies, but for those who have not had prophylactic mastectomies, is controversial.

Other cancer associated with *BRCA1/2* PVs include pancreatic and melanoma skin cancer. Current guidelines from the International Cancer of the Pancreas Screening (CAPS) consortium recommend pancreatic cancer screening starting at age 45, or 10 years younger than the youngest affected blood relative with use of endoscopic ultrasound (EUS) and/or MRI/magnetic resonance cholangiopancreatography (MRCP) [93]. Regarding melanoma risk prevention, consensus recommendations call for yearly full-body skin exams (but still unclear when to initiate screening). No specific recommendations for colorectal cancer screening exist for *BRCA* mutation carriers.

Adjuvant Treatment Considerations for Hereditary Breast Cancer

Breast cancer patients with evidence of germline *BRCA1* and *BRCA2* mutations benefit from use of poly(adenosine diphosphate [ADP]–ribose) polymerase (PARP) inhibitors. These medications deliver a "second knock" to the already defective DNA repair mechanism of the breast cancer cell and induce apoptosis. Currently olaparib is the only PARP inhibitor approved in the adjuvant setting for breast cancer patients with *BRCA* germline mutations and evidence of residual disease post neoadjuvant/adjuvant therapy. The phase 3 Olympia trial showed that patients receiving adjuvant olaparib had higher distant disease-free survival (87.5% versus 80.4% with placebo) and was associated with fewer deaths. Common toxicity associated with use of PARP inhibitors include nausea, vomiting, fatigue, anemia, and decreased WBC [77].

In the advanced/metastatic disease setting, two PARP inhibitors, olaparib and talazoparib, are approved for patients with germline *BRCA* mutations. These drugs can be used as early as second line therapy in HER2 negative locally advanced or metastatic breast cancer based on improvement in progression free survival (PFS) compared to physician's choice of chemotherapy [94, 95].

Fertility Preservation and Timing of Future Conception

The possibility of treatment-related infertility should be discussed with all premenopausal women of reproductive age. Current fertility preservation modalities include cryopreservation of embryos, oocytes, and ovarian tissue and use of gonadotropin-releasing hormone (GnRH) agonist treatment before and during chemotherapy to reduce the risk of premature ovarian insufficiency. Prompt referral to a fertility specialist is recommended [96].

Most recently, the POSITIVE trial enrolled ER+ breast cancer patients that completed between 18 to 30 months of adjuvant ET and wished to pause their endocrine therapy to achieve pregnancy. The rates of conception and childbirth were on par with or higher than rates in the general public. The trial also showed a similar three-year rate of breast cancer recurrence between those that pause endocrine therapy and the external control cohort that continues endocrine blockers from the SOFT/TEXT trials (8.9% versus 9.2%). For women desiring pregnancy, a minimum of 18 months of endocrine therapy should be completed and a three month "wash-out" of tamoxifen is recommended prior to unprotected intercourse [97].

Premenopausal patients receiving adjuvant tamoxifen should use reliable nonhormonal methods of contraception as tamoxifen is teratogenic. Similarly, use of trastuzumab has a risk of oligo and/or anhydramnios and unknown long-term sequalae on the fetus [98].

Other Toxicities and Special Considerations

There are multiple considerations in the short- and long-term management of breast cancer patients that warrant further discussion:

1. Body image issues: the long-term psychological effects of the surgical approach (segmental versus total mastectomy) may lead to some patients feeling less feminine and less confident. Patients should be offered consultation with a plastic surgery team to discuss best timing and modality for tissue rearrangement if undergoing lumpectomy or reconstruction modalities if undergoing mastectomy.

2. Alopecia: hair loss is a common toxicity associated with multiple chemotherapies that is usually temporal but may become permanent in up to 10% of patients [99]. The use of scalp cooling devices protects the hair follicles by reducing the delivery of chemotherapy to the scalp. This approach reduced the rates of temporal alopecia in patients receiving docetaxel from historic 100% down to 11%, with minimal associated headaches and discomfort from wearing the device. The efficacy of scalp cooling in patients receiving anthracyclines is significantly lower, with 53% of patients still experiencing residual temporal alopecia despite the use of the cooling device [100]. Based on these numbers, we do not recommend using a scalp cooling device on patients receiving an anthracycline based regimen. Use of adjuvant endocrine therapies with aromatase

inhibitors also produces hair thinning and may increase rate of hair loss, but this toxicity tends to be limited and reverts upon discontinuation of the endocrine blocker.

3. Neuropathy: Chemotherapy-induced peripheral neuropathy is a common adverse effect that can have a profound impact on patient's quality of life and survivorship. Agents associated with the highest incidence of peripheral neuropathy include use of platinum drugs (carboplatin, cisplatin) as well as taxanes (docetaxel, paclitaxel). Use of cryotherapy (i.e. frozen socks and gloves) over hands and feet 15 minutes before, during, and 15 minutes after the infusion of the chemotherapy agent induces vasoconstriction and reduces the delivery and toxicity over nerve endings in hands and feet, preventing direct nerve damage and neuropathy, although data is limited [101].

4. Lymphedema: risk factors for lymphedema include axillary lymph node dissection, adjuvant radiation therapy, local infection, and obesity. Sentinel lymph node biopsy instead of axillary lymph node dissection has dramatically decreased risk of secondary lymphedema. Other noninvasive interventions like lymphatic massage therapy and use of garments and compression devices may help prevent further deterioration, but require constant daily use. The role of lymph node reconstruction and lympho-venous bypass surgery to treat lymphedema are under active investigation.

5. Vaginal dryness and dyspareunia are direct consequences of adjuvant endocrine therapy. Their risk is lower with use of tamoxifen compared to use of aromatase inhibitors. Recent studies have shown that for highly symptomatic patients with dyspareunia and decreased libido, use of a vaginal estriol ring does not increase blood concentration of estradiol and significantly improves vaginal health (decreased dryness, improved turgor and elasticity) and increased sexual satisfaction scores. The long-term effects in the risk of recurrence for breast cancer patients has not been described yet [102].

6. Psychosocial health: Most survivors will experience psychosocial distress at a level that is significant but does not meet criteria for a psychiatric disorder. This includes fear of recurrence, depression, anxiety, emotional, financial, and spiritual distress among others. Mindfulness and relaxation techniques like introspection and yoga can help better deal with some of the stressors.

Breast Cancer Survivorship

Patients with a history of breast cancer should undergo regular follow-up including history and physical examination every six months (or sooner as needed based on symptoms), surveillance mammography, and evaluation and management of treatment-related late effects, including assessment of psychosocial distress. Breast cancer survivors should also receive ongoing age-appropriate screening studies (papanicolaou smears, screening colonoscopies beginning at age 45, tobacco cessation) and preventive care, consistent with recommendations for the general population.

We recommend against repeat monitoring using tumor markers and serial screening CT or bone scans to detect early asymptomatic relapses, as they do not change the natural course of the disease or help improve overall survival. Use of newer technologies like detection of circulating tumor cells (CTCs) and circulating tumor DNA (ctDNA) appear to have strong prognostic value to diagnose early relapses but its clinical utility is under investigation at this time.

Case Resolution

BW has stage IIB (cT2N1M0) triple negative breast cancer of the right breast. Upfront staging scans are negative for distant metastatic disease. Considering her strong family history and young age of diagnosis, she undergoes genetic testing and is found to have a germline *BRCA1* mutation. She received neoadjuvant chemo-immunotherapy (four cycles of carboplatin/paclitaxel/pembrolizumab followed by four cycles of doxorubicin/cyclophosphamide/pembrolizumab) and underwent a right modified radical mastectomy with axillary lymph node dissection.

The final pathology report shows a residual tumor bed measuring 6x8 mm with 10% residual cellularity and 3 out of 16 axillary lymph nodes with evidence of chemotherapy effect and no viable cancer. She receives comprehensive postmastectomy radiotherapy to the chest wall and undissected draining lymphatics, to include the internal mammary, level III axilla, and supraclavicular nodes, to a dose of 4005 cGy in 15 fractions using 3D conformal radiation, followed by a boost to the mastectomy flaps. Considering she has evidence of residual disease (did not achieve pCR) and *gBRCA1* mutation, she completes nine cycles of adjuvant pembrolizumab as well as a year of adjuvant Olaparib.

Upon completion of adjuvant therapy, she undergoes a prophylactic contralateral left mastectomy and prophylactic bilateral salpingo-oophorectomy. She continues on active surveillance, currently entering her second year postdiagnosis with no evidence of recurrence.

Take Home Points

- Breast cancer is the most common diagnosed cancer in women in the USA (excluding skin cancer). Its incidence continues to increase and now affects one in every eight women during their lifetime.
- Risk factors associated with developing breast cancer include advanced age, race, dense breast tissue, obesity, use of alcohol, use of HT, family history of breast cancer, and presence of germline mutations.
- Screening mammograms allow for an early diagnosis and save lives. For women without pathogenic variants, they should begin by age 40. Use of breast ultrasound may be considered for women with dense breast tissue.
- Women with pathogenic variants (ex. germline *BRCA1/2* mutations, *PALB2* or *CHEK2* mutations) should start self-breast exams beginning at age 18 to become aware of morphologic changes. Screening breast MRI should start by age 25, while screening mammograms with tomosynthesis can start at age 30. Prophylactic mastectomy is indicated for *BRCA1* and *BRCA2* pathogenic variant carriers.
- Initial workup of a breast mass should include physical examination of breast and axilla, diagnostic mammogram, dedicated ultrasound of breast and nodal basin, as well as tissue biopsy. Pathologic features including tumor grade, receptor status (estrogen, progesterone, and HER2 expression) and measurement of Ki-67 help inform treatment options.
- Staging scans including CT of the chest/abdomen/pelvis and bone scan are recommended to exclude distant metastatic disease for patients with breast masses larger than 5 cm or with 3 or more positive lymph nodes.

- The management of breast cancer is multidisciplinary and includes surgical resection, systemic therapy, and adjuvant radiation. Systemic therapy options include chemotherapy, endocrine treatment, targeted agents, antibodies, and antibody drug conjugates.
- Nearly all patients undergoing lumpectomy will require radiation, although omission is reasonable in pT1N0 ER+ HER2- patients over 65 years of age or in patients with low-risk DCIS.
- Mastectomy patients who meet criteria for regional nodal irradiation should undergo postmastectomy radiation to the chest wall and nodes.
- Cytotoxic chemotherapy can be given as neoadjuvant treatment (before surgery) to help reduce size of tumor, achieve negative resection margins, and to prove sensitivity of the tumor to therapy.
- Use of endocrine therapy varies based on menopausal status, final pathological staging, and comorbidities. For younger premenopausal women with high-risk features, suppression of ovarian function further decreases the risk of local and distant relapse and improves overall survival.
- Inflammatory breast cancer is an aggressive clinical presentation that can be mistaken with cellulitis or abscess and requires a high index of clinical suspicion, prompt workup and early treatment to improve outcomes.
- Fertility preservation and referral to oncofertility specialist should be discussed with all patients of reproductive age. Endocrine therapy can be interrupted after 18 months of use to pursue pregnancy without increasing the risk of breast cancer recurrence.
- For women desiring pregnancy, a minimum of a three month "wash-out" of tamoxifen is recommended prior to unprotected intercourse.
- Other treatment related toxicities include body image issues, alopecia, neuropathy, lymphedema, vaginal dryness, decreased libido, and psychosocial well-being. It is important to address these issues on an ongoing basis and refer to adequate specialists as needed.

References

1. Giaquinto A. N., Sung H., Miller K. D., et al. Breast cancer statistics, 2022. *CA: A Cancer Journal for Clinicians.* 2022;**72**(6):524–41.

2. DeSantis C. E., Ma J., Gaudet M. M., et al. Breast cancer statistics, 2019. *CA: A Cancer Journal for Clinicians.* 2019;**69**(6):438–51.

3. Rossouw J. E., Anderson G. L., Prentice R. L., et al. Risks and benefits of estrogen plus progestin in healthy postmenopausal women: Principal results from the Women's Health Initiative randomized controlled trial. *Jama.* 2002;**288**(3):321–33.

4. Taskforce UPS. www.uspreventiveservices taskforce.org/uspstf/sites/default/files/file/su pporting_documents/breast-cancer-screen ing-draft-rec-bulletin.pdf. Published 2023.

5. Holm J., Humphreys K., Li J., et al. Risk factors and tumor characteristics of interval cancer by mammographic density. *J Clin Oncol.* 2015;**33**(9):1030–7.

6. Surveillance, Epidemiology, and End Results (SEER) Program (www.seer.cancer.gov) SEER*Stat Database: Populations - Total U.S. (2015–2019).

7. Le-Petross H. T., Whitman G. J., Atchley D. P., et al. Effectiveness of

alternating mammography and magnetic resonance imaging for screening women with deleterious BRCA mutations at high risk of breast cancer. *Cancer.* 2011;**117**(17):3900–7.

8. Kauff N. D., Satagopan J. M., Robson M. E., et al. Risk-reducing salpingo-oophorectomy in women with a BRCA1 or BRCA2 mutation. *N Engl J Med.* 2002;**346**(21):1609–15.

9. Giuliano A. E., Connolly J. L., Edge S. B., et al. Breast Cancer: Major changes in the American Joint Committee on Cancer eighth edition cancer staging manual. *CA Cancer J Clin.* 2017;**67**(4):290–303.

10. (NCCN). NCCN. NCCN Clinical Practice Guidelines in Oncology. www.nccn.org. Published 2023.

11. Amin M. B., Edge S. B., Greene F. L., et al. *AJCC cancer staging manual.* Vol **1024**: Springer; 2017.

12. Fisher B., Anderson S., Bryant J., et al. Twenty-year follow-up of a randomized trial comparing total mastectomy, lumpectomy, and lumpectomy plus irradiation for the treatment of invasive breast cancer. *The New England Journal of Medicine.* 2002;**347**(16):1233–41.

13. Veronesi U., Cascinelli N., Mariani L., et al. Twenty-year follow-up of a randomized study comparing breast-conserving surgery with radical mastectomy for early breast cancer. *The New England Journal of Medicine.* 2002;**347**(16):1227–32.

14. Agarwal S., Pappas L., Neumayer L., Kokeny K., Agarwal J. Effect of breast conservation therapy vs mastectomy on disease-specific survival for early-stage breast cancer. *JAMA Surg.* 2014;**149**(3):267–74.

15. Hartmann-Johnsen O. J., Kåresen R., Schlichting E., Nygård J. F. Survival is better after breast conserving therapy than mastectomy for early stage breast cancer: A registry-based follow-up study of Norwegian women primary operated between 1998 and 2008. *Ann Surg Oncol.* 2015;**22**(12):3836–45.

16. Schumacher J. R., Wiener A. A., Greenberg C. C., et al. Local/regional recurrence rates after breast conserving therapy in patients enrolled in legacy trials of the Alliance for Clinical Trials in Oncology (AFT-01). *Ann Surg.* 2022;**277**(5):841–5.

17. van Maaren M. C., de Munck L., de Bock G. H., et al. 10 year survival after breast-conserving surgery plus radiotherapy compared with mastectomy in early breast cancer in the Netherlands: A population-based study. *Lancet Oncol.* 2016;**17**(8):1158–70.

18. Carter S. A., Lyons G. R., Kuerer H. M., et al. Operative and oncologic outcomes in 9861 patients with operable breast cancer: Single-institution analysis of breast conservation with oncoplastic reconstruction. *Ann Surg Oncol.* 2016;**23**(10):3190–8.

19. Clough K. B., Benyahi D., Nos C., Charles C., Sarfati I. Oncoplastic surgery: Pushing the limits of breast-conserving surgery. *Breast J.* 2015;**21**(2):140–6.

20. Domchek S. M., Friebel T. M., Singer C. F., et al. Association of risk-reducing surgery in BRCA1 or BRCA2 mutation carriers with cancer risk and mortality. *Jama.* 2010;**304**(9):967–75.

21. Metcalfe K. A., Cil T. D., Semple J. L., et al. Long-term psychosocial functioning in women with bilateral prophylactic mastectomy: Does preservation of the nipple-areolar complex make a difference? *Ann Surg Oncol.* 2015;**22**(10):3324–30.

22. Smith B. L., Coopey S. B. Nipple-sparing mastectomy. *Adv Surg.* 2018;**52**(1):113–26.

23. Macadam S. A., Bovill E. S., Buchel E. W., Lennox P. A. Evidence-based medicine: Autologous breast reconstruction. *Plast Reconstr Surg.* 2017;**139**(1):204e–229e.

24. Baker J. L., Dizon D. S., Wenziger C. M., et al. "Going flat" after mastectomy: Patient-reported outcomes by online survey. *Ann Surg Oncol.* 2021;**28**(5):2493–505.

25. Gipponi M., Bassetti C., Canavese G., et al. Sentinel lymph node as a new marker for therapeutic planning in breast cancer patients. *J Surg Oncol.* 2004;**85**(3):102–11.

26. Albertini J. J., Lyman G. H., Cox C., et al. Lymphatic mapping and sentinel node biopsy in the patient with breast cancer. *Jama*. 1996;**276**(22):1818–22.

27. Kim T., Giuliano A. E., Lyman G. H. Lymphatic mapping and sentinel lymph node biopsy in early-stage breast carcinoma: A metaanalysis. *Cancer*. 2006;**106**(1):4–16.

28. Krag D. N., Anderson S. J., Julian T. B., et al. Sentinel-lymph-node resection compared with conventional axillary-lymph-node dissection in clinically node-negative patients with breast cancer: Overall survival findings from the NSABP B-32 randomised phase 3 trial. *Lancet Oncol*. 2010;**11**(10):927–33.

29. Galimberti V., Cole B. F., Viale G., et al. Axillary dissection versus no axillary dissection in patients with breast cancer and sentinel-node micrometastases (IBCSG 23-01): 10-year follow-up of a randomised, controlled phase 3 trial. *Lancet Oncol*. 2018;**19**(10):1385–93.

30. Giuliano A. E., McCall L., Beitsch P., et al. Locoregional recurrence after sentinel lymph node dissection with or without axillary dissection in patients with sentinel lymph node metastases: The American College of Surgeons Oncology Group Z0011 randomized trial. *Ann Surg*. 2010;**252**(3):426–32.

31. Caudle A. S., Yang W. T., Krishnamurthy S., et al. Improved axillary evaluation following neoadjuvant therapy for patients with node-positive breast cancer using selective evaluation of clipped nodes: Implementation of targeted axillary dissection. *J Clin Oncol*. 2016;**34**(10):1072–8.

32. Fisher B., Anderson S., Bryant J., et al. Twenty-year follow-up of a randomized trial comparing total mastectomy, lumpectomy, and lumpectomy plus irradiation for the treatment of invasive breast cancer. *New England Journal of Medicine*. 2002;**347**(16):1233–41.

33. de Boniface J., Szulkin R., Johansson A. L. V. Survival after breast conservation vs mastectomy adjusted for comorbidity and socioeconomic status:

A Swedish national 6-Year follow-up of 48 986 women. *JAMA Surg*. 2021;**156**(7):628–37.

34. Hwang E. S., Lichtensztajn D. Y., Gomez S. L., Fowble B., Clarke C. A. Survival after lumpectomy and mastectomy for early stage invasive breast cancer: The effect of age and hormone receptor status. *Cancer*. 2013;**119**(7):1402–11.

35. Abdulkarim B. S., Cuartero J., Hanson J., et al. Increased risk of locoregional recurrence for women with T1-2N0 triple-negative breast cancer treated with modified radical mastectomy without adjuvant radiation therapy compared with breast-conserving therapy. *J Clin Oncol*. 2011;**29**(21):2852–8.

36. Mouabbi J. A., Chand M., Asghar I. A., et al. Lumpectomy followed by radiation improves survival in HER2 positive and triple-negative breast cancer with high tumor-infiltrating lymphocytes compared to mastectomy alone. *Cancer Med*. 2021;**10**(14):4790–5.

37. Darby S., McGale P., Correa C., et al. Effect of radiotherapy after breast-conserving surgery on 10-year recurrence and 15-year breast cancer death: Meta-analysis of individual patient data for 10,801 women in 17 randomized trials. *Lancet*. 2011;**378**(9804):1707–16.

38. Kunkler I. H., Williams L. J., Jack W. J. L, Cameron D. A., Dixon J. M. Breast-conserving surgery with or without irradiation in early breast cancer. *New England Journal of Medicine*. 2023;**388**(7):585–94.

39. Hughes K. S., Schnaper L. A., Bellon J. R., et al. Lumpectomy plus tamoxifen with or without irradiation in women age 70 years or older with early breast cancer: Long-term follow-up of CALGB 9343. *Journal of Clinical Oncology*. 2013;**31**(19):2382–7.

40. Hughes L. L., Wang M., Page D. L., et al. Local excision alone without irradiation for ductal carcinoma in situ of the breast: A trial of the Eastern Cooperative Oncology Group. *J Clin Oncol*. 2009;**27**(32):5319–24.

41. McCormick B., Winter K. A., Woodward W., et al. Randomized phase III trial evaluating radiation following surgical excision for good-risk ductal carcinoma in situ: Long-term report from NRG Oncology/RTOG 9804. *J Clin Oncol.* 2021;**39**(32):3574–82.

42. Whelan T. J., Pignol J. P., Levine M. N., et al. Long-term results of hypofractionated radiation therapy for breast cancer. *N Engl J Med.* 2010;**362**(6):513–20.

43. Haviland J. S., Owen J. R., Dewar J. A., et al. The UK Standardisation of Breast Radiotherapy (START) trials of radiotherapy hypofractionation for treatment of early breast cancer: 10-year follow-up results of two randomised controlled trials. *Lancet Oncol.* 2013;**14**(11):1086–94.

44. Smith B. D., Bellon J. R., Blitzblau R., et al. Radiation therapy for the whole breast: Executive summary of an American Society for Radiation Oncology (ASTRO) evidence-based guideline. *Pract Radiat Oncol.* 2018;**8**(3):145–52.

45. Murray Brunt A., Haviland J. S., Wheatley D. A., et al. Hypofractionated breast radiotherapy for 1 week versus 3 weeks (FAST-Forward): 5-year efficacy and late normal tissue effects results from a multicentre, non-inferiority, randomised, phase 3 trial. *Lancet.* 2020;**395**(10237):1613–26.

46. Krug D., Baumann R., Combs S. E., et al. Moderate hypofractionation remains the standard of care for whole-breast radiotherapy in breast cancer: Considerations regarding FAST and FAST-Forward. *Strahlenther Onkol.* 2021;**197**(4):269–80.

47. Vicini F. A., Cecchini R. S., White J. R., et al. Long-term primary results of accelerated partial breast irradiation after breast-conserving surgery for early-stage breast cancer: A randomised, phase 3, equivalence trial. *Lancet.* 2019;**394**(10215):2155–64.

48. Whelan T. J., Julian J. A., Berrang T. S., et al. External beam accelerated partial breast irradiation versus whole breast irradiation after breast conserving surgery in women with ductal carcinoma in situ and node-negative breast cancer (RAPID): A randomised controlled trial. *Lancet.* 2019;**394**(10215):2165–72.

49. Coles C. E., Griffin C. L., Kirby A. M., et al. Partial-breast radiotherapy after breast conservation surgery for patients with early breast cancer (UK IMPORT LOW trial): 5-year results from a multicentre, randomised, controlled, phase 3, non-inferiority trial. *Lancet.* 2017;**390**(10099):1048–60.

50. Meattini I., Marrazzo L., Saieva C., et al. Accelerated partial-breast irradiation compared with whole-breast irradiation for early breast cancer: Long-term results of the randomized phase III APBI-IMRT-Florence Trial. *Journal of Clinical Oncology.* 2020;**38**(35):4175–83.

51. Correa C., Harris E. E., Leonardi M. C., et al. Accelerated partial breast irradiation: Executive summary for the update of an ASTRO evidence-based consensus statement. *Pract Radiat Oncol.* 2017;**7**(2):73–9.

52. Whelan T. J., Olivotto I. A., Parulekar W. R., et al. Regional nodal irradiation in early-stage breast cancer. *N Engl J Med.* 2015;**373**(4):307–316.

53. Poortmans P. M., Weltens C., Fortpied C., et al. Internal mammary and medial supraclavicular lymph node chain irradiation in stage I-III breast cancer (EORTC 22922/10925): 15-year results of a randomised, phase 3 trial. *Lancet Oncol.* 2020;**21**(12):1602–10.

54. McGale P., Taylor C., Correa C., et al. Effect of radiotherapy after mastectomy and axillary surgery on 10-year recurrence and 20-year breast cancer mortality: Meta-analysis of individual patient data for 8135 women in 22 randomised trials. *Lancet.* 2014;**383**(9935):2127–35.

55. Recht A., Comen E. A., Fine R. E., et al. Postmastectomy radiotherapy: An American Society of Clinical Oncology, American Society for Radiation Oncology, and Society of Surgical Oncology Focused Guideline Update. *Ann Surg Oncol.* 2017;**24**(1):38–51.

56. Wang S.-L., Fang H., Song Y.-W., et al. Hypofractionated versus conventional fractionated postmastectomy radiotherapy for patients with high-risk breast cancer: A randomised, non-inferiority, open-label, phase 3 trial. *The Lancet Oncology.* 2019;**20**(3):352–60.

57. Clarke M., Collins R., Darby S., et al. Effects of radiotherapy and of differences in the extent of surgery for early breast cancer on local recurrence and 15-year survival: an overview of the randomised trials. *Lancet.* 2005;**366**(9503):2087–2106.

58. Darby S. C., Ewertz M., McGale P., et al. Risk of ischemic heart disease in women after radiotherapy for breast cancer. *N Engl J Med.* 2013;**368**(11):987–98.

59. Freislederer P., Kügele M., Öllers M., et al. Recent advances in Surface Guided Radiation Therapy. *Radiat Oncol.* 2020;**15**(1):187.

60. Mutter R. W., Choi J. I., Jimenez R. B., et al. Proton therapy for breast cancer: A consensus statement from the particle therapy cooperative group breast cancer subcommittee. *Int J Radiat Oncol Biol Phys.* 2021;**111**(2):337–59.

61. Sparano J. A., Gray R. J., Makower D. F., et al. Adjuvant chemotherapy guided by a 21-gene expression assay in breast cancer. *New England Journal of Medicine.* 2018;**379**(2):111–21.

62. Kalinsky K., Barlow W. E., Gralow J. R., et al. 21-gene assay to inform chemotherapy benefit in node-positive breast cancer. *New England Journal of Medicine.* 2021;**385**(25):2336–47.

63. Braybrooke J., Bradley R., Gray R., et al. Anthracycline-containing and taxane-containing chemotherapy for early-stage operable breast cancer: a patient-level meta-analysis of 100 000 women from 86 randomised trials. *The Lancet.* 2023;**401**(10384):1277–92.

64. Blum J. L., Flynn P. J., Yothers G., et al. Anthracyclines in early breast cancer: The ABC Trials—USOR 06-090, NSABP B-46-I/USOR 07132, and NSABP B-49 (NRG Oncology). *Journal of Clinical Oncology.* 2017;**35**(23):2647–55.

65. Alba E., Calvo L., Albanell J., et al. Chemotherapy (CT) and hormonotherapy (HT) as neoadjuvant treatment in luminal breast cancer patients: Results from GEICAM/2006-03, a multicenter, randomized, phase-II study. *Ann Oncol.* 2012;**23**(12):3069–74.

66. Spring L. M., Gupta A., Reynolds K. L., et al. Neoadjuvant endocrine therapy for estrogen receptor–positive breast cancer: A systematic review and meta-analysis. *JAMA Oncology.* 2016;**2**(11):1477–86.

67. Davies C., Godwin J., Gray R., et al. Relevance of breast cancer hormone receptors and other factors to the efficacy of adjuvant tamoxifen: Patient-level meta-analysis of randomised trials. *Lancet.* 2011;**378**(9793):771–84.

68. Francis P. A., Regan M. M., Fleming G. F., et al. Adjuvant ovarian suppression in premenopausal breast cancer. *New England Journal of Medicine.* 2015;**372**(5):436–46.

69. Pagani O., Regan M. M., Walley B. A., et al. Adjuvant exemestane with ovarian suppression in premenopausal breast cancer. *New England Journal of Medicine.* 2014;**371**(2):107–18.

70. Johnston S. R., Harbeck N., Hegg R., et al. Abemaciclib combined with endocrine therapy for the adjuvant treatment of HR+, HER2−, node-positive, high-risk, early breast cancer (monarchE). *Journal of Clinical Oncology.* 2020;**38**(34):3987.

71. Pan H., Gray R., Braybrooke J., et al. 20-year risks of breast-cancer recurrence after stopping endocrine therapy at 5 years. *New England Journal of Medicine.* 2017;**377**(19):1836–46.

72. Davies C., Pan H., Godwin J., et al. Long-term effects of continuing adjuvant tamoxifen to 10 years versus stopping at 5 years after diagnosis of oestrogen receptor-positive breast cancer: ATLAS, a randomised trial. *The Lancet.* 2013;**381**(9869):805–16.

73. Rugo H. S., Lerebours F., Ciruelos E., et al. Alpelisib plus fulvestrant in PIK3CA-mutated, hormone receptor-positive advanced breast cancer after a CDK4/6 inhibitor (BYLieve): One

cohort of a phase 2, multicentre, open-label, non-comparative study. *The Lancet Oncology.* 2021;**22**(4):489–98.

74. Schettini F., Chic N., Brasó-Maristany F., et al. Clinical, pathological, and PAM50 gene expression features of HER2-low breast cancer. *NPJ breast cancer.* 2021;**7**(1):1.

75. Rugo H. S., Bardia A., Tolaney S. M., et al. TROPiCS-02: A Phase III study investigating sacituzumab govitecan in the treatment of HR+/HER2-metastatic breast cancer. *Future Oncology.* 2020;**16**(12):705–15.

76. Schmid P., Cortes J., Pusztai L., et al. Pembrolizumab for early triple-negative breast cancer. *New England Journal of Medicine.* 2020;**382**(9):810–21.

77. Tutt A. N., Garber J. E., Kaufman B., et al. Adjuvant olaparib for patients with BRCA1-or BRCA2-mutated breast cancer. *New England Journal of Medicine.* 2021;**384**(25):2394–405.

78. Cortes J., Rugo H. S., Cescon D. W., et al. Pembrolizumab plus chemotherapy in advanced triple-negative breast cancer. *New England Journal of Medicine.* 2022;**387**(3):217–26.

79. Bardia A., Hurvitz S. A., Tolaney S. M., et al. Sacituzumab govitecan in metastatic triple-negative breast cancer. *N Engl J Med.* 2021;**384**(16):1529–41.

80. Modi S., Jacot W., Yamashita T., et al. Trastuzumab deruxtecan in previously treated HER2-low advanced breast cancer. *New England Journal of Medicine.* 2022;**387**(1):9–20.

81. Tolaney S. M., Tarantino P., Graham N., et al. Adjuvant paclitaxel and trastuzumab for node-negative, HER2-positive breast cancer: Final 10-year analysis of the open-label, single-arm, phase 2 APT trial. *The Lancet Oncology.* 2023;**24**(3):273–85.

82. Schneeweiss A., Chia S., Hickish T., et al. Pertuzumab plus trastuzumab in combination with standard neoadjuvant anthracycline-containing and anthracycline-free chemotherapy regimens in patients with HER2-positive early breast cancer: A randomized phase II cardiac safety study (TRYPHAENA). *Annals of oncology.* 2013;**24**(9):2278–84.

83. Von Minckwitz G., Huang C.-S., Mano M. S., et al. Trastuzumab emtansine for residual invasive HER2-positive breast cancer. *New England Journal of Medicine.* 2019;**380**(7):617–28.

84. Swain S. M., Baselga J., Kim S.-B., et al. Pertuzumab, trastuzumab, and docetaxel in HER2-positive metastatic breast cancer. *New England Journal of Medicine.* 2015;**372**(8):724–34.

85. Cortés J., Kim S.-B., Chung W.-P., et al. Trastuzumab deruxtecan versus trastuzumab emtansine for breast cancer. *New England Journal of Medicine.* 2022;**386**(12):1143–54.

86. Murthy R. K., Loi S., Okines A., et al. Tucatinib, trastuzumab, and capecitabine for HER2-positive metastatic breast cancer. *New England Journal of Medicine.* 2020;**382**(7):597–609.

87. Hance K. W., Anderson W. F., Devesa S. S., Young H. A., Levine P. H. Trends in inflammatory breast carcinoma incidence and survival: The surveillance, epidemiology, and end results program at the National Cancer Institute. *JNCI: Journal of the National Cancer Institute.* 2005;**97**(13):966–75.

88. Dawood S., Merajver S. D., Viens P., et al. International expert panel on inflammatory breast cancer: Consensus statement for standardized diagnosis and treatment. *Annals of Oncology.* 2011;**22**(3):515–23.

89. Mylavarapu S., Das A., Roy M. Role of BRCA mutations in the modulation of response to platinum therapy. *Frontiers in Oncology.* 2018;**8**:16.

90. Kuchenbaecker K. B., Hopper J. L., Barnes D. R., et al. Risks of breast, ovarian, and contralateral breast cancer for BRCA1 and BRCA2 mutation carriers. *JAMA.* 2017;**317**(23):2402–16.

91. Meijers-Heijboer H., van Geel B., van Putten W. L., et al. Breast cancer after prophylactic bilateral mastectomy in women with a BRCA1 or BRCA2 mutation. *New England Journal of Medicine.* 2001;**345**(3):159–64.

92. Rebbeck T. R., Friebel T., Lynch H. T., et al. Bilateral prophylactic mastectomy reduces breast cancer risk in BRCA1 and BRCA2 mutation carriers: The PROSE Study Group. *Journal of Clinical Oncology.* 2004;**22**(6):1055–62.

93. Goggins M., Overbeek K. A., Brand R., et al. Management of patients with increased risk for familial pancreatic cancer: Updated recommendations from the International Cancer of the Pancreas Screening (CAPS) Consortium. *Gut.* 2020;**69**(1):7–17.

94. Robson M., Im S.-A., Senkus E., et al. Olaparib for metastatic breast cancer in patients with a germline BRCA mutation. *New England Journal of Medicine.* 2017;**377**(6):523–33.

95. Litton J. K., Rugo H. S., Ettl J., et al. Talazoparib in patients with advanced breast cancer and a germline BRCA mutation. *New England Journal of Medicine.* 2018;**379**(8):753–63.

96. Oktay K., Harvey B. E., Partridge A. H., et al. Fertility preservation in patients with cancer: ASCO Clinical Practice Guideline Update. *J Clin Oncol.* 2018;**36**(19):1994–2001.

97. Partridge A. H., Niman S. M., Ruggeri M., et al. Interrupting endocrine therapy to attempt pregnancy after breast cancer. *New England Journal of Medicine.* 2023;**388**(18):1645–56.

98. Zagouri F., Sergentanis T. N., Chrysikos D., et al. Trastuzumab administration during pregnancy: A systematic review and meta-analysis. *Breast Cancer Research and Treatment.* 2013;**137**:349–57.

99. Martín M., de la Torre-Montero J. C., López-Tarruella S., et al. Persistent major alopecia following adjuvant docetaxel for breast cancer: Incidence, characteristics, and prevention with scalp cooling. *Breast Cancer Research and Treatment.* 2018;**171**(3):627–34.

100. Gianotti E., Razzini G., Bini M., et al. Scalp cooling in daily clinical practice for breast cancer patients undergoing curative chemotherapy: A multicenter interventional study. *Asia-Pacific Journal of Oncology Nursing.* 2019;**6**(3):277–82.

101. Hanai A., Ishiguro H., Sozu T., et al. Effects of cryotherapy on objective and subjective symptoms of paclitaxel-induced neuropathy: Prospective self-controlled trial. *JNCI: Journal of the National Cancer Institute.* 2017;**110**(2):141–8.

102. Melisko M. E., Goldman M. E., Hwang J., et al. Vaginal testosterone cream vs estradiol vaginal ring for vaginal dryness or decreased libido in women receiving aromatase inhibitors for early-stage breast cancer: A randomized clinical trial. *JAMA Oncology.* 2017;**3**(3):313–19.

Chapter 15

Cervical Cancer

Mary Katherine Anastasio, Anuja Jhingran, and Travis T. Sims

Case Presentation

A 30-year-old G0 patient with no pertinent medical history presents to her gynecologist with postcoital bleeding. Pelvic exam is unremarkable, and the cervix is normal appearing without masses or lesions. A Papanicolaou smear is collected which reveals high-grade squamous intraepithelial lesion (HSIL). Colposcopy and biopsy reveal cervical intra-epithelial neoplasia (CIN) 3, and cold knife conization reveals invasive squamous cell carcinoma confined to the cervix with stromal invasion depth of 2 mm. Lymphovascular space invasion is not present. The patient strongly desires fertility sparing treatment. What are the next steps?

Epidemiology

Incidence and Long-Term Prognosis

Worldwide, cervical cancer is the fourth most common cancer in females with an estimated 604,000 new cases and 342,000 deaths in 2020 [1]. Higher incidences are found in resource-limited countries; almost 85% of cervical cancer cases were reported in developing countries [2]. In the United States, there are approximately 14,000 new cases of cervical cancer diagnosed and 4,000 deaths each year [3]. Compared to other gynecologic cancer, cervical cancer is most frequently diagnosed in younger women between ages 35–44 years, and the average age at diagnosis is 50 years [4]. In the United States, cervical cancer incidence is highest among American Indian/Alaska Native (10.1 per 100,000 population) and Hispanic (10/100,000) females followed by Non-Hispanic Black (9/100,000) and Non-Hispanic White (7.1/100,000) females [5].

Accurate cervical cancer staging using the International Federation of Gynecology and Obstetrics (FIGO) staging system is crucial, as FIGO stage (Table 15.1) is a significant prognostic factor [6]. Additionally, tumor size is an important prognostic factor and is associated with risk of parametrial and nodal spread [7, 8]. Stage I tumors are strictly confined to the cervix, with stage IA tumors having a maximum depth of invasion of ≤ 5mm and IB tumors having a maximum depth of invasion > 5mm. Stage II tumors invade beyond the uterus but do not extend to the lower third of the vagina or the pelvic wall. Stage III tumors involve the following areas: lower third of the vagina, pelvic wall, pelvic and/or paraaortic lymph nodes, or tumors causing hydronephrosis or a nonfunctioning kidney. Stage IV tumors extend beyond the true pelvis or involve the bladder or rectum [9, 10]. Using FIGO 2018 staging, five-year survival rates were 92–97% for stage IA tumors and 76–92% for stage IB tumors [11]. Additionally, lymph node involvement is associated with worse prognosis with five-year survival rates near 40–60% [11].

Table 15.1 2018 International Federation of Gynecology and Obstetrics (FIGO) staging of cervical cancer

Stage	Description
I	Carcinoma strictly confined to cervix
IA	Invasive carcinoma, diagnosed only by microscopy, with maximum depth of invasion < 5 mm
IA1	Stromal depth of invasion < 3 mm
IA2	Stromal depth of invasion ≥ 3 mm and < 5 mm
IB	Invasive carcinoma, with deepest invasion ≥ 5 mm, lesion limited to cervix
IB1	Stromal depth of invasion ≥ 5 mm, tumor < 2 cm in greatest dimension
IB2	Tumor ≥ 2 cm and < 4 cm in greatest dimension
IB3	Tumor ≥ 4 cm in greatest dimension
II	Carcinoma invades beyond the uterus but has not extended to the lower third of the vagina or pelvic wall
IIA	Involvement of the upper two-third of the vagina without parametrial involvement
IIA1	Tumor < 4 cm in greatest dimension
IIA2	Tumor ≥ 4 cm in greatest dimension
IIB	Parametrial involvement but not up to the pelvic wall
III	Carcinoma involves lower third of vagina, and/or extends to pelvic wall, and/or causes hydronephrosis or nonfunctioning kidney, and/or involves pelvic and/or para-aortic lymph nodes
IIIA	Carcinoma involves lower third of vagina, no extension to pelvic wall
IIIB	Extension to pelvic wall and/or hydronephrosis or nonfunctioning kidney
IIIC	Involvement of pelvic and/or para-aortic lymph nodes, irrespective of tumor size and extent
IIIC1	Pelvic lymph node involvement only
IIIC2	Para-aortic lymph node involvement
IV	Carcinoma extends beyond the true pelvis or has involved the mucosa of the bladder or rectum
IVA	Spread to adjacent pelvic organs
IVB	Spread to distant organs

Adapted from FIGO staging of cancer of the cervix uterine 2018 [9]

Etiology and Risk Factors

Human papillomavirus (HPV) is the primary etiologic infectious agent, and HPV infection is associated with 99.7% of cervical cancer [12]. Oncogenic HPV subtypes infect the epithelium at the cervical transformation zone. While most females readily clear HPV, persistent infection can lead to preinvasive dysplastic cervical lesions and development of invasive carcinoma [13]. Additional risk factors associated with HPV exposure through sexual intercourse include multiple sexual partners, younger age at first intercourse, increased parity, high-risk sexual partners, history of sexually transmitted infections, and immunosuppression (e.g., HIV infection) [14].

While HPV infection is the most significant risk factor, there are several additional risk factors unrelated to HPV. Current cigarette smoking is associated with significantly increased risk of squamous cell carcinoma of the cervix [14, 15]. Increasing duration of oral contraceptive use is associated with increased rates of both adenocarcinoma and squamous cell carcinoma [16]. Patients with lower socioeconomic status have significantly higher rates of cervical cancer [17]. Genetic factors contributing to the development of cervical cancer are not well-established, but studies suggest an increased incidence of cervical cancer within families [18]. Patients with Peutz-Jeghers syndrome are at increased risk of adenocarcinoma of the cervix and are recommended to initiate annual screening starting at age 25 years [19]. In contrast to germline mutations found in hereditary gynecologic cancer such as ovarian and endometrial cancer, polymorphisms in a wide variety of genes related to the immune system have been associated with cervical cancer [20, 21]. Additional work is needed to determine genetic factors associated with cervical cancer.

Squamous cell carcinoma is the most common histologic subtype of cervical cancer. It arises from the ectocervix and comprises approximately 70% of cases. Adenocarcinoma is the second most common histologic subtype. It arises from the endocervical columnar cells and accounts for approximately 25% of cases [22]. Over the past 30 years, incidence of squamous cell carcinoma has declined while the incidence of adenocarcinoma has increased [22, 23]. Other histologic subtypes are quite rare and often highly aggressive. They include adenosquamous carcinomas, neuroendocrine or small cell carcinomas, sarcomas, and malignant lymphomas among others [24]. Cervical cancer spreads by direct extension or by hematogenous or lymphatic dissemination. The presence of lymphovascular space invasion (LVSI) is associated with increased risk of lymph node metastasis and is an important negative prognostic factor [25]. Tumor expression of programmed cell death ligand 1 (PD-L1) is associated with worse survival in solid tumors, and patients with cervical cancer with tumor expression of PD-L1 may benefit from immune therapy against PD-L1 [26].

Fertility Considerations/Consultation Prior to Treatment

As previously discussed, cervical cancer is most often diagnosed in younger females who may not have completed childbearing at the time of diagnosis [4]. Therefore, pretreatment counseling on fertility-sparing treatment options and fertility concerns associated with cervical cancer treatment is crucial. First, a patient must undergo preoperative assessment to determine whether fertility-sparing treatment is feasible. Thorough pre-operative assessment includes staging, which typically involves frozen section analysis of pelvic lymph nodes, pelvic magnetic resonance imaging (MRI) to determine the extent of disease, and thorough pathology review of the excisional specimen [27, 28]. Pretreatment counseling includes a detailed discussion of criteria which must be met for a patient to be considered for fertility sparing treatment including low risk for recurrence, desire for future fertility and reproductive age group.

For patients with locally advanced disease, where chemotherapy and radiation therapy are primary treatment, fertility cannot be spared. Patients who desire to have future children should be counseled regarding expedited oocyte or ovarian tissue cryopreservation. An option to maintain ovarian function after treatment is ovarian transposition which also needs to be performed prior to treatment. The success rate of this procedure however varies markedly. If pelvic radiation is utilized, pregnancy is typically contraindicated (even with donor gametes) in light of adverse obstetric outcomes. For a detailed discussion regarding fertility preservation please refer to Chapter 1.

Diagnosis and Workup

Signs and Symptoms

Patients with early-stage cervical cancer are often asymptomatic at the time of diagnosis. Others may present with blood-tinged or watery vaginal discharge, postcoital bleeding, or heavy bleeding in more advanced cases [29].

Physical Exam Findings

A thorough pelvic examination including visualization of the cervix on speculum exam should be performed. The cervix may appear grossly normal in cases of microinvasive disease. Visible disease may appear as exophytic or endophytic growth, a polypoid mass, ulceration, necrotic tissue, or a barrel-shaped cervix. If cancer is suspected, a rectovaginal exam with assessment of vaginal or parametrial involvement, and palpation of the groin and supraclavicular areas for lymph node involvement should also be performed.

Diagnostic Tests

In the United States, cervical cancer screening methods include collection of cervical cytology with the Papanicolaou (Pap) test, HPV testing, and cotesting with cervical cytology and HPV [30]. Recommendations for cervical cancer screening are typically based on a patient's age, and several different guidelines exist with slightly different approaches. According to the United States Preventive Services Task Force (USPSTF) guidelines, cervical cancer screening is recommended every 3 years starting at age 21 with cervical cytology alone. Between ages 30 and 65, one of the following methods is recommended with no preference for one method over another: HPV testing every 5 years, Pap and HPV testing every 5 years, or Pap alone every 3 years [31] (see Chapter 7).

If cervical cytology results are abnormal, colposcopy and cervical biopsy are recommended based on current American Society for Colposcopy and Cervical Pathology (ASCCP) guidelines [32]. The ASCCP Risk-Based Management Consensus Guidelines have been streamlined using an app and web application to aid providers with uncomplicated, evidence-based management guidelines at their fingertips. Colposcopy is a diagnostic procedure used to identify precancerous or cancer lesions, and cervical biopsy may be obtained if invasive disease is suspected. Histologic evaluation of a cervical biopsy is the primary method used to diagnose cervical cancer. If malignancy is suspected based on exam findings, a cervical biopsy of the suspicious lesion should be obtained [33].

Imaging Studies

Historically, cervical cancer has been staged clinically. The current FIGO staging system (Table 15.1) now incorporates physical examination, cervical biopsy results, radiologic studies, cystoscopy, and proctoscopy into staging of cervical cancer, but these are not all required for diagnosis if resources are not available. Imaging studies are now incorporated into FIGO staging and can be important for accurate evaluation and treatment planning as treatment options differ by stage [34]. Radiologic studies include computed tomography (CT) scan or positron emission tomography (PET-CT) to assess lymph node involvement, MRI to assess tumor size and extent of disease, and chest radiograph to assess for metastatic disease [35].

Treatment Options and Surveillance

Treatment recommendations vary by stage, tumor factors, and patient factors. Treatment options for patients with early-stage (stages I–II) cervical cancer include hysterectomy with or without pelvic lymph node sampling or dissection, fertility-sparing surgery, and radiation therapy alone or in combination with chemotherapy [36]. Hysterectomy is typically recommended over primary radiation therapy for early-stage disease, and the type of hysterectomy (simple versus radical) depends on the specific disease stage. A simple (extra-fascial) hysterectomy involves removing the fascia of the cervix and lower uterine segment. A modified radical hysterectomy involves ligating the uterine artery where it crosses over the ureter, resecting the upper third of the vagina, separating both the uterosacral and cardinal ligaments halfway between their attachments to the uterus and the sacrum/pelvic sidewall (Figure 15.1). The ovaries may remain in situ if unaffected in premenopausal patients as ovarian metastases are uncommon [37], but the fallopian tubes and ovaries should be removed in postmenopausal patients. Patients with stage IA1 cancer without LVSI on conization specimen may undergo a simple hysterectomy. For those with stage IA1 disease with LVSI or stage IA2 disease, a modified radical hysterectomy with lymphadenectomy is recommended [36].

If a patient desires and is a candidate for fertility-sparing treatment, options include cold knife conization, simple trachelectomy, or radical trachelectomy [36]. The type of procedure is determined based on the disease stage, location and size of lesion, and surgeon preference. Cold knife conization is the most conservative approach and involves resecting a cone-shaped specimen from the cervix with a scalpel. A simple trachelectomy is performed vaginally and involves resecting the cervix as a cylinder-shaped specimen. A radical trachelectomy is the most invasive approach and involves resecting the cervix along with 1–2 cm of

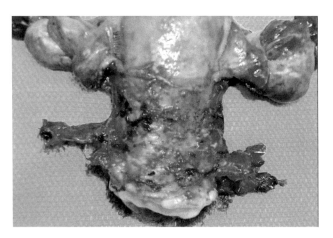

Figure 15.1 Radical hysterectomy specimen with parametrial margins

vaginal mucosa and proximal parametrial tissue. Radical trachelectomies may be performed vaginally, abdominally, laparoscopically, or robotically. A permanent cerclage is often placed during a radical trachelectomy to improve obstetric outcomes. A recent international retrospective study on open versus minimally invasive radical trachelectomy in patients with early-stage cervical cancer found no difference in disease-free or overall survival rates between groups [38]. Patients with stage IA1 disease without LVSI and no high-risk features may undergo cold knife conization. For patients with stage IA1 disease with LVSI and negative lymph nodes, stage IA2, or stage IB1 disease, radical trachelectomy with pelvic sentinel lymph node biopsy or lymph node dissection is most commonly performed worldwide. However, a trend toward more conservative surgery with conization or simple trachelectomy is evolving [39].

Patients with early-stage disease may require adjuvant therapy with chemoradiation or radiation therapy alone to reduce the risk of recurrence and death if they have specific pathologic risk factors [40, 41]. Risk factors include tumor size, stromal invasion, the presence of LVSI, positive surgical margins, lymph node involvement, or parametrial involvement [40–43].

Patients with locally advanced cervical cancer (IB3 to IVA) have a higher rate of recurrence, thus primary surgery is not recommended as it is unlikely to be curative and patients often require adjuvant treatment. Primary treatment recommendations for patients with stage IB3 to IVA disease include a combination of pelvic external beam radiation therapy (EBRT) with concurrent platinum-containing chemotherapy (e.g. cisplatin) and brachytherapy. EBRT is used to treat lymph nodes in the pelvic and para-aortic chains. A meta-analysis of several randomized controlled trials demonstrated that pelvic radiation therapy combined with platinum-based chemotherapy is superior to radiation therapy alone in patients with locally advanced disease [44]. Brachytherapy, an integral component of definitive chemoradiation, safely delivers high doses of radiation to the tumor while sparing surrounding normal tissue.

Those with stage IVB disease that is amenable to local treatment may receive chemoradiation, while distant metastatic disease not amenable to local treatment may be treated with systemic therapy [39]. Systemic therapy for this patient population typically includes carboplatin or cisplatin, paclitaxel, and bevacizumab. In a randomized, phase 3 trial on patients with metastatic, recurrent, or persistent cervical cancer comparing chemotherapy with or without bevacizumab, chemotherapy with bevacizumab resulted in significantly improved overall survival and progression-free survival. Patients who received chemotherapy with bevacizumab experienced increased incidence of hypertension, thromboembolic events, and gastrointestinal fistulas [45]. For patients with persistent, recurrent, or metastatic cervical cancer with PD-L1 positive tumors, the addition of pembrolizumab to chemotherapy with or without bevacizumab led to significantly longer progression-free and overall survival [26].

Surveillance after primary treatment (surgery versus chemoradiation) with curative intent is recommended for early detection of recurrence and prompt treatment. Patients should have a history and physical exam every 6 months for 2 years, then every 6–12 months for up to 5 years followed by annually [36]. When obtaining a history, providers should inquire about vaginal bleeding or discharge, urinary or bowel symptoms, and abdominopelvic pain as these raise concern for recurrence [46]. Exam findings suspicious for recurrence include raised or friable vaginal lesions, enlarged lymph nodes, palpable nodularity or masses in the rectovaginal septum or pelvis. Patients who opt for fertility-sparing surgery should follow up with a gynecologic oncologist long-term with cervical cytology, HPV cotesting, and colposcopic examination every three to four months for three years, every six months for the following two years, and then yearly [47].

Contraception/Hormone Therapy

Rationale

Cervical cancer is not hormone-dependent. Therefore, if needed, hormone therapy (HT) for the treatment of menopausal symptoms is not contraindicated [48, 49]. Ovarian failure is common in patients who undergo pelvic radiation therapy, and premenopausal aged patients may experience menopausal symptoms [50]. While the ovaries are typically left in situ during surgery, patients may still experience menopausal symptoms if perfusion to the ovaries is impaired [51].

Options

HT is recommended over nonhormonal treatment for menopausal symptoms. Data suggest that use of HT is safe with no increased risk of recurrence and similar five-year survival rates compared to those who do not use HT [48]. Systemic or vaginal formulations are suitable; estrogen alone may be given if the uterus has been removed, whereas combined therapy (estrogen in combination with a progestogen) should be given if the uterus remains in situ.

Contraindications

General contraindications to HT include a history of venous thromboembolism or stroke, coronary heart disease, history of breast cancer, and active liver disease [52].

Screening Recommendations after Cancer

Pap/HPV

For patients who underwent primary surgery only, annual cervical cytology should be obtained. For those who underwent radiation therapy, cytology is not recommended as it is often not accurate [53]. For patients who opted for fertility-sparing treatment, cervical cytology, HPV cotesting, and colposcopy are recommended every three to four months for three years, every six months for the next two years, and yearly thereafter [47].

HPV Vaccination

In the United States, the human papillomavirus 9-valent (types 6, 11, 16, 18, 31, 33, 45, 52, 58) vaccine is the only vaccine available. HPV vaccination is recommended for patients with a history of cervical cancer or cervical dysplasia within the recommended age range (up to age 45 years), regardless of history of prior HPV infection [54]. While a patient may have a history of one strain of HPV infection, the vaccine will still provide immunity against additional strains of HPV. Cervical cancer rates have decreased significantly at a population level in the United States since the approval of the HPV vaccine [55].

Special Considerations

Frequent Gynecologic Concerns During and After Treatment

Cervical cancer survivors may experience an array of symptoms during and after definitive treatment, as their surgery and/or chemoradiation can lead to significant sequelae. Treatment related sequelae should be considered when approaching the care of cervical cancer survivors. Patients who undergo radical hysterectomy are more likely to have long-term side effects than those who undergo a simple hysterectomy. Disruption of the autonomic nervous system during a radical hysterectomy can result in bladder and/or bowel dysfunction in the form of urinary urgency, urinary incontinence, fecal incontinence, incomplete stool evacuation, or constipation [56]. Additionally, patients may experience lymphedema following pelvic lymphadenectomy, vaginal shorting after resection of the upper vagina, and menopausal symptoms if there is disruption of ovarian perfusion [57, 58].

Chemotherapy and radiation also can lead both to short- and long-term side effects. Patients can experience urinary and bowel dysfunction, fatigue, bone fractures and sexual dysfunction following radiation therapy [59]. Bladder dysfunction is a common long-term side effect for patients treated with radiation and may present as urinary frequency, urinary urgency, dysuria, hematuria, cystitis, or incontinence due to vesicovaginal fistula [60–62]. Bowel dysfunction is also common and may present as nausea, vomiting, diarrhea, fecal urgency, fecal leakage, proctitis, enteritis, or incontinence due to rectovaginal or enterovaginal fistula [63–66]. Fractures occur in about 10–20% of patients treated with pelvic radiation therapy and usually occur within the first two years after treatment and are seen most typically in postmenopausal women. They are usually managed with bedrest and analgesia but sometimes surgical intervention may be indicated. Preventive management is important including replacing low Vitamin D and weight-bearing exercise [67]. Improved treatment techniques such as intensity-modulated radiation therapy (IMRT) have been used to minimize radiation exposure to normal tissues and therefore reduce toxicities.

Sexual Toxicity

Sexual toxicity caused by radiation include decreased sexual desire, arousal, enjoyment, and satisfaction as well as vaginal pain, dryness, and decreased length of the vagina [68]. Radiation-induced vaginal mucosal changes and grading are very well described in Chapter 12. Common alterations after radiation therapy include vaginal mucositis, atrophy, telangiectasia, reduced lubrication, adhesions, and fibrosis leading to vaginal stenosis and shortening. In rare situations, ulcerations, necrosis, and fistulae are seen. Degree of changes is correlated with length of vagina treated, total dose delivered to vagina and tumor extension into the vagina. Physician reported morbidity markedly underreports patients' symptoms, highlighting the importance of incorporating patient reported outcomes while managing patients post-treatment [69]. The incidence of vaginal toxicities from patient reported data include 35% moderate/severe lack of lubrication, 55% mild/severe dyspareunia, 30% dissatisfaction with sexual intercourse, 26% moderate/substantial reduction in vaginal length, 23% moderate/substantial reduction in vaginal elasticity and 26% reporting "much distress" with regards to vaginal changes and problems with intercourse [70, 71].

Vaginal stenosis is the most prevalent complication with an incidence that varies from 1.2% to 88% [72]. Vaginal dilation is recommended as a best practice guideline to help prevent or decrease this morbidity by preventing and separating adhesions that form between the walls of the vagina and by stretching the vaginal tissue. The vaginal dilator treatment should start 2–6 weeks post brachytherapy treatment and should be used minimally 3 times a week for 5–10 minutes per session for a duration of greater than 12 months after radiation treatment. [73]

Vaginal dryness is another common side effect in female cancer survivors and is usually multifactorial due to effects from surgery, chemotherapy, age, and radiation therapy. Vaginal lubricants without additives should be used with sexual intercourse as well as dilator therapy. Besides lubricants, vaginal moisturizers such as hyaluronic acid-based products should also be used as they help restore the pH of the vagina and add moisture to the vaginal/vulvar mucosa which assist epithelial regeneration [74]. Moisturizers should be used 3–5 times a week but results will not be noticed for 2–3 months from the start of treatment [75]. Hormone-containing vaginal creams will also help with atrophy and dryness and promote healing the of the vaginal wall.

Survivors of pelvic cancer may exhibit pelvic floor dysfunction including urinary frequency, urge/stress incontinence, incomplete emptying, stool incontinence and pelvic pain. The incidence of pelvic pain has been reported as high as 38% in survivors of cervical cancer [76] and the pathophysiology of the pain is not well understood. (Internal scarring and adhesions from surgery and radiation therapy may be potential etiologies.) Pelvic floor physical therapists should be consulted for patients with pelvic floor dysfunction. Pelvic floor therapy including pelvic floor strengthening, relaxation exercises and massage may increase tissue flexibility, improve blood circulation in the paravaginal tissues and improve pelvic floor strength. Pelvic floor strength training has led to improved sexual function, particularly in regards to arousal and orgasm [78].

Case Resolution

Cold knife conization is recommended for this patient with stage IA1 squamous cell carcinoma and negative LVSI who desires fertility-sparing treatment. The patient should follow up with a gynecologic oncologist long-term with cervical cytology, HPV cotesting, and colposcopic examination every three to four months for three years, every six months for the following two years, and then annually. HPV vaccination is recommended for patients with a history of cervical cancer or cervical dysplasia within the recommended age range (up to age 45 years), regardless of history of prior HPV infection.

Take Home Points

- Cervical cancer incidence in the United States is decreasing due to improved access to screening with Pap smears and prevention with the HPV vaccine.
- HPV infection is the cause of almost all cervical cancer.
- Fertility-sparing treatment for cervical cancer may be recommended for optimal candidates with low risk of recurrence.
- Cervical cancer treatment-related sequelae including urinary, bowel or sexual dysfunction as well as menopausal symptoms must be considered in cervical cancer survivors.

References

1. Sung H., Ferlay J, Siegel R. L., et al., Global Cancer Statistics 2020: GLOBOCAN estimates of incidence and mortality worldwide for 36 cancer in 185 countries. *CA Cancer J Clin*. 2021;**71**(3):209–49.

2. Torre L. A., Bray F., Siegel, R. L., et al., Global cancer statistics, 2012. *CA Cancer J Clin*. 2015;**65**(2):87–108.

3. Siegel R. L., Miller K. D., Wagle N. S., et al., Cancer statistics, 2023. *CA Cancer J Clin*, 2023;**73**(1):17–48.

4. Howlader N., Noone A., Krapcho M., et al. *SEER Cancer Statistics Review, 1975–2016.* 2019; https://seer.cancer.gov/csr/1975_2016/ based on November 2018 SEER data submission, posted to the SEER web site, April 2019.

5. Surveillance E., and End Results Program, *Cancer stat facts: Cervical cancer.* 2022.

6. Yan D. D., Tang Q., Chen J. H., et al., Prognostic value of the 2018 FIGO staging system for cervical cancer patients with surgical risk factors. *Cancer Manag Res.* 2019;**11**:5473–80.

7. Kubota S., Kobayashi E., Kakuda M., et al., Retrospective analysis for predictors of parametrial involvement in IB cervical cancer. *J Obstet Gynaecol Res.* 2019;**45**(3):679–85.

8. Melamed A., Margul D. J., Chen L., et al., Survival after minimally invasive radical hysterectomy for early-stage cervical cancer. *N Engl J Med.* 2018;**379**(20):1905–14.

9. Bhatla N., Aoki D., Sharma D. N., et al., Cancer of the cervix uteri. *Int J Gynaecol Obstet*. 2018;**143** Suppl 2:22–36.

10. Bhatla N., Berek J. S., Cuello Fredes M., et al., Revised FIGO staging for carcinoma of the cervix uteri. *Int J Gynaecol Obstet*. 2019;**145**(1):129–35.

11. Wright J. D., Matsuo K., Huang Y., et al., Prognostic performance of the 2018 International Federation of Gynecology and Obstetrics Cervical Cancer Staging Guidelines. *Obstet Gynecol.* 2019;**134**(1):49–57.

12. Walboomers J. M., Jacobs M. V., Manos M. M., et al., Human papillomavirus is a necessary cause of invasive cervical cancer worldwide. *J Pathol*. 1999;**189**(1):12–19.

13. Schiffman M., Castle P. E., Jeronimo J., et al., Human papillomavirus and cervical cancer. *Lancet*. 2007;**370**(9590):890–907.

14. International Collaboration of Epidemiological Studies of Cervical Cancer, Comparison of risk factors for invasive squamous cell carcinoma and adenocarcinoma of the cervix: collaborative reanalysis of individual data on 8,097 women with squamous cell carcinoma and 1,374 women with adenocarcinoma from 12 epidemiological studies. *Int J Cancer*. 2007;**120**(4):885–91.

15. International Collaboration of Epidemiological Studies of Cervical Cancer, et al., Carcinoma of the cervix and tobacco smoking: collaborative reanalysis of individual data on 13,541 women with carcinoma of the cervix and 23,017 women without carcinoma of the cervix from 23 epidemiological studies. *Int J Cancer*. 2006;**118**(6):1481–95.

16. International Collaboration of Epidemiological Studies of Cervical Cancer, et al., Cervical cancer and hormonal contraceptives: collaborative reanalysis of individual data for 16,573 women with cervical cancer and 35,509 women without cervical cancer from 24 epidemiological studies. *Lancet*. 2007;**370**(9599):1609–21.

17. Singh G. K., Miller B. A., Hankey B. F., et al., Persistent area socioeconomic disparities in U.S. incidence of cervical cancer, mortality, stage, and survival, 1975–2000. *Cancer*. 2004;**101**(5):1051–7.

18. Hemminki K., Chen B. Familial risks for cervical tumors in full and half siblings: etiologic apportioning. *Cancer Epidemiol Biomarkers Prev.* 2006;**15**(7):1413–14.

19. Syngal S., Brand R. E., Church J. M., et al., ACG clinical guideline: Genetic testing and management of hereditary gastrointestinal

cancer syndromes. *Am J Gastroenterol.* 2015;**110**(2):223–62; quiz 263.

20. Craveiro R., Bravo I., Catarino R., et al., The role of p73 G4C14-to-A4T14 polymorphism in the susceptibility to cervical cancer. *DNA Cell Biol.* 2012;**31**(2):224–9.

21. Liu L., Yang X., Chen X., et al., Association between TNF-alpha polymorphisms and cervical cancer risk: A meta-analysis. *Mol Biol Rep.* 2012;**39**(3):2683–8.

22. Adegoke O., Kulasingam S., Virnig B., Cervical cancer trends in the United States: a 35-year population-based analysis. *J Womens Health (Larchmt).* 2012;**21**(10):1031–7.

23. Smith H. O., Tiffany M. F., Qualls C. R., et al., The rising incidence of adenocarcinoma relative to squamous cell carcinoma of the uterine cervix in the United States: A 24-year population-based study. *Gynecol Oncol.* 2000;**78**(2):97–105.

24. Vinh-Hung V., Bourgain C., Vlastos G., et al., Prognostic value of histopathology and trends in cervical cancer: a SEER population study. *BMC Cancer.* 2007;**7**:164.

25. Sevin B. U., Lu Y., Bloch D. A., et al., Surgically defined prognostic parameters in patients with early cervical carcinoma. A multivariate survival tree analysis. *Cancer.* 1996;**78**(7):1438–46.

26. Colombo N., Dubot C., Lorusso D., et al., Pembrolizumab for persistent, recurrent, or metastatic cervical cancer. *N Engl J Med.* 2021;**385**(20):1856–67.

27. Hauspy J., Beiner M., Harley I., et al., Sentinel lymph nodes in early stage cervical cancer. *Gynecol Oncol.* 2007;**105**(2):285–90.

28. Noel P., Dube M., Plante M., et al., Early cervical carcinoma and fertility-sparing treatment options: MR imaging as a tool in patient selection and a follow-up modality. *Radiographics.* 2014;**34**(4):1099–119.

29. Arbyn M., Xu L., Simoens C., et al., Prophylactic vaccination against human papillomaviruses to prevent cervical cancer and its precursors. *Cochrane Database Syst Rev.* 2018;**5**(5):CD009069.

30. Fontham E. T. H., Wolf A. M. D., Church T. R., et al., Cervical cancer screening for individuals at average risk: 2020 guideline update from the American Cancer Society. *CA Cancer J Clin.* 2020;**70**(5):321–46.

31. Kim J. J., Burger E. A., Regan C., et al., Screening for cervical cancer in primary care: A decision analysis for the US Preventive Services Task Force. *JAMA.* 2018;**320**(7):706–14.

32. Saslow D., Solomon D., Lawson H. W., et al., American Cancer Society, American Society for Colposcopy and Cervical Pathology, and American Society for Clinical Pathology screening guidelines for the prevention and early detection of cervical cancer. *CA Cancer J Clin.* 2012;**62**(3):147–72.

33. Partridge E. E., Abu-Rustum N. R., Campos S. M., et al., Cervical cancer screening. *J Natl Compr Canc Netw.* 2010;**8**(12):1358–86.

34. Pecorelli S., Zigliani L., Odicino F. Revised FIGO staging for carcinoma of the cervix. *Int J Gynaecol Obstet.* 2009;**105**(2):107–8.

35. Benedet J. L., Bender H., Jones H., et al., FIGO staging classifications and clinical practice guidelines in the management of gynecologic cancer. FIGO Committee on Gynecologic Oncology. *Int J Gynaecol Obstet.* 2000;**70**(2):209–62.

36. Network, N.C.C. *NCCN Clinical Practice Guidelines in Oncology. Cervical cancer.* . 2023 3/10/2023]; www.nccn.org/profes sionals/physician_gls/pdf/cervical.pdf.

37. Shimada M., Kigawa J., Nishimura R., et al., Ovarian metastasis in carcinoma of the uterine cervix. *Gynecol Oncol.* 2006;**101**(2):234–7.

38. Salvo G., Ramirez P. T., Leitao M. M., et al., Open vs minimally invasive radical trachelectomy in early-stage cervical cancer: International Radical Trachelectomy Assessment Study. *Am J Obstet Gynecol.* 2022;**226**(1):e1–97.

39. Koh W. J., Abu-Rustum N. R., Bean S., et al., Cervical Cancer, Version 3.2019, NCCN Clinical Practice Guidelines in

Oncology. *J Natl Compr Canc Netw.* 2019;**17**(1):64–84.

40. Rotman M., Sedlis A., Piedmonte M. R., et al., A phase III randomized trial of postoperative pelvic irradiation in Stage IB cervical carcinoma with poor prognostic features: Follow-up of a gynecologic oncology group study. *Int J Radiat Oncol Biol Phys.* 2006;**65**(1):169–76.

41. Sedlis A., Bundy B. N., Rotman M. Z. et al., A randomized trial of pelvic radiation therapy versus no further therapy in selected patients with stage IB carcinoma of the cervix after radical hysterectomy and pelvic lymphadenectomy: A Gynecologic Oncology Group Study. *Gynecol Oncol.* 1999;**73**(2):177–83.

42. Monk B. J., Wang J., Im S., et al., Rethinking the use of radiation and chemotherapy after radical hysterectomy: A clinical-pathologic analysis of a Gynecologic Oncology Group/ Southwest Oncology Group/Radiation Therapy Oncology Group trial. *Gynecol Oncol.* 2005;**96**(3):721–8.

43. Peters W. A., 3rd, Liu P. Y., Barrett R. J., 2nd, et al., Concurrent chemotherapy and pelvic radiation therapy compared with pelvic radiation therapy alone as adjuvant therapy after radical surgery in high-risk early-stage cancer of the cervix. *J Clin Oncol.* 2000;**18**(8):1606–13.

44. Chemoradiotherapy for Cervical Cancer Meta-analysis, Reducing uncertainties about the effects of chemoradiotherapy for cervical cancer: Individual patient data meta-analysis. *Cochrane Database Syst Rev.* 2010;**2010**(1):CD008285.

45. Tewari K. S., Sill M. W., Long H. J., 3rd, et al., Improved survival with bevacizumab in advanced cervical cancer. *N Engl J Med.* 2014;**370**(8):734–43.

46. Elit L., Fyles A. W., Devries M. C., et al., Follow-up for women after treatment for cervical cancer: A systematic review. *Gynecol Oncol.* 2009;**114**(3):528–35.

47. Shepherd J. H., Uterus-conserving surgery for invasive cervical cancer. *Best Pract Res Clin Obstet Gynaecol.* 2005;**19**(4):577–90.

48. Ploch E., Hormonal replacement therapy in patients after cervical cancer treatment. *Gynecol Oncol.* 1987;**26**(2):169–77.

49. Singh P., Oehler M. K., Hormone replacement after gynaecological cancer. *Maturitas.* 2010;**65**(3):190–7.

50. Baker T. G., Radiosensitivity of mammalian oocytes with particular reference to the human female. *Am J Obstet Gynecol.* 1971;**110**(5):746–61.

51. Feeney D. D., Moore D. H., Look K. Y. et al., The fate of the ovaries after radical hysterectomy and ovarian transposition. *Gynecol Oncol.* 1995;**56**(1):3–7.

52. Stuenkel C. A., Davis S. R., Gompel A., et al., Treatment of symptoms of the menopause: An Endocrine Society Clinical Practice Guideline. *J Clin Endocrinol Metab.* 2015;**100**(11):3975–4011.

53. Salani R., Backes F. J., Fung M. F., et al., Posttreatment surveillance and diagnosis of recurrence in women with gynecologic malignancies: Society of Gynecologic Oncologists recommendations. *Am J Obstet Gynecol.* 2011;**204**(6):466–78.

54. Markowitz L. E., Dunne E. F., Saraiya M., et al., Human papillomavirus vaccination: recommendations of the Advisory Committee on Immunization Practices (ACIP). *MMWR Recomm Rep.* 2014;**63** (RR-05):1–30.

55. Liao C. I., Francoeur A. A., Kapp D. S., et al., Trends in human papillomavirus-associated cancer, demographic characteristics, and vaccinations in the US, 2001–2017. *JAMA Netw Open.* 2022;**5**(3): e222530.

56. Brooks R. A., Wright J. D., Powell M. A., et al., Long-term assessment of bladder and bowel dysfunction after radical hysterectomy. *Gynecol Oncol.* 2009;**114**(1):75–9.

57. Ferrandina G., Mantegna G., Petrillo M., et al., Quality of life and emotional distress in early stage and locally advanced cervical cancer patients: A prospective, longitudinal study. *Gynecol Oncol.* 2012;**124**(3):389–94.

58. Pieterse Q. D., Maas C. P., ter Kuile M. M., et al., An observational longitudinal study

to evaluate miction, defecation, and sexual function after radical hysterectomy with pelvic lymphadenectomy for early-stage cervical cancer. *Int J Gynecol Cancer.* 2006;**16**(3):1119–29.

59. Frumovitz M., Sun C. C., Schover L. R., et al., Quality of life and sexual functioning in cervical cancer survivors. *J Clin Oncol.* 2005;**23**(30):7428–36.

60. Denton A. S., Clarke N. W., Maher E. J., Non-surgical interventions for late radiation cystitis in patients who have received radical radiotherapy to the pelvis. *Cochrane Database Syst Rev.* 2002;**2002**(3): CD001773.

61. Parkin D. E., Davis J. A., Symonds R. P., Long-term bladder symptomatology following radiotherapy for cervical carcinoma. *Radiother Oncol.* 1987;**9**(3):195–9.

62. Parkin D. E., Davis J. A., Symonds R. P., Urodynamic findings following radiotherapy for cervical carcinoma. *Br J Urol.* 1988;**61**(3):213–17.

63. Bjelic-Radisic V., Jensen P. T., Vlasic K. K. et al., Quality of life characteristics inpatients with cervical cancer. *Eur J Cancer.* 2012;**48**(16):3009–18.

64. Klee M., Thranov I., Machin D., Life after radiotherapy: The psychological and social effects experienced by women treated for advanced stages of cervical cancer. *Gynecol Oncol.* 2000;**76**(1):5–13.

65. Velji K., Fitch M., The experience of women receiving brachytherapy for gynecologic cancer. *Oncol Nurs Forum.* 2001;**28**(4):743–51.

66. Yeoh E., Sun W. M., Russo A., et al., A retrospective study of the effects of pelvic irradiation for gynecological cancer on anorectal function. *Int J Radiat Oncol Biol Phys.* 1996;**35**(5):1003–10.

67. Schmeler K. M., Jhingran A., Iyer R. B., et al. Pelvic fractures after radiotherapy for cervical cancer: implications for survivors. *Cancer.* 2010;**116**:625–30.

68. Suvaal I., Kirchheiner K., Nout R. A., et al. Vaginal changes, sexual functioning and distress of women with locally advanced

cervical cancer treated in the EMBRACE vaginal morbidity substudy. *Gyn Onc.* 2023;**170**;123–32.

69. Chin C., Damast S . Brachytherapy inpacts on sexual function: An integrative review of literature focusing on cervical cancer. *Brachytherapy.* 2023;**22**:30–46.

70. Jensen P. T., Klee M. C., Thranov I., Groenvld M. *Psychooncology.* 2004;**8**:577–92.

71. Bergmark K., Avall-Lundqvist E., Dickman P. W., et al. Vaginal changes and sexuality in women with a history of cervical cancer. *N Engl J Med.* 1999;**18**:1383–9.

72. Hartman P., Diddle A. W. Vaginal stenosis following irradiation therapy for carcinoma of the cervix uteri. *Cancer.* 1972;**30**:426–42.

73. Damast S., Jeffery D. D., Son C. H., et al. Literature review of vaginal stenosis and dilator use in radiation. *Pract Radiat Oncol.* 2019;**9**:479–91.

74. Chin C., Damast S. Brachytherapy impacts on sexual function: An integrative review of the literature focusing on cervical cancer. *Brachytherapy.* 2022;**17**:27.

75. Carter J., Baser R. E., Goldfrank D. J., et al. A single-arm, prospective trial investigating the effectiveness of a non-hormonal vaginal moisturizer containing hyaluronic acid in postmenopausal cancer survivors. *Support Care Cancer.* 2021;**29**:311–22.

76. Vistad I., Cvancarova M., Kristensen G. B., Fossa S. D. A study of chronic pelvic pain after radiotherapy in survivors of locally advanced cervical cancer. *J Cancer Surviv.* 2011;**5**:208–16.

77. Alappattu M. J. Pain and psychological outcomes after rehabilitative treatment for a woman with chronic pelvic pain with stage III cervical cancer: A case report. *J Womens Health Hys Therap.* 2013;**37**:97–102.

78. Lowenstein L., Gruenwald I., Gartman I., et al. Can stronger pelvic muscle floor improve sexual function? *Int Urogynecol J.* 2010;**21**:553–6.

Endometrial Cancer

Anuja Jhingran and Travis T. Sims

Case Presentation

A 65-year-old female presents with one episode of postmenopausal bleeding. The speculum exam reveals a normal appearance to the cervix and normal vagina without erythema, inflammation or lesions. The bimanual exam reveals a normal uterus with no adnexal masses appreciated. Pelvic ultrasound is significant for an endometrial echostripe of 12.6 mms with a heterogeneous appearance. What is your next best step?

Epidemiology

Incidence and Long-Term Prognosis

Endometrial cancer is the sixth most common cancer in women worldwide, and the average age of diagnosis is 63 years [1]. Women with a normal body-mass index (BMI) have a 3% lifetime risk of endometrial cancer [2]. Approximately 60% of all endometrial cancer are attributable to obesity and with every 5-unit increase in the BMI, a women's risk of endometrial cancer increases by more than 50% [1, 2]. In the United States, an estimated 65,950 new cases and 12,550 associated deaths are expected [3] for 2022. 75% of patients with endometrial cancer have International Federation of Gynecologic and Obstetrics (FIGO) stage I disease, and for this early-stage disease 5-year overall survival rates exceed 90% [1]. Consequently, despite being the fourth leading cause of cancer, endometrial cancer is only the sixth leading cause of cancer deaths among women in the United States.

Pathophysiology and Risk Factors

Endometrial carcinoma arises from the lining of the uterus and is categorized based on histology as type I (endometrioid) or type II (nonendometriod) endometrial cancer. Endometrioid endometrial cancer (type I) comprises 80% of patients, while nonendometrioid endometrial cancer (type II) which includes serous, clear cell adenocarcinoma and carcinosarcoma, represents the remaining 20% of patients.

Type I – endometrioid endometrial carcinomas are associated with relative estrogen excess, which includes obesity, the use of unopposed estrogen for hormone-replacement therapy, and exposure to estrogen-producing tumors (e.g., ovarian granulosa-cell tumors). In obese women, excess adipose tissue leads to the peripheral aromatization of androstenedione to estrone resulting in a surplus of estrone. In post-menopausal women, this means the endometrium is exposed to nearly continuous estrogen stimulation without an ensuing progestational effect; hence no menstrual shedding occurs. The relative excess estrogen exposure results in the development of a precancerous lesion called complex atypical hyperplasia (CAH). Endometrioid carcinomas are graded on a three-tiered FIGO system according to the relative proportion of the glandular and solid-tumor components. Grade 1 lesions have a solid-tumor component of less than 6%; grade 2, have a solid-tumor component between 6 and 50%; and grade 3, have a solid-tumor component of more than 50%. Grade 1 and grade 2 tumors are considered low grade, are characteristically indolent, have little tendency to spread outside the uterus or recur, and are associated with good prognosis. Grade 3 tumors are associated with an intermediate-to-poor prognosis given their increased potential for myometrial invasion and nodal/distant metastasis.

Type II – nonendometrioid endometrial carcinomas, in contrast, have no known precancer lesion and have a hormone-independent pathogenesis. They typically arise from the atrophic endometrium of older postmenopausal women. Nonendometrioid endometrial carcinomas include endometrial serous carcinoma, clear-cell carcinoma, and carcinosarcoma.

Endometrial serous carcinoma is the most common of the nonendometrioid tumors, accounting for 5 to 10% of endometrial cancer, are highly aggressive and are typically associated with a poor prognosis [4, 5]. These tumors at times are found to be confined within an endometrial polyp with no evidence for spread, however, up to 37% of women with no evidence of endometrial stromal or myometrial invasion will have extrauterine disease [5, 6].

Endometrial clear cell adenocarcinomas are similar to endometrial serous carcinoma in that they tend to be high-grade, deeply invasive tumors, and overall confer a worse prognosis [7, 8].

Carcinosarcomas (or malignant mixed müllerian tumors) are a biphasic malignant neoplasm composed of both malignant epithelial (carcinomatous) and malignant mesenchymal (sarcomatous) elements. In the past, carcinosarcomas were classified as a type of uterine sarcoma, but its pattern of metastasis and recurrence reflects carcinoma rather than sarcoma. Molecular studies have shown that most carcinosarcomas are monoclonal and driven by their epithelial component [9, 10]. At the time of diagnosis, approximately 40% of patients diagnosed with a carcinosarcoma are stage I, 10% stage II, 25% stage III, and 25% stage IV disease, which confers a worse prognosis than endometrioid, clear-cell, and serous carcinomas [11–13]. Additional risk factors include older age and family history.

Women with Lynch syndrome have an elevated lifetime risk of endometrial and colon cancer [14, 15]. This autosomal-dominant syndrome is diagnosed on the basis of a germline mutation in the mismatch-repair genes, *MLH1*, *MSH2*, *MSH6*, and *PMS2* [16, 17]. During DNA replication base mismatches are common, hence a defect with the DNA repair system due to these gene mutations promotes carcinogenesis. Women with Lynch syndrome have a lifetime risk of endometrial cancer ranging from 40 to 60%, with a median age at onset of 48 years, and the risk for endometrial cancer actually exceeds that for colorectal cancer [10, 17, 18, 20]. Of all endometrial cancer cases, three percent are attributable to Lynch syndrome, and in women under the age of 50 years, nine percent of endometrial cancer are attributable to Lynch syndrome, which occurs substantially earlier than sporadic endometrial cancer [21–23]. A risk reducing option for women with Lynch syndrome is hystectomy, however the decision and timing of surgery should be tailored to the individual patient [24].

Increased parity and oral contraceptive use are factors that confer protection against endometrial cancer [25]. Combination oral contraceptive (COC) use for at least one year (ideally greater than five years) decreases the risk of endometrial cancer up to 40% and lasts years after cessation [26]. Tamoxifen use approximately doubles the risk of developing endometrial cancer given its progestogenic effects in the uterus [27]. Tamoxifen increases the risk of both endometrioid and nonendometrioid types of endometrial cancer but affects postmenopausal women almost exclusively. Endometrial cancer rates increase with the duration of tamoxifen use, increasing fourfold when tamoxifen duration exceeds five years [27–29].

Evaluation

Postmenopausal bleeding or abnormal uterine bleeding (in premenopausal women) often prompt patients to seek care and should trigger evaluation. Approximately 90% of patients with endometrial carcinoma present with abnormal uterine bleeding or postmenopausal bleeding. In older women, abnormal vaginal discharge may be the presenting symptom. Physicians should have a high index of suspicion when evaluating these women, particularly if the patient has associated risk factors. Diagnosis is often made with in-office endometrial biopsy [30] and is usually adequate for treatment planning. Of note, endometrial biopsies have a false-negative rate of approximately 10% even in women with months or years of heavy, irregular bleeding. Thus, a persistently symptomatic patient with a negative endometrial biopsy should undergo dilation and curettage (D&C) under anesthesia to rule out invasive disease [31]. Complex atypical hyperplasia (CAH) on endometrial biopsy is associated with a high risk of endometrial cancer at time of hysterectomy (40–50%).

In women who have a diagnosis of low grade endometrioid endometrial cancer, consideration of chest imaging (chest x-ray) to rule out obvious metastatic disease is recommended, but additional imaging can be considered based on clinical symptoms, physical findings, or abnormal laboratory findings. With high risk histologies, imaging tests such as computed tomography (CT) or magnetic resonance (MR) or PET/CT may be used to evaluate disease extent and to exclude metastatic disease [32]. In patients with extrauterine disease, a serum CA-125 assay may be helpful in monitoring clinical response [33].

Staging

Uterine cancer are surgically staged according to an FIGO staging classification (Table 16.1). Surgical staging historically includes removal of the uterus and cervix, and/or pelvic/paraaortic lymph node assessment. Contemporary surgical intervention typically consists of a minimally invasive total hysterectomy, bilateral salpingo-oophorectomy, sentinel lymph node mapping and biopsy, and possible pelvic and para-aortic lymph node dissection. The type and extent of post-operative therapy is based upon the intraoperative findings and final pathology report.

Screening

At this time, routine screening of low or average risk women for hyperplasia or endometrial cancer is not supported. Postmenopausal patients should be counseled regarding signs and symptoms and factors that increase risk of endometrial cancer and providers should encourage their patients to report postmenopausal bleeding or spotting [14, 15].

Table 16.1 FIGO staging classification for endometrial cancer

STAGE	CRITERIA
I	**Tumor confined to the corpus uteri.**
IA	Limited to the endometrium or less than half myometrial invasion.
IB	Invasion equal to or more than half of the myometrium.
II	**Tumor invades cervical stroma but does not extend beyond the uterus.**
III	**Local and/or regional spread of the tumor.**
IIIA	Tumor invades the serosa of the corpus uteri and/or adnexae.
IIIB	Vaginal and/or parametrial involvement.
IIIC	Metastases to pelvic and/or para-aortic lymph nodes.
IIIC1	Positive pelvic nodes.
IIIC2	Positive paraaortic lymph nodes with or without positive pelvic lymph nodes.
IV	**Tumor invades bladder and/or bowel mucosa, and/or distant metastases.**
IVA	Tumor invasion of bladder and/or bowel mucosa.
IVB	Distant metastases, including intraabdominal metastases and/or inguinal lymph nodes.

Patients with Inherited Cancer Syndromes

Due to the high 40–60% lifetime risk of endometrial cancer in Lynch syndrome patients, risk-reducing salpingo-oophorectomy (RRSO) and hysterectomy at approximately ages 40–45 or upon completion of childbearing should be considered. Endometrial biopsy either in the clinic or as a combined procedure with colonoscopy termed combined screening (CS), on an annual basis, or every one to two years is recommended with annual transvaginal ultrasound a consideration. Due to the elevated risk of ovarian cancer associated with Lynch syndrome, ovarian cancer assessment using yearly transvaginal ultrasound, with yearly pelvic exam should also be recommended. CA-125 is not routinely recommended but can be considered [34]. However, these screening modalities have not been proven to detect ovarian cancer at early stages, or to decrease mortality of ovarian cancer.

Treatment

Surgical

For women with endometrial cancer, the mainstay of treatment is a minimally invasive hysterectomy and staging performed by a gynecologic oncologist. Data has shown equivalent oncologic outcomes with a minimally invasive compared to an open approach [35]. Historically, complete lymphadenectomy of the pelvic and paraaortic lymph nodes was part of the initial staging of endometrial cancer. However complete lymphadenectomy is accompanied with significant morbidity, including irreversible lymphedema [36]. Fortunately, sentinel lymph node (SLN) mapping and biopsy has replaced lymphadenectomy as the main strategy to evaluate lymphatic spread in women with endometrial cancer [37]. The first lymph node to receive tumor lymphatic drainage is designated the sentinel lymph node. Thus, a sentinel lymph node mapping procedure devoid of disease infers absent lymph node metastases within the entire lymph node chain.

Advanced Stage and Recurrent Disease

For all advanced stage or recurrent endometrial cancer, combination chemotherapy with carboplatin and paclitaxel has been considered the standard of care [38]. The role of surgery in advanced or recurrent endometrial cancer is less clear, but typically patients with metastatic multifocal disease are not considered ideal candidates for surgery. The molecular characterization of endometrial tumors is critical in directing treatment for advanced or recurrent disease. This includes the tumors estrogen receptor (ER)/progesterone receptor (PR) status and microsatellite instability-high (MSI-H) or mismatch repair deficient (dMMR) status. Immunotherapy, such as pembrolizumab, is approved for patients who are not candidates for curative surgery or radiation therapy and who have disease that is MSI-H or dMMR. This approval is based on findings from the KEYNOTE-158 trial [39]. Lenvatinib, a multiple kinase inhibitor, in combination with pembrolizumab is approved for the treatment of advanced endometrial cancer based on the KEYNOTE-775 trial that reported an objective response rate of 30.3% in tumors that are not MSI-H or dMMR and progressed following prior therapy [40].

Recently, two large randomized controlled trials suggested a benefit in adding immunotherapy to the above chemotherapy combination, regardless of MSI/MMR status. In the first trial, the randomized, blinded, phase III, NRG Oncology NRG-GY-018 trial, 816 patients with stage III, IVA, IVB, or recurrent endometrial cancer were randomly assigned to receive either pembrolizumab plus chemotherapy or placebo plus chemotherapy across six cycles, followed by up to 14 cycles of maintenance pembrolizumab or placebo [41]. Progression-free survival in the dMMR patients was 74% in the pembrolizumab group and 38% in the placebo group. Furthermore, in the non dMMR endometrial cancer cohort, patients who received pembrolizumab and chemotherapy experienced progression-free survival of 11.7 months versus 8.7 months among those receiving chemotherapy alone. In the second trial the randomized, blinded, phase III ENGOT-EN6-NSGO/GOG-3031/RUBY trial, 494 patients with first recurrent or primary advanced stage III or IV endometrial cancer were randomly assigned to receive immunotherapy with dostarlimab plus chemotherapy followed by monotherapy or placebo plus chemotherapy followed by monotherapy [42]. Among the 245 patients who received treatment with both dostarlimab and chemotherapy, there was a statistically significant and clinically meaningful progression-free survival benefit compared with the patients who received chemotherapy alone.

Molecular Classification and Prognosis

Molecularly, endometrioid carcinoma, endometrial serous carcinoma, and, to a lesser extent, carcinosarcoma have been characterized in the Cancer Genome Atlas database and can be broadly categorized based on genomic alterations [43]. These four groups include POLE-ultramutated; microsatellite instability-high (MSI-H); copy number–low; and copy number–high. Cancer with POLE mutations, have the highest number of mutations (ultramutated) and significantly longer survival. The MSI-H group of cancer comprise primarily endometrioid carcinomas with a high mutation rate, but not as high as that of the *POLE* group. The copy-number–low group accounts for the majority of cases and is composed primarily of microsatellite-stable endometrioid carcinomas. Endometrial serous carcinoma are characterized by *TP53* mutations, low mutation rate, frequent copy-number alterations ("copy-number–high" group) and generally have a poor prognosis [43].

Radiation

Depending on risk factors and pathological stage, adjuvant radiation therapy may be recommended. The most common radiation therapy employed is vaginal brachytherapy (internal radiation treatment) either alone or in conjunction with systemic therapy. The use of vaginal brachytherapy for stage I and stage II disease depends on tumor grade, histology, depth of myometrial invasion, age of patient and presence of lymphovascular space invasion. The most common site of recurrence in patients with early-stage endometrial cancer treated with surgery alone is the vaginal apex, and vaginal brachytherapy for patients with high risk factors reduces recurrence [44, 45, 46]. Vaginal brachytherapy is an outpatient procedure providing localized radiation to the vaginal apex. Typically the top 3–5 cm of the vagina are treated using a vaginal cylinder (Figure 16.1). Each treatment duration is approximately 3–5 minutes depending on the activity of the radiation source. Total doses and fractions vary but range from 5.5–6 Gy in 5 fractions ("divided doses"), given every other day to a total of 7 Gy in 3 fractions given once a week. Vaginal brachytherapy has minimal side effects especially when prescribed to the vaginal surface, as there is minimal radiation delivered to the rectum and bladder. The most common fractionation is 7 Gy prescribed to 5 mm of vaginal depth and this fractionation has a slightly higher incidence of acute diarrhea and risk of vaginal atrophy. One study found rates of vaginal atrophy at three years to be 26% (grade 1 mild, assymptomatic), 10% (grade 2 moderate, symptomatic), and 1.4% (grade 3 severe) [47]. However, the most

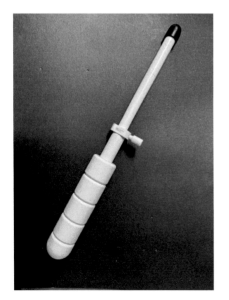

Figure 16.1 Vaginal cylinder utilized for vaginal brachytherapy

common side effects of vaginal brachytherapy is increased dryness at the top of the vagina and risk of vaginal scarring or fibrosis. Many physicians recommend consistent use of vaginal dilators after treatment (see Chapter 12 and Chapter 15 for further discussion of vaginal atrophy and the use of vaginal dilator therapy).

For more advanced stage disease (particularly Stage IIIC1 and IIIC2) the addition of external beam radiation reduces local recurrence [48, 49]. External beam radiation is administered using intensity modulated radiation therapy (IMRT) as a randomized trial found IMRT reduced both acute and long term side effects compared to 3-D conformal therapy [50]. External beam radiation may be given with concurrent chemotherapy, before or after full dose systemic therapy. Doses for external beam radiation range from 45 Gy in 25 daily fractions to 50.4 Gy in 28 fractions. Side effects are definitively increased with the use of external beam radiation and include both acute and chronic sequelae. Acute side effects include diarrhea, fatigue, nausea, vomiting, and urinary symptoms. Chronic side effects include risk of proctitis, cystitis, premature ovarian insufficiency, and fractures. Presently, with new molecular testing and the increased use of immunotherapy, the role of external beam in endometrial cancer is evolving.

Fertility-Sparing Approach

Endometrial cancer is frequently detected in young, obese women who desire fertility. A conservative alternative to hysterectomy for highly selected women with grade 1, Stage IA (noninvasive) disease is the use of oral progestins or a progestin-containing intrauterine device such as the levonorgesterel intrauterine system (LNG-IUS). A recent prospective study evaluating progestin-containing IUDs found at 12 months postinsertion approximately 50% of women with endometrial cancer had a complete response [51]. Patients who undergo fertility-sparing therapy should be counseled that hysterectomy plus bilateral salpingo-oophorectomy (BSO) with surgical staging is still recommended if there is evidence of disease progression or upon completion of childbearing. Fertility-sparing therapy is not recommended for women with high-grade type I endometrioid adenocarcinomas or type II histologies.

The initial work-up to determine if a patient is an appropriate candidate for conservative management includes hysteroscopy D&C to confirm grade and histology, and a pelvic MRI (or pelvic transvaginal ultrasound if MRI is contraindicated) to evaluate local disease extent and to exclude myometrial invasion. A chest x-ray is indicated to exclude metastatic disease.

Referral to a fertility expert should be considered prior to offering fertility-sparing management. A realistic assessment of the patient's future fertility potential should be provided based on maternal age and ovarian reserve parameters (e.g. antral follicle count and anti mullerian hormone level). Discussion should include weight optimization (if needed) and options available for third party reproduction such as use of a gestational carrier and/or donor gametes.

There is no consensus on ovarian preservation at the time of surgical staging, however per National Comprehensive Cancer Network (NCCN) guidelines, ovarian preservation may be safe in select premenopausal patients with stage I endometrioid cancer, normal-appearing ovaries, and no family history of breast or ovarian cancer or Lynch syndrome. Bilateral salpingectomy is recommended.

Recommendations After Cancer Therapy

Most endometrial cancer is cured with surgical management. For most patients, if their disease recurs, it will recur within the first three years of initial treatment. It is recommended that patients be followed with pelvic examination every 3 to 6 months for the first 2 years and then every 6 to 12 months for 3 years for a total of 5 years. Although routine imaging is not typically recommended, in patients with treated Stage III/IV disease, imaging with chest/abdominal/pelvic CT may be helpful in the detection of recurrence with consideration given to imaging every 6 months during the first 3 years of surveillance, then every 6 to 12 months for an additional 2 years. Most patients with a recurrence will be symptomatic. Symptoms include bleeding (vaginal, bladder, or rectal), weight loss, decreased appetite, pain, cough, shortness of breath, and swelling (in the abdomen or legs). Papanicolaou testing is not a recommended part of surveillance unless a patient has a history of cervical dysplasia [52]. Serum CA-125 measurements may be valuable, particularly for high grade histologies and/or if the level was elevated at the time of diagnosis.

Gynecologic Considerations After Treatment

Contraception/Hormone Therapy

In premenopausal women following hysterectomy and bilateral salpingo-oophorectomy for endometrial cancer, hormone therapy (HT) is often considered. HT can minimize hot flushes, mood lability, vaginal dryness, osteoporosis, and may lower risk of cardiovascular disease. As endometrial carcinoma is associated with relative estrogen excess and due to the fear of recurrence, many women have been denied HT. However, HT has not been shown to increase rates of recurrence. In one randomized trial evaluating women with early-stage endometrial cancer, women were randomly assigned to receive either estrogen or placebo. Although the enrollment target was not reached, after 35.7 months, the authors did not find an increased rate of recurrence [53]. At this time, the NCCN states that HT can be considered for endometrial cancer patients who are at low risk for recurrence, but treatment should be individualized and risk should be discussed in detail with the patient [54].

Case Resolution

Endometrial biopsy revealed endometrial cancer and she was referred to a gynecologic oncologist. The patient underwent a robot-assisted total laparoscopic hysterectomy with bilateral salpingo-oophorectomy, bilateral sentinel lymph node mapping and biopsies. Her final pathology was consistent with a FIGO Stage 1B, Grade 2, endometrioid adenocarcinoma of the uterus (depth of invasion >50% of myometrium (3.6/4.0 cm), with positive lymphovascular involvement, and bilateral sentinel lymph nodes negative for disease. Further recommendation by radiation oncology was for vaginal cuff brachytherapy.

Take Home Points

- All postmenopausal uterine bleeding warrants evaluation.
- Premenopausal women reporting persistent abnormal uterine bleeding or changes in menses should be evaluated.

- Complex atypical hyperplasia (CAH) with atypia on endometrial biopsy is associated with a high risk of endometrial cancer at time of hysterectomy (40–50%).
- Surgery is the mainstay of initial management of endometrial cancer, but a conservative alternative to hysterectomy for low grade, noninvasive disease, is the use of an oral progestin or a progestin-containing intrauterine device (IUD), until definitive surgery is performed.
- National Comprehensive Cancer Network guidelines states that HT can be considered for endometrial cancer patients who are at low risk for recurrence (early-stage disease), but treatment should be individualized and risk should be discussed in detail with the patient.
- Vaginal brachytherapy is often used to reduce vaginal recurrence, which is the most common site of recurrence following surgery.
- Most patients with recurrences will be symptomatic, and routine physical examination continues to be the best method for detecting recurrent disease.

References

1. Lu K. H., Broaddus R. R. Endometrial cancer. *The New England Journal of Medicine*. 2020;**383**(21):2053–64. https://doi.org/10.1056/NEJMRA1514010

2. Renehan A. G., Tyson M., Egger M., Heller R. F., Zwahlen M. Body-mass index and incidence of cancer: A systematic review and meta-analysis of prospective observational studies. *The Lancet*. 2008;**371**(9612);569–78. https://doi.org/10.1016/S0140-6736(08)60269-X

3. Siegel R. L., Miller K. D., Fuchs H. E., Jemal A. Cancer statistics, 2022. *CA: A Cancer Journal for Clinicians*. 2022;**72**(1):7–33. https://doi.org/10.3322/CAAC.21708

4. Jordan L. B., Abdul-Kader M., Al-Nafussi, A. Uterine serous papillary carcinoma: Histopathologic changes within the female genital tract. *International Journal of Gynecological Cancer: Official Journal of the International Gynecological Cancer Society*. 2001;**11**(4):283–9. https://doi.org/10.1046/J.1525-1438.2001.011004283.

5. Slomovitz B. M., Burke T. W., Eifel P. J., et al. Uterine papillary serous carcinoma (UPSC): A single institution review of 129 cases. *Gynecologic Oncology*. 2003;**91**(3):463–9. https://doi.org/10.1016/j.ygyno.2003.08.018

6. Carcangiu M. L., Chambers J. T. Uterine papillary serous carcinoma: A study on 108 cases with emphasis on the prognostic significance of associated endometrioid carcinoma, absence of invasion, and concomitant ovarian carcinoma. *Gynecologic Oncology*. 1992;**47**(3):298–305. https://doi.org/10.1016/0090-8258(92)90130-B

7. Cirisano F. D., Robboy S. J., Dodge R. K., et al. Epidemiologic and surgicopathologic findings of papillary serous and clear cell endometrial cancer when compared to endometrioid carcinoma. *Gynecologic Oncology*. 1999;**74**(3):385–94. https://doi.org/10.1006/GYNO.1999.5505

8. Hamilton C. A., Cheung M. K., Osann K., et al. Uterine papillary serous and clear cell carcinomas predict for poorer survival compared to grade 3 endometrioid corpus cancer. *British Journal of Cancer*. 2006;**94**(5):642–6. https://doi.org/10.1038/SJ.BJC.6603012

9. Jin Z., Ogata S., Tamura G., et al. Carcinosarcomas (malignant mullerian mixed tumors) of the uterus and ovary: A genetic study with special reference to histogenesis. *International Journal of Gynecological Pathology*. 2003;**22**(4):368–73. https://doi.org/10.1097/01.pgp.0000092134.88121.56

10. Sreenan J. J., Hart W. R. Carcinosarcomas of the female genital tract. A pathologic study of 29 metastatic tumors: Further evidence for the dominant role of the epithelial component and the conversion theory of histogenesis. *The American Journal of Surgical Pathology.* 1995;**19**(6):666–74. https://doi.org/10.1097/00000478-199506000-00007

11. George E., Lillemoe T. J., Twiggs L. B., Perrone T. Malignant mixed müllerian tumor versus high-grade endometrial carcinoma and aggressive variants of endometrial carcinoma: A comparative analysis of survival. *International Journal of Gynecological Pathology: Official Journal of the International Society of Gynecological Pathologists.* 1995;**14**(1):39–44. https://doi.org/10.1097/00004347-199501000-00007

12. Sartori E., Bazzurini L., Gadducci A., et al. Carcinosarcoma of the uterus: a clinicopathological multicenter CTF study. *Gynecologic Oncology.* 1997;**67**(1):70–5. https://doi.org/10.1006/GYNO.1997.4827

13. Vaidya A. P., Horowitz N. S., Oliva E., Halpern E. F., Duska L. R. Uterine malignant mixed mullerian tumors should not be included in studies of endometrial carcinoma. *Gynecologic Oncology.* 2006;**103**(2):684–7. https://doi.org/10.1016/J.YGYNO.2006.05.009

14. Hemminki K., Bermejo J. L., Granström C. Endometrial cancer: Population attributable risks from reproductive, familial and socioeconomic factors. *European Journal of Cancer.* 2005;**41**(14):2155–9. https://doi.org/10.1016/J.EJCA.2005.03.031

15. Møller P., Seppälä T. T., Bernstein I., et al. Cancer risk and survival in path_MMR carriers by gene and gender up to 75 years of age: A report from the Prospective Lynch Syndrome Database. *Gut.* 2018;**67**(7):1306–16. https://doi.org/10.1136/GUTJNL-2017-314057

16. Bansal N., Yendluri V., Wenham R. M. The molecular biology of endometrial cancer and the implications for pathogenesis, classification, and targeted therapies.

Cancer Control: Journal of the Moffitt Cancer Center. 2009;**16**(1):8–13. https://doi.org/10.1177/107327480901600102

17. Møller P., Seppälä T. T., Bernstein I., et al. Cancer risk and survival in path-MMR carriers by gene and gender up to 75 years of age: A report from the Prospective Lynch Syndrome Database. *Gut.* 2018b;**67**(7):1306–16. https://doi.org/10.1136/GUTJNL-2017-314057

18. Aarnio M., Sankila R., Pukkala E., et al. Cancer risk in mutation carriers of dna-mismatch-repair genes. *J. Cancer.* 1999;**81**:214–18. https://doi.org/10.1002/(SICI)1097-0215(19990412)81:2

19. Delin J. B., Miller D. S., Coleman R. L. Other primary malignancies in patients with uterine corpus malignancy. *American Journal of Obstetrics and Gynecology.* 2004;**190**(5):1429–31. https://doi.org/10.1016/j.ajog.2004.01.075

20. Ryan N. A. J., Morris J., Green K., et al. Association of mismatch repair mutation with age at cancer onset in lynch syndrome implications for stratified surveillance strategies. *JAMA Oncology.* 2017;**3**(12):E1–E5. https://doi.org/10.1001/JAMAONCOL.2017.0619

21. Hampel H., Frankel W., Panescu J., et al. Screening for Lynch syndrome (hereditary nonpolyposis colorectal cancer) among endometrial cancer patients. *Cancer Research.* 2006;**66**(15):7810–17. https://doi.org/10.1158/0008-5472.CAN-06-1114

22. Lu K. H., Schorge J. O., Rodabaugh K. J., et al. Prospective determination of prevalence of Lynch syndrome in young women with endometrial cancer. *Journal of Clinical Oncology.* 2007;**25**(33):5158–64. https://doi.org/10.1200/JCO.2007.10.8597

23. Resnick K. E., Hampel H., Fishel R., Coh D. E. Current and emerging trends in Lynch syndrome identification in women with endometrial cancer. *Gynecologic Oncology.* 2009;**114**(1):128–34. https://doi.org/10.1016/J.YGYNO.2009.03.003

24. Schmeler K. M., Lynch H. T., Chen L., et al. Prophylactic surgery to reduce the risk of

gynecologic cancer in the Lynch syndrome. *New England Journal of Medicine*. 2006;**354**(3):261–9. https://doi.org/10.1056/NEJMOA052627

25. Brinton L. A., Berman M. L., Mortel R., et al. Reproductive, menstrual, and medical risk factors for endometrial cancer: Results from a case-control study. *American Journal of Obstetrics and Gynecology*. 1992;**167**(5):1317–25. https://doi.org/10.1016/S0002-9378(11)91709-8

26. Stanford J. L., Brinton L. A., Hoover R. N., et al. Oral contraceptives and endometrial cancer: Do other risk factors modify the association? *International Journal of Cancer*. 1993;**54**(2):243–8. https://doi.org/10.1002/IJC.2910540214

27. Bernstein L., Deapen D., Cerhan J. R., et al. Tamoxifen therapy for breast cancer and endometrial cancer risk. *Journal of the National Cancer Institute*. 1999;**91**(19):1654–62. https://doi.org/10.1093/JNCI/91.19.1654

28. Fisher B., Costantino J. P., Wickerham D. L., et al. Tamoxifen for prevention of breast cancer: report of the National Surgical Adjuvant Breast and Bowel Project P-1 Study. *Journal of the National Cancer Institute*. 1998;**90**(18):1371–88. https://doi.org/10.1093/JNCI/90.18.1371

29. Swerdlow A. J., Jones M. E., Brewster D. H., et al. Tamoxifen treatment for breast cancer and risk of endometrial cancer: A case-control study. *Journal of the National Cancer Institute*. 2005;**97**(5):375–84. https://doi.org/10.1093/JNCI/DJI057

30. McCluggage W. G. My approach to the interpretation of endometrial biopsies and curettings. *Journal of Clinical Pathology*. 2006;**59**(8):801–12. https://doi.org/10.1136/JCP.2005.029702

31. Leitao M. M., Kehoe S., Barakat R. R., et al. Comparison of D&C and office endometrial biopsy accuracy in patients with FIGO grade 1 endometrial adenocarcinoma. *Gynecologic Oncology*. 2009;**113**(1):105–8. https://doi.org/10.1016/J.YGYNO.2008.12.017

32. Lee J. H., Dubinsky T., Andreotti R. F., et al. ACR appropriateness Criteria® pretreatment evaluation and follow-up of endometrial cancer of the uterus. *Ultrasound Quarterly*. 2011;**27**(2):139–45. https://doi.org/10.1097/RUQ.0B013E31821B6F73

33. Duk J. M., Aalders J. G., Fleuren G. J., de Bruijn H. W. A. CA 125: A useful marker in endometrial carcinoma. *American Journal of Obstetrics and Gynecology*. 1986;**155**(5):1097–102. https://doi.org/10.1016/0002-9378(86)90358-3

34. Ryan N. A. J., Snowsill T., McKenzie E., Monahan K. J., Nebgen D. Should women with Lynch syndrome be offered gynaecological cancer surveillance? *BMJ (Clinical Research Ed.)*. 2021;**374**. https://doi.org/10.1136/BMJ.N2020

35. Walker J. L., Piedmonte M. R., Spirtos N. M., et al. Recurrence and survival after random assignment to laparoscopy versus laparotomy for comprehensive surgical staging of uterine cancer: Gynecologic Oncology Group LAP2 Study. *Journal of Clinical Oncology: Official Journal of the American Society of Clinical Oncology*. 2012;**30**(7):695–700. https://doi.org/10.1200/JCO.2011.38.8645

36. Carlson J. W., Kauderer J., Hutson A., et al. GOG 244-The lymphedema and gynecologic cancer (LEG) study: Incidence and risk factors in newly diagnosed patients. *Gynecologic Oncology*. 2020;**156**(2):467–74. https://doi.org/10.1016/J.YGYNO.2019.10.009

37. Holloway R. W., Abu-Rustum N. R., Backes F. J., et al. Sentinel lymph node mapping and staging in endometrial cancer: A Society of Gynecologic Oncology literature review with consensus recommendations. *Gynecologic Oncology*. 2017;**146**(2):405–15. https://doi.org/10.1016/J.YGYNO.2017.05.027

38. Miller D. S., Filiaci V. L., Mannel R. S., et al. Carboplatin and paclitaxel for advanced endometrial cancer: Final overall survival and adverse event analysis of a phase III trial (NRG Oncology/GOG0209). *Journal of Clinical Oncology: Official Journal of the*

American Society of Clinical Oncology. 2020;38(33):3841–50. https://doi.org/10.1200/JCO.20.01076

39. O'Malley D. M., Bariani G. M., Cassier P. A., et al. Pembrolizumab in patients with microsatellite instability-high advanced endometrial cancer: Results from the KEYNOTE-158 Study. *Journal of Clinical Oncology: Official Journal of the American Society of Clinical Oncology.* 2022;**40** (7):752–61. https://doi.org/10.1200/JCO.21.01874

40. Makker V., Colombo N., Casado Herráez A., et al. Lenvatinib plus pembrolizumab for advanced endometrial cancer. *The New England Journal of Medicine.* 2022;**386** (5):437–48. https://doi.org/10.1056/NEJMOA2108330

41. Eskander R. N., Sill M. W., Beffa L., et al. Pembrolizumab plus chemotherapy in advanced endometrial cancer. *The New England Journal of Medicine.* 2023;**388** (23):2159–70. https://doi.org/10.1056/NEJMOA2302312

42. Mirza M. R., Chase D. M., Slomovitz B. M., et al. Dostarlimab for primary advanced or recurrent endometrial cancer. *The New England Journal of Medicine.* 2023;**388** (23):2145–58. https://doi.org/10.1056/NEJMOA2216334

43. Getz G., Gabriel S. B., Cibulskis K., et al. Integrated genomic characterization of endometrial carcinoma. *Nature.* 2013;**497** (7447):67–73. https://doi.org/10.1038/nature12113

44. Keys H. M., Roberts J. A., Brunetto V. L., et al. A phase III trial of surgery with and without adjunctive external pelvic radiation therapy in intermediate risk endometrial adenocarcinoma: A Gynecologic Oncology Group study. *Gyn Onc.* 2004;**92**:744–51.

45. Creutzberg C., Nout R. A., Lybeert M. L. M., et al. Fifteen-year radiotherapy outcomes of the randomized PORTEC-1 trial for endometrial carcinoma. *Int J RAdiat Oncol Biol Phys.* 2011;**81**:631–8.

46. Wortman B. G., Creutzberg C. L., Putter H., et al. Ten-year results of the PORTEC-2 trial for high-intermediate risk endometrial carcinoma: Improving patient selection for adjuvant therapy. *British Journal of Cancer.* 2018;**119**(9):1067–74. doi:10.1038/s41416-018-0310-8

47. Nout R. A., Smit V. T., Potter H, et al. Vaginal brachytherapy versus pelvic external beam radiotherapy for patients with endometrial cancer of high-intermediate risk (PORTEC 2), opem-label, non-inferiority, randomized trial. *Lancet.* 2010; **2010**:816–23.

48. De Boer S. M., Powell M. E., Mileshkin L., et al. Adjuvant chemoradiotherapy versu radiotherapy in high-risk endometrial cancer (PORTEC-3): Patterns of recurrence and ad hoc survival analysis of a randomized phase 3 trial. *Lancet.* 2019;**9**:1273–58.

49. Matei D., Filiaci V., Randall M., et al. Adjuvant chemotherapy plus radiation for locally advanced endometrial cancer. *N Engl J Med.* 2019;**13**: 2317–26.

50. Klopp A., Yeung A. R., Deshmukh S., et al. Patient-reported toxicity during pelvic intensity modulated radiation therapy: NRG Oncologyg- RTOG 1203. *J Clin Oncol.* 2018;**36**:2538–44.

51. Westin S. N., Fellman B., Sun C. C., et al. Prospective phase II trial of levonorgestrel intrauterine device: Nonsurgical approach for complex atypical hyperplasia and early-stage endometrial cancer. *American Journal of Obstetrics and Gynecology.* 2021;**224** (2):191.e1–191.e15. https://doi.org/10.1016/J.AJOG.2020.08.032

52. Cooper A. L., Dornfeld-Finke J. M., Banks H. W., Davey D. D., Modesitt S. C. Is cytologic screening an effective surveillance method for detection of vaginal recurrence of uterine cancer? *Obstetrics and Gynecology.* 2006;**107**(1):71–6. https://doi.org/10.1097/01.AOG.0000194206.38105.C8

53. Barakat R. R., Bundy B. N., Spirtos N. M., et al. Randomized double-blind trial of estrogen replacement therapy versus placebo in stage I or II endometrial cancer: A Gynecologic Oncology Group Study. *Journal of Clinical Oncology: Official Journal of the American Society of Clinical* *Oncology*. 2006;**24**(4):587–92. https://doi.org/10.1200/JCO.2005.02.8464

54. McMillian N., Motter A., Frederick P., et al. (2021). NCCN Guidelines Version 1.2022 Uterine Neoplasms Current NCCN Guidelines. www.nccn.org

Head and Neck Cancer

Caitlin M. Coviello, Erich M. Sturgis,
and Kristina R. Dahlstrom

Case Presentation

A 50-year-old woman (lifelong nonsmoker) presents with a painless neck mass that she noticed 2 months ago, without any recent upper respiratory infection. Her history is significant for prior high-grade cervical intraepithelial neoplasia and prior hysterectomy for fibroids. Her primary care doctor treated her with antibiotics for two weeks with no improvement and then referred her to an otolaryngologist-head and neck surgeon. Examination including flexible fiberoptic examination of the pharynx and larynx, demonstrated fullness of the left base of tongue (BOT) and a left level II (upper neck) 3 cm mass. CT scan (Figure 17.1) with contrast revealed 2 necrotic lymph nodes adjacent to one another along the left upper jugular vein as well as a 4.5 cm enhancing mass of the left BOT and a suspicious contralateral level II lymph node. Biopsy of the base of tongue was consistent with an HPV-related cancer (p16 positive by immunohistochemistry). PET-CT scan was consistent with a left BOT cancer with bilateral neck metastases but without evidence of distant metastatic disease. Her TNM staging was T3N2M0, Stage II. Circulating HPV16 DNA testing with a clinical-grade digital droplet PCR assay revealed more than 1,000 fragments/milliliter of plasma. A radiation oncologist and a medical oncologist, both with significant experience in head and neck cancer care evaluated the patient. The patient was presented along with pathology and imaging at a multidisciplinary treatment planning conference, and the recommendation was for concurrent cisplatin with radiation therapy. She was evaluated by a dentist experienced in caring for cancer patients requiring head and neck radiation, and the dentist declared her dental health to be adequate to proceed to radiation. A protective fluoride formulation was provided for daily use.

Introduction

The term "head and neck cancer" traditionally refers to tobacco and alcohol associated squamous cell carcinomas of the upper aerodigestive tract (mouth [oral cavity], throat [pharynx], and voice box [larynx]). However, today's head and neck surgeons and oncologists deal with a more diverse group of malignancies, dominated by thyroid carcinoma, melanoma and nonmelanoma skin cancer, and human papillomavirus (HPV)-related oropharyngeal (tonsils and base of tongue) cancer (OPC). As compared to men, some of these cancer have clear differences in risks (both modifiable and fixed) for women, as well as associations with other malignancies in women. For instance, thyroid cancer are about three times more common in women than in men, and while radiation exposure as a child or young adult is a clear risk factor, very few thyroid cancer patients report such exposure. Increased risk for second primary breast cancer among thyroid cancer survivors is reported, but alterations to

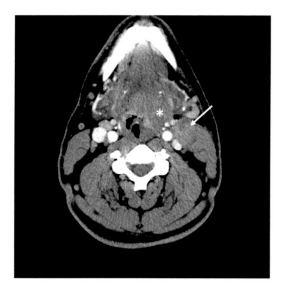

Figure 17.1 CT scan showing a 4.5 cm enhancing lesion of the left base of tongue (*) with two necrotic lymph nodes along the left upper jugular vein (arrow) and a suspicious contralateral level II lymph node

United States Preventive Services Task Force (USPSTF) breast cancer screening recommendations are not endorsed. Melanoma and nonmelanoma skin cancer are more common in men with sun exposure, tanning bed exposure, and skin type being well-understood modifiable and fixed risk factors. Sun protection and screening for subsequent second primary skin cancer are well-accepted survivorship practices for skin cancer patients.

Cigarette smoking and alcohol abuse have also been more prevalent in men than in women and as expected squamous cell carcinomas of the upper aerodigestive tract are two to three times more common in men, with some exceptions. Laryngeal cancer are much more common in men (fivefold), while oral tongue cancer in those under 40 years of age and gingivobuccal oral cavity cancer in those over 70 years of age are more common in women. Reasons for these differences are not fully explained by different exposure frequencies, in fact these cancer (particularly in the young and very old) are often not associated with tobacco and alcohol use. Regardless, treatment of these cancer often requires complex and intensive multidisciplinary care (surgery, radiation, and systemic therapy) with high morbidity and major detriments to the processes of everyday life including: eating, speaking, swallowing, breathing, neck/shoulder function, dental/mouth care, appearance/self-image, chronic pain, and distress/depression/anxiety. Survivorship care is complex and best managed when patients have access to an experienced and engaged multidisciplinary team with full ancillary services in support. Second malignancies are very common for those cured of their initial tobacco-associated head and neck cancer and most commonly identified at tobacco-exposed sites: upper aerodigestive tract, esophagus, lungs, and bladder. Screening of these sites is typically symptom-directed, with only routine screening for lung cancer supported by a USPSTF recommendation. However, when such patients are in formal survivorship follow-up, periodic head and neck examination is a national standard, and such exams will occasionally find a second primary earlier than would have been found waiting for symptoms. For those with tobacco-related head and neck cancer, neither routine urinalysis nor serial esophageal endoscopy is endorsed by the field, and no evidence supports any alterations to USPSTF breast/cervix cancer screening recommendations in women.

Globally, HPV is a leading cause of cancer and cancer-related death in women, overwhelmingly attributed to rates of cervical cancer in low and middle-income countries. However, in the USA, HPV-related OPC has surpassed cervical cancer as the most common HPV-related cancer, though it is much more common (fivefold) in men than women. Similar to other head and neck cancer, HPV-related OPCs typically require complex multidisciplinary treatments often with major lifelong sequelae. However, HPV-related OPCs have much better cancer cure rates and lower second primary malignancy rates than tobacco-related head and neck cancer. Unique patterns of second primary malignancies, related to HPV exposures, are often a concern for female patients. This chapter will focus on HPV-related OPC, its associations with other malignancies in women, and prevention/screening recommendations and potentials for women with HPV-related OPC.

Epidemiology

Anatomic Site Distinctions

The upper aerodigestive tract is a passageway to the lower aerodigestive tract. These areas are broadly divided into the oral cavity (mouth), the pharynx (throat), and the larynx (voice box). The pharynx can be further divided into the nasopharynx, oropharynx, and hypopharynx (Figure 17.2). The nasopharynx is immediately behind the nasal cavity and extends from the skull base superiorly to the soft palate inferiorly. The oropharynx is immediately behind the oral cavity and extends from the soft palate to the level of the hyoid bone inferiorly. The hypopharynx is behind and to the sides of the larynx and extends from the hyoid bone to the esophageal inlet inferiorly. The oral cavity and oropharynx are separated by the hard-soft palate junction superiorly, the anterior tonsillar pillars laterally, and the circumvallate papillae of the tongue inferiorly (Figure 17.2). The oropharynx is composed of the following subsites: soft palate (including the uvula),

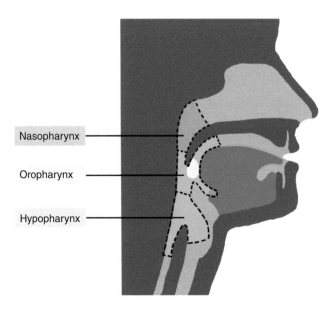

Figure 17.2 Sagittal view of the pharynx, which can be divided into the nasopharynx, oropharynx, and hypopharynx. The oropharynx consists of the soft palate, palatine tonsils, tonsillar pillars, lingual tonsils/base of tongue, and posterior and lateral pharyngeal walls

Nasopharynx

Oropharynx

Hypopharynx

palatine tonsils, tonsillar pillars, lingual tonsils/BOT, and the posterior and lateral pharyngeal walls [1]. The distinction of cancer site between oral cavity and oropharynx is critical as cancer arising from the oral cavity have different etiologies, management, and outcomes from those of the oropharynx. Oral cavity cancer are typically related to tobacco and alcohol use, while OPC (especially those of the tonsils and BOT) are most commonly related to prior HPV infection and relatively rarely (25% or less in the USA) caused by tobacco [2, 3]. Oral cavity cancer are treated with surgery with or without adjuvant postoperative radiation (with concurrent chemoradiotherapy for those with positive margins or extranodal extension), while OPC are most commonly treated with definitive concurrent chemoradiotherapy with transoral surgery alone, radiation alone, or transoral surgery with postoperative radiation (some requiring postoperative chemoradiation) for selected cases. Finally, and as relevant to this chapter, prevention and screening concepts among patients with HPV-related OPC are unique from patients with tobacco and alcohol associated head and neck cancer.

Incidence Trends

Historically, almost all head and neck cancer were associated with tobacco and alcohol exposures, and the incidence of head and neck cancer began to plateau or decline in the 1980s along with other smoking-related cancer as a consequence of lower smoking rates resulting from effective public health messaging initiated with the Surgeon General's warning about the dangers of tobacco in 1965 [4]. However, unlike the incidence of other head and neck cancer, which have continued to decline, the incidence of OPC continues to increase [5, 6]. This increase is attributed to the increase in proportion of HPV-related OPC, from 16% during the 1980s to 73% during the 2000s [5] and likely higher now. HPV-related OPC has now replaced cervical cancer as the most common HPV-related cancer in the US [7]. The annual number of HPV-related OPC cases in 2019 was 21,567, projected to increase to 30,629 by 2029 [6, 8].

Demographic Characteristics

HPV-related OPC is most commonly seen in middle-aged non-Hispanic white men often of middle to higher socioeconomic status (SES) [6, 9]. It is the eighth most commonly diagnosed cancer in men as of 2022 [10]. While men are five times more likely to develop HPV-related OPC than women, there are estimated 4,000–6,000 new cases annually among women [10]. Over the last 20 years, the age of diagnosis appears to be increasing with a large single institution study reporting age at diagnosis of patients with HPV-related OPC versus HPV-negative OPC showing the mean age of diagnosis of patients with HPV-related OPC to have increased from 51.6 in 2002–7 to 58.5 in 2014–17 [11]. As of 2022, the CDC reports the median age of diagnosis of HPV-related OPC to be 63 in women and 61 in men [12]. HPV-related OPC most commonly affects non-Hispanic whites, followed by African Americans and Asian/Pacific islanders [13, 14]. HPV-related OPC is more commonly seen in those of higher SES than is HPV-negative OPC [15]. Similar to other head and neck cancer disparities, survival for patients with HPV-related OPC appears worse for African Americans and those with lower SES [16].

Behavioral Risks

While no inherited or genetic risk factor for HPV-related OPC has been identified, several behavioral risk factors have been elucidated. Both oral and genital HPV infection are transmitted from mucosal contact, and HPV infection rates are linked to frequency of sexual behaviors [17]. The overall point prevalence among the North American population is 7% for oral HPV and 40% for genital HPV with more than 80% of individuals acquiring an infection by age 45 [18–20]. Individuals with a higher number of sexual partners are at an increased risk of HPV infection [19, 21].

The prevalence of oral HPV-infection is threefold higher in men than in women, even when controlling for number of sexual partners [21]. Analysis of US population-based data showed that the association between oral HPV infection and sexual behaviors appears to be stronger among men than women [21]. Specifically, increased prevalence on a per-partner basis was three to four times greater among men than women and plateaued with fewer partners for women than men. There is evidence from several studies that the rate of transmission is higher from female-to-male than vice versa [21–23]. The reasons for this are still unknown but are likely multi-factorial. It is possible that women have a lower oral HPV prevalence because they have some protection against oral HPV exposures due to a stronger immune response and memory from prior genital HPV infections [17, 22]. Additionally, as stated above, transmission through oral sex performed on a woman is thought to be higher compared to oral sex performed on a man, possibly because HPV viral load is higher at the cervix than the penis [23]. A population-based study in England showed a significantly higher five-year prevalence of OPC among lesbian and bisexual women as compared to heterosexual women with an opposite but nonsignificant trend for gay and bisexual men, supporting the likelihood of greater risk of transmission in oral-vaginal sex than oral-penile [24]. Finally, similar to other HPV-related cancer, patients with HIV/AIDS are at increased risk of developing oral HPV infection and HPV-related OPC [25].

While tobacco and alcohol use are primarily risk factors for development of HPV-negative head and neck cancer, tobacco use has also been reported as a modifiable risk factor for HPV-related OPC, though this is an area of controversy. Active smoking may promote persistence of oral HPV infection. Some studies have shown an independent association of tobacco use with oral HPV infection [26, 27] while others have not found this association [28]. Marijuana use has also been hypothesized as a risk factor, though there is no conclusive evidence of an association [29]. It is also possible that marijuana and tobacco smoking are markers of risky behavior such as more sex partners and thus confounding such associations.

Second Primary Cancer Risks Among Patients with an HPV-Related OPC

Traditionally, patients with head and neck cancer are considered at high risk of developing secondary primary malignancies (SPM). Multiple studies have shown that patients with head and neck cancer have a 2–3% annual risk (10–15% at five years) of developing a SPM [30, 31]. This historically high rate, however, is largely seen in HPV-negative head and neck cancer and is consistent with the typical prolonged history of tobacco use. These patients are at an increased risk for developing other tobacco-related malignancies – most commonly in the head and neck, lung, or esophagus [32].

However, patients with HPV-related OPC have a relatively low risk of developing a SPM. In a large study utilizing Surveillance, Epidemiology, and End Results (SEER) data, patients with OPC were found to have a lower three-year SPM rate (5.2%) than their non-OPC counterparts (8.3%) [14]. Of note, HPV-related OPC patients with a history of smoking have SPM risks that are similar to patients with HPV-negative OPC [14]. While HPV-related OPC patients do have a reduced risk of SPMs, studies have examined the relationship and possible increased risk of developing another HPV-related cancer (typically at anogenital sites, though a separate HPV-related cancer at another head and neck site is also possible). In addition to OPC, HPV can cause carcinomas of the cervix [33], vulva [34], vagina, anus [35], penis [36], and very rarely at other sites in the head and neck region (nasopharynx, hypopharynx, and larynx). Sikora et al. demonstrated a significant increased incidence of anal cancer in men with OPC and an elevated, but not significant risk of penile cancer [37]. Given the lower incidence of women with HPV-related OPC, there is a paucity of data on women with HPV-related OPC and their site-specific risk of SPM. Rietbergen et al. examined a cohort of women diagnosed with HPV-related OPC and found a significant association with HPV-related OPC and suspicious cervical Papanicolaou (Pap) smear results [38]. These studies demonstrate that an association exists between HPV-related OPC and subsequent development of other HPV-related malignancies; however, more research is needed to provide precision to the risk estimates.

HPV-Related OPC Risk in Patients with Cancer at Anogenital Sites

As stated above, HPV is a well-established cause of cervical, vulvar, vaginal, anal, and penile carcinomas. Multiple population-based studies have estimated OPC risks in patients with high-grade cervical pre-cancerous lesions and cervical cancer. All have shown an increased incidence of OPC in patients previously diagnosed with high-grade cervical pre-cancerous lesions and cervical cancer. This increased risk persists even 10–20 years after diagnosis of cervical pathology [39,40].

In a population-based study of SEER, patients diagnosed with anal squamous cell carcinoma also appear to have an increased risk of developing OPC compared to the general population. While multiple mucosal sites of HPV exposure are consistent with these SPM risks, the authors note that HIV infection and associated immunocompromise may also contribute to this increased risk [41]. The risk of HPV-related OPC as SPM among women with vulvar and vaginal cancer has also been shown [42].

A systematic review by Gilbert et al. examined the risk of developing a second HPV-related malignancy after diagnosis of any preinvasive or invasive HPV-associated cancer. Eight of the studies evaluated risk of OPC development, demonstrating that all primary HPV-related malignancy sites had an increased risk of secondary OPC development. Overall, patients with a primary HPV associated malignancy had a five-fold increased risk of secondary HPV-associated malignancy compared to unaffected individuals [43].

HPV-Related Cancer Risks Among Partners of Patients with HPV-Related OPC

Multiple studies have examined the risk of concomitant HPV infection in partners of patients with HPV-related OPC. A case-control study of 198 couples found a 15% rate of oral HPV infection in partners of patients with HPV-related OPC, suggesting a higher oral HPV prevalence in this population [43]. However, other studies with similar methodologies have shown prevalence of oral HPV infection in partners of patients with HPV-related OPC to be similar to the general population [44]. A systematic review showed a small, increased absolute risk of HPV-related cancer of 1–3%, for partners of patients with HPV-related OPC [45]. While prospective studies are needed to better understand risks for partners, comprehensively identifying and following both current and past partners of patients with HPV-related OPC will be methodologically difficult.

Prevention and Screening

HPV Vaccination

Several vaccines that offer protection against infection with the most common HPV types are available. Three of these, Gardasil (Merck), Cervarix (GlaxoSmithKline), and Gardasil 9 (Merck), have been licensed by the Food and Drug Administration (FDA) for use in the USA, although distribution has been limited to Gardasil 9 since 2016 [46]. The Centers for Disease Control and Prevention Advisory Committee on Immunization Practices initially limited their recommendation to females aged 9–26 years but has since expanded it to include males and adults up to age 45 years [46, 47]. The currently recommended vaccine, Gardasil 9, offers protection against the seven most common oncogenic HPV types (16, 18, 31, 33, 45, 52, and 58) as well as the two types that cause anogenital warts or laryngeal papillomatosis (6 and 11) [48]. HPV vaccines have been shown to be highly efficacious in preventing anogenital HPV infections and associated premalignant lesions in vaccine trials [49], and this is now supported by real-world evidence from several countries with population-based vaccination programs [50–52].

Although designed for use in primary prevention of HPV infection, vaccination as a secondary prevention measure, specifically as an adjuvant to surgical treatment for cervical high-grade intraepithelial lesions (HSIL), has also been evaluated [53]. Several studies have reported decreased recurrence rates of HSIL among women who were vaccinated shortly before or after surgical excision. While the mechanism of action is unclear, these results likely represent prevention of a new infection or viral reactivation rather than a therapeutic effect on the malignant process because current prophylactic HPV vaccines target capsid proteins that are unlikely to be present by the time cancer treatment occurs [54]. There are currently no licensed therapeutic vaccines to treat HPV-related cancer available although several candidates are in various phases of clinical trials [55].

Oral HPV Testing

Cervical cancer screening includes detection of oncogenic HPV DNA on cervical swabs; additionally, HPV DNA detection is a valid biomarker for anal cancer screening among high-risk individuals [56]. Development of a premalignant lesion or cancer at an anogenital site is known to be preceded by a persistent oncogenic HPV infection [57], and this association with precedent persistent HPV infection is presumed to be the case for HPV-related OPC as well. The precise risk for developing HPV-related OPC among those with a persistent oral oncogenic HPV infection is currently unknown. Regardless, prevalent or incident oral oncogenic HPV DNA is not considered ideal as the sole marker for a population-based screening program as the prevalence in the general population is too high to be reliably used to select a high-risk population (6.6% among men and 1.5% among women) [21]. The incidence of a new oral oncogenic HPV infection was estimated to be 1.7% at one year among men participating in the HPV in Men (HIM) study, a large population-based study investigating the natural history of HPV [58]. In a cohort study of 447 individuals at risk for HPV-related OPC (73% HIV-positive) with up to 7 years of follow-up, persistence of oral HPV16 was 58% at 1 year and 32% at 5 years, and was significantly associated with older age and male sex [59]. A large multinational natural history study is currently underway to further understand oral HPV infection (PROGRESS study) [60].

Emerging Blood Biomarkers

Liquid biopsies are among the emerging tools for minimally invasive cancer screening and early detection. Serum antibodies to HPV16 early (E) oncoproteins and circulating tumor tissue-modified (ctm) HPV DNA are two biomarkers that offer better sensitivity and specificity than oral HPV DNA for predicting risk of HPV-related cancer as well as recurrence of OPC. Development of antibodies to the viral capsid proteins may occur as a natural consequence of an infection, but development of antibodies to the oncogenic HPV E proteins are rare among those without an HPV-related cancer. The association between E antibodies and HPV-related OPC appears to be stronger than for other HPV-related cancer. The elevated risk of HPV-related OPC among seropositive individuals has been shown in several large case-control studies [61–64].

Two case-control studies that were nested within large prospective cohorts found that seropositivity to HPV16 E oncoproteins were associated with extreme risk (odds ratio [OR] > 140 and > 270) [63, 64]. Another case-control study showed a strong association between seropositivity and HPV-positive OPC when applying a previously defined binary classifier derived from the combination of all HPV16 E antibodies (OR > 450; $p < 0.001$; sensitivity = 83% and specificity = 99%) [61, 62]. The high sensitivity and specificity for HPV16 E seropositivity (83% and 95%, respectively) was confirmed in a meta-analysis [65]. Analysis of data from the HPV Cancer Cohort Consortium estimated that the 10-year cumulative risk for OPC following a positive HPV16 E serologic test for a 60-year-old is 27% for men and 6% for women [66].

The other biomarker, ctmHPVDNA, is detectable in peripheral blood of patients with HPV-related cancer. This marker has been shown to be especially useful during post-treatment monitoring of patients with HPV-related OPC as it is possible to detect recurrences earlier than with the traditional methods of clinical examination or imaging. The possibility of early detection additionally makes ctmHPVDNA suitable as a potential screening marker for diagnosis of HPV-related cancer [67, 68]. In a study of 103 patients diagnosed with OPC, 84 were found to have detectable ctmHPVDNA prior to diagnosis, corresponding to 84% sensitivity and 97% specificity [67]. Additionally, the same group has shown that patients who clear their ctmHPVDNA during or after treatment have a favorable prognosis compared to patients who do not [67, 68]. Another group found circulating HPV16 DNA in the archived plasma samples of 3 out of 7 patients up to 43 months before their diagnosis with HPV-related OPC while none was found among 5 patients with non-oropharyngeal head and neck cancer [69].

Ongoing Screening Trials

To date, two prospective cohort studies designed to evaluate the use of biomarkers as screening tools for OPC are ongoing, the Throat and Other HPV-Related Cancer in Men: Identifying Them Early (TRINITY; ClinicalTrials.gov Identifier: NCT02897427) study [56] and the Men and Women Offering Understanding of Throat HPV (MOUTH; ClinicalTrials.gov Identifier: NCT03644563) study [70]. Both studies are evaluating antibodies to HPV16 E antigens and oral rinse oncogenic HPV DNA as markers for development of OPC; the TRINITY study is additionally evaluating ctmHPVDNA. The TRINITY study is limited to middle-aged men (50 to 64 years) while the MOUTH study includes adult men and women. Additionally, the Study of Prevention of Anal Cancer (SPANC), a cohort study of anal HPV among MSM (men who have sex with men) in Australia, evaluated HPV16 E serostatus among 603 men. Nine of 12 seropositive men underwent a head and neck exam with positron emission tomography-computed tomography (PET-CT) scan and one was diagnosed with an asymptomatic T1N1 HPV-related OPC (one additional seropositive man had history of a OPC prior to study enrollment and subsequently developed metastatic OPC recurrence) [71]. Based on these encouraging findings, the same group included the first 5,000 participants of a population-based prospective cohort study, the Hamburg City Health Study, in an analysis of serum HPV16 E antibodies (E1, E2, E6, and E7) for detection of OPC. Of the 4,424 participants with an evaluable sample, 35 (0.8%) were HPV16 E6-positive. Of these 35, 11 (0.3%) were also positive for at least one additional HPV16 E antibody type. and were invited to attend regular follow-up screening. Three of nine who participated were subsequently diagnosed with stage I HPV-related OPC, one with incident early disease and the remaining two with advanced disease [72]. Although these studies will provide valuable information on identification of high-risk individuals, much larger population-based trials will be required before any screening programs are broadly instituted.

Risk Stratification for Screening Selection

Risk prediction models are useful for personalized risk assessments to select individuals for more extensive screening. The benefits of early detection and improved prognosis must be weighed against the harms of overdiagnosis and high health-care costs and are among the most important considerations for instituting a screening program. There is currently no formal screening process for OPC, but because of the low incidence in the general population, risk stratification would necessarily be a key part of any future screening program. A risk stratification model could include demographic and behavioral factors as well as one or more biomarkers. One such model predicted mean one-year absolute risk for OPC and found that increased risk was associated with older age, male sex, smoking, heavy alcohol use, and prevalent oral oncogenic HPV DNA [73]. Additionally, this modeling study estimated that to detect one case of OPC, 12,195 individuals from the general US population would need to be screened, although this was decreased to 323 when including only individuals in the 1% highest predicted risk group. It is likely that a combination of several biomarkers, such as serum antibodies to HPV16 E oncoproteins and ctmHPVDNA, would be needed to maximize accuracy of a risk prediction model.

Treatment and Outcomes

Clinical Presentation

HPV-related OPC often has an insidious onset. Symptoms are frequently vague and nonspecific, though can include difficulty swallowing (dysphagia), pain with swallowing (odynophagia), foreign body sensation (globus), or generalized throat pain. Referred pain may also exist and can include ear pain (otalgia). However, cancer arising at the tonsils and BOT are often called "silent primaries," and thus the most common presenting symptom of HPV-related OPC is a neck mass (Figure 17.3), indicating nodal metastasis [74]. HPV-related OPC most commonly metastasizes to the upper neck lymph nodes along the jugular vein (levels 2 and 3), but any neck mass in an adult should raise concern for malignancy. For this reason, it is imperative to refer any adult with a neck mass to an otolaryngologist for further evaluation.

Diagnosis and Staging

The otolaryngologist evaluation will include a focused history and physical examination. Examination of the larynx and oropharynx will be performed, either using a mirror or more typically through fiberoptic examination with a rigid or flexible scope. This office-based procedure obtains visualization of areas that are inadequately seen directly through the open mouth; particularly the BOT and inferior aspect of the tonsils. Additionally, the flexible fiberoptic scope allows examination of the nasopharynx, hypopharynx, and larynx (all three are sites which can be impacted by an HPV-related OPC or as a location of a primary malignancy, typically tobacco/alcohol related though rarely viral-associated). Biopsy of any lesion is necessary to confirm the diagnosis and can be done in the office or operating room depending on tumor location and patient factors. As most patients present with lymph node metastases, ultrasound-guided fine needle aspiration biopsy is a more convenient and comfortable means of pathologic diagnosis, though circulating HPV DNA analysis is rapidly becoming a means of not only HPV confirmation but also formal diagnosis. Patients should undergo CT neck with contrast to evaluate tumor burden and presence of nodal metastases and PET-CT (or CT chest in some cases) is used to rule out distant metastatic disease.

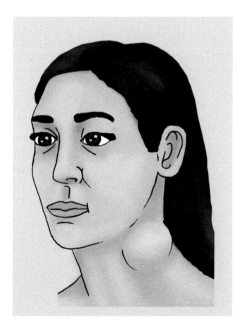

Figure 17.3 Left sided level II neck mass in an otherwise asymptomatic patient. Any neck mass in an adult should raise concern for malignancy and prompt further evaluation with an otolaryngologist

Multiple studies have demonstrated dramatically and consistently improved locorregional control and overall survival for patients with HPV-related OPC compared to those with HPV-negative OPC [75, 76]. As a consequence of such evidence, HPV-related OPC is considered a disease unique from HPV-negative, tobacco/alcohol associated OPC and thus was given its own separate staging system in 2018. Clinical TNM staging based upon the eighth edition of the American Joint Committee on Cancer guidelines [77]. Tables 17.1–17.3 should be documented in all patients to assist in treatment decision making, to provide prognostic information, and for fully informing patients. Pathologic TNM staging should be used postoperatively, if surgical intervention is performed.

Treatment and Toxicities

HPV-related OPC can be treated with a combination of surgery, chemotherapy, and radiation therapy depending on the extent of disease. While many current and recent past clinical trial efforts have focused on the possibility of treatment de-escalation to reduce treatment toxicity with mixed results [78, 79] herein we present the current accepted standard of care. T1–T2 lesions with clinically negative neck (N0) can be treated with primary surgery or definitive radiation

Table 17.1 Classification of tumor size based American Joint Committee on Cancer (AJCC) guidelines

Tumor (T) definition

T0	No tumor identified, but p16+ cervical node involvement
Tis	Carcinoma in situ
T1	Tumor ≤ 2 cm
T2	Tumor >2 and ≤ 4 cm
T3	Tumor >4 cm or extension to lingual surface of epiglottis
T4	Moderately advanced local disease; tumor invades larynx, extrinsic muscles of tongue, medial pterygoid, hard palate, mandible, and beyond

Table 17.2 Clinical assessment of regional lymph nodes based on American Joint Committee on Cancer (AJCC) guidelines

Clinical assessment of regional lymph nodes (cN)

cNX	Regional lymph nodes cannot be assessed
cN0	No regional lymph node metastasis
cN1	One or more ipsilateral lymph nodes ≤ 6 cm
cN2	Contralateral or bilateral lymph nodes ≤ 6 cm
cN3	Lymph node(s) > 6 cm

Table 17.3 AJCC clinical staging groups. The white boxes indicate stage 1 disease, which is considered T1–2 with N0–1 disease. The light grey boxes indicate stage 2 disease, which is considered T3 and N0–2, or any T1–2 lesion with N2 disease. The dark grey boxes indicate stage 3, which is any T4 lesion or any N3 disease.

	T1	T2	T3	T4
N0				
N1		Stage 1		
N2		Stage 2		
N3		Stage 3		

therapy, though proper selection of patients for transoral surgery with neck dissection requires significant experience and is critical to avoiding surgical misadventure and/or need for postoperative radiotherapy. Larger lesions (T3–T4) or patients with multiple neck metastases typically are treated with concurrent chemoradiation, though selected cases may be treated with transoral surgery with neck dissection typically followed by radiation therapy (or chemoradiation). Induction chemotherapy is rarely used but may be required in extremely advanced cases and/or in cases of major concern of distant metastasis risk. Controversy between a surgery first approach and a definitive concurrent chemoradiation approach may arise in cases of moderate size primaries without nodal disease (T3N0) and those early primaries with minimal nodal disease (T1–2 early N1), and while both are accepted, experienced multidisciplinary evaluation and recommendation is critical and clinical trial options should be offered if available. If a patient elects to undergo surgical intervention, they must be made aware that certain pathologic features (unknown to the surgeon or to the patient before surgery) of the surgical specimen may warrant post-operative radiation and/or concurrent chemoradiation therapy [80]. Choice of treatment is complex, requires experienced multidisciplinary input, and ultimately must be a shared decision between the patient and treatment team.

Regardless of treatment type, all modalities are associated with toxicities having the potential of major impact on one's quality of life or even death. Toxicities of radiation therapy to the head and neck region include dysphagia, dry mouth (xerostomia), mucositis, change in taste (dysgeusia), accelerated atherosclerotic disease of the carotid system, and both soft tissue radionecrosis and osteoradionecrosis [81]. Surgical intervention can also cause dysphagia and shoulder dysfunction, and rare cases of life-threatening hemorrhage and death are reported after transoral surgery. Chemotherapeutic regimens most commonly include cisplatin, which has nephro-, oto- and digestive toxicity. All treatment modalities have a risk of dysphagia, which may become severe enough to require gastrostomy tube placement. Gastrostomy tube dependence is common during and shortly after treatment, with reported rates anywhere from 40–80%. Long term risk of gastrostomy tube dependence is significantly lower at 10–15%, although many patients continue to experience some degree of dysphagia [82]. These long-term impacts on swallowing are significant and ultimately lead to chronic pulmonary problems and along with accelerated atherosclerotic disease of the carotid system are likely the main reasons for early non-cancer death in patients with history of HPV-related OPC. Within a large cohort of patients cured of OPC (N=1699) by definitive radiation or chemoradiation, 15-year mortality was fourfold higher than expected for a similar population without OPC history [83].

While pregnancy in a woman presenting with an HPV-related OPC is very rare, all women with an HPV-related OPC should have a pregnancy test if not having had prior hysterectomy or confirmed as postmenopausal. Cisplatin is a FDA pregnancy category D medication, meaning that it could be harmful to the fetus [84]. Radiation exposure is also harmful to a fetus [85], and this cannot be fully mitigated with lead shielding due to internal scatter from a head and neck treatment. Surgery may be a reasonable approach in these rare cases, after obstetric consultation and careful consideration of timing.

Screening for Second HPV-Related Cancer Among Patients with HPV-Related OPC and Their Partners

The associations amongst HPV-related malignancies as presented above in the Epidemiology Section and the opportunity to diagnose cancer earlier through screening of groups at high risk raises three questions:

(1) Should women with HPV-related OPC have screening for cancer at anogenital sites? Certainly, these women should follow current USPSTF recommendations for cervical cancer screening, but there is not sufficient evidence (including costs and harms analysis) at this time to support more frequent cervical cancer screening or for expanding screening to include anal cancer screening.

(2) Should women with anogenital cancer be screened for HPV-related OPC? Unfortunately, standardized OPC screening does not currently exist and is unlikely to be effective or efficient without better selection of a high-risk group through emerging biomarker testing as discussed above in the Prevention and Screening Section.

(3) Should partners of women with HPV-related OPC undergo screening for HPV-related cancer? Female partners of these women should follow current evidenced-based recommendations for cervical cancer screening. There is not sufficient evidence to support more frequent cervical cancer screening or for expanding screening to include anal cancer screening, and standardized OPC screening for either women or men does not exist, though emerging biomarker-directed screening is discussed above.

Case Resolution

The patient underwent concurrent cisplatin with radiotherapy consisting of cisplatin 100 mg/m2 every 3 weeks (at week 0, 3, and 6). Radiotherapy was administered 5 days a week for 35 fractions to a total dose of 70 gray (2 gray/fraction) to the primary and gross nodal disease, 60 gray to the high-risk subclinical regions, and 54 gray to the low-risk subclinical regions including the bilateral neck nodal levels. She did not require a feeding tube during therapy but did experience expected acute odynophagia and dysphagia during treatment. While she had a normal pretreatment audiogram, she did experience posttreatment mild sensorineural hearing loss in high frequencies, and tinnitus when in quiet environments. After treatment, she complained of xerostomia, dysgeusia, and mild dysphagia requiring some alterations in her diet. Her posttreatment baseline PET-CT imaging revealed complete resolution of her cancer and repeat of circulating HPV16 DNA assay was negative with no fragments detected. Approximately six months from the end of treatment, she began to have odynophagia with left otalgia and dysphagia, which worsened over one month. On exam, she had an ulcer of the left BOT. CT

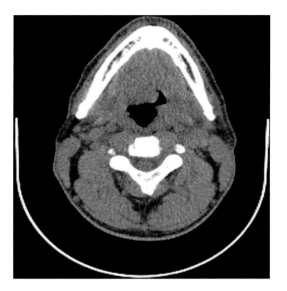

Figure 17.4 Post treatment CT scan showing ulceration along the left base of tongue. There is no longer an enhancing mass or lymphadenopathy present, suggesting good treatment response

scan with contrast (Figure 17.4) revealed an ulcer of the left BOT without an associated enhancing mass or lymphadenopathy. PET-CT showed no significant metabolic activity at the BOT, nor evidence of any metastatic adenopathy or distant disease. Repeat circulating HPV16 DNA assay remained negative. With a presumptive diagnosis of soft tissue radionecrosis of the BOT, the patient underwent hyperbaric oxygen (HBO) therapy for 20 dives over a 4-week period. One month after completion of HBO the patient was without pain and exam of the left BOT ulcer had healed as a scarred but mucosalized defect. Imaging and circulating HPV16 DNA assay were both negative, and thus the patient continued on to routine serial follow-up.

Take Home Points

- Virtually all HPV-related cancer are preventable through childhood HPV vaccination. It is a tragedy that HPV vaccination rates remain below public health goals 16 years after FDA approval, and current projections do not show a major impact on HPV-related oropharyngeal cancer incidence until 2060 [86]. HPV vaccination must be implemented more broadly as the cornerstone to preventing deaths and suffering from HPV-related cancer and their treatment.
- While screening does not currently exist for HPV-related oropharyngeal cancer, adults with signs of a potential oropharyngeal cancer (a neck mass or throat symptoms) need to be assessed by an otolaryngologist/head and neck surgeon without delay.
- For oropharyngeal cancer patients, a multidisciplinary team is critical to effective work-up, treatment, and survivorship.
- Patients with a primary HPV associated malignancy have a five-fold increased risk of secondary HPV-associated malignancy compared to unaffected individuals.
- The pattern of potential second primary cancer in women with an HPV-related oropharyngeal cancer are unique, and with the exception of those in a palliative situation, such women should continue USPSTF recommended cancer screenings.

- Emerging research will likely provide primary screening opportunities for HPV-related oropharyngeal cancer, and these approaches may also improve detection of second HPV-related cancer at other sites.

Financial and competing interests disclosure: Dr. Sturgis received research reagents from Roche Diagnostics, in 2021 served as the Board Chair for The Immunization Partnership (a nonprofit organization) and served on the Medical Advisory Board Member of The Prevent Cancer Foundation (a nonprofit organization). Dr. Dahlstrom received research reagents from Roche Diagnostics. No other authors have any interests to declare, including financial interests or relationships or affiliations that are relevant to the subject of this manuscript.

Funding: This work was supported in part by the Cancer Prevention & Research Institute of Texas (RP200025 [EMS]).

Acknowledgments: The authors thank Colin Coviello for his artistic work in creating Figures 17.2 and 17.3.

References

1. Mourad W. F., Hu K. S., Choi W. H., et al. General Principles and Management Cancer of the Oropharynx. In Harrison L. B., Sessions R. B., Kies M. S. (Eds.), *Head and Neck Cancer: A Multidisciplinary Approach*. Wolters Kluwer; 2013, pp. 373–440.

2. Kreimer A. R., Clifford G. M., Boyle P., Franceschi S. Human papillomavirus types in head and neck squamous cell carcinomas worldwide: A systematic review. *Cancer Epidemiol Biomarkers Prev*. 2005;**14**:467–75. https://doi.org/10.1158/1055-9965.EPI-04-0551.

3. Syrjänen S., Lodi G., von Bültzingslöwen I., et al. Human papillomaviruses in oral carcinoma and oral potentially malignant disorders: A systematic review. *Oral Dis*. 2011;**17**:58–72. https://doi.org/10.1111/J.1601-0825.2011.01792.X.

4. Sturgis E. M., Cinciripini P. M. Trends in head and neck cancer incidence in relation to smoking prevalence: An emerging epidemic of human papillomavirus-associated cancer? *Cancer*. 2007;**110**:1429–35. https://doi.org/10.1002/CNCR.22963.

5. Chaturvedi A. K., Engels E. A., Pfeiffer R. M., et al. Human papillomavirus and rising oropharyngeal cancer incidence in the United States. *J Clin Oncol*. 2011;**29**:4294–301. https://doi.org/10.1200/JCO.2011.36.4596.

6. Tota J. E., Best A. F., Zumsteg Z. S., et al. Evolution of the oropharynx cancer epidemic in the United States: Moderation of increasing incidence in younger individuals and shift in the burden to older individuals. *Journal of Clinical Oncology* 2019;**37**:1538–46. https://doi.org/10.1200/JCO.19.00370.

7. Van Dyne E. A., Henley S. J., Saraiya M., et al. *Trends in Human Papillomavirus–Associated Cancer – United States, 1999-2015*. Morbidity and Mortality Weekly Report: US Department of Health and Human Services, CDC 2018;67.

8. U.S. Cancer Statistics Working Group. U.S. Cancer Statistics Data Visualizations Tool, based on 2021 submission data (1999–2019): U.S. Department of Health and Human Services, Centers for Disease Control and Prevention and National Cancer Institute; www.cdc.gov/cancer/dataviz, released in June 2022. n.d. https://gis.cdc.gov/Cancer/USCS/#/RiskFactors/ (accessed October 10, 2022).

9. Dahlstrom K. R., Bell D., Hanby D., et al. Socioeconomic characteristics of patients with oropharyngeal carcinoma according to tumor HPV status, patient smoking status, and sexual behavior. *Oral Oncol*. 2015;**51**:832–8. https://doi.org/10.1016/j.oraloncology.2015.06.005.

10. Siegel R. L., Miller K. D., Fuchs H. E., Jemal A. Cancer Statistics, 2022. *CA Cancer J Clin.* 2022;**72**:7–33.

11. Rettig E. M., Fakhry C., Khararjian A., Westra W. H. Age profile of patients with oropharyngeal squamous cell carcinoma. *JAMA Otolaryngology–Head & Neck Surgery.* 2018;**144**:538–9. https://doi.org/10.1001/JAMAOTO.2018.0310.

12. HPV-Associated Cancer Diagnosis by Age | CDC n.d. www.cdc.gov/cancer/hpv/statistics/age.htm (accessed September 16, 2022).

13. Mahal B. A., Catalano P. J., Haddad R. I., et al. Incidence and demographic burden of HPV-associated oropharyngeal head and neck cancer in the United States. *Cancer, Epidemiology, Biomarkers, and Prevention.* 2019;**28**:1660–7. https://doi.org/10.1158/1055-9965.EPI-19-0038.

14. Gan S. J., Dahlstrom K. R., Peck B. W., et al. Incidence and pattern of second primary malignancies in patients with index oropharyngeal cancer versus index nonoropharyngeal head and neck cancer. *Cancer.* 2013:2593–601. https://doi.org/10.1002/cncr.28107.

15. Dahlstrom K. R., Bell D., Hanby D., et al. Socioeconomic characteristics of patients with oropharyngeal carcinoma according to tumor HPV status, patient smoking status, and sexual behavior. *Oral Oncol.* 2015;**51**(9):832–8. https://doi.org/10.1016/j.oraloncology.2015.06.005.

16. Rotsides J. M., Oliver J. R., Moses L. E., et al. Socioeconomic and racial disparities and survival of human papillomavirus-associated oropharyngeal squamous cell carcinoma. *Otolaryngology-Head and Neck Surgery.* 2021;**164**:131–8. https://doi.org/10.1177/0194599820935853.

17. Souza G. d', Wentz A., Kluz N., et al. Sex differences in risk factors and natural history of oral human papillomavirus infection. *J Infect Dis.* 2016;**213**:1893–6. https://doi.org/10.1093/infdis/jiw063.

18. Lewis R. M., Gargano J. W., Unger E. R., Querec T. D., Markowitz L. E. Genital human papillomavirus prevalence over the lifespan among females and males in a national cross-sectional survey, United States, 2013–2016. *Sex Transm Dis.* 2021;**48**:855–63. https://doi.org/10.1097/OLQ.0000000000001447.

19. Chesson H. W., Dunne E. F., Hariri S., Markowitz L. E. The estimated lifetime probability of acquiring human papillomavirus in the United States. *Sex Transm Dis.* 2014;**41**:660–4. https://doi.org/10.1097/OLQ.0000000000000193.

20. Chaturvedi A. K., Graubard B. I., Broutian T., et al. Prevalence of oral HPV infection in unvaccinated men and women in the United States, 2009–2016. *JAMA – Journal of the American Medical Association.* 2019;**322**:977–9. https://doi.org/10.1001/JAMA.2019.10508.

21. Chaturvedi A. K., Graubard B. I., Broutian T., et al. NHANES 2009–2012 findings: Association of sexual behaviors with higher prevalence of oral oncogenic human papillomavirus infections in U.S. men. *Cancer Res.* 2015;**75**:2468–77. https://doi.org/10.1158/0008-5472.CAN-14-2843.

22. Giuliano A. R., Nyitray A. G., Kreimer A. R., et al. EUROGIN 2014 roadmap: differences in human papillomavirus infection natural history, transmission and human papillomavirus-related cancer incidence by gender and anatomic site of infection. *Int J Cancer.* 2015;**136**:2752–60. https://doi.org/10.1002/IJC.29082.

23. Bleeker M. C. G., Hogewoning C. J. A., Berkhof J., et al. Concordance of specific human papillomavirus types in sex partners is more prevalent than would be expected by chance and is associated with increased viral loads. *Clinical Infectious Diseases.* 2005;**41**:612–20. https://doi.org/10.1086/431978/2/41-5-612-TBL005.GIF.

24. Saunders C. L., Meads C., Abel G. A., Lyratzopoulos G. Associations between sexual orientation and overall and site-specific diagnosis of cancer: Evidence from two national patient surveys in England. *J Clin Oncol.* 2017;**35**:3654–61. https://doi.org/10.1200/JCO.

25. Gillison M. L. Oropharyngeal cancer: A potential consequence of concomitant HPV and HIV infection. *Curr Opin Oncol.*

2009;**21**:439–44. https://doi.org/10.1097/CCO.0B013E32832F3E1B.

26. Gillison M. L., Broutian T., Pickard R. K. L., et al. Prevalence of oral HPV infection in the United States, 2009–2010. *JAMA*. 2012;**307**:693–703. https://doi.org/10.1001/JAMA.2012.101.

27. Smith E. M., Rubenstein L. M., Haugen T. H., Hamsikova E., Turek L. P. Tobacco and alcohol use increases the risk of both HPV-associated and HPV-independent head and neck cancer. *Cancer Causes Control*. 2010;**21**:1369–78. https://doi.org/10.1007/S10552-010-9564-Z.

28. Applebaum K. M., Furniss C. S., Zeka A., et al. Lack of association of alcohol and tobacco with HPV16-associated head and neck cancer. *J Natl Cancer Inst*. 2007;**99**:1801–10. https://doi.org/10.1093/JNCI/DJM233.

29. Marks M. A., Chaturvedi A. K., Kelsey K., et al. Association of marijuana smoking with oropharyngeal and oral tongue cancer: Pooled analysis from the INHANCE consortium. *Cancer, Epidemiology, Biomarkers, & Prevention*. 2014;**23**:160–71. https://doi.org/10.1158/1055-9965.EPI-13-0181.

30. Morris L. G. T., Sikora A. G., Patel S. G., Hayes R. B., Ganly I. Second primary cancer after an index head and neck cancer: Subsite-specific trends in the era of human papillomavirus – Associated oropharyngeal cancer. *Journal of Clinical Oncology*. 2011;**29**:739–46. https://doi.org/10.1200/JCO.2010.31.8311.

31. Sturgis E. M., Miller R. H. Second primary malignancies in the head and neck cancer patient. *Rhinology & Laryngology*. 1995;**104**:946. https://doi.org/0.1177/000348949510401206.

32. Do K. -A., Johnson M. M., Lee J. J., et al. Longitudinal study of smoking patterns in relation to the development of smoking-related secondary primary tumors in patients with upper aerodigestive tract malignancies. *Cancer*. 2004;**101**:2837–42. https://doi.org/10.1002/cncr.20714.

33. Walboomers J. M., Jacobs M. v., Manos M., et al. Human papillomavirus is a necessary cause of invasive cervical cancer worldwide. *Journal of Pathology*. 1999;**189**:12–19. https://doi.org/10.1002/(SICI)1096-9896(199909)189:1<2::aid-path431>3.0.CO;2-F.

34. Sutton B. C., Allen R. A., Moore W. E., Dunn S. T. Distribution of human papillomavirus genotypes in invasive squamous carcinoma of the vulva. *Modern Pathology*. 2008;**21**:3:45–54. https://doi.org/10.1038/modpathol.3801010.

35. Steenbergen R. D. M., de Wilde J., Wilting S. M., et al. HPV-mediated transformation of the anogenital tract. *Journal of Clinical Virology* 2005;**32**:25–33. https://doi.org/10.1016/J.JCV.2004.11.019.

36. Tornesello M. L., Duraturo M. L., Losito S., et al. Human papillomavirus genotypes and HPV16 variants in penile carcinoma. *Int J Cancer*. 2008;**122**:132–7. https://doi.org/10.1002/ijc.23062.

37. Sikora A. G., Morris L. G., Sturgis E. M. Bidirectional association of anogenital and oral cavity/pharyngeal carcinomas in men. *Arch Otolaryngol Head Neck Surg*. 2009;**135**:402–5. https://doi.org/10.1001/archoto.2009.19.

38. Rietbergen M. M., van Bokhoven A. A. J. D., Lissenberg-Witte B. I., et al. Epidemiologic associations of HPV-positive oropharyngeal cancer and (pre)cancerous cervical lesions. *Int J Cancer*. 2018;**143**:283–8. https://doi.org/10.1002/ijc.31315.

39. Ebisch R. M. F., Rutten D. W. E., IntHout J., et al. Long-lasting increased risk of human papillomavirus–related carcinomas and premalignancies after cervical intraepithelial neoplasia grade 3: A population-based cohort study. *Journal of Clinical Oncology*. 2017;**35**:2542–50. https://doi.org/10.1200/JCO.2016.71.4543.

40. Ragin C. C. R., Taioli E. Second primary head and neck tumor risk in patients with cervical cancer: SEER data analysis. *Head Neck*. 2007;**30**:58–66. https://doi.org/10.1002/hed.20663.

41. Jani K. S., Lu S.-E., Murphy J. D., et al. Malignancies diagnosed before and after anal squamous cell carcinomas: A SEER registry analysis. *Cancer Med*.

2021;**10**:3575–83. https://doi.org/10.1002/cam4.3909.

42. Suk R., Mahale P., Sonawane K., et al. Trends in risks for second primary cancer associated with index human papillomavirus-associated cancer. *JAMA Netw Open.* 2018;**1**:e181999. https://doi.org/10.1001/jamanetworkopen.2018.1999.

43. Tsao A. S., Papadimitrakopoulou V., Lin H., et al. Concordance of oral HPV prevalence between patients with oropharyngeal cancer and their partners. *Infect Agent Cancer.* 2016;**11**:1–9. https://doi.org/10.1186/s13027-016-0066-9.

44. D'Souza G., Gross N. D., Pai S. I., et al. Oral Human Papillomavirus (HPV) infection in HPV-positive patients with oropharyngeal cancer and their partners. *Journal of Clinical Oncology.* 2014;**32**:2408–15. https://doi.org/10.1200/JCO.2014.55.1341.

45. Mirghani H., Strugis E. M., Auperin A., Monsonego J., Blanchard P. Is there an increased risk of cancer among spouses of patients with HPV-related cancer: A systematic Review. *Oral Oncol.* 2017;**67**:138–45. https://doi.org/10.1016/j.oraloncology.2017.02.024.

46. Meites E., Szilagyi P. G., Chesson H. W., et al. Human papillomavirus vaccination for adults: Updated recommendations of the Advisory Committee on Immunization Practices. *American Journal of Transplantation.* 2019;**19**:3202–6. https://doi.org/10.1111/ajt.15633.

47. FDA approves expanded use of Gardasil 9 to include individuals 27 through 45 years old | FDA n.d. www.fda.gov/news-events/press-announcements/fda-approves-expanded-use-gardasil-9-include-individuals-27-through-45-years-old (accessed August 21, 2022).

48. Petrosky E., Bocchini J. A., Hariri S., et al. Use of 9-valent human papillomavirus (HPV) vaccine: Updated HPV vaccination recommendations of the advisory committee on immunization practices. *MMWR Morb Mortal Wkly Rep.* 2015;**64**:300–4.

49. Lehtinen M., Dillner J. Clinical trials of human papillomavirus vaccines and

beyond. *Nat Rev Clin Oncol.* 2013;**10**:400–10. https://doi.org/10.1038/nrclinonc.2013.84.

50. Drolet M., Bénard É., Pérez N., et al. Population-level impact and herd effects following the introduction of human papillomavirus vaccination programmes: Updated systematic review and meta-analysis. *The Lancet.* 2019;**394**:497–509. https://doi.org/10.1016/S0140-6736(19)30298-3.

51. Brisson M., Kim J. J., Canfell K., et al. Impact of HPV vaccination and cervical screening on cervical cancer elimination: A comparative modelling analysis in 78 low-income and lower-middle-income countries. *The Lancet.* 2020;**395**:575–90. https://doi.org/10.1016/S0140-6736(20)30068-4.

52. Markowitz L. E., Naleway A. L., Lewis R. M., et al. Declines in HPV vaccine type prevalence in women screened for cervical cancer in the United States: Evidence of direct and herd effects of vaccination. *Vaccine.* 2019;**37**:3918–24. https://doi.org/10.1016/j.vaccine.2019.04.099.

53. Michalczyk K., Misiek M., Chudecka-Głaz A . Can adjuvant HPV vaccination be helpful in the prevention of persistent/recurrent cervical dysplasia after surgical treatment? A literature review. *Cancer.* 2022;**14**:4352. https://doi.org/10.3390/CANCER14184352.

54. di Donato V., Caruso G., Petrillo M., et al. Adjuvant HPV vaccination to prevent recurrent cervical dysplasia after surgical treatment: A meta-analysis. *Vaccines (Basel).* 2021;**9(5)**:410. https://doi.org/10.3390/VACCINES9050410.

55. Tang J., Li M., Zhao C., et al. Therapeutic DNA vaccines against HPV-related malignancies: Promising leads from clinical trials. *Viruses.* 2022;**14(2)**: 239. https://doi.org/10.3390/V14020239.

56. Dahlstrom K. R., Anderson K. S., Guo M., et al. Screening for HPV-related oropharyngeal, anal, and penile cancer in middle-aged men: Initial report from the HOUSTON clinical trial. *Oral Oncol.* 2021;**120**. https://doi.org/10.1016/j.oraloncology.2021.105397.

57. Bosch F. X., Broker T. R., Forman D., et al. Comprehensive control of human papillomavirus infections and related diseases. *Vaccine*. 2013;**31** Suppl 7:H1–31. https://doi.org/10.1016/j.vaccine.2013.10.003.

58. Kreimer A. R., Pierce Campbell C. M., Lin H. Y., et al. Incidence and clearance of oral human papillomavirus infection in men: The HIM cohort study. *The Lancet* 2013;**382**:877–87. https://doi.org/10.1016/S0140-6736(13)60809-0.

59. D'Souza G., Clemens G., Strickler H. D., et al. Long-term Persistence of oral HPV over 7 years of follow-up. *JNCI Cancer Spectr*. 2020;**4**(5):pkaa047. https://doi.org/10.1093/JNCICS/PKAA047.

60. Morais E., Kothari S., Roberts C., et al. Oral human papillomavirus (HPV) and associated factors among healthy populations: The design of the PROGRESS (PRevalence of Oral hpv infection, a Global aSSessment) study. *Contemp Clin Trials*. 2022;**115**. https://doi.org/10.1016/J.CCT.2021.106630.

61. Anderson K. S., Dahlstrom K. R., Cheng J. N., et al. HPV16 antibodies as risk factors for oropharyngeal cancer and their association with tumor HPV and smoking status. *Oral Oncol*. 2015;**51**. https://doi.org/10.1016/j.oraloncology.2015.04.011.

62. Dahlstrom K. R., Anderson K. S., Field M. S., et al. Diagnostic accuracy of serum antibodies to human papillomavirus type 16 early antigens in the detection of human papillomavirus–related oropharyngeal cancer. *Cancer*. 2017;**123**. https://doi.org/10.1002/cncr.30955.

63. Kreimer A. R., Johansson M., Waterboer T., et al. Evaluation of human papillomavirus antibodies and risk of subsequent head and neck cancer. *J Clin Oncol* 2013;**31**:2708–15. https://doi.org/10.1200/JCO.2012.47.2738.

64. Kreimer A. R., Johansson M., Yanik E. L., et al. Kinetics of the human papillomavirus type 16 E6 antibody response prior to oropharyngeal cancer. *J Natl Cancer Inst*. 2017;**109**. https://doi.org/10.1093/JNCI/DJX005.

65. Hibbert J., Halec G., Baaken D., Waterboer T., Brenner N. Sensitivity and specificity of human papillomavirus (HPV) 16 early antigen serology for HPV-driven oropharyngeal cancer: A systematic literature review and meta-analysis. *Cancer (Basel)*. 2021;**13**:3010.

66. Robbins H. A., Ferreiro-Iglesias A., Waterboer T., et al. Absolute risk of oropharyngeal cancer after an HPV16-E6 serology test and potential implications for screening: Results from the human papillomavirus cancer cohort consortium. *J Clin Oncol*. 2022;**JCO2101785**. https://doi.org/10.1200/JCO.21.01785.

67. Chera B. S., Kumar S., Beaty B. T., et al. Rapid clearance profile of plasma circulating tumor HPV type 16 DNA during chemoradiotherapy correlates with disease control in HPV-associated oropharyngeal cancer. *Clinical Cancer Research*. 2019;**25**:4682–90.

68. Chera B. S., Kumar S., Shen C., et al. Plasma circulating tumor HPV DNA for the surveillance of cancer recurrence in HPV-associated oropharyngeal cancer. *Journal of Clinical Oncology*. 2020;**38**:1050–8. https://doi.org/10.1200/JCO.19.02444.

69. Rettig E. M., Faden D. L., Sandhu S., et al. Detection of circulating tumor human papillomavirus DNA before diagnosis of HPV-positive head and neck cancer. *Int J Cancer*. 2022;**151**:1081–5. https://doi.org/10.1002/ijc.33996.

70. Scott-Wittenborn N., D'Souza G., Aygun N., et al. Feasibility of clinical evaluation of individuals with increased risk for HPV-associated oropharynx cancer. *Head Neck*. 2022. https://doi.org/10.1002/HED.27212.

71. Waterboer T., Brenner N., Gallagher R., et al. Early detection of human papillomavirus–driven oropharyngeal cancer using serology from the study of prevention of anal cancer. *JAMA Oncol*. 2020;**6**:1806–8. https://doi.org/10.1001/JAMAONCOL.2020.4527.

72. Busch C. J., Hoffmann A. S., Viarisio D., et al. Detection of stage I HPV-driven oropharyngeal cancer in asymptomatic

individuals in the Hamburg City Health Study using HPV16 E6 serology: A proof-of-concept study. *EClinicalMedicine.* 2022;**53**. https://doi.org/10.1016/J.ECLINM.2022.101659.

73. Tota J. E., Gillison M. L., Katki H. A., et al. Development and validation of an individualized risk prediction model for oropharynx cancer in the US population. *Cancer.* 2019;**125**:4407–16. https://doi.org/10.1002/CNCR.32412.

74. McIlwain W. R., Sood A. J., Nguyen S. A., Day T. A. Initial symptoms in patients with HPV-positive and HPV-negative oropharyngeal cancer. *JAMA Otolaryngol Head Neck Surg.* 2014;**140**:441–7. https://doi.org/10.1001/jamaoto.2014.141.

75. Ang K., Harris J., Wheeler R., et al. Human papillomavirus and survival of patients with oropharyngeal cancer. *N Engl J Med.* 2010;**363**:24–35. https://doi.org/10.1056/NEJMoa0912217.

76. Fakhry C., Westra W. H., Li S., et al. Improved survival of patients with human papillomavirus-positive head and neck squamous cell carcinoma in a prospective clinical trial. *Journal National Cancer Institute.* 2008;**100**:261–9.

77. Amin M. B., Edge S. B., Greene F. L., et al. (Eds.). *AJCC Cancer Staging Manual.* 8th ed. Springer; 2017.

78. Petrelli F., Luciana A., Ghidini A., et al. Treatment de-escalation for HPV+ oropharyngeal cancer: A systematic review and meta-analysis. *Head Neck.* 2022;**44**:1255–66.

79. Mehanna H., Robinson M., Hartley A., et al. Articles radiotherapy plus cisplatin or cetuximab in low-risk human papillomavirus-positive oropharyngeal cancer (De-ESCALaTE HPV): An open-label andomized controlled phase 3 trial. *The Lancet.* 2019;**393**:51–60. https://doi.org/10.1016/S0140-6736(18)32752-1.

80. NCCN Guidelines Version 2.2022. National Comprehensive Cancer Network 2022. www.nccn.org/professionals/physician_gls/pdf/head-and-neck.pdf (accessed September 26, 2022).

81. Quan D. L., Sukari A., Nagasaka M., et al. Gastrostomy tube dependence and patient-reported quality of life outcomes based on type of treatment for human papillomavirus-associated oropharyngeal cancer: Systematic review and meta-analysis. *Head Neck.* 2021;**43**:3681–98. https://doi.org/10.1002/hed.26829.

82. Martin A., Murray L., Sethugavalar B., et al. Changes in patient-reported swallow function in the long term after chemoradiotherapy for oropharyngeal carcinoma. *Clin Oncol (R Coll Radiol).* 2018;**30**:756–63. https://doi.org/10.1016/J.CLON.2018.06.013.

83. Dahlstrom K. R., Song J., Thall P. F., et al. Conditional survival among patients with oropharyngeal cancer treated with radiation therapy and alive without recurrence 5 years after diagnosis. *Cancer.* 2021;**127**:1228–37.

84. Mir O., Berveiller P., Ropert S., Goffinet F. F., Goldwasser F. F. Use of platinum derivatives during pregnancy. *Cancer.* 2008;**113**:3069–74. https://doi.org/10.1002/cncr.23935.

85. Hepner A., Negrini D., Hase A., et al. Cancer during pregnancy: The oncologist overview. *Review World J Oncol.* 2019;**10**:28–34. https://doi.org/10.14740/wjon1177.

86. Zhang Y., Fakhry C., D'Souza G. Projected association of human papillomavirus vaccination with oropharynx cancer incidence in the US, 2020–2045. *JAMA Oncol.* 2021;**7**. https://doi.org/10.1001/JAMAONCOL.2021.2907.

Chapter 18

Leukemia: Acute and Chronic

Sai Prasad Desikan, Sara Bresser, and Alessandra Ferrajoli

Introduction

Leukemias encompass a diverse range of bone marrow disorders characterized by genetic changes (mutations, translocations etc.) resulting in proliferation of blood cells. Acute leukemias are defined by cessation of maturation in addition to proliferation with a blast (immature precursor cells) percentage of 20% or more in the blood or bone marrow. Chronic leukemias are a result of proliferation of mature cells. In chronic myeloid leukemia (CML), the Philadelphia translocation (defined in the CML section) results in proliferation of mature myeloid cells. In chronic lymphocytic leukemia (CLL), mature, monoclonal B lymphocytes expand in the marrow and lymph nodes. Leukemias and their treatments pose unique obstetric and gynecologic challenges, often requiring a multidisciplinary approach. In this chapter we discuss the pathogenesis, treatment, and gynecologic challenges, as well as our approach to addressing these challenges.

Acute Leukemias

Case Presentation

A 19-year-old female presents after a syncopal episode and heavy menstrual bleeding. The patient initially thought this was secondary to heavy menses; however, the bleeding continued after her normal menses should have stopped. Her fatigue continued to worsen, especially with exertion. She is a college student and had to sit down while walking from her classes to her dormitory. After the syncopal episode she was taken to the emergency department. Systolic blood pressure was 90 mmHg with a heart rate of 120. Blood counts on presentation were significant for a white blood cell count of 50 K/μL (normal range: 4.5–11.0 x 10^9/L) with circulating immature cells, a hemoglobin of 7.5 g/dL (normal range: 12.0–16.0 g/dL), and a platelet count of 15 K/μL (normal range 140–440 K/μL). The patient was admitted to the hospital. What are the appropriate next steps?

Pathophysiology of Acute Leukemias

Hematopoiesis is the process by which immature hematopoietic stem cells replicate and differentiate to form mature blood constituents: lymphocytes, granulocytes, megakaryocytes, monocytes, and erythrocytes. Self-renewal in this system is limited to hematopoietic stem and progenitor cells. Under normal conditions, these cells are quiescent. Acute leukemias develop after a series of mutations in early stem or progenitor cells results in cessation of differentiation and expansion of blasts (leukemic counterpart to progenitor or stem cells) [1]. Acute leukemias (characterized by 20% or more blasts in the peripheral blood or bone marrow) can be divided into two categories: acute myeloid leukemia (AML) and acute lymphoblastic leukemia (ALL) [2, 3].

AML is a result of mutations or chromosomal changes in myeloid progenitor cells, termed myeloblasts, that impede maturation and promote uncontrolled growth. These immature cells are committed to the granulocytic, monocytic, erythroid, or megakaryocytic lineages and are morphologically subclassified accordingly. Importantly, these cells can continue to accrue genetic changes throughout the disease process and treatment [4]. AML is characterized by over 20% myeloblasts in the bone marrow or in the peripheral blood with characteristic expression of myeloid markers (MPO, CD34, HLA-DR, CD33 etc.). While most patients develop AML de novo, prior chemotherapy exposure (often anthracyclines and alkylating agents), prior ionizing radiation, history of tobacco usage, and significant prior benzene exposure can increase the risk of AML. Certain genetic abnormalities like trisomy 21 and Fanconi's anemia predispose to the development of AML. Familial germline mutations such as *DDX41*, *RUNX1*, and *CEBPA* have been associated with the development of AML [3, 5].

ALL is characterized by the arrest of lymphoid maturation with expansion of either T or B lymphoblasts via the presence or absence of certain chromosomal abnormalities and the acquisition of mutations in oncogenes and tumor suppressors genes. Classification is based on lineage (T or B-lineages) and on which stage of development the arrest occurs. Cytofluorimetric analyses of peripheral blood, bone marrow or lymphoid tissue is required for the diagnosis of ALL and allows further subclassification together with cytogenetic and molecular analyses. The findings and ability to further subclassify ALL have additional prognostic and therapeutic implications particularly in patients with Burkitt's lymphoma and Philadelphia positive ALL [6–8]. Without prompt recognition and treatment acute leukemias are almost universally fatal.

Epidemiology

According to the Surveillance, Epidemiology and End Results (SEER) program data published in 2022, AML makes up 1% of all new cancer cases with 20,050 new cases annually, and 2% of all cancer-related deaths annually. Most patients are elderly with a median age of 68 at diagnosis. The incidence in the general population is 4.1 per 100,000 with an incidence of 5.1 and 3.4 per 100,000 in men and women respectively. When analyzed based on race, AML is most common among Caucasians with an incidence of 4.3 per 100,000. The incidence amongst other races is 3 to 4 per 100,000. While incidence in the entire population remains relatively low, five-year relative survival is poor at 30.5% [9].

ALL has a bimodal distribution, primarily impacting children younger than 20 years of age and adults older than 55 years. The incidence is 1.8 per 100,000 in the general population with an incidence among men and women of 2.1 and 1.6 per 100,000. Incidence is highest among Hispanics and Caucasians with an incidence of 2.7 and 1.6 per 100,000, respectively [9]. With advances in therapy, survival has improved with 5-year survival prior to 1990 of 51% improving to 72% after 2010. Socioeconomic factors continue to play a role with African American patients, Hispanic patients, and patients in lower income households having lower rates of survival [10].

Presentation and Evaluation

Patients with acute leukemias have a variety of clinical presentations. Some patients are asymptomatic and are found incidentally to have cytopenias on laboratory evaluation, while others can present in critical condition due to coagulopathy, respiratory failure, renal failure, and shock [11]. At our institution, all patients with a newly diagnosed acute leukemia are admitted to the hospital for monitoring and treatment. A bone marrow biopsy should be performed in stable patients; however, if unable to obtain biopsy, the peripheral blood can be used preliminarily in some patients to guide initial management [12].

Acute leukemias primarily impact the bone marrow, resulting in fatigue secondary to anemia. However bruising or mucosal bleeding related to thrombocytopenia and infections due to neutropenia can be seen, and a thorough review of systems is needed as any organ could be impacted. While CNS infiltration is more frequent in ALL, patients with either type of acute leukemia can present with headaches or neurologic deficits. Due to the release of cytokines secondary to the malignancy (common in monocytic disease, a subtype of AML), patients may present complaining of shortness of breath secondary to pulmonary edema, weight gain, or lower extremity swelling. Hepatosplenomegaly and lymphadenopathy, which are more common with ALL, may result in early satiety and weight loss. A thorough skin exam looking for lesions or subcutaneous nodules, which would be concerning for extramedullary disease should be performed, in addition to cardiovascular and respiratory examinations [11, 13].

Concerns for acute leukemias usually arise after an initial complete blood count demonstrates cytopenias or increase in the percentage of blasts. An electrolyte panel should be checked as many patients present with acute kidney injury secondary to rapid cell turnover with associated hyperkalemia, hyperphosphatemia, and/or hyperuricemia. Patients with acute leukemia can present with coagulopathies (particularly in the AML subtype of acute promyelocytic leukemia), compounding their risk of bleeding in conjunction with thrombocytopenia. Coagulation studies (prothrombin time with international normalized ratio, activated partial thromboplastin time, and fibrinogen) must be obtained on presentation [11, 13]. A chest x-ray allows for evaluation of potential infiltrates and mediastinal masses. An echocardiogram allows for evaluation of cardiac reserve, an important metric in regard to volume as many patients receive numerous blood product transfusions and intravenous fluids. Additionally, an understanding of the patient's baseline cardiac reserve is important when considering the incorporation of anthracyclines and other agents in the planned treatment.

Acute Management

The acute management of these patients is related to their presentation. Patients with elevated WBC and those with hyperleukocytosis, defined as WBC greater than 50 K/μL, should be managed aggressively with cytoreduction. Initial management involves careful cytoreduction typically with hydroxyurea or cytarabine in patients with AML [14, 15]. In patients with ALL, steroids can be given as part of the initial management, once the diagnosis has been confirmed. These patients should have close monitoring for tumor lysis syndrome. The assistance of nephrology specialists is needed for patients experiencing tumor lysis syndrome, a result of rapid cell lysis or apoptosis with release of uric acid, phosphorous, and potassium, which can result in significant renal injury and end-organ damage [15]. Rasburicase, recombinant urate oxidase that converts uric acid to allantoin, is indicated in patients with significant elevation in uric acid on presentation and allopurinol should be administered to all patients without contraindications [16]. Sevelamer, a phosphate binder, may prevent accumulation of phosphorous [17].

Monitoring and correction of coagulopathies are key components of management. Fresh frozen plasma is indicated in patients with sequelae of bleeding and elevated INR. Cryoprecipitate should be considered for patients with decreased fibrinogen [15, 18]. Aminocaproic acid can be administered for patients with mucosal bleeding, except in cases of hematuria as clots can result in bladder outlet obstruction. Patients with acute leukemia receive numerous blood product transfusions as well as intravenous medications, hence fluid status must be monitored carefully, and diuretics given to prevent fluid overload.

Management and Long-Term Considerations

After initial bone marrow biopsy with concomitant cytomolecular workup, patients are assigned prognostic categories that aid in the determination of appropriate treatment strategies.

Acute Myeloid Leukemia

Current AML risk stratification is based on cytomolecular characteristics (Figure 18.1). Favorable risk patients have either core binding factor rearrangements (inversion 16 [inv[16]] or translocation 8;21 t[8;21]), mutations in *NPM1*, or in-frame mutations involving the b-zip portion of *CEBPA*. These patients usually respond well to standard chemotherapy-based regimens and do not usually require stem cell transplantation. Intermediate risk patients have mutations impacting *FLT3*, translocation 9;11 t(9;11), or cytogenetic or molecular abnormalities that cannot be further classified as favorable or adverse. These patients should be evaluated for stem cell transplant. Patients with particular chromosomal changes (inversion 3 [inv[3]], deletion 7 (-7), deletion 17 (-17), deletion 5 (-5) to name a few), complex karyotypes, or particular predefined mutations including but not limited to *ASXL1*, specific MDS-related mutations and *TP53* have poor/adverse risk AML and a guarded prognosis. These patients should be considered candidates for further consolidation with stem cell transplantation [3].

Induction and consolidation regimens are dictated by the underlying fitness of the patients and their unique disease characteristics (Figure 18.1). Younger, fit patients are often treated with intensive regimens typically consisting of cytarabine with or without other nucleotide analogues and an anthracycline. These intensive regimens consist of an induction portion consisting of high dose cytarabine (defined as 2 grams per meter squared or greater) in combination with other agents followed by a consolidation portion in patients that have achieved a remission. Consolidation utilizes lower doses of chemotherapy to eradicate residual disease. Further consolidation of therapy is achieved with stem cell transplants in which patients receive conditioning chemotherapy (intensive chemotherapy with intent to eliminate all cells in the bone marrow) followed by allogeneic (from another individual) stem cell transplant. Older, unfit patients or patients with bi-allelic *TP53* mutations are managed with lower intensity regimens, primarily utilizing hypomethylating agents, followed by maintenance (lower doses of therapy for a prolonged period of time) [3, 19]. Venetoclax, a *BCL-2* inhibitor, in combination with azacitidine has been FDA approved since 2020 for the treatment of AML [19, 20]. Stem cell transplantation should be discussed with select older (65 and older) patients based on performance status.

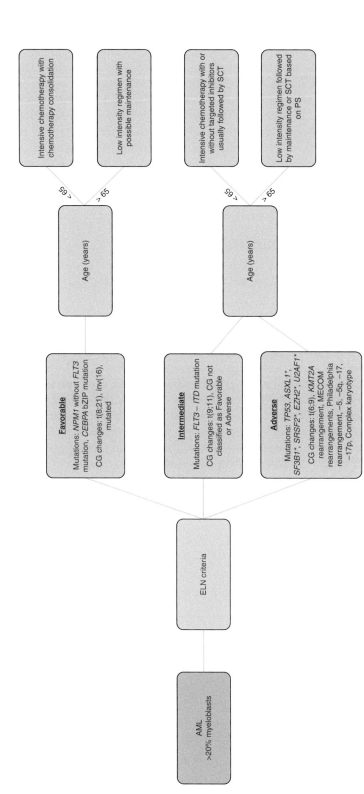

Figure 18.1 Current AML risk stratification based on cytomolecular characteristics

Acute myelogenous leukemia (AML), European Leukemia Net (ELN), Cytogenetic (CG), Stem-cell transplant (SCT), Performance Status (PS), translocation 8;21 [t(8;21)], inversion [16] [inv[16]], translocation 9;11 [t(9;11)], translocation 6;9 [t(6;9)], Deletion of chromosome 5 [-5], Deletion of q arm of chromosome 5 [-5q], Deletion of chromosome 17 [-17], Deletion of p arm of chromosome 17 [-17p]

*At this time these mutations are not considered adverse if they occur in the setting of favorable mutations or cytogenetic changes

Some mutations involved in AML (*FLT3*, *IDH1*, *IDH2*) have targeted inhibitor therapies available [3, 21–24]. These inhibitors are primarily used in conjunction with other agents to optimize outcomes including rates of response, depth of remission, and relapse free survival.

Acute Lymphoblastic Leukemia

ALL can be separated into B-cell ALL (B-ALL) and T-cell ALL (T-ALL) comprising 75% and 25% of cases respectively.

B-Cell Acute Lymphoblastic Leukemia

B-ALL patients can be divided into three broad categories: Philadelphia-positive (Ph+) with a BCR::ABL translocation on FISH, Philadelphia-negative (Ph-), and Philadelphia-like (Ph-like), a newer category with a gene expression profile similar to Ph+ALL without the associated translocation. At this time, most regimens utilize a chemotherapy platform that consist of a multitude of agents: cyclophosphamide, vincristine, an anthracycline, methotrexate, cytarabine, and dexamethasone [25, 26].

Ph + ALL results from the translocation of the proto-oncogene Abelson (*ABL*) tyrosine kinase on chromosome 9 with the breakpoint cluster region (*BCR*) on chromosome 21. There are 2 isoforms: a 190 kilobase isoform and a 210 kilobase isoform. In contrast to patients with chronic myelogenous leukemia, the 190 kilobase isoform is the predominant isoform represented in Ph + ALL. The resulting fusion gene BCR::ABL results in a fusion protein with constitutive kinase activity, promoting uncontrolled proliferation and resistance to apoptosis. Ph + ALL was previously considered a poor prognostic indicator; however, with the advent of targeted inhibitors that inhibit the fusion kinase (imatinib, dasatinib, nilotinib, ponatinib) in conjunction with chemotherapy, patients with Ph+ ALL now have improved outcomes [27, 28].

In the setting of Ph -ALL or Ph -Like ALL, chemotherapy-based regimens remain the standard of care. The use of conjugated antibodies (inotuzumab, ozogamicin) and bispecific T-cell engagers (blinatumomab) in combination with chemotherapy-based regimens have shown promise in clinical trials [29–33]. Currently, both inotuzumab and blinatumomab are FDA approved in the relapsed or refractory setting as monotherapy [34].

T-Cell Acute Lymphoblastic Leukemia

T-ALL utilizes a similar chemotherapy backbone to B-ALL. Unfortunately, the development of novel agents for T-ALL has proven difficult [25]. Nelarabine, a nucleoside analog, utilized in combination with other chemotherapy regimens is the only drug that is FDA approved specifically for the treatment of T-ALL [35]. Recently, however, anti-apoptotic inhibitors have shown promise in specific subsets of T-ALL [25, 36].

Regardless of the type of ALL, all patients receive intrathecal chemotherapy to prevent CNS disease, consisting of cytarabine alternating with methotrexate.

Obstetric and Gynecologic Considerations

Women diagnosed and treated for acute leukemia face multiple challenges regarding loss of fertility, abnormal uterine bleeding, hormone dysregulation, early menopause, and sexual dysfunction.

Gynecologic Considerations with Acute Leukemia

Cytopenias in Patients with a History of Platinum-Based Therapy

All cytopenias, even mild, should be carefully investigated. Many gynecologic cancer treatments and other cancer treatments utilize platinum-based agents, which are known to cause clonal hematopoiesis (CH), potentially leading to "therapy-related myeloid neoplasms" (a diagnostic qualifier encompassing patients who have had exposure to cytotoxic or radiation therapy for an unrelated neoplasm with development of AML or myelodysplasia). It has been shown that there is a dose-dependent relationship between *PPM1D-* and *TP53*-mutated clonal hematopoiesis and exposure to platinum-based therapy [37]. If a patient has a cytopenia that is out of proportion to her current treatment or chemotherapy cycle a bone marrow biopsy should be performed. Along with evaluation by morphology, cytogenetics, and immunophenotype, it is recommended to also perform next generation sequencing (NGS) searching for leukemia-related mutations. If a mutation is detected with a variant allele frequency (VAF) greater than or equal to 2% that is inconsistent with the patient's gynecologic cancer, then the gynecologic oncologist should be concerned about a clonal cytopenia of undetermined significance (CCUS) or a clonal hematopoiesis of indeterminate potential (CHIP), prompting referral to a hematologist oncologist to rule out development of a myeloid neoplasm [38].

Abnormal Uterine Bleeding (AUB)

Significant thrombocytopenia occurs in almost all patients receiving treatment for acute leukemia. For premenopausal patients, menorrhagia secondary to severe thrombocytopenia is common [39]. Additionally, many patients with acute leukemias develop coagulopathies which could further exacerbate bleeding. Controlling AUB consists of two components: prevention of menses and management of thrombocytopenia and coagulopathies.

There are multiple strategies that can be utilized to prevent menses. One strategy involves suppression of menses prior to initiation of treatment. GnRH analogues, such as leuprolide, prophylactically prevents the onset of menses. This was demonstrated in multiple retrospective analyses in which premenopausal women were administered leuprolide prior to stem cell transplant. Leuprolide, although variable, resulted in 73% to 97% of patients achieving amenorrhea. Timing is important, however, as leuprolide can initially worsen bleeding due to an initial "flare effect" soon after starting therapy. Ideal administration is two weeks to one month before anticipated thrombocytopenia, to avoid a transient two week increase in estradiol levels (Leuprolide "flare") [40–45]. In patients presenting with acute leukemia, thrombocytopenia on presentation is anticipated; therefore, leuprolide is not ideal as monotherapy for the acute management of AUB. For these patients, combining leuprolide with combination oral contraceptive pills or progesterone therapy is beneficial to attenuate the transient rise in estradiol. In subsequent cycles in which thrombocytopenia and the potential for menorrhagia can be anticipated, leuprolide is a viable option. At our institution a treatment algorithm guides the clinicians in the prevention and management of abnormal uterine bleeding (see Chapter 2).

Currently oral contraceptives are the treatment of choice for patients with active uterine bleeding. In the setting of acute AUB, combined oral contraceptives with ethinyl estradiol

(30–35 µg) are started as daily dosing, but can be increased to twice or three times daily if needed for further control [46]. In a randomized controlled trial comparing oral medroxyprogesterone to combined oral contraceptives, both treatments were deemed effective [47].

Data concerning intrauterine devices and implants in patients with acute leukemia are inadequate currently. There are numerous studies documenting the safety of these devices in patients with human immunodeficiency virus; however, at this time there are no published studies concerning these devices in the setting of neutropenia [48–52]. Due to significant risk of bleeding, the placement of these devices should be avoided upon initial presentation in the context of thrombocytopenia. If intrauterine devices are present at the time of diagnosis, a consultation with the gynecological service is recommended to discuss appropriate management.

In a patient with active menstrual bleeding in the context of acute leukemia, appropriate transfusion support and correction of coagulopathy are key factors in controlling the bleeding. At our institution patients are transfused to a platelet count of 50 K/µL. Due to demonstrated efficacy in menorrhagia, the addition of oral tranexamic acid is often considered [53–57]. Studies in patients with menorrhagia have demonstrated the efficacy of tranexamic acid in the reduction of blood loss with recommended dosing of 4 grams/day for 4 to 5 days or until resolution [53]. Finally, coagulation studies allow correction via fresh frozen plasma for elevated PT or aPTT and cryoprecipitate for patients with reduced fibrinogen.

Fertility Considerations

Data regarding infertility in patients treated for acute leukemia are limited. In one study regarding adults who received treatments for acute leukemia as a child, approximately 26% and 29% of patients with ALL and AML developed suspected infertility [58]. Unfortunately, due to the nature of the disease processes, acute leukemias require aggressive treatment soon after diagnosis. Fertility preservation in this population is difficult as treatment is initiated on an emergent basis as soon as the diagnosis is made. Fertility consultations should be offered immediately upon diagnosis for patients of child-bearing age. Additionally, as many medications utilized during therapy can be teratogenic, exclusion of pregnancy is required in reproductive aged women prior to treatment initiation and during therapy.

Fertility preservation includes a diverse range of options: hormone therapies (GnRH agonists), oocyte and embryo cryopreservation, and ovarian tissue cryopreservation with subsequent reimplantation [59]. In a single-center retrospective analysis in which patients with acute leukemia who were eligible for fertility preservation, only one out of 44 female patients was able to undergo ovarian tissue cryopreservation [60]. Additionally, reimplantation of previously cryopreserved ovarian tissue may have the unfortunate consequence of reintroduction of leukemic cells. Cryopreserved ovarian tissue from 12 patients with ALL was obtained, and ten patients had leukemic molecular markers that were monitored. Of these 10, 7 samples were positive for leukemic markers and mice engrafted with samples from these patients developed intraperitoneal leukemic lesions [61].

While there are case reports of successful pregnancy after ovarian tissue cryopreservation, the risk of the procedure needs to be carefully assessed. In the context of cytopenias, general anesthesia and abdominal surgery may pose an unacceptably high risk. In addition, ovarian tissue can contain malignant cells [61–63].

The administration of gonadotropin releasing hormone (GnRH) agonists or antagonists utilized during conditioning therapy has been attempted with patients with lymphoma deriving benefit in fertility preservation; however, patients with leukemia did not derive benefit [64].

Pediatric regimens utilizing lower doses of cyclophosphamide and anthracyclines are being considered for patients between 15 and 45 with ALL. While these regimens are still effective, lower doses of cyclophosphamide and anthracyclines will hopefully reduce long term sequalae such as reproductive and cardiac toxicities [65].

Treatment Induced Gonadotoxicity and Subsequent Premature Ovarian Insufficiency

The risk of premature ovarian insufficiency ("menopause" prior to age 40) is increased in premenopausal women undergoing treatment for acute leukemia, even if stem cell transplantation is not utilized. Unfortunately, the risk is difficult to predict in light of variability in regards to patient age, baseline status of ovarian function, and type of treatment protocol. Premature ovarian insufficiency is associated with sexual dysfunction, infertility, vasomotor symptoms, increased risk of poor bone health, and cardiovascular disease. Even in the setting of regular menses, premenopausal women who have received chemotherapy for leukemia may have compromised ovarian reserve as indicated by decreased antimullerian hormone levels and antral follicle counts [65b]. For a detailed discussion regarding specific chemotherapy agents that impact fertility and options for fertility preservation please refer to Chapter 1. For a detailed discussion regarding diagnosis and sequelae of premature ovarian insufficiency, please see Chapter 5. All reproductive-aged women with a new leukemia cancer diagnosis should be aware of the potential adverse impact on ovarian function.

Acute Leukemia During Pregnancy

The development of acute leukemia in pregnant patients is rare occurring in 1 in 10,000 to 1 in 75,000 pregnancies [66, 67]. Survival in pregnant and nonpregnant patients in the context of standard chemotherapy for AML are similar [68–70]. However, the treatment of patients that are diagnosed with acute leukemias during pregnancy remains challenging and immediate involvement of a maternal fetal medicine specialist is required to decide the best course of action regarding maternal and fetal health (see Chapter 10).

The main factors that dictate the management of pregnant patients with leukemia are gestational age at time of presentation, the placental physiology and the therapeutic agents utilized. Many agents utilized for the treatment of acute leukemia are teratogenic. We will discuss the different stages of pregnancy and the role of the placenta in preventing exposure of the fetus to teratogenic agents.

For the two weeks immediately after conception, the fetal circulation has not yet been established and the fetus is thought to be resistant to teratogens [71–73]. After this narrow window of time, fetal exposure to chemotherapy will often result in spontaneous abortion. Starting the fifth week of gestation, organogenesis begins with damage to the embryo potentially resulting in fetal malformations. As a result, spontaneous abortions and malformations are highest with first trimester chemotherapy exposure [72]. After 12 weeks and as the fetus progresses into the second trimester, the risk of chemotherapy related congenital malformations decreases as most organs have developed. Rates of spontaneous abortions also decrease as the fetus progresses to the second and third trimester [74]. However, the central nervous system continues to develop through the second trimester and intrauterine growth restriction may occur. Finally, as the pregnancy progresses into the third trimester and towards delivery, the timing of chemotherapy administration is important to reduce perinatal myelosuppression [75].

Throughout the pregnancy, the placenta plays an important role in regulating which substances come in contact with the fetus. Substances less than 500 daltons, that are lipophilic and unbound to proteins can cross the placenta; however, larger, hydrophilic, substances bound to proteins have more difficulty entering fetal circulation. Additionally, the placenta has multiple enzymes and transporters that metabolize or excrete potentially teratogenic substances. As a result, small agents that are not metabolized by the placenta can come in direct contact with the fetus, potentially exerting teratogenic effects [76].

Pregnancy Related Considerations in AML

In patients of younger age, intensive therapies utilizing higher doses of cytarabine in combination with an anthracycline are often recommended. While traditional regimens utilize cytarabine with an anthracycline exclusively, other regimens incorporate a nucleotide analogue, usually fludarabine or cladribine, to augment the effect of cytarabine. Cytarabine is a smaller molecule at 243 daltons and is not metabolized by the placenta. Animal models have demonstrated that cytarabine can cross the placental barrier with resulting skeletal defects, retinal dysplasia, and renal changes [77]. Similarly, cladribine and fludarabine have both shown embryo lethality. As a result, these antimetabolites have been categorized as pregnancy risk category D by the FDA (Food and Drug Administration) in which human studies have demonstrated harm to the fetus) [78]. Of these agents, cytarabine has been the most studied. In a literature review conducted by Chang and coll., pregnancy outcomes in 83 mothers with AML were reported. All patients received cytarabine in combination with other agents. Of eight mothers that received induction chemotherapy in the first trimester, there were five births and three miscarriages. Of the 62 fetuses that were exposed in the second trimester, there were 56 births and 6 fetal deaths. Of the 15 fetuses exposed to cytarabine in the third trimester, there were 15 births and no deaths. This pattern demonstrates that there is increased fetal toxicity in the first and second trimester as compared to the third. The most common side effects impacting newborns were anemia and myelosuppression; however, there were cases of acral cyanosis, hyaline membrane disease, meningeal hemorrhage, and growth defects [78]. In a study by Chelghoum et al., 37 pregnant patients who were diagnosed with acute leukemia, with 31 having AML, were studied. All six patients in the first trimester had either spontaneous or therapeutic abortions. Of the 10 patients that received therapy in the second trimester, 6 had therapeutic or spontaneous abortions and 4 had live births. Comparatively, all 15 patients exposed in the third trimester had live births [79]. Of note, in both above studies cytarabine was combined with other agents.

While there are no studies with cladribine or fludarabine in patients who were pregnant with AML, cladribine has been studied in patients with multiple sclerosis (MS) who were pregnant. Data from 10 studies were summarized in a report by Giovannoni and colleagues. In this study, 70 patients with MS were evaluated and compared to a control group consisting of 62 patients who had received placebo. The rates of spontaneous abortions were comparable in the cladribine and the placebo cohorts: 22.4% and 23.8% respectively [80]. However, it must be noted that the doses of cladribine were much lower in the treatment of MS as compared to AML.

Anthracyclines, like nucleotide analogues, are key components of AML treatment regimens; however, there are some notable differences in how they may impact pregnancies. Unlike nucleotide analogues which are smaller molecules, anthracyclines are larger than 500 daltons, hydrophilic, and are metabolized by P-glycoprotein in the placental membrane. As a result, this class of drug does not readily pass the placenta. The transplacental transport of therapy measured via animal models demonstrated that fetal anthracycline levels were much lower than the maternal levels, suggesting limited transport across the placenta. However, idarubicin, unlike other anthracyclines, is lipophilic, small, and not metabolized by P-glycoprotein, hence the current recommendation to avoid idarubicin in pregnancy. Fetal death rate was 6.4% versus 12.5 % for patients who received daunorubicin and cytarabine compared to those who received idarubicin and cytarabine [76].

Hypomethylating agents such as azacytidine and decitabine are at times utilized in lower intensity regimens and or during consolidation treatment. These agents have not been extensively studied in pregnant patients. Hypomethylating agents in rat models demonstrated a reduction in placental weight, a surrogate for trophoblast growth, when compared to placebo [81]. While there are case reports of patients receiving hypomethylating agents and successfully completing pregnancies, there is not enough data to make definitive conclusions concerning the safety of these agents during pregnancy [82–85].

In summary, the underlying aggressive nature of the disease and the intensity of treatment need to be discussed with the patient. If the patient is in the first trimester and if it is legal in the state of practice, the possibility of a therapeutic abortion should be discussed with the patient, due to the higher likelihood of a spontaneous abortion or fetal teratogenicity. Chemotherapeutic regimens appear better tolerated in subsequent trimesters; however, the underlying risks of proceeding with treatment to the mother and the fetus need to be discussed. Both cytarabine and anthracyclines appear to be relatively safe in the second and third trimester. Additionally, in the context of a rapidly increasing white count, the emergent requirement of cytarabine or hydroxyurea and the inherent risks to the fetus needs to be discussed with pregnant patients. Unfortunately, little is known about the impact of hypomethylating agents or targeted inhibitors on pregnant patients. If there is therapeutic necessity for any of these drugs, as an example progression with a new *FLT3* (a targetable mutation with FDA approved inhibitors) mutation, patients must be informed of both the risks of delaying treatment of progressive AML and the potential harm to the fetus of initiating such treatments.

Pregnancy Related Considerations in ALL

ALL regimens involve a multitude of agents typically organized into induction and consolidation followed by either maintenance or stem cell transplant. There are many regimens with varying doses, however the chemotherapies utilized most are: cyclophosphamide, vincristine, anthracyclines, cytarabine, methotrexate, and a steroid (usually dexamethasone). During the induction and consolidation phases, patients will also typically receive intrathecal therapies for CNS prophylaxis [86]. Some patients may require stem cell transplant. Maintenance regimens consist of 6-mercaptopurine, vincristine, methotrexate and prednisone and last up to two years. For patients with Philadelphia positive ALL, the treatment plan will include BCR::ABL1 inhibitors [87–89]. The conjugated antibody and the bispecific antibody, inotuzumab and blinatumomab have been FDA approved for relapsed or refractory disease [34].

The teratogenic potential of cyclophosphamide, an agent that results in DNA cross-linking, has been established and is assigned pregnancy risk category D (FDA category in which there is investigational evidence of potential risk to human fetus). Cyclophosphamide can cross the placental membrane with fetal concentration of the active agent at 25% of that of the mother [90, 91]. Multiple case reports have been published in which patients with systemic lupus erythematosus received cyclophosphamide in the first trimester and delivered infants with congenital anomalies including severe hydrocephalus, radial aplasia, micrognathia, cleft palate, microcephaly, hypotelorism, short palpebral fissure, and hypoplastic digits [92–94].

Methotrexate is a pregnancy category X agent (FDA pregnancy category in which there is significant evidence of risk to fetus and risk of harm to the patient are substantially higher than benefit). It inhibits dihydrofolate reductase and prevents thymidine synthesis [95]. Numerous case reports and case series demonstrate that methotrexate exposure, especially in the first trimester, results in congenital malformations, particularly neural tube defects (hydrocephaly, anencephaly, spina bifida), skeletal abnormalities (absent ossification, micrognathia, syndactyly, hypoplastic digits), and congenital heart defects (atrial or ventricular septal defects and tetralogy of Fallot). Malformations have also been reported in patients that received low dose methotrexate at 7.5 mg per week. While uncommon, third trimester exposure has resulted in intellectual disability. At this time, methotrexate is contraindicated at any time during pregnancy [96–99].

While therapies like cyclophosphamide and methotrexate have accumulated clinical data in pregnancy, vincristine has limited clinical data concerning teratogenicity. Animal models have suggested that fetuses can develop malformations after exposure to vincristine, hence it is assigned a pregnancy risk category of D [100, 101]. Congenital anomalies have been noted in offspring exposed to vincristine, albeit in combination treatment regimens [102]. Conversely, data from patients who received R-CHOP for non-Hodgkins lymphoma suggest that this combination, including vincristine, is safe starting in the second trimester [103].

Information regarding tyrosine kinase inhibitor use in pregnancy is limited to the CML setting with a few case reports in ALL. Imatinib and dasatinib are both pregnancy risk category D with reports in patients with CML describing congenital abnormalities [104, 105].

There is exceedingly limited data available concerning blinatumomab or inotuzumab in pregnant patients. Rituximab, a CD20 antibody utilized in some ALL regimens, is pregnancy risk category C with limited data suggesting that it could be safe in pregnancy. In a study of 231 pregnant patients that received rituximab for lymphoma, autoimmune hemolytic anemia, thrombotic thrombocytopenia and idiopathic thrombocytopenia purpura, most patients had uncomplicated live births. Notably, first trimester pregnancy loss was higher than in the general population at 21% (normal 10–15%); however, some patients received rituximab in the context of combination regimens and the underlying rate of first trimester pregnancy loss in autoimmune conditions is unknown [106].

While there are fewer reported cases of pregnancy with ALL as compared to AML, retrospective analyses do provide some consideration regarding ALL management. Chelghoum et al. reported on three pregnant women with ALL that chose to continue their pregnancies. One was diagnosed late in the second trimester and two were diagnosed in early-third trimester. All three women delivered prematurely: two via c-section and one by spontaneous vaginal delivery [79]. In a subset analysis of a large cooperative study (RALL-2009 trial), 15 patients were either enrolled while pregnant or were found to be pregnant while on trial. Induction occurred in two separate phases. In the first phase, patients received steroids, daunorubicin, and vincristine. In the second phase, patients received cyclophosphamide, cytarabine, and 6- mercaptopurine. Methotrexate and L-asparaginase were delayed until after delivery. Intrathecal therapies were limited to cytarabine. Three patients diagnosed in the first trimester elected to terminate the pregnancy. Three patients diagnosed in the third trimester proceeded with delivery prior to treatment. Of the remaining nine patients, five were in the second trimester and four were in the third trimester. Four patients received one cycle and five patients received multiple rounds of therapy. All 9 patients delivered at or after 35 weeks and all 9 children developed normally, however 4 had neonatal cerebral ischemia, 1 was small for gestational age, and 1 infant had a strangulated small bowel obstruction 2 weeks after delivery [107].

These studies in conjunction with characteristics of individual drugs provide guidance on how to approach these challenging patients. For pregnant patients with AML, medical abortions in the first trimester should be considered as this expands the drugs available for use including methotrexate, antibody therapy, and tyrosine kinase inhibitors. Steroids, cyclophosphamide, daunorubicin, and cytarabine appear safe in the second trimester. However, it must be noted that most patients in these limited series were treated later in the second trimester. Discussions with patients must include shared decision making including a multidisciplinary team (often including social workers and ethic consultants). If a patient has relapsed ALL or is refractory to therapy, discussion regarding the addition of tyrosine kinase inhibitors in Philadelphia positive disease, antibodies (rituximab, blinatumomab, inotuzumab), or other chemotherapies (methotrexate and asparaginase) must take place.

Case Resolution

This 19-year-old female presented with significant bleeding and peripheral blood counts consistent with an acute leukemia. The first priority was to stabilize her with blood product support. As she had significant uterine bleeding, the gynecology team was consulted and combined oral contraceptives were initiated. In order to administer her first injection of leuprolide 11.25 mg intramuscular, she was transfused platelets to achieve a count > 50 K. She was initially treated with dexamethasone for cytoreduction. A screening β-hCG was negative. Bone marrow assessment was performed and was consistent with B-ALL. Within five days of presentation, the patient started induction therapy with a combination chemotherapy regimen. The oncofertility team was consulted, however fertility preservation was declined secondary to the need to expedite therapy. Uterine bleeding resolved a week after admission. The patient subsequently obtained remission with count recovery after the first cycle. After completion of eight cycles of therapy, she completed a maintenance regimen and has maintained a disease-free remission.

Take Home Points: Acute Leukemia

- Acute leukemias are defined by blasts >20% and are fatal without treatment.
- The foundation of management of acute abnormal uterine bleeding in acute leukemias is controlling the bleeding and cessation of menses.
- Oral contraceptives (if no contraindications) and leuprolide are the treatment of choice for abnormal uterine bleeding. (See Chapter 2).
- Fertility consultations should be offered to women of child-bearing age upon diagnosis of acute leukemia.

- Outcomes regarding response to therapy and survival are similar in pregnant and nonpregnant women.
- Fetal mortality and defects are highest with chemotherapy exposure in the first trimester, as opposed to second or third trimester exposures.
- Discussions with pregnant patients with acute leukemia must include shared decision making and involvement of a multidisciplinary team.
- In the context of relapsed or refractory acute leukemia that may benefit from novel therapies, the risks and benefits of these therapies must be discussed with the patient regarding ongoing pregnancy and risk of infertility.
- Even if stem cell transplantation is not utilized, women undergoing treatment for acute leukemia are at risk for diminished ovarian reserve and premature ovarian insufficiency.

Chronic Leukemias

Chronic Myeloid Leukemia

Case Presentation

A 56-year-old female with obesity presented to her primary care physician with complaints of fatigue, weight loss, early satiety, and intermittent abdominal pain. She was found to have a white blood cell count of 56.0 K/μL (normal range: 4.5 to 11.0 x 10^9/L), differential showed an increased number of neutrophils, hemoglobin 13.5 g/dL (normal range: 12.0–16.0 g/dL), and platelet count of 120 K/μL (normal range 140–440 K/μL). Physical exam was unremarkable except for marked splenomegaly and mild hepatomegaly. The physician ordered a liver and hepatitis panel which was unremarkable and an abdominal ultrasound that showed no hepatomegaly. However, the exam was notable for an enlarged spleen with a maximum diameter of 17 cm. What is the next best step?

Pathophysiology and Epidemiology of CML

CML is a hematologic malignancy that arises from uncontrolled proliferation of a clonal population of a mature myeloid cell. It is associated with the fusion of two genes, the BCR and ABL1 gene, resulting from the translocation between chromosome 22 and chromosome 9. This translocation causes the presence of an abnormal chromosome 22, known as the Philadelphia-chromosome. The BCR::ABL1 fusion gene codes for a deregulated tyrosine kinase protein. The disease has a slight male predominance, it is usually diagnosed during the sixth decade of life and the estimated annual incidence is 0.7–1.0/100,000 persons [108, 109].

Presentation and Evaluation of CML

CML can present in three different phases at diagnosis: chronic phase (most common in ~85% of new cases), accelerated phase, and blast phase. Chronic phase CML (CML-CP) is by far the most common form of the disease with an indolently progressing leukocytosis with marked neutrophilia generally found incidentally on routine blood work. However, CML-CP can later progress to accelerated or blast phase. The World Health Organization (WHO) defines accelerated phase CML (CML-AP) as 10–19% blasts in the bone marrow, while blast phase CML (CML-BP) will have more than 20% blasts or present with extramedullary

Table 18.1 Phases of chronic myeloid leukemia

Chronic Phase	Accelerated Phase	Blast Phase
≤10% blasts	10–19% blasts	≥20% blasts +/- extramedullary disease
Asymptomatic to mild symptoms ↔ Progressive/constitutional symptoms		

disease (Table 18.1). Patients can be asymptomatic. However, common symptoms include fatigue, night sweats, and signs and symptoms relating to splenomegaly, including left upper quadrant pain, abdominal fullness, early satiety, and weight loss. Patients can also have bleeding or thrombosis due to platelet dysfunction. The accelerated and blast phases can present similar to acute leukemia with constitutional symptoms including fever, chills, night sweats, infections, headaches, and bone pain [110]. The diagnosis is confirmed with a bone marrow biopsy which should include cytogenetic testing, fluorescence in situ hybridization (FISH), and/or polymerase chain reaction (PCR) testing to confirm the Philadelphia chromosome (BCR::ABL1 fusion gene). The bone marrow biopsy will also show granulocytic hyperplasia meaning an increased production of granulocytes.

Management of CML

Leukoreduction with hydroxyurea may be needed on initial diagnosis. However, the mainstay of treatment for CML is an oral tyrosine kinase inhibitor (TKI), since the Philadelphia chromosome BCR::ABL1 fusion gene codes for a deregulated tyrosine kinase protein. Selection of a specific TKI is based on the patient's comorbidities, phase of CML, and cost. There are several second-generation TKIs that have improved side effect profiles with less incidence of nausea, vomiting, diarrhea, myalgias, bone pain, fatigue, and rashes. Response to therapy is monitored, first, by improvement in the patient's symptoms and normalization of peripheral blood counts (complete hematologic response [CHR]) and, second, by cytomolecular testing with well-defined milestones in terms of achieving disappearance (complete cytogenetic response) of the Philadelphia chromosome and reduction of the percentage of BCR::ABL1 with the goal of achieving a at least a major molecular response (BCR::ABL1/ABL 0.1% of baseline) [111, 112]. Effective therapy can prevent the progression to accelerated and blast phase and significantly improve survival. Patients with CML treated with TKIs have more than an 80% overall survival probability [113].

Patient should continue to follow with their primary care provider for appropriate age-related health maintenance. Comorbidities can limit selection and tolerability of certain TKIs.

Special Considerations in CML

Females who are pregnant or trying to conceive should not use TKIs as they are teratogenic. Alternative therapies or a treatment-free interval should be discussed prior to pregnancy depending on the current status of their CML and their response to treatment. Reliable methods of contraception are recommended during therapy for reproductive aged women. For women wanting to conceive while unable to discontinue CML-directed therapy, a consultation regarding use of a gestational carrier is recommended [114]. While more studies are needed, retrospective data indicates that the risk of teratogenicity is much lower for male partners on TKI therapy.

Case Resolution

She was referred to a hematologist/oncologist and presented 3 weeks later to her consult with laboratory evaluation showing a white blood cell count of 186.0 K/μL (normal range: 4.5 to 11.0 x 10^9/L), absolute neutrophil count 78.00 K/μL (normal range: 1.70–7.30 K/μL), hemoglobin 11.7 g/dL (normal range: 12.0–16.0 g/dL), and platelets of 90 K/μL (normal range 140–440 K/μL) with 2% peripheral blasts. She was admitted to the hospital for a diagnostic bone marrow biopsy and leukoreduction. The bone marrow biopsy showed 4% blasts with granulocytic hyperplasia. The BCR::ABL1 fusion transcript was detected by PCR to a level greater than 100%. She was initiated on hydroxyurea for leukoreduction for several days while admitted and, subsequently, started on therapy with the TKI dasatinib. At her six-month follow-up appointment, her laboratory parameters had normalized, and PCR detected the BCR::ABL1 at 8.6% or CML – chronic phase (CP).

Take Home Points: CML

- Most chronic phase CML patients are asymptomatic but diagnosed incidentally on routine blood work.
- The diagnosis of CML requires the presence of the Philadelphia chromosome (BCR-ABL gene fusion).
- The BCR-ABL1 oncogene codes for a dysregulated tyrosine kinase protein, so the mainstay of treatment for CML is with tyrosine kinase inhibitors (TKIs).
- Individuals with chronic phase CML are expected to achieve a near-normal life expectancy with treatment.

Chronic Lymphocytic Leukemia

Case Presentation

A 65-year-old female with past medical history of hypertension and hyperlipidemia presented to her primary care provider (PCP) for routine follow-up. Her labs showed a white blood cell count of 30,000 K/μL (normal range: 4.5 to 11.0 x 109/L), absolute lymphocyte count 23.0 K/μL (normal range: 1.00–4.80 K/μL), hemoglobin 13.2 g/dL (normal range: 12.0–16.0 g/dL), and platelets of 160 K/μL (normal range: 140–440 K/μL). Physical exam revealed palpable supraclavicular and cervical adenopathy but no splenomegaly. She was referred to a hematologist/oncologist who diagnosed her with CLL based on flow cytometry from peripheral blood showing a monoclonal B cell population. A computerized tomography (CT) scan of the neck, chest, abdomen, and pelvis revealed diffusely enlarged cervical, supraclavicular, and mediastinal adenopathy but no splenomegaly. Since she was asymptomatic, active surveillance was recommended and a follow-up in three months was planned since her prognostic testing revealed an unmutated immunoglobulin heavy chain variable region, (IGHV), del17 by FISH testing and cytogenetics, and an *ATM* mutation by next generation sequencing (NGS).

Pathophysiology and Epidemiology of CLL

CLL and small lymphocytic lymphoma (SLL) are malignancies of mature B cells. B cells are a key part of our immune system. Healthy, functioning B cells produce antibodies and antigen-presenting cells that will bind to foreign cells such as toxins or viruses to eliminate them. Thus, a malignancy of B cells will also cause immune system dysfunction.

Together CLL and SLL are the most prevalent forms of leukemia in Western countries, accounting for 25 to 35% of all leukemias in the United States. CLL and SLL have identical pathologic and immunophenotypic features. The key difference is that in CLL there is a significant number of abnormal lymphocytes found in peripheral blood circulation as well as involvement of bone marrow and lymphoid tissues, while in SLL, the malignant cells primarily aggregate in lymphoid tissues (WHO classification) [115]. The median age at diagnosis of CLL is 71 years, it has a male predominance with a male:female ratio of 2:1 and most of the patients are white [116]. Although CLL is incurable, some patients will have an indolent clinical course with a subgroup never requiring CLL-directed therapy. Other patients, however, can have rapidly progressive disease and require immediate treatment. CLL/SLL can transform into an aggressive type of non-Hodgkin lymphoma (NHL), termed Richter's syndrome with an approximate incidence rate of 0.5% per year [117, 118].

Evaluation and Prognosis in CLL

The clinical presentation of CLL is typically characterized by an elevated lymphocyte count, enlarged lymphadenopathy and in more advanced disease, with systemic symptoms such as fevers, night sweats, fatigue, and weight loss. Progressive infiltration of bone marrow and splenomegaly can lead to cytopenias. Enlarged lymph nodes may become symptomatic or impair adjacent organ function. Treatment for CLL is not usually initiated until these signs and symptoms of advanced disease (worsening anemia/thrombocytopenia, splenomegaly, or lymph node burden) are present, as defined by the International Working Group on CLL (IWCLL) guidelines. Autoimmune hemolytic anemia and other autoimmune manifestations can occur in about 10% of cases. CLL can be staged using the Rai or Binet Staging systems (Table 18.2) [119]. The Table 18.2 includes disease characteristics and median survival if left untreated.

Diagnosis is based on laboratory findings, including a CBC with differential demonstrating lymphocytosis and, in some patients, hypogammaglobinemia and elevated beta-2 microglobulinemia and lactate dehydrogenase (LDH). Immunophenotype by flow cytometry from peripheral blood, bone marrow aspirate, or lymph node biopsy should show a monoclonal B cell population with co-expression of CD19 and CD5 antigens, CD20 (diminished), CD23 expression and light chain restriction. Differential diagnosis of lymphocytosis includes infectious causes and other hematologic lymphoid malignancies that should be excluded. Imaging should be performed based on clinical presentation to assess for the presence of lymphadenopathy and splenomegaly [115].

Prognostic factors in CLL help predict clinical behavior and guide treatment selection. Prognostic markers that are widely available and frequently used include: status of the immunoglobulin heavy chain variable region (IGHV) gene mutation, cytogenetic abnormalities by FISH, CpG-stimulated karyotyping, cell surface markers expression, beta2microglobulin, LDH serum levels and gene mutations by whole genome sequencing. High risk prognostic factors include unmutated IGHV, deletion of chromosome 17 del [17], and the presence of *TP53* abnormalities, *BCL2*, or *NOTCH1* mutations on NGS. Whereas mutated IGHV and deletion of chromosome 13 by FISH are associated with more indolent disease course [120, 121]. See Table 18.3.

Table 18.2 Staging systems for CLL

Staging System	Stage	Characteristics	Median Survival (months)
Rai Staging System	Rai Stage 0	Lymphocytosis	150
	Rai Stage I	Lymphocytosis + enlarged lymph nodes	101
	Rai Stage II	Lymphocytosis + enlarged spleen	71
	Rai Stage III	Lymphocytosis + anemia (Hemoglobin <11 g/dL)	19
	Rai Stage IV	Lymphocytosis + thrombocytopenia (platelets <100 K/μL)	19
Binet Staging System	Binet Stage A (corresponds to Rai Stages 0, I, & II)	<3 areas of lymphoid tissue enlarged without anemia or thrombocytopenia	N/A
	Binet Stage B (corresponds to Rai Stages I & II)	≥3 areas of lymphoid tissue enlarged without anemia or thrombocytopenia	N/A
	Binet Stage C (corresponds to Rai Stages III & IV)	Anemia +/- thrombocytopenia	N/A

Table 18.3 Prognostic indicators for CLL

Favorable Prognostic Indicators	Unfavorable Prognostic Indicators
IGHV mutated	IGHV un-mutated
del[13]	del[17]
	NGS showing *TP53*, *BCL2*, or *NOTCH1*

Management of CLL

A unique feature of CLL is that not all patients require treatment at the time of diagnosis. Patients without symptoms and Rai stage 0-II or Binet stages A and B are candidates for a period of "watch and wait" since the disease can have an indolent course. Furthermore, early intervention trials have not resulted in a survival advantage. A period of observation can, therefore, be appropriate for lower risk patients while also optimizing health maintenance. The length of this period of observation without treatment can vary from months to years depending on the patient's prognostic factors. For patients requiring treatment, the most used therapies for CLL are treatment with first or second-generation Bruton's Tyrosine Kinase (BTK) inhibitors or treatment with the BCL2 inhibitor venetoclax, either as monotherapy or in combination with monoclonal antibodies against CD20. Antiviral prophylaxis with acyclovir or valacyclovir is frequently used for patients undergoing treatment, whereas antibiotic and antifungal prophylaxis are only used in special circumstances.

While these medications are generally well tolerated, they can cause immunosuppression and increase the risk of bleeding. In female patients, increased bleeding can present as abnormal uterine bleeding due to thrombocytopenia and/or treatment with agents that can interact with platelet function, such as BTK inhibitors. Maintaining adequate platelet levels with transfusions and holding therapy prior to and immediately following surgical procedures are ways to mitigate bleeding risk. However, therapies should not be frequently held (i.e. during monthly menstruation) as patients can develop resistance mutations to therapy. Menstrual suppression with leuprolide combined with OCP or progestins, or continuous OCP or progestins alone can be considered after consultation with a gynecologist (see Chapter 2).

Life expectancy in CLL when adjusted for sex and age has been increasing in the last 30 years due to improvements in therapy. However, further population-based studies are needed to determine if CLL infers a normal or decreased life expectancy [122].

Special Considerations in CLL

Patients with CLL should follow routine age-appropriate health maintenance, including annual exams with their primary care provider, mammograms, and colonoscopy. They should be especially vigilant with (at least) annual full body skin cancer surveys based on their Fitzpatrick skin level since patients with CLL are at increased risk of skin cancer. CLL, even in the absence of current therapy, can cause immunosuppression, hence patients should also remain up to date on immunizations including the Herpes Zoster and pneumococcal vaccines [123].

It should be noted that approximately 2–9% of patients with CLL can evolve to a more aggressive histology, most commonly diffuse large B cell lymphoma (DLBCL), via a process called Richter's transformation (RT). Patients who develop lymphoma via Richter's transformation have poor prognoses compared to patient who develop DLBCL without the antecedent CLL/SLL. Less than 20% of patients with Richter's transformation achieve long-term survival with chemoimmunotherapy [124]. However, both autologous and allogeneic stem cell transplants have shown durable remissions in nearly half of patients with DLBCL Richter's transformation [125]. Risk factors for Richter's transformation have yet to be conclusively identified but are theorized to include younger age at initial diagnosis, multiple prior lines of therapy, advanced stage of disease at diagnosis, and certain genetic mutations such as TP53 and NOTCH1 [123].

Patients with CLL can be at increased risk for infections due to their immune dysfunction regardless of current treatment. The female patient will be at a particularly increased risk of UTIs which should be promptly treated with appropriate antibiotic therapy. Urine cultures should be obtained for recurrent infections [126]. In addition, patients with CLL may not mount an appropriate immune response to certain vaccines due to their impaired immune function, this includes the human papillomavirus (HPV) vaccine. Patients should be encouraged to stay current with cervical cancer screening [126].

Inguinal lymph nodes can be present in patients with CLL so should be included on the differential of a female patient with enlarged inguinal lymphadenopathy and a full body lymph node survey should be performed. In patients with gynecologic cancer, a biopsy can be performed to differentiate the involvement of lymph nodes by CLL versus a gynecologic cancer.

Therapies for CLL are considered teratogenic and should be avoided during conception and pregnancy.

Reliable methods of contraception are recommended during therapy for reproductive aged women. If pregnancy is desired, a discussion of the risks and benefits of temporarily discontinuing treatment prior to conception and during pregnancy should take place [127].

Case Resolution

The patient returns three months later for her CLL follow-up visit. Laboratory results reveal a WBC of 41.0 K/μL (normal range: 4.5 to 11.0 x 109/L), Absolute Lymphocyte Count 33.0 K/μL (normal range: 1.00–4.80 K/μL), Hemoglobin 12.5 g/dL (normal range: 12.0–16.0 g/dL), and Platelets of 71 K/μL μL (normal range 140–440 K/μL). She also complains of early satiety. Physical exam is significant for enlarging cervical, supraclavicular and inguinal lymph nodes and a palpable spleen 3 cm below the left costal margin. Her physician reports that her disease has progressed from Rai Stage I to Rai Stage IV and therapy is initiated.

Take Home Points: CLL

- Lymphocytosis, lymphadenopathy, splenomegaly, anemia, and thrombocytopenia are common symptoms of CLL.
- CLL can progress at a variable pace. In fact, a small subgroup of patients may never require therapy.
- Patients with CLL should be encouraged to stay current with cervical cancer screening and they may not mount an appropriate immune response to human papillomavirus vaccination.
- The three main areas of therapy for CLL are BTK inhibitors, the BCL2 inhibitor venetoclax, and monoclonal antibodies against CD20.
- CLL patients will have some degree of immunosuppression due to both the nature of their disease and CLL-directed therapies.
- Therapies for CLL are considered teratogenic and should be avoided during conception and pregnancy. Reliable methods of contraception are recommended during therapy for reproductive aged women.
- Development of a Richter's transformation is seen in approximately 2–9% of patients with CLL and confers a poor prognosis.

References

1. Pinho S., Frenette P. S. Haematopoietic stem cell activity and interactions with the niche. *Nature Reviews Molecular Cell Biology*. 2019;**20**(5):303–20.

2. Brown P. A., Shah B., Advani A., et al. Acute Lymphoblastic Leukemia, Version 2.2021, NCCN Clinical Practice Guidelines in

Oncology. *J Natl Compr Canc Netw.* 2021;**19**(9):1079–109.

3. Döhner H., Wei A. H., Appelbaum F. R., et al. Diagnosis and management of AML in adults: 2022 recommendations from an international expert panel on behalf of the ELN. *Blood.* 2022;**140**(12):1345–77.

4. Stelmach P., Trumpp A. Leukemic stem cells and therapy resistance in acute myeloid leukemia. *Haematologica.* 2023;**108**(2):353–66.

5. Brunner A. M., Graubert T. A. Chapter 58 – Pathobiology of Acute Myeloid Leukemia. In: Hoffman R., Benz E. J., Silberstein L. E., et al., editors. *Hematology* (7th ed.). Elsevier; 2018. pp. 913–23.

6. Burns M., Armstrong S. A., Gutierrez A. Chapter 64 – Pathobiology of Acute Lymphoblastic Leukemia. In: Hoffman R., Benz E. J., Silberstein L. E., et al., editors. *Hematology* (7th ed.). Elsevier; 2018. pp. 1005–19.e11.

7. Inaba H., Mullighan C. G. Pediatric acute lymphoblastic leukemia. *Haematologica.* 2020;**105**(11):2524–39.

8. Swaminathan S., Klemm L., Park E., et al. Mechanisms of clonal evolution in childhood acute lymphoblastic leukemia. *Nature Immunology.* 2015;**16**(7):766–74.

9. Surveillance, Epidemiology, and End Results (SEER) *Program Populations (1969-2020).* National Cancer Institute. 2022.

10. Sasaki K., Jabbour E., Short N. J., et al. Acute lymphoblastic leukemia: A population-based study of outcome in the United States based on the surveillance, epidemiology, and end results (SEER) database, 1980–2017. *American Journal of Hematology.* 2021;**96**(6):650–8.

11. Faderl S., Kantarjian H. M. Chapter 59 – Clinical Manifestations and Treatment of Acute Myeloid Leukemia. In: Hoffman R., Benz E. J., Silberstein L. E. et al., editors. *Hematology* (7th ed.) Elsevier; 2018. pp. 924–43.

12. de Haas V., Ismaila N., Advani A., et al. Initial diagnostic work-up of acute leukemia: ASCO Clinical Practice Guideline Endorsement of the College of American Pathologists and American Society of Hematology Guideline. *Journal of Clinical Oncology.* 2018;**37**(3):239–53.

13. Dinner S., Gurbuxani S., Jain N., Stock W. Chapter 66 – Acute Lymphoblastic Leukemia in Adults. In: Hoffman R., Benz E. J., Silberstein L. E. et al., editors. *Hematology* (7th ed.) Elsevier; 2018. Pp. 1029–54.e2.

14. Porcu P., Cripe L. D., Ng E. W., et al. Hyperleukocytic leukemias and leukostasis: A review of pathophysiology, clinical presentation and management. *Leukemia & Lymphoma.* 2000;**39** (1–2):1–18.

15. Macaron W., Sargsyan Z., Short N. J. Hyperleukocytosis and leukostasis in acute and chronic leukemias. *Leukemia & Lymphoma.* 2022;**63**(8):1780–91.

16. Dinnel J., Moore B. L., Skiver B. M., Bose P. Rasburicase in the management of tumor lysis: An evidence-based review of its place in therapy. *Core Evid.* 2015;**10**:23–38.

17. Kahlon D. K., Dinand V., Yadav S. P., Sachdeva A. Sevelamer is an effective drug in treating hyperphosphatemia due to tumor lysis syndrome in children: A developing world experience. *Indian J Hematol Blood Transfus.* 2016;**32**(1):78–82.

18. Bewersdorf J. P., Zeidan A. M. Hyperleukocytosis and leukostasis in acute myeloid leukemia: Can a better understanding of the underlying molecular pathophysiology lead to novel treatments? *Cells.* 2020;**9**(10).

19. Kadia T. M., Ravandi F., Borthakur G., et al. Long-term results of low-intensity chemotherapy with clofarabine or cladribine combined with low-dose cytarabine alternating with decitabine in older patients with newly diagnosed acute myeloid leukemia. *American Journal of Hematology.* 2021;**96**(8):914–24.

20. DiNardo C. D., Jonas B. A., Pullarkat V., et al. Azacitidine and venetoclax in previously untreated acute myeloid leukemia. *New England Journal of Medicine.* 2020;**383**(7):617–29.

21. Senapati J., Kadia T. M. Which FLT3 inhibitor for treatment of AML? *Curr Treat Options Oncol.* 2022;**23**(3):359–80.

22. DiNardo C. D., Stein E. M., de Botton S., et al. Durable remissions with ivosidenib in IDH1-mutated relapsed or refractory AML. *New England Journal of Medicine.* 2018;**378**(25):2386–98.

23. Venugopal S., Takahashi K., Daver N., et al. Efficacy and safety of enasidenib and azacitidine combination in patients with IDH2 mutated acute myeloid leukemia and not eligible for intensive chemotherapy. *Blood Cancer Journal.* 2022;**12**(1):10.

24. Desikan S. P., Daver N., DiNardo C., et al. Resistance to targeted therapies: Delving into FLT3 and IDH. *Blood Cancer J.* 2022;**12**(6):91.

25. Short N. J., Kantarjian H., Jabbour E. Optimizing the treatment of acute lymphoblastic leukemia in younger and older adults: New drugs and evolving paradigms. *Leukemia.* 2021;**35**(11):3044–58.

26. Jain N., Roberts K. G., Jabbour E., et al. Ph-like acute lymphoblastic leukemia: A high-risk subtype in adults. *Blood.* 2017;**129**(5):572–81.

27. Foà R., Chiaretti S. Philadelphia chromosome–positive acute lymphoblastic leukemia. *New England Journal of Medicine.* 2022;**386**(25):2399–411.

28. Thomas X. Philadelphia chromosome-positive leukemia stem cells in acute lymphoblastic leukemia and tyrosine kinase inhibitor therapy. *World J Stem Cells.* 2012;**4**(6):44–52.

29. Desikan S. P., Senapati J., Jabbour E., et al. Outcomes of adult patients with relapsed/refractory CRLF2 rearranged B-cell acute lymphoblastic leukemia. *Am J Hematol.* 2023;**98**(6):E142–e4.

30. Jabbour E., Patel K., Jain N., et al. Impact of Philadelphia chromosome-like alterations on efficacy and safety of blinatumomab in adults with relapsed/refractory acute lymphoblastic leukemia: A post hoc analysis from the phase 3 TOWER study.

31. Jabbour E., Sasaki K., Short N. J., et al. Long-term follow-up of salvage therapy using a combination of inotuzumab ozogamicin and mini–hyper-CVD with or without blinatumomab in relapsed/refractory Philadelphia chromosome-negative acute lymphoblastic leukemia. *Cancer.* 2021;**127**(12):2025–38.

32. Jabbour E. J., Sasaki K., Ravandi F., et al. Inotuzumab ozogamicin in combination with low-intensity chemotherapy (mini-HCVD) with or without blinatumomab versus standard intensive chemotherapy (HCVAD) as frontline therapy for older patients with Philadelphia chromosome-negative acute lymphoblastic leukemia: A propensity score analysis. *Cancer.* 2019;**125**(15):2579–86.

33. Kantarjian H., Haddad F. G., Jain N., et al. Results of salvage therapy with mini-hyper-CVD and inotuzumab ozogamicin with or without blinatumomab in pre-B acute lymphoblastic leukemia. *Journal of Hematology & Oncology.* 2023;**16**(1):44.

34. Kantarjian H., Jabbour E. Incorporating immunotherapy into the treatment strategies of B-cell adult acute lymphoblastic leukemia: The role of blinatumomab and inotuzumab ozogamicin. *American Society of Clinical Oncology Educational Book.* 2018 (38):574–8.

35. Cohen M. H., Johnson J. R., Justice R., Pazdur R. FDA drug approval summary: nelarabine (Arranon) for the treatment of T-cell lymphoblastic leukemia/lymphoma. *Oncologist.* 2008;**13**(6):709–14.

36. Pullarkat V. A., Lacayo N. J., Jabbour E., et al. Venetoclax and navitoclax in combination with chemotherapy in patients with relapsed or refractory acute lymphoblastic leukemia and lymphoblastic lymphoma. *Cancer Discov.* 2021;**11**(6):1440–53.

37. Takahashi K. Untangling the relationship between clonal hematopoiesis and ovarian cancer therapies. *J Natl Cancer Inst.* 2022;**114**(4):487–8.

Note: reference 30 concludes with "*American Journal of Hematology.* 2021;**96**(10):E379–E83." and reference 35 appears accordingly.

38. DeZern A. E., Malcovati L., Ebert B. L. CHIP, CCUS, and other acronyms: Definition, implications, and impact on practice. *Am Soc Clin Oncol Educ Book.* 2019;**39**:400–10.

39. Nebgen D. R., Rhodes H. E., Hartman C., Munsell M. F., Lu K. H. Abnormal uterine bleeding as the presenting symptom of hematologic cancer. *Obstet Gynecol.* 2016;**128**(2):357–63.

40. Purisch S. E., Shanis D., Zerbe C., et al. Management of uterine bleeding during hematopoietic stem cell transplantation. *Obstet Gynecol.* 2013;**121**(2 Pt 2 Suppl 1):424–7.

41. Quaas A. M., Ginsburg E. S. Prevention and treatment of uterine bleeding in hematologic malignancy. *Eur J Obstet Gynecol Reprod Biol.* 2007;**134**(1):3–8.

42. Ghalie R., Porter C., Radwanska E., et al. Prevention of hypermenorrhea with leuprolide in premenopausal women undergoing bone marrow transplantation. *Am J Hematol.* 1993;**42**(4):350–3.

43. Laufer M. R., Townsend N. L., Parsons K. E., et al. Inducing amenorrhea during bone marrow transplantation. A pilot study of leuprolide acetate. *J Reprod Med.* 1997;**42**(9):537–41.

44. Chiusolo P., Salutari P., Sica S., et al. Luteinizing hormone-releasing hormone analogue: Leuprorelin acetate for the prevention of menstrual bleeding in premenopausal women undergoing stem cell transplantation. *Bone Marrow Transplant.* 1998;**21**(8):821–3.

45. Lhommé C., Brault P., Bourhis J. H., et al. Prevention of menstruation with leuprorelin (GnRH agonist) in women undergoing myelosuppressive chemotherapy or radiochemotherapy for hematological malignancies: A pilot study. *Leuk Lymphoma.* 2001;**42**(5):1033–41.

46. Chang K., Merideth M. A., Stratton P. Hormone use for therapeutic amenorrhea and contraception during hematopoietic cell transplantation. *Obstet Gynecol.* 2015;**126**(4):779–84.

47. Munro M. G., Mainor N., Basu R., Brisinger M., Barreda L. Oral medroxyprogesterone acetate and combination oral contraceptives for acute uterine bleeding: A randomized controlled trial. *Obstet Gynecol.* 2006;**108**(4):924–9.

48. Kakaire O., Byamugisha J. K., Tumwesigye N. M, Gemzell-Danielsson K. Intrauterine contraception among women living with human immunodeficiency virus: A randomized controlled trial. *Obstet Gynecol.* 2015;**126**(5):928–34.

49. Kakaire O., Tumwesigye N. M., Byamugisha J. K., Gemzell-Danielsson K. Acceptability of intrauterine contraception among women living with human immunodeficiency virus: A randomised clinical trial. *Eur J Contracept Reprod Health Care.* 2016;**21**(3):220–6.

50. Achilles S. L., Creinin M. D., Stoner K. A., et al. Changes in genital tract immune cell populations after initiation of intrauterine contraception. *Am J Obstet Gynecol.* 2014;**211**(5):489.e1–9.

51. Morrison C. S., Hofmeyr G. J., Thomas K. K., et al. Effects of depot medroxyprogesterone acetate, copper intrauterine devices, and levonorgestrel implants on early HIV disease progression. *AIDS Res Hum Retroviruses.* 2020;**36**(8):632–40.

52. Stringer E. M., Kaseba C., Levy J., et al. A randomized trial of the intrauterine contraceptive device vs hormonal contraception in women who are infected with the human immunodeficiency virus. *Am J Obstet Gynecol.* 2007;**197**(2):144. e1–8.

53. Bonnar J., Sheppard B. L. Treatment of menorrhagia during menstruation: Randomised controlled trial of ethamsylate, mefenamic acid, and tranexamic acid. *BMJ.* 1996;**313**(7057):579–82.

54. Kriplani A., Kulshrestha V., Agarwal N., Diwakar S. Role of tranexamic acid in management of dysfunctional uterine bleeding in comparison with medroxyprogesterone acetate. *J Obstet Gynaecol.* 2006;**26**(7):673–8.

55. Kouides P. A., Byams V. R., Philipp C. S., et al. Multisite management study of

menorrhagia with abnormal laboratory haemostasis: A prospective crossover study of intranasal desmopressin and oral tranexamic acid. *Br J Haematol.* 2009;**145**(2):212–20.

56. Lukes A. S., Freeman E. W., Van Drie D., Baker J., Adomako T. L. Safety of tranexamic acid in women with heavy menstrual bleeding: An open-label extension study. *Womens Health (Lond).* 2011;**7**(5):591–8.

57. Preston J. T., Cameron I. T., Adams E. J., Smith S. K. Comparative study of tranexamic acid and norethisterone in the treatment of ovulatory menorrhagia. *Br J Obstet Gynaecol.* 1995;**102**(5):401–6.

58. Balcerek M., Reinmuth S., Hohmann C., Keil T., Borgmann-Staudt A. Suspected infertility after treatment for leukemia and solid tumors in childhood and adolescence. *Dtsch Arztebl Int.* 2012;**109**(7):126–31.

59. Jadoul P., Kim S. S. Fertility considerations in young women with hematological malignancies. *J Assist Reprod Genet.* 2012;**29**(6):479–87.

60. Noetzli J., Voruz S., Wunder D., et al. Ten-year single-centre experience in fertility preservation of 459 patients suffering from acute leukaemia. *Br J Haematol.* 2019;**184**(6):969–73.

61. Dolmans M. M., Marinescu C., Saussoy P., et al. Reimplantation of cryopreserved ovarian tissue from patients with acute lymphoblastic leukemia is potentially unsafe. *Blood.* 2010;**116**(16):2908–14.

62. Rodriguez-Wallberg K. A., Milenkovic M., Papaikonomou K., et al. Successful pregnancies after transplantation of ovarian tissue retrieved and cryopreserved at time of childhood acute lymphoblastic leukemia: A case report. *Haematologica.* 2021;**106**(10):2783–7.

63. Salama M., Anazodo A., Woodruff T. K. Preserving fertility in female patients with hematological malignancies: A multidisciplinary oncofertility approach. *Annals of Oncology.* 2019;**30**(11):1760–75.

64. Blumenfeld Z., Patel B., Leiba R., Zuckerman T. Gonadotropin-releasing hormone agonist may minimize premature ovarian failure in young women undergoing autologous stem cell transplantation. *Fertil Steril.* 2012;**98**(5):1266–70.e1.

65. Rytting M. E., Jabbour E. J., O'Brien S. M., Kantarjian H. M. Acute lymphoblastic leukemia in adolescents and young adults. *Cancer.* 2017;**123**(13):2398–403.

66. Rossi B. V., Missmer S., Correia K. F., Wadleigh M., Ginsburg E. S. Ovarian reserve in women treated for acute lymphocytic leukemia or acute myeloid leukemia with chemotherapy, but not stem cell transplantation. *ISRN Oncol.* 2012;**2012**:956190.

67. McCormick A., Peterson E. Cancer in pregnancy. *Obstetrics and Gynecology Clinics of North America.* 2018;**45**(2):187–200.

68. Shapira T., Pereg D., Lishner M. How I treat acute and chronic leukemia in pregnancy. *Blood Rev.* 2008;**22**(5):247–59.

69. Chelghoum Y., Vey N., Raffoux E., et al. Acute leukemia during pregnancy. *Cancer.* 2005;**104**(1):110–17.

70. Fracchiolla N. S., Sciumè M., Dambrosi F., et al. Acute myeloid leukemia and pregnancy: Clinical experience from a single center and a review of the literature. *BMC Cancer.* 2017;**17**(1):442.

71. Wang P., Yang Z., Shan M., et al. Maternal and fetal outcomes of acute leukemia in pregnancy: A retrospective study of 52 patients. *Front Oncol.* 2021;**11**:803994.

72. Arnon J., Meirow D., Lewis-Roness H., Ornoy A. Genetic and teratogenic effects of cancer treatments on gametes and embryos. *Hum Reprod Update.* 2001;**7**(4):394–403.

73. Buekers T. E., Lallas T. A. Chemotherapy in pregnancy. *Obstet Gynecol Clin North Am.* 1998;**25**(2):323–9.

74. Haram K., Mortensen J. H., Myking O., et al. Early development of the human placenta and pregnancy complications. *The Journal of Maternal-Fetal & Neonatal Medicine.* 2020;**33**(20):3538–45.

75. Elshazzly M., Lopez M. J., Reddy V., Caban O. *Embryology, Central Nervous*

System. StatPearls. Treasure Island (FL): StatPearls Publishing Copyright © 2023, StatPearls Publishing LLC.; 2023.

76. Esposito S., Tenconi R., Preti V., Groppali E., Principi N. Chemotherapy against cancer during pregnancy: A systematic review on neonatal outcomes. *Medicine (Baltimore).* 2016;**95**(38):e4899.

77. Framarino-Dei-Malatesta M., Sammartino P., Napoli A. Does anthracycline-based chemotherapy in pregnant women with cancer offer safe cardiac and neurodevelopmental outcomes for the developing fetus? *BMC Cancer.* 2017;**17**(1):777.

78. Triarico S., Rivetti S., Capozza M. A., et al. Transplacental passage and fetal effects of antineoplastic treatment during pregnancy. *Cancer (Basel).* 2022;**14**(13).

79. Chang A., Patel S. Treatment of acute myeloid leukemia during pregnancy. *Annals of Pharmacotherapy.* 2015;**49**(1):48–68.

80. Chelghoum Y., Vey N., Raffoux E., et al. Acute leukemia during pregnancy: A report on 37 patients and a review of the literature. *Cancer.* 2005;**104**(1):110–17.

81. Giovannoni G., Galazka A., Schick R., et al. Pregnancy outcomes during the clinical development program of cladribine in multiple sclerosis: An integrated analysis of safety. *Drug Saf.* 2020;**43**(7):635–43.

82. Serman L., Vlahović M., Sijan M., et al. The impact of 5-azacytidine on placental weight, glycoprotein pattern and proliferating cell nuclear antigen expression in rat placenta. *Placenta.* 2007;**28**(8–9):803–11.

83. Karagiannis P., Alsdorf W., Tallarek A. C., et al. Treatment of refractory acute myeloid leukaemia during pregnancy with venetoclax, high-dose cytarabine and mitoxantrone. *Br J Haematol.* 2021;**192**(2):e60–e3.

84. Alrajhi A. M., Alhazzani S. A., Alajaji N. M., et al. The use of 5-azacytidine in pregnant patient with Acute Myeloid Leukemia (AML): A case report. *BMC Pregnancy Childbirth.* 2019;**19**(1):394.

85. Lee B. S., Sathar J., Ong T. C. Teratogenic effect of decitabine in a pregnant patient with acute myeloid leukemia: A case report. *Hematol Transfus Cell Ther.* 2022;**44**(3):429–32.

86. Mahdi A. J., Gosrani D., Chakraborty M., et al. Successful molecular targeted treatment of AML in pregnancy with Azacitidine and Sorafenib with no adverse fetal outcomes. *Br J Haematol.* 2018;**180**(4):603–4.

87. Terwilliger T., Abdul-Hay M. Acute lymphoblastic leukemia: A comprehensive review and 2017 update. *Blood Cancer J.* 2017;**7**(6):e577.

88. Ravandi F., O'Brien S. M., Cortes J. E., et al. Long-term follow-up of a phase 2 study of chemotherapy plus dasatinib for the initial treatment of patients with Philadelphia chromosome-positive acute lymphoblastic leukemia. *Cancer.* 2015;**121**(23):4158–64.

89. Daver N., Thomas D., Ravandi F., et al. Final report of a phase II study of imatinib mesylate with hyper-CVAD for the front-line treatment of adult patients with Philadelphia chromosome-positive acute lymphoblastic leukemia. *Haematologica.* 2015;**100**(5):653–61.

90. Jabbour E., Short N. J., Ravandi F., et al. Combination of hyper-CVAD with ponatinib as first-line therapy for patients with Philadelphia chromosome-positive acute lymphoblastic leukaemia: Long-term follow-up of a single-centre, phase 2 study. *Lancet Haematol.* 2018;**5**(12):e618–e27.

91. Meirow D., Epstein M., Lewis H., Nugent D., Gosden R. G. Administration of cyclophosphamide at different stages of follicular maturation in mice: effects on reproductive performance and fetal malformations. *Human Reproduction.* 2001;**16**(4):632–7.

92. D'Incalci M., Sessa C., Colombo N., et al. Transplacental passage of cyclophosphamide. *Cancer Treat Rep.* 1982;**66**(8):1681–2.

93. Rengasamy P. Congenital malformations attributed to prenatal exposure to cyclophosphamide. *Anticancer Agents Med Chem.* 2017;**17**(9):1211–27.

94. Vaux K. K., Kahole N. C. O., Jones K. L. Cyclophosphamide, methotrexate, and cytarabine embropathy: Is apoptosis the common pathway? *Birth Defects Research Part A: Clinical and Molecular Teratology.* 2003;**67**(6):403–8.

95. Paladini D., Vassallo M., D'Armiento M. R., Cianciaruso B., Martinelli P. Prenatal detection of multiple fetal anomalies following inadvertent exposure to cyclophosphamide in the first trimester of pregnancy. *Birth Defects Res A Clin Mol Teratol.* 2004;**70**(2):99–100.

96. Rushworth D., Mathews A., Alpert A., Cooper L. J. Dihydrofolate reductase and thymidylate synthase transgenes resistant to methotrexate interact to permit novel transgene regulation. *J Biol Chem.* 2015;**290**(38):22970–6.

97. Lloyd M. E., Carr M., McElhatton P., Hall G. M., Hughes R. A. The effects of methotrexate on pregnancy, fertility and lactation. *Qjm.* 1999;**92**(10):551–63.

98. Hyoun S. C., Običan S. G., Scialli A. R. Teratogen update: methotrexate. *Birth Defects Res A Clin Mol Teratol.* 2012;**94**(4):187–207.

99. Dawson A. L., Riehle-Colarusso T., Reefhuis J., Arena J. F. Maternal exposure to methotrexate and birth defects: A population-based study. *Am J Med Genet A.* 2014;**164a**(9):2212–16.

100. Verberne E. A., de Haan E., van Tintelen J. P., Lindhout D., van Haelst M. M. Fetal methotrexate syndrome: A systematic review of case reports. *Reprod Toxicol.* 2019;**87**:125–39.

101. Courtney K. D., Valerio D. A. Teratology in the Macaca mulatta. *Teratology.* 1968;**1**(2):163–72.

102. Joneja M., Ungthavorn S. Teratogenic effects of vincristine in three lines of mice. *Teratology.* 1969;**2**(3):235–40.

103. Mulvihill J. J., McKeen E. A., Rosner F., Zarrabi M. H. Pregnancy outcome in cancer patients. Experience in a large cooperative group. *Cancer.* 1987;**60**(5):1143–50.

104. Brenner B., Avivi I., Lishner M. Haematological cancer in pregnancy. *Lancet.* 2012;**379**(9815):580–7.

105. Cortes J. E., Abruzzese E., Chelysheva E., et al. The impact of dasatinib on pregnancy outcomes. *Am J Hematol.* 2015;**90**(12):1111–15.

106. Madabhavi I., Sarkar M., Modi M., Kadakol N. Pregnancy outcomes in chronic myeloid leukemia: A single center experience. *J Glob Oncol.* 2019;**5**:1–11.

107. Chakravarty E. F., Murray E. R., Kelman A., Farmer P. Pregnancy outcomes after maternal exposure to rituximab. *Blood.* 2011;**117**(5):1499–506.

108. Parovichnikova E. N., Troitskaya V. V., Gavrilina O. A., et al. The outcome of Ph-negative acute lymphoblastic leukemia presenting during pregnancy and treated on the Russian prospective multicenter trial RALL-2009. *Leuk Res.* 2021;**104**:106536.

109. Sampaio M. M., Santos M. L. C., Marques H. S., et al. Chronic myeloid leukemia-from the Philadelphia chromosome to specific target drugs: A literature review. *World J Clin Oncol.* 2021;**12**(2):69–94.

110. Faderl S., Talpaz M., Estrov Z., et al. The biology of chronic myeloid leukemia. *New England Journal of Medicine.* 1999;**341**(3):164–72.

111. Jabbour E., Kantarjian H. Chronic myeloid leukemia: 2020 update on diagnosis, therapy and monitoring. *American Journal of Hematology.* 2020;**95**(6):691–709.

112. Haznedaroğlu İ. C., Kuzu I., İlhan O. WHO 2016 definition of chronic myeloid leukemia and tyrosine kinase inhibitors. *Turk J Haematol.* 2020;**37**(1):42–7.

113. Deininger M. W., Shah N. P., Altman J. K., et al. Chronic myeloid leukemia, Version 2.2021, NCCN Clinical Practice Guidelines in Oncology. *J Natl Compr Canc Netw.* 2020;**18**(10):1385–415.

114. Pfirrmann M., Baccarani M., Saussele S., et al. Prognosis of long-term survival considering disease-specific death in

patients with chronic myeloid leukemia. *Leukemia.* 2016;**30**(1):48–56.

115. Rambhatla A., Strug M. R., De Paredes J. G., Cordoba Munoz M. I., Thakur M. Fertility considerations in targeted biologic therapy with tyrosine kinase inhibitors: A review. *J Assist Reprod Genet.* 2021;**38**(8):1897–908.

116. Hernández J. A., Land K. J., McKenna R. W. Leukemias, myeloma, and other lymphoreticular neoplasms. *Cancer.* 1995;**75**(1 Suppl):381–94.

117. Siegel R. L., Miller K. D., Wagle N. S., Jemal A. Cancer statistics, 2023. *CA Cancer J Clin.* 2023;**73**(1):17–48.

118. Burger J. A. Treatment of chronic lymphocytic leukemia. *New England Journal of Medicine.* 2020;**383**(5):460–73.

119. Vitale C., Ferrajoli A. Richter syndrome in chronic lymphocytic leukemia. *Curr Hematol Malig Rep.* 2016;**11**(1):43–51.

120. Binet J. L., Leporrier M., Dighiero G., et al. A clinical staging system for chronic lymphocytic leukemia: Prognostic significance. *Cancer.* 1977;**40**(2):855–64.

121. Tausch E., Schneider C., Robrecht S., et al. Prognostic and predictive impact of genetic markers in patients with CLL treated with obinutuzumab and venetoclax. *Blood.* 2020;**135**(26):2402–12.

122. Döhner H., Stilgenbauer S., Benner A., et al. Genomic aberrations and survival in chronic lymphocytic leukemia. *N Engl J Med.* 2000;**343**(26):1910–16.

123. van der Straten L., Maas C., Levin M. D., et al. Long-term trends in the loss in expectation of life after a diagnosis of chronic lymphocytic leukemia: A population-based study in the Netherlands, 1989–2018. *Blood Cancer J.* 2022;**12**(4):72.

124. Sinisalo M., Aittoniemi J., Käyhty H., Vilpo J. Vaccination against infections in chronic lymphocytic leukemia. *Leuk Lymphoma.* 2003;**44**(4):649–52.

125. Thompson P. A., Siddiqi T. Treatment of Richter's syndrome. *Hematology.* 2022;**2022**(1):329–36.

126. Herrera A. F., Ahn K. W., Litovich C., et al. Autologous and allogeneic hematopoietic cell transplantation for diffuse large B-cell lymphoma-type Richter syndrome. *Blood Adv.* 2021;**5**(18):3528–39.

127. Rivera D., Ferrajoli A. Managing the risk of infection in chronic lymphocytic leukemia in the era of new therapies. *Curr Oncol Rep.* 2022;**24**(8):1003–14.

128. Zhang C., Tian B. Nonclinical safety assessment of zanubrutinib: A novel irreversible BTK inhibitor. *International Journal of Toxicology.* 2020;**39**(3):232–40.

Chapter 19

Lung Cancer

Maria Azhar, Lara Bashoura, and Saadia A. Faiz

Case Presentation

S.K. is a 48-year-old woman who underwent imaging after a motor vehicle accident and was incidentally found to have a 1.6 cm right upper lobe nodule without any mediastinal lymphadenopathy. She underwent CT guided biopsy which revealed adenocarcinoma of the lung which was EGFR (epidermal growth factor receptor) positive. She underwent right upper lobectomy with negative margins and no visceral, pleural, or lymphatic involvement, and classified as Stage IA. She was treated with a tyrosine kinase inhibitor (afatinib) and was doing well with close surveillance. However, two years later she was found to have a 2 cm right lower paratracheal lymph node. Bronchoscopy with endobronchial ultrasound transbronchial needle aspiration revealed lung adenocarcinoma with PD-L1 (programmed cell death-ligand 1) expression level of 50%. MRI of the brain was negative for metastatic disease. What could be considered next?

Introduction

Although previously considered a disease predominantly affecting men, lung cancer has emerged as a significant malignancy in women [1, 2]. A dramatic increase in lung cancer incidence and mortality ensued in women when tobacco use garnered social acceptance after World War II [3]. In fact, by 1987 lung cancer surpassed breast cancer as the leading cause of cancer death in American women. Although tobacco use is a major contributor, lung cancer is more common in never-smoking women than men, thus highlighting potential sex-based differences influencing carcinogenesis [4]. The landscape of lung cancer has been evolving with earlier detection and improved survival, so recognition of the salient features of diagnosis, treatment options and sequelae are paramount to those taking care of this cohort. The purpose of this chapter is to provide an overview of lung cancer, highlight gender differences, and review therapy-related sequelae and its impact on the patient's health.

Epidemiology

Lung cancer is the third most common cancer in women worldwide (after breast and colorectal), and the second leading cause of cancer death in women [5]. Within developing countries, the proportion of lung cancer incidence among women increased from 31% to 50% over the past 20 years [6]. Although shifts in the global distribution of lung cancer reflects the temporal change of tobacco use, an estimated 15% of lung cancer in men and 53% in women are attributable to factors other than tobacco use, so lung cancer in never smokers is also a significant concern in women [6].

Within the United States, lung cancer is the second most common cancer but the leading cause of cancer-related death in women. In general, the age-standardized incidence and mortality associated with lung cancer has been lower in women than among men; however recent data reveals a higher lung cancer incidence in young women compared to young men in the United States [7]. According to the cancer registry data from 1995 to 2014, the incidence of lung cancer in non-Hispanic whites in the 30- to 49-year age group is higher in women than men. The reversal in trends is not accounted for by gender differences in smoking behaviors. Within the white 40- to 44- year age group, female-to-male incidence rate ratio increased from 0.88 (95% confidence interval (CI), 0.84 to 0.92) during the 1995 to 1999 period to 1.17 (95% CI, 1.11 to 1.23) during the 2010 to 2014 period [7]. Thus, the incidence rates in women are increasing at an alarming rate and in younger age, so lung cancer may present in women during years of reproductive potential.

Lung Cancer Classification

Lung cancer is a heterogenous disease with a wide spectrum of clinical and pathologic findings. It is broadly classified into non-small cell lung cancer (NSCLC, 85% of total diagnosis) and small cell lung cancer (SCLC, 15% of total diagnosis). The two most common histological subtypes of NSCLC are adenocarcinomas followed by squamous-cell carcinomas [1]. All histological types are associated with smoking, but SCLC and squamous cell carcinoma are more commonly associated with smoking than adenocarcinoma [6]. Lung cancer in never smokers occurs consistently more frequently in women than men, and this characteristic is noted globally [6]. Adenocarcinoma is the most common lung cancer histological subtype among never smokers, often with driver mutations which allow targeted therapies.

SCLC has similar rates between men and women (14.8% in women and 13% among men). Case control studies have reported a higher odds ratio of SCLC among women smokers than squamous cell carcinoma [2]. However, female gender was reported to be a favorable prognostic factor in SCLC [8].

Risk Factors

There are many risk factors for lung cancer. Although tobacco use is the main risk factor in those that smoke, women never-smokers have a unique set of risk factors compared to men (Figure 19.1). Risk factors for lung cancer in never smokers include environmental tobacco smoke, residential radon, cooking oil vapors, indoor coal and wood burning, genetic factors, and viral infections [6, 9].

- *Cigarette smoke.* More preventable deaths are associated with lung cancer than any other malignancy, with cigarette smoking as the main culprit [10]. Public health efforts have helped decrease tobacco use in many countries, but the rate of decline for both smoking rates and lung cancer incidence occurred later and has been slower in women compared to men [9]. Several thousand chemicals including over 60 identified as carcinogens are contained in cigarette smoke, and the most potent carcinogens are the polycyclic aromatic hydrocarbons (PAH, such as benzo[a]pyrene and the tobacco-specific nitrosamine) [6]. It remains controversial whether female smokers have higher susceptibility to tobacco carcinogens when compared to male counterparts with studies showing mixed results [4].

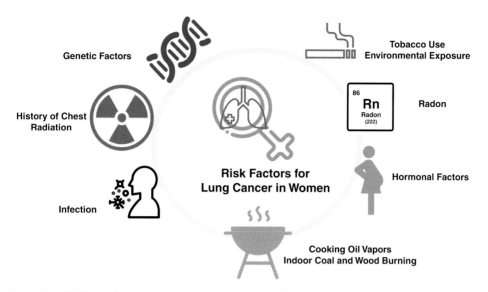

Genetic Factors

Tobacco Use
Environmental Exposure

History of Chest
Radiation

86
Rn
Radon
(222)

Radon

Infection

Risk Factors for
Lung Cancer in Women

Hormonal Factors

Cooking Oil Vapors
Indoor Coal and Wood Burning

Figure 19.1 Risk factors for lung cancer in women. Sex-based differences in lung cancer exist, and compared to men, women are more likely to be diagnosed at a younger age and with adenocarcinoma, lack a smoking history or have a genetic predisposition. Specific environmental exposures also increase their risk for lung cancer.

- *Environmental tobacco smoke (ETS).* ETS includes a mixture of sidestream smoke released by the burning of the cigarette or smoking device as well as the mainstream smoke exhaled by the smoker. Analyses of data pooled from larger studies as well as by the United States Environmental Protection Agency supports spousal and workplace exposure to ETS is associated with a 20 to 25% excess risk of lung cancer [6].
- *Radon.* Radon is a colorless odorless naturally occurring radioactive soil gas produced from the process of radioactive decay of radium, thorium and uranium in soils and rocks throughout the world. The "radon progeny," the active products that radon degrades into, can attach themselves to particulate matter in the air, adhere to the respiratory epithelium and further decay and directly damage DNA [6]. Residential radon exposure is associated with a small increase in the risk of lung cancer for both smokers and never smokers, but the risk for lung cancer is greater among smokers due to a synergy in lung cancer development [3].
- *Cooking oil vapors, indoor coal and wood burning.* Exposure to cooking oil fumes is associated with a significantly increased risk of lung cancer in never smokers based on epidemiological studies from mainland China, Taiwan, and Singapore [6]. Use of indoor coal burning without adequate ventilation in China is another risk factor, with one study demonstrating that women who cook with coal have five times increased odds of developing lung cancer [9]. Lack of ventilation and cooking practices compound inhalation of fume from volatile substances containing mutagenic and carcinogenic PAHs [11].
- *Hormonal factors.* The higher proportion of lung cancer in female never smokers suggests that hormones could play a role in lung cancer [2–4, 6]. Estrogen plus

progestin therapy is associated with an increased risk of lung cancer in large randomized studies [12–14]. A lower incidence of lung cancer has been reported in patients with breast cancer treated with tamoxifen [2]. On a biological level, the exact role of estrogen and its involvement with lung cancer remains unclear, but several possible mechanisms may include its role in: gene regulation; modulation of gene expression in tumor cells; direct carcinogenesis via formation of DNA adducts; growth factor gene activation; stimulating angiogenesis; and accelerating metabolism of smoking-related carcinogens [2]. Progesterone inhibits cell proliferation, induces apoptosis in NSCLC and inhibits cell migration. A meta-analysis of 66 studies with 20 distinct reproductive factors concluded higher parity (OR 0.83, 95% CI 0.72–0.96), longer menstrual cycle length (OR 0.79, 95% CI 0.65–0.96) and older age at first birth (OR 0.85, 95% CI 0.74–0.98) were associated with a lower risk of overall lung cancer [15]. Nonnatural menopause (after surgical intervention) was associated with a higher lung cancer risk (OR 1.52, 95% CI 1.25–1.86) [15]. Further studies on the role of estrogen and other hormones in lung cancer are needed, for investigations have yielded conflicting results thus their role remains controversial [6].

- *Genetic factors.* The genetic inheritance of lung cancer includes family history and possibly involves low-penetrance oncogenes or tumor suppressor genes [6]. This may also alter cancer susceptibility including metabolism of carcinogens, DNA repair, apoptosis, angiogenesis, and other features of cancer [11]. Women are also at an increased risk of developing lung cancer with a driver mutation including epidermal growth factor receptor (EGFR), anaplastic lymphoma kinase (ALK), and Kirsten RAt Sarcoma mutations (KRAS) [9].

- *Infection.* The two most common infectious risk factors for pathogenesis of lung cancer includes human papillomavirus (HPV) and mycobacterial infections (both tuberculosis and non-tuberculosis mycobacterium) [9].

   o HPV has been associated with several different cancer notably cervical cancer, but it may also play a role in lung cancer. High-risk HPV may lead to genomic instability that can lead to malignant transformation. A large meta-analysis reported a 24.5% worldwide incidence of HPV in lung cancer [3]. Significant geographic variation likely exists especially in women never smokers in Asia [3, 16]. A study from Taiwan noted women never smokers with lung cancer had a significantly higher prevalence of infection with oncogenic variants (HPV16 and HPV18), and they proposed this accounted for their country's high lung cancer prevalence and death rates [17]. Within the United States, HPV infection rates in tumors have been lower and associated with squamous cell as opposed to adenocarcinoma [3]. The risk of chronic scarring to the lung from granulomatous disease may also potentially contribute [9].

   o One meta-analysis suggested a 1.7-fold increased relative risk of developing lung cancer in patients with a history of tuberculosis, although it is not clear if this is higher in women [9]. Smaller studies have also suggested an association of non-tuberculosis mycobacteria in woman with lung cancer, and they hypothesized the chronic inflammatory microenvironment may predispose to the development of lung cancer [2].

- **Radiation therapy.** Exposure to radiation to the chest from previous cancer treatments (Hodgkin's lymphoma, breast cancer) have a higher risk of developing a second primary lung cancer, and incidence is increased in smokers [9, 18, 19].

Lung Cancer Screening

Lung cancer screening, in at risk individuals, has now become standard of care across the United States. The goal of lung cancer screening is to identify malignant disease at an early curable stage. Both the United States' National Lung Screening Trial (NLST) and the European Dutch-Belgian Randomized Lung Cancer Screening Trial (NELSON) are large randomized trials which have demonstrated clear reduction in lung cancer mortality with low-dose computed tomography (CT) of the chest for screening [1]. Annual low-dose CT was recommended by the US Preventive Services Task Force (USPSTF) in 2021 for patients aged 50 to 80 years with a 20 pack-year history of smoking within 15 years (similar to previous recommendation) [20]. The mortality benefit from low-dose CT screening has been shown to be more favorable in women than in men (39%–61% versus 26%, respectively) [2]. Unfortunately current screening guidelines only capture smoking history and therefore may underestimate the risk in women and minorities [9, 21].

Lung Cancer Symptoms

Symptoms of lung cancer are often nonspecific, and typically manifest in advanced stage of disease. In a large consecutive cohort of NSCLC treated over 25 years, the most common symptoms were: cough (54.7%); dyspnea (45.3%); tumor pain (37.8%); weight loss (35.9%); night sweats (20.0%); incidental diagnosis (18.3%); hemoptysis (17.4%); pneumonia (15.9%); fever (10.4); neurologic symptoms (9.6%); symptoms suspicious for tuberculosis (7.4%); and hoarseness (4.0%) [22]. Coughing is common among smokers, however, change in character of cough, both in frequency and strength, should raise suspicion. Chest pain can be attributed to involvement of the pleura, chest wall or mediastinum. Dyspnea is also frequently seen with NSCLC and may develop due to other manifestations of disease including malignant pleural effusion, central airway obstruction with tumor, or post-obstructive pneumonia due to tracheobronchial abnormalities. Other processes including superior vena cava syndrome, pulmonary embolism or other paraneoplastic syndromes can herald lung cancer diagnosis.

Imaging Studies in Lung Cancer

Imaging studies often detect findings concerning for lung cancer (Figure 19.2). A pulmonary nodule may be the initial finding, especially in those undergoing low-dose CT chest. A pulmonary nodule is defined as a discrete radiographic opacity that is less than 3 cm, surrounded by normal lung parenchyma, and a pulmonary mass is larger than 3 cm. Other findings including mediastinal adenopathy, pleural effusion, nonresolving parenchymal abnormality or pleural nodularity can also signal possible malignant disease.

Chest imaging is often the initial work up for nonspecific respiratory symptoms or it may be part of initial screening tool in at risk individuals. Chest radiograph is frequently the most common initial imaging modality ordered in primary care setting for various respiratory symptoms. However, this imaging modality lacks the resolution to differentiate between benign and malignant disease processes and has low sensitivity to rule out lung cancer.

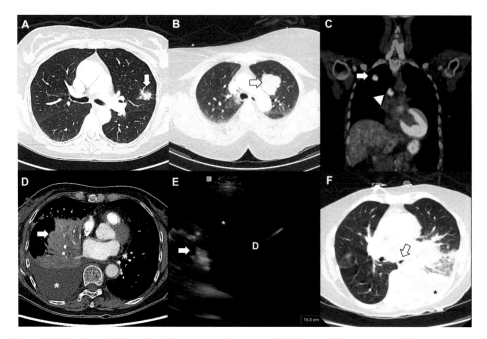

Figure 19.2 Radiographic imaging of lung cancer in women. Clinical stage of lung cancer guides treatment and prognosis. A) Stage Ia (cT1b, cN0, M0) in a woman recently diagnosed with left intraductal breast carcinoma found to have incidental partially solid left upper lobe nodule 1.8 cm without lymphadenopathy consistent with adenocarcinoma. B) Stage IIa (cT2b, cN0, cM0) with 4.2 cm mass in the left upper lobe and an 8 mm right hilar lymph node with biopsy positive for poorly differentiated adenocarcinoma. C) Stage IIIA adenocarcinoma of the lung with a hypermetabolic spiculated lesion in the right upper lobe (2.5 cm, SUV of 8.7, arrow) and hypermetabolic right lower paratracheal node (1.5 cm, SUV of 10.5, arrowhead). D) Metastatic lung adenocarcinoma with increasing soft tissue density in the right perihilar region with adjacent nodal metastatic disease, new obstruction of the bronchi to the middle lobe and right lower lobe (arrow), and new moderate right pleural effusion (asterisk). E) Metastatic lung cancer with pleural effusion (asterisk), lung mass (arrow) and diaphragm (D) on ultrasound F) Metastatic lung cancer with narrowing of left mainstem bronchus (arrow) due to extrinsic compression and left pleural effusion (asterisk)

CT chest is the standard imaging modality for patients with suspected lung cancer. Often CT chest will be obtained for another reason, and incidental findings are concerning for malignant disease. It can also be part of the initial screening process, prompted by evaluation of symptoms or follow up after an abnormality on initial scan. Other features concerning for malignant disease include: lesions with an irregular or spiculated border; thick-walled cavity without infection; nodules containing a solid component and a less dense ground-glass component; pure ground glass lesions; or multiple nodules or masses. Once a lung nodule is suspected as malignant on CT chest, the next steps involve both obtaining the tissue diagnosis and categorizing the stage of lung cancer.

Fluorodeoxyglucose-PET (FDG-PET) is used with CT for staging lung cancer. It has a reported sensitivity of 58–94% and specificity of 76–96% for mediastinal lesions greater than 1 cm [1]. FDG-PET with CT allows identification of involved mediastinal lymph nodes as well as distant metastases, so it allows reliable identification of patients with resectable disease and minimization of unnecessary thoracotomies.

Biomarker Testing

Over the past decade, predictive biomarkers (Figure 19.3) have allowed new therapeutic options with targeted therapy and immunotherapy. These targetable, driver mutations are rare, yet important to identify in NSCLC as the impact of targeted drug therapy changes outcomes, both in terms of survival and prognosis.

- **Tumor PD-L1 expression.** Tumor programmed death-ligand 1 (PD-L1) expression should be assessed in all patients with newly diagnosed advanced NSCLC, to help guide therapy for the potential use of immune checkpoint inhibitors (ICIs) [1]. Immunohistochemistry is used to detect PD-L1 expression by tumor cells.

- **Molecular markers.** Current guidelines also recommend molecular testing for all newly diagnosed advanced lung adenocarcinoma [23, 24]. Oncogenic driver mutations are mutations in cellular pathways that result in tumor proliferation and confer survival advantages to the tumor cells while maintaining clonal preservation. Somatic activating mutation in EGFR was the first to be identified as a driver mutation in NSCLCs leading to utilization of tyrosine-kinase inhibitors (TKIs) as an important targeted therapy [25]. These targetable, driver mutations are rare, yet important to identify in NSCLC as the impact of targeted drug therapy changes outcomes, both in terms of survival and prognosis. It is now known that driver mutations can be found in any lung cancer histology, irrespective of age and smoking history, and identification allows for targeted and personalized therapy.

- **Liquid biopsies.** Tumor sampling or liquid biopsy (blood sample analyzed for circulating tumor DNA by sequencing) for mutation testing should be performed both at the initial diagnosis as well as with disease progression. Of note, the frequency of NSCLC mutations varies by patient population. It is estimated that about 50% of non-squamous NSCLC patients have some form of driver mutation [1].

Lung Cancer Staging

The tumor, node, metastasis (TNM) staging system for lung cancer (Figure 19.3) allows characterization of the extent of disease [26]. It is an internationally accepted system, facilitates communication among medical providers, guides treatment decisions, and serves as a prognostic indicator.

Prognostic factors associated with good outcomes include good performance status, early stage of cancer, younger age, female gender, and absence of weight loss. Women are diagnosed at a less-advanced stage of disease and have better treatment outcomes [27]. Other factors include presence or absence of symptoms related to site of metastasis, absence of smoking, smoking cessation, and NSCLC subtype (squamous slightly better than non-squamous histology) [28–30]. Predictive factors along with use of biomarker data can help identify appropriate treatment. Significant expression in tumor of PD-L1 predicts benefits of ICI therapy [31]. In advanced NSCLC treated with platinum-based chemotherapy, absence of KRAS gene mutation and low or no expression of the DNA excision repair protein ERCC1 is associated with improved prognosis. In a meta-analysis, KRAS mutations were associated with poorer survival, particularly in adenocarcinoma [32].

Female gender also accounts for a survival benefit and better treatment outcomes among women at all cancer stages, particularly, in local stage disease. In a retrospective, single institution study from Japan, women with adenocarcinoma demonstrated the most

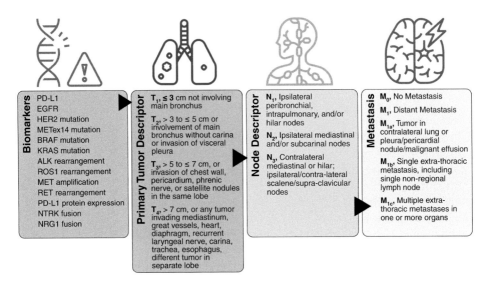

Figure 19.3 Lung cancer biomarkers and staging [1, 26]. In clinical practice, lung cancer staging along with molecular features of the tumor guide prognostic assessment and treatment selections. Lung cancer staging includes primary tumor description (T) [T_x, Tumor in sputum but not in imaging or bronchoscopy; T_0, No evidence of tumor; T_{is}, Carcinoma in situ], node descriptor (N) and metastasis descriptor (M).

*Legend for figure: Abbreviations: EGFR: epidermal growth factor receptor; HER2: human epidermal growth factor receptor 2; ALK: anaplastic lymphoma kinase; PCR: polymerase chain reaction; PD-L1: programmed cell death-ligand 1; NTRK: neurotrophic receptor tyrosine kinase; NRG1: neuregulin 1.

favorable prognosis. Furthermore, multivariate analysis of the same study confirmed female gender to be an independent, favorable prognostic factor [33]. Overall, multiple studies have shown that women with any lung cancer have higher survival rates than men [33–35]. The etiology for survival benefit in women remains elusive, but potentially could include superior baseline health, less comorbidities or plausibly hormonal influences, however, further studies are needed.

Treatment of Lung Cancer

Treatments for lung cancer are tailored based on tumor history, mutation testing, immune inhibition, performance status, and comorbid conditions.

- **Surgery.** The treatment of choice for clinical stage I and stage II disease, without evidence of mediastinal involvement is surgical resection. Selection of surgery often requires absence of tumor involvement of the mediastinal lymph nodes with either mediastinoscopy or endobronchial ultrasound guided transbronchial needle aspiration (EBUS-TBNA). Surgery may also be an option in some Stage IIIA (T3N1) if technically feasible after negative mediastinal staging [1]. Although clinical staging is performed prior to surgical resection, patients are restaged pathologically following surgery, and further interventions including radiation and other adjuvant treatments may be warranted. Stage I disease has a 5-year survival rate of about 80% while stage II and III have a 5-year survival of 13–60% [1].

o Lobectomy continues to be the gold standard in the treatment for stage I and stage II NSCLC. Video-assisted thoracoscopic surgery (VATS) is a minimal invasive approach for surgical resection, and it has been associated with better postoperative recovery, less pain, shorter length of stay, improved quality of life, and similar long term oncological outcomes compared to thoracotomy [36, 37]. Postoperative percent predicted forced expiratory volume in 1 second (FEV1) or diffusion capacity less than 40% predict higher morbidity and mortality following lung cancer surgery.

o Women are likely to be diagnosed with lung cancer at an earlier stage than men, and sex-based differences in outcomes of surgical resection demonstrate lower 30-day mortality, less post-operative complication and better survival rates [9].

- **Radiotherapy.** Stereotactic body radiotherapy (SBRT) is now the preferred treatment for patients with medically inoperable stage I disease. SBRT is a technique that uses precise and accurate delivery method of highly conformal and dose-intensive radiation to small-volume targets. When compared to conventional fractionated radiotherapy, SBRT spares normal lung tissue by precise stereotactic localization, image guidance, motion management and delivery of a higher biologic effective dose. Long term follow-up with SBRT has shown 5-year local control of 93%, lobar control 80%, distant failure rate of 31%, and overall survival of 40% [38]. Overall, it was well tolerated with minimal side effects including grade 2 pneumonitis and chest wall pain. There is no benefit to postoperative radiotherapy in completely resected stage II and IIB NSCLC [1].

o Sex-specific survival data for patients receiving definitive SBRT with curative intent is limited. However, a larger retrospective study in adults over age 70 undergoing SBRT versus observation alone for early-stage lung cancer revealed women treated with SBRT did have slightly improved survival rates compared to women who underwent observation [9].

o **Neoadjuvant and adjuvant therapy.** Neoadjuvant treatment may be an option in those with potentially resectable disease, and those eligible include single station mediastinal nodal involvement or superior sulcus tumors or chest wall invasion in the setting of N1 nodal involvement. For carefully selected Stage III patients, surgery may be indicated with or without neoadjuvant chemotherapy or chemoradiotherapy or immunotherapy [39]. In general for Stage III disease, a combined approach using concurrent chemoradiotherapy is generally preferred, with subsequent immunotherapy if there is no progression [1].

o There are sex-based differences in the development of side effects of systemic therapy, and some data suggest women may develop more immune-mediated adverse events [9]. Some have suggested differences in the gut microbiome may predisposition to side effects, but difference in immunotherapy response rates has not been confirmed [9].

- **Metastatic disease.** Stage IV NSCLC treatment should be guided by histology, molecular pathology, age, comorbidities, performance status, and patient preferences. In general, patients with Stage IV disease are treated with palliative systemic therapy, immunotherapy or symptom-based palliative approach. In patients with NSCLC without driver oncogenic mutations (EGFR, ALK, etc.) and low PD-L1 expression, platinum-based doublet chemotherapy is used as first line therapy. However, despite lower PD-L1 staining (PD-L1 < 50%), combination therapy with platinum-based chemotherapy and immunotherapy is now emerging as preferred therapy due to superiority of results. For PD-L1 staining greater than 50%, immunotherapy alone is now the standard of care.

o A pooled analysis in 2010 of five randomized trials of platinum-based chemotherapy in advanced NSCLC found that women had a higher response rate (42% versus 40%) and a longer overall survival (9.6 versus 8.6 months) [9]. More recent landmark trials (FLAURA trial with osimertininb compared to first generation EGFR; alectinib versus crizotinib) have not shown an outcome difference between men and women [9].

- **Oligometastatic disease.** Oligometastatic disease includes those with metastases limited in number and organ sites, and these patients may benefit from a radical ablative therapy of both the primary lesion and all metastatic sites [40]. Interventions should be based on multi-disciplinary assessment and restricted to brain, lung and adrenal metastases [40].

Lung Cancer Survivorship

A lung cancer survivor is a person who has been diagnosed with cancer, starting the day of their diagnosis until the end of life [41]. In those undergoing treatment, significant symptom burden related both to the treatment as well as the disease may occur. In long term survivors, those that have completed their therapy living five years after diagnosis, symptoms such as fatigue and dyspnea may persist.

- **Cancer-related fatigue.** Cancer-related fatigue is understudied in lung cancer survivors, and it encompasses physical, emotional and/or cognitive tiredness due to the cancer and its treatments [42]. Treatments include both pharmacologic and non-pharmacologic interventions, and pharmacologic treatments address comorbid mood disorders, anxiety and pain. A recent research agenda from the American Thoracic Society has emphasized a role for enhancing physical activity and detecting sleep disruption in this cohort [43].
- **Reproductive counseling.** With every cancer diagnosis, it is imperative to address fertility goals, preservation, and overall impact of potential oncological treatments on the reproductive health of women. American Society of Clinical Oncology (ASCO) guideline recommends that before initiation of any cancer therapy, physicians should address the impact of all therapies on fertility, options of fertility preservation including work up and procedures and appropriate timely referrals to reproductive specialists [44].
- **Lung cancer and pregnancy.** Cancer during pregnancy is rare, and lung cancer in pregnancy has been described in less than 70 case reports in the medical literature [45]. For lung cancer, there is no data evaluating molecular and genomic characteristics of disease in women [46]. Nonsmoking pregnant women comprise more than 40% in those reported [46]. In a single institution cohort of NSCLC diagnosed and treated between 2009 and 2015, 160 women of reproductive age (out of 2422) were identified, and 8 of these had NSCLC diagnosed during pregnancy [47]. All of the pregnant patients had stage IV disease, were never-smokers or light smokers, and all had a targetable molecular alteration (6 with *ALK*

translocation and 2 with *EGFR* mutation) [47]. They concluded testing for targetable molecular alterations was imperative. The care of pregnant women with lung cancer requires a multi-disciplinary approach and treatment must weigh risks and benefits for both the fetus and mother. Further prospective and multi-center studies are needed.

- **ICI therapy.** There is a lack of data on the potential adverse effects of immune check point inhibitors on fertility, pregnancy, or impact on sexual life after this line of therapy. Primary hypogonadism which results in ovarian or testicular dysfunction may occur in the setting of ICI therapy. Although there are reports of orchitis, epididymal-orchitis and azoospermia in men after ICI therapy, data is scarce for primary hypogonadism in women [48]. Secondary hypogonadism in the setting of hypophysitis and panhypopituitarism may occur, but these endocrinopathies may be underestimated due to lack of routine sex hormone testing [49].

- **Sexual health.** Sexual health may be a significant concern for women, and sexual dysfunction is becoming a common side effect of cancer therapies [50]. In a study of lung cancer patients, self-reported sexual concerns were prevalent, and they were significantly related to physical and emotional symptoms [51]. Simple tools incorporated into clinical practice including knowledge, diagnosis and sexual counseling, may help identify and ameliorate symptoms [50].

- **Sleep disruption.** Sleep disruption is common in cancer patients. In a study of cancer patients undergoing chemotherapy, lung cancer survivors (12%) had the highest prevalence of sleep disturbance (fatigue, use of sleeping pills, daytime hypersomnia, insomnia) [52]. In a small polysomnography study, lung cancer survivors under-reported sleep difficulties and had sleep patterns like otherwise healthy insomniacs [53]. Sleep-disordered breathing related to pulmonary dysfunction, concomitant cardiac dysfunction and use of pain medications may also occur in this cohort [43]. Data on sleep disturbances and disorders in lung cancer patient is limited; further study is needed.

- **Symptom clusters.** Lung cancer patients have significant symptom burden, which include fatigue, dyspnea, pain, cough, insomnia, impaired cognitive function and psychological distress and may persist as late- and long-term effects of treatment [41]. Symptom clusters in lung cancer encompasses concurrent physical and/or psychosocial symptoms. These may be impacted by tumor histology, cancer stage, therapeutic interventions, and other comorbidities. Symptoms clusters in lung cancer patients typically include psychoneurological (fatigue, mood changes, pain, anxiety, cognitive and sleep disturbances), respiratory (cough, dyspnea, wheezing) and gastrointestinal (nausea, vomiting, lack of appetite) [43].

- **Therapy-related complications.** As with all interventions, risks and benefits exist with each treatment. Long-term sequelae from chemotherapy often include neuropathy, hearing loss, and neurocognitive changes. Immunotherapy has been associated with fatigue as well as many immune-mediated adverse events that can affect any organ system. Radiation can manifest with both acute and chronic lung injury, and it can exacerbate respiratory symptoms. Even surgical patients may have residual pain, dyspnea, and respiratory limitations requiring oxygen.

Sex-based differences occur across the continuum of lung cancer from risk factors to screening and diagnosis to outcomes and mortality. With the evolving demographics of lung cancer among women, it is important to promptly recognize risk factors, symptoms and radiographic findings concerning for lung cancer. Prompt staging, diagnosis and molecular characterization are needed to facilitate proper treatment. Lung cancer portends significant symptom burden during and after treatment, and eliciting patients' concerns can facilitate interventions to ameliorate symptom burden.

Case Resolution

She then underwent concurrent chemoradiation therapy with systemic carboplatin and paclitaxel and radiation directed towards site of recurrence. She was initiated on immuno-therapy maintenance (durvalumab) with a total of 12 cycles. She developed flank pain and was found to have pancreatitis. Immunotherapy was stopped due to an immune-related adverse event. She was treated with steroid therapy with resolution of symptoms. She continues to follow in cancer survivorship clinic, and imaging four years after last treatment shows chronic changes from radiation and no new findings.

Take Home Points

- Women have unique risk factors for lung cancer.

  o Exogenous factors include primary tobacco use, secondhand smoke, radon, radiation to chest wall, and infections.

  o Endogenous factors include hormones and genetic polymorphisms.

  o Nonsmoking women are at a higher risk for lung cancer compared with nonsmoking men.

- Current lung cancer screening guidelines center around tobacco use, so women never-smokers may be missed.

  o Inclusion of women in landmark screening trials has been low.

  o Results from several studies suggest larger reduction in lung cancer mortality in women than men related to screening.

- There is higher likelihood of adenocarcinoma histology in women compared with men.
- Women are more likely to be diagnosed with lung cancer at an earlier age.
- Women have better five-year lung cancer survival, regardless of age, stage, and treatment.

References

1. Thai A. A., Solomon B. J., Sequist L. V., Gainor J. F., Heist R. S. Lung cancer. *Lancet.* 2021;398(10299):535–54.

2. MacRosty C. R., Rivera M. P. Lung cancer in women: A modern epidemic. *Clin Chest Med.* 2020;41(1):53–65.

3. Kligerman S., White C. Epidemiology of lung cancer in women: Risk factors, survival, and screening. *AJR Am J Roentgenol.* 2011;196(2):287–95.

4. Tanoue L. T. Women and lung cancer. *Clin Chest Med.* 2021;42(3):467–82.

5. Sung H., Ferlay J., Siegel R. L., et al. Global Cancer Statistics 2020: GLOBOCAN estimates of incidence and mortality worldwide for 36 cancer in 185 countries. *CA Cancer J Clin.* 2021;71(3):209–49.

6. Sun S., Schiller J. H., Gazdar A. F. Lung cancer in never smokers: A different disease. *Nat Rev Cancer.* 2007;7(10):778–90.

7. Jemal A., Miller K. D., Ma J., et al. Higher lung cancer incidence in young women than young men in the United States. *N Engl J Med.* 2018;**378**(21):1999–2009.

8. Fu J. B., Kau T. Y., Severson R. K., Kalemkerian G. P. Lung cancer in women: Analysis of the national Surveillance, Epidemiology, and End Results database. *Chest.* 2005;**127**(3):768–77.

9. Ragavan M., Patel M. I. The evolving landscape of sex-based differences in lung cancer: A distinct disease in women. *Eur Respir Rev.* 2022;**31**(163):210100.

10. Thun M. J., Carter B. D., Feskanich D., et al. 50-year trends in smoking-related mortality in the United States. *N Engl J Med.* 2013;**368**(4):351–64.

11. Novello S., Vavala T. Lung cancer and women. *Future Oncol.* 2008;**4**(5):705–16.

12. Slatore C. G., Chien J. W., Au D. H., Satia J. A., White E. Lung cancer and hormone replacement therapy: Association in the vitamins and lifestyle study. *J Clin Oncol.* 2010;**28**(9):1540–6.

13. Chlebowski R. T., Schwartz A. G., Wakelee H., et al. Oestrogen plus progestin and lung cancer in postmenopausal women (Women's Health Initiative trial): A post-hoc analysis of a randomised controlled trial. *Lancet.* 2009;**374**(9697):1243–51.

14. Heiss G., Wallace R., Anderson G. L., et al. Health risks and benefits 3 years after stopping randomized treatment with estrogen and progestin. *JAMA.* 2008;**299**(9):1036–45.

15. Yin X., Zhu Z., Hosgood H. D., Lan Q., Seow W. J. Reproductive factors and lung cancer risk: A comprehensive systematic review and meta-analysis. *BMC Public Health.* 2020;**20**(1):1458.

16. Fei Y., Yang J., Hsieh W. C., et al. Different human papillomavirus 16/18 infection in Chinese non-small cell lung cancer patients living in Wuhan, China. *Jpn J Clin Oncol.* 2006;**36**(5):274–9.

17. Cheng Y. W., Chiou H. L., Sheu G. T., et al. The association of human papillomavirus 16/18 infection with lung cancer among nonsmoking Taiwanese women. *Cancer Res.* 2001;**61**(7):2799–803.

18. Kaufman E. L., Jacobson J. S., Hershman D. L., Desai M., Neugut A. I. Effect of breast cancer radiotherapy and cigarette smoking on risk of second primary lung cancer. *J Clin Oncol.* 2008;**26**(3):392–8.

19. Travis L. B., Gospodarowicz M., Curtis R. E., et al. Lung cancer following chemotherapy and radiotherapy for Hodgkin's disease. *J Natl Cancer Inst.* 2002;**94**(3):182–92.

20. Force USPST, Krist A. H., Davidson K. W., et al. Screening for lung cancer: US Preventive Services Task Force Recommendation Statement. *JAMA.* 2021;**325**(10):962–70.

21. Pinsky P. F., Lau Y. K., Doubeni C. A. Potential disparities by sex and race or ethnicity in lung cancer screening eligibility rates. *Chest.* 2021;**160**(1):341–50.

22. Kocher F., Hilbe W., Seeber A., Pircher, et al. Longitudinal analysis of 2293 NSCLC patients: A comprehensive study from the TYROL registry. *Lung Cancer.* 2015;**87**(2):193–200.

23. Kalemkerian G. P., Narula N., Kennedy E. B., et al. Molecular testing guideline for the selection of patients with lung cancer for treatment with targeted tyrosine kinase inhibitors: American Society of Clinical Oncology Endorsement of the College of American Pathologists/International Association for the Study of Lung Cancer/Association for Molecular Pathology Clinical Practice Guideline Update. *J Clin Oncol.* 2018;**36**(9):911–19.

24. Lindeman N. I., Cagle P. T., Aisner D. L., et al. Updated molecular testing guideline for the selection of lung cancer patients for treatment with targeted tyrosine kinase inhibitors: Guideline from the College of American Pathologists, the International Association for the Study of Lung Cancer, and the Association for Molecular Pathology. *J Thorac Oncol.* 2018;**13**(3):323–58.

25. Lynch T. J., Bell D. W., Sordella R., et al. Activating mutations in the epidermal growth factor receptor underlying

responsiveness of non-small-cell lung cancer to gefitinib. *N Engl J Med.* 2004;**350**(21):2129–39.

26. Detterbeck F. C., Boffa D. J., Kim A. W., Tanoue L. T. The Eighth Edition Lung Cancer Stage Classification. *Chest.* 2017;**151**(1):193–203.

27. Sagerup C. M., Smastuen M., Johannesen T. B., Helland A., Brustugun O. T. Sex-specific trends in lung cancer incidence and survival: A population study of 40,118 cases. *Thorax.* 2011;**66**(4):301–7.

28. Nakamura H., Ando K., Shinmyo T., et al. Female gender is an independent prognostic factor in non-small-cell lung cancer: A meta-analysis. *Ann Thorac Cardiovasc Surg.* 2011;**17**(5):469–80.

29. Husain Z. A., Kim A. W., Yu J. B., Decker R. H., Corso C. D. Defining the high-risk population for mortality after resection of early stage NSCLC. *Clin Lung Cancer.* 2015;**16**(6):e183–7.

30. Chang M. Y., Mentzer S. J., Colson Y. L., et al. Factors predicting poor survival after resection of stage IA non-small cell lung cancer. *J Thorac Cardiovasc Surg.* 2007;**134**(4):850–6.

31. Reck M., Rodriguez-Abreu D., Robinson A. G., et al. Pembrolizumab versus chemotherapy for PD-L1-Positive non-small-cell lung cancer. *N Engl J Med.* 2016;**375**(19):1823–33.

32. Mascaux C., Iannino N., Martin B., et al. The role of RAS oncogene in survival of patients with lung cancer: A systematic review of the literature with meta-analysis. *Br J Cancer.* 2005;**92**(1):131–9.

33. Alexiou C., Onyeaka C. V., Beggs D., et al. Do women live longer following lung resection for carcinoma? *Eur J Cardiothorac Surg.* 2002;**21**(2):319–25.

34. Ferguson M. K., Wang J., Hoffman P. C., et al. Sex-associated differences in survival of patients undergoing resection for lung cancer. *Ann Thorac Surg.* 2000;**69**(1):245–9; discussion 249–50.

35. Yoshino I., Baba H., Fukuyama S., et al. A time trend of profile and surgical results in 1123 patients with non-small cell lung cancer. *Surgery.* 2002;**131**(1 Suppl):S242–8.

36. Yang C. J., Kumar A., Klapper J. A., et al. A national analysis of long-term survival following thoracoscopic versus open lobectomy for stage I non-small-cell lung cancer. *Ann Surg.* 2019;**269**(1):163–71.

37. Bendixen M., Jorgensen O. D., Kronborg C., Andersen C., Licht P. B. Postoperative pain and quality of life after lobectomy via video-assisted thoracoscopic surgery or anterolateral thoracotomy for early stage lung cancer: A randomised controlled trial. *Lancet Oncol.* 2016;**17**(6):836–44.

38. Timmerman R., Paulus R., Galvin J., et al. Stereotactic body radiation therapy for inoperable early stage lung cancer. *JAMA.* 2010;**303**(11):1070–6.

39. Kozower B. D., Larner J. M., Detterbeck F. C., Jones D. R. Special treatment issues in non-small cell lung cancer: Diagnosis and management of lung cancer, 3rd ed: American College of Chest Physicians evidence-based clinical practice guidelines. *Chest.* 2013;**143**(5 Suppl):e369S–e99S.

40. Eichhorn F., Winter H. How to handle oligometastatic disease in nonsmall cell lung cancer. *Eur Respir Rev.* 2021;**30** (159):200234.

41. Pozo C. L., Morgan M. A., Gray J. E. Survivorship issues for patients with lung cancer. *Cancer Control.* 2014;**21**(1):40–50.

42. Bower J. E. Cancer-related fatigue: Mechanisms, risk factors, and treatments. *Nat Rev Clin Oncol.* 2014;**11**(10):597–609.

43. Bade B. C., Faiz S. A., Ha D. M., et al. Cancer-related fatigue in lung cancer: A research agenda: An Official American Thoracic Society Research Statement. *Am J Respir Crit Care Med.* 2023;**207**(5): e6–e28.

44. Loren A. W., Mangu P. B., Beck L. N., et al. Fertility preservation for patients with cancer: American Society of Clinical Oncology clinical practice guideline update. *J Clin Oncol.* 2013;**31**(19):2500–10.

45. Bellido C., Barbero P., Forcen L., et al. Lung adenocarcinoma during pregnancy:

Clinical case and literature review. *J Matern Fetal Neonatal Med.* 2019;**32**(19):3300–2.

46. Rothschild S. I. Lung cancer in pregnancy: A forgotten disease entity. *J Thorac Oncol.* 2016;**11**(9):1376–8.

47. Dagogo-Jack I., Gainor J. F., Porter R. L., et al. Clinicopathologic features of NSCLC diagnosed during pregnancy or the peripartum period in the era of molecular genotyping. *J Thorac Oncol.* 2016;**11**(9):1522–8.

48. Rabinowitz M. J., Kohn T. P., Pena V. N., et al. Onset of azoospermia in man treated with ipilimumab/nivolumab for BRAF negative metastatic melanoma. *Urol Case Rep.* 2021;**34**:101488.

49. de Filette J., Andreescu C. E., Cools F., Bravenboer B., Velkeniers B. A systematic review and meta-analysis of endocrine-related adverse events associated with immune checkpoint inhibitors. *Horm Metab Res.* 2019;**51**(3):145–56.

50. Del Pup L., Villa P., Amar I. D., Bottoni C., Scambia G. Approach to sexual dysfunction in women with cancer. *Int J Gynecol Cancer.* 2019;**29**(3):630–4.

51. Reese J. B., Shelby R. A., Abernethy A. P. Sexual concerns in lung cancer patients: An examination of predictors and moderating effects of age and gender. *Support Care Cancer.* 2011;**19**(1):161–5.

52. Davidson J. R., MacLean A. W., Brundage M. D., Schulze K. Sleep disturbance in cancer patients. *Soc Sci Med.* 2002;**54**(9):1309–21.

53. Silberfarb P. M., Hauri P. J., Oxman T. E., Schnurr P. Assessment of sleep in patients with lung cancer and breast cancer. *J Clin Oncol.* 1993;**11**(5):997–1004.

Chapter 20

Pelvic Mass and Ovarian Cancer

Mary Katherine Anastasio and Travis T. Sims

Pelvic Mass

Case Presentation

A 55-year-old postmenopausal female presents with left lower quadrant pain, abdominal fullness, and early satiety. Pelvic ultrasound reveals a 10 cm unilocular cyst with solid components and two papillary projections. CA-125 value of 50 units/mL. What are the next best steps in management?

Epidemiology

Incidence and Long-Term Prognosis

Adnexal masses are found in up to 35% of premenopausal patients and 17% of postmenopausal patients [1, 2]. In a large, prospective study including 4,848 patients with a persistent adnexal mass that required surgery, 66% of masses were benign and 34% were malignant [3]. Among postmenopausal women who underwent surgery for a suspicious adnexal mass, 36–59% of masses were malignant [4]. The prognosis of the mass varies significantly based on the final pathology results. For most benign masses, surgical excision leads to complete resolution. However, the prognosis of malignancy is poor unless diagnosed and treated at an early stage (stages I–II). In the United States, ovarian cancer is the fifth leading cause of cancer-related death in females [5].

Etiology and Risk Factors

The differential diagnosis of an adnexal mass is broad and includes both benign and malignant lesions as well as gynecologic and nongynecologic lesions. While diagnosis must be made with histopathology, imaging characteristics may help differentiate the mass. Gynecologic lesions include those of the ovary, fallopian tube, and uterus. Simple appearing gynecologic masses include follicular cysts, corpus luteal cysts, serous or mucinous cystadenomas, and hydrosalpinx. Complex appearing gynecologic masses include endometriomas, cystic teratomas, hemorrhagic cysts, abscesses, and malignant ovarian cancer. Solid masses include fibromas, fibroids, thecomas, and primary ovarian malignancies. In a large, prospective study of approximately 5,000 patients with a persistent adnexal mass that required surgery, the most common benign lesions included endometriomas (17.4%), cystic teratomas (10.6%), and simple cysts (5.9%). The most common malignant tumors included primary invasive stage III tumors (13.6%), borderline stage I tumors

(5.1%) and primary invasive stage I tumors (4.6%) [3]. In addition, nongynecologic lesions can be described as adnexal masses and include gastrointestinal abscesses, ureteral diverticula, bladder diverticula, and pelvic kidney among others. Malignant, nongynecologic pelvic masses include gastrointestinal cancer, metastatic cancer and retroperitoneal sarcomas [6].

Several risk factors for ovarian cancer have been identified. The most significant independent risk factor for ovarian cancer in the general population is age; incidence significantly increases after menopause [7]. The mean age at diagnosis of ovarian cancer in the United States population is 63 years [8]. The most important personal risk factor for the development of ovarian cancer is a strong family history of breast and/or ovarian cancer [9]. Patients at high risk for epithelial ovarian and fallopian tube, or primary peritoneal cancer include those with genetic predisposition including *BRCA1* and *BRCA2* mutations, hereditary nonpolyposis colorectal cancer (Lynch syndrome), and mutations in *BRIP1*, *RAD51C*, and *RAD51D* [10]. Patients with *BRCA1* mutations have a 41–46% lifetime risk of ovarian, fallopian tube, or primary peritoneal cancer (hereafter referred to as ovarian cancer) by age 70, and those with *BRCA2* mutations have a 10–27% lifetime risk of ovarian, fallopian tube or primary peritoneal cancer by age 70 [11–14]. Additional risk factors for ovarian cancer include nulliparity, early menarche, late menopause, and endometriosis [15–17].

Of note, there are no conclusive data to support an association between talc use and ovarian cancer. A systematic review and meta-analysis evaluating the association between perineal talc use and ovarian cancer risk found that talc use was associated with an increased risk of ovarian cancer in case control studies but not in cohort studies [18]. However, one main limitation of case control studies is a risk of recall bias. A subsequent prospective cohort study found no association between perineal talc use and ovarian cancer [19]. It is important to note that infertility and infertility treatments are not independent risk factors for ovarian cancer. However, both infertility and endometriosis can result in nulliparity, which is a risk factor for ovarian cancer. A large meta-analysis evaluating the risk of ovarian cancer in patients treated with ovulation stimulating drugs for infertility found no evidence of an increased risk of invasive ovarian cancer with fertility drug treatment [20].

Diagnosis and Workup

Signs and Symptoms

Most patients with adnexal masses are asymptomatic. However, in patients with symptoms, pelvic or abdominal pain is common [21]. Pressure or fullness in the abdomen and/or pelvis may result from the bulk of the cyst or stretch of the ovarian capsule [21]. Dysmenorrhea, dyspareunia, or abnormal uterine bleeding may be associated with endometriomas [22]. While less common, patients may present with acute pain, nausea, and vomiting with torsion of either benign or malignant adnexal masses [23, 24]. Tubo-ovarian abscesses may present with fever and abdominal or pelvic pain [25, 26]. Persistent bloating, generalized abdominal pain, and early satiety may be signs of malignancy [27]. Postmenopausal bleeding may be seen with granulosa cell tumors due to estrogen production [28]. Virilization may be seen with androgen-producing adnexal tumors [29].

Physical Exam Findings

If the mass is palpable on physical exam and/or pelvic exam, the size, consistency, and mobility of the mass can be assessed. Physical signs of virilization or androgen excess including acne, hirsutism, deepening voice, alopecia, clitoromegaly, and menstrual irregularities may be found in patients with androgen-producing tumors [29]. Physical exam findings that are concerning for malignancy include fixed and irregular masses, posterior cul-de-sac nodularity, and the presence of ascites [30].

Diagnostic Tests

Serum tumor markers can be used to assess the likelihood of malignancy (Table 20.1). Cancer antigen 125 (CA-125), the most studied tumor marker, is a protein associated with epithelial ovarian malignancies as well as other benign and malignant ovarian tumors. CA-125 can also be elevated in other benign conditions including pregnancy, endometriosis, cirrhosis, and pelvic inflammatory disease [31]. Human Epididymis 4 (HE4) is a protein that has a sensitivity and specificity of detecting ovarian cancer similar to that of CA-125, and HE4 is less frequently positive in postmenopausal patients with benign masses [32]. Carcinoembryonic antigen (CEA) is a protein that may by elevated in gastrointestinal tract tumors or mucinous ovarian cancer [33]. Cancer antigen 19-9 (CA 19-9) is a protein that may be elevated in epithelial ovarian cancer but is more often used for cancer of the gastrointestinal tract including gastric, pancreatic, and gallbladder cancer [34–36]. Other serum markers that may be secreted by germ cell or sex cord stromal tumors include: inhibin A and B – granulosa cell tumors, LDH – dysgerminomas, hCG – choriocarcinomas, and AFP and LDH – yolk sac tumors [37–40]. While a tissue sample is needed for diagnosis, biopsy is often not recommended to avoid intraabdominal spillage and subsequent upstaging of a possible cancer [30].

Imaging Studies

Transvaginal ultrasound is the most used imaging technique for evaluating adnexal masses [6]. Characteristics assessed on ultrasound include the size, composition (cystic, solid, mixed); and

Table 20.1 Serum tumor markers can be used to assess the likelihood of malignancy associated with a pelvic mass

Serum tumor marker	Associated malignancy or tumor
CA-125	Ovarian cancer
HE-4	Ovarian cancer
CEA	Gastrointestinal tract tumors, mucinous ovarian cancer
CA 19-9	Epithelial ovarian cancer, gastrointestinal tract cancer (gastric, pancreatic, gallbladder)
Inhibin A and B	Granulosa cell tumors
LDH	Dysgerminoma, yolk sac tumors
hCG	Choriocarcinoma
AFP	Yolk sac tumors

presence of septations, nodules, papillary excrescences, free fluid, or Doppler color flow. There are several proposed ultrasound classification systems to determine the risk for malignancy. Two of the most common tools include the International Ovarian Tumor Analysis (IOTA) Simple Rules and the Ovarian-Adnexal Reporting and Data System (O-RADS). The IOTA Simple Rules are a classification system with 5 benign and 5 malignant ultrasound features of adnexal masses. Benign features include unilocular cysts, presence of solid components < 7 mm, presence of acoustic shadows, smooth multilocular tumors < 10 cm, and no doppler blood flow. Malignant features include irregular solid tumors, presence of ascites, at least 4 papillary structures, irregular multilocular solid tumors ≥ 10 cm, and high doppler blood flow. Masses are considered benign if only benign features are seen or considered malignant if only malignant features are seen. If both benign and malignant features are seen, the mass is inconclusive [41]. The IOTA Simple Rules have a sensitivity of 93% and specificity of 81% for predicting whether an adnexal mass is benign or malignant preoperatively [42]. The O-RADS system, published in 2018, is the most recent risk stratification and management system. This system provides a standardized glossary with definitions for all ultrasound characteristics of normal ovaries and adnexal masses [43]. It is the most detailed risk stratification system and was designed to decrease ambiguity and increase consistency of imaging interpretations. It divides imaging findings into six different risk categories and has a high probability of accuracy in assigning risk of malignancy (Table 20.2). In a retrospective study comparing the ability of O-RADS and IOTA Simple Rules to detect malignancy, O-RADS had higher sensitivity than IOTA Simple Rules with relatively similar specificity and reliability [44].

MRI can be a useful secondary imaging modality to better characterize large masses, or those with indeterminate features on ultrasound [45]. CT is not commonly used for assessment of an adnexal mass. However, CT is frequently used as a diagnostic tool for patients with suspected or known ovarian cancer to assess for extent of disease and presence of peritoneal carcinomatosis [46–48].

Treatment Options and Surveillance

Masses Requiring Emergent Intervention

One of the first priorities of management is to identify patients with adnexal masses who require prompt intervention to avoid significant morbidity due to hemorrhage, sepsis, or loss of ovarian function. Examples of masses which require timely intervention include adnexal torsion, ectopic pregnancy, tubo-ovarian abscesses, and ruptured or hemorrhagic cysts causing hemodynamic instability.

Masses Concerning for Malignancy

The likelihood of malignancy should be determined based on imaging characteristics of the adnexal mass, serum tumor markers and patient risk factors such as a genetic predisposition. A referral to gynecologic oncology is recommended as surgery by gynecologic oncologists improves outcomes for patients with ovarian cancer [49–53] . If a mass is considered high-risk (O-RADS 5) regardless of menopausal status, surgery is often required for appropriate diagnosis and treatment. Postmenopausal patients with intermediate-risk masses (O-RADS 4) and symptoms concerning for malignancy or additional risk factors for ovarian cancer also require surgery. Premenopausal patients with intermediate-risk masses (O-RADS 4) and elevated

Table 20.2 O-RADS Risk Stratification System

O-RADS Score	Risk Category	Positive Predictive Value for Malignancy	Description
0	Incomplete evaluation	N/A	N/A
1	Normal ovaries	N/A	No ovarian lesion, ≤3 cm simple follicle, hemorrhagic cyst, or corpus luteum in premenopausal woman
2	Almost certainly benign	<0.5%	Unilocular cysts, dilated fallopian tubes, or paraovarian cysts with simple fluid, smooth and thin walls, no enhancing solid tissue, with or without wall enhancement
3	Low risk	~5%	Unilocular cysts, multilocular cysts, or dilated fallopian tubes with complex fluid, no enhancing solid tissue, and smooth enhancing walls; lesions with solid tissue with low risk time intensity curve (assessment of signal intensity over time)
4	Intermediate risk	~50%	Lesions with solid tissue with intermediate risk time intensity curve, lesion with lipid content and large volume enhancing solid tissue
5	High risk	~90%	Lesion with solid tissue with high risk intensity curve; peritoneal, mesenteric or omental nodularity or irregular thickening with or without ascites

Adapted from [87]

serum tumor markers, or those with suspicion for germ cell or sex cord-stromal tumors also require surgery.

Benign Masses

Once acute processes and malignancy are excluded, management of a benign lesion is determined based on several factors including a patient's age, fertility desires, persistent symptoms, and preferences regarding surgery.

Surgical Approach

Open (via laparotomy) surgery may be performed for known malignancy with metastatic disease, large masses, or indeterminate masses with concern for intraoperative rupture. However, minimally invasive surgery is the preferred approach for adnexal masses that are presumed benign [54]. Compared to open surgery, a minimally invasive approach is associated with decreased hospital stay, cost, postoperative pain, and postoperative complications [55]. One risk of minimally invasive surgery is the potential for cyst rupture, intraabdominal spillage of cyst contents, and upstaging of possible cancer [56]. However, minimally invasive techniques have even been proposed for management of large adnexal masses with low probability of malignancy [57, 58]. For example, laparoscopic retrieval bags have been used to allow for extraction of even large (up to 20 cm) pelvic masses using laparoscopy. The edges of the bag are typically pulled up through an incision, and controlled drainage is performed to avoid leakage or spillage of cyst contents into the peritoneal cavity. If malignancy is suspected, laparoscopic removal should be avoided.

Procedure

In postmenopausal patients, appropriate surgical staging is performed for malignant masses. This often includes total hysterectomy, bilateral salpingo-oophorectomy, and omentectomy in addition to lymph node sampling in some cases. This can be done through an open or minimally invasive approach depending on the extent of disease. If an adnexal mass is benign appearing or is benign on intraoperative frozen section assessment, a unilateral salpingo-oophorectomy or bilateral salpingo-oophorectomy, particularly in postmenopausal patients, may be performed to reduce the risk of ovarian cancer.

In premenopausal patients, the extent of surgical staging for malignant masses depends on a patient's extent of disease and desire for future childbearing. If an adnexal mass is benign appearing or is benign on intraoperative frozen section assessment, an ovarian cystectomy may be performed.

Surveillance

If a patient does not meet criteria for surgery, management with surveillance is recommended. There is no consensus on the optimal approach for surveillance, but an interval pelvic ultrasound with or without serum tumor markers is typically performed. The frequency with which pelvic ultrasounds are repeated depends on the patient's menopausal status and the mass features on imaging. For small simple cysts regardless of menopausal status, no follow up is recommended. For masses that appear almost certainly benign on ultrasound (O-RADS 2), follow up is typically recommended in 8–12 weeks for premenopausal patients and in 1 year for postmenopausal patients [45]. While recommendations vary, a repeat transvaginal ultrasound may be performed in three to six months for patients with low-risk masses (O-RADS 3) regardless of menopausal status. For patients with intermediate-risk masses (O-RADS 4), a pelvic ultrasound should be repeated in six weeks for premenopausal patients, and a pelvic ultrasound plus CA-125 level should be repeated in six weeks for postmenopausal patients. During management with surveillance, it is important to counsel the patient on when surveillance may be discontinued. If a mass resolves, remains unchanged in size or decreases in size and if CA-125 remains normal, surveillance can be discontinued when the planned discontinuation point is reached.

Ovarian Cancer

Background

Ovarian cancer is the second most common gynecologic malignancy after uterine carcinoma and is the deadliest gynecologic cancer in the United States. Approximately 95% of ovarian cancer arise from the epithelial cells and include high grade serous, low grade serous, endometrioid, clear cell, and mucinous carcinoma. Serous carcinomas are the most common and make up 75% of epithelial carcinomas [59]. Less common types of ovarian cancer include germ cell and sex cord stromal tumors. Germ cell tumors include dysgerminoma, yolk sac tumor, embryonal carcinoma, and immature teratoma. Sex cord stromal tumors include granulosa cell and Sertoli-Leydig cell tumors. For this discussion, ovarian, fallopian tube, and primary peritoneal carcinomas will be referred to collectively as "ovarian cancer."

Clinical Presentation

Most patients have advanced staged disease at the time of ovarian cancer diagnosis. A major contributor to this is the subacute nature of the clinical presentation of ovarian cancer. Most patients present with vague abdominal pain, bloating, or gastrointestinal symptoms. Alternatively, patients may present with an incidental finding of an adnexal mass discovered at the time of imaging performed for a different indication. Patients may have a more acute presentation of ovarian cancer if they present with symptoms from complications of advanced disease such as a pleural effusion or a bowel obstruction.

Histologic Subtypes

While ovarian carcinoma is typically discussed as a single entity, it is made up of a heterogenous group of histologic subtypes. Epithelial ovarian cancer arise from the surface epithelium of the ovary, germ cell tumors arise from the primordial germ cells of the ovary, and sex cord stromal tumors arise from the sex cord cells of the ovary. Accurate diagnosis of a specific subtype is important, as each subtype has different molecular biology, prognosis, and treatment options.

Epithelial Carcinomas

Epithelial carcinomas are the most common histologic type of ovarian cancer and consist of high grade serous, low grade serous, endometrioid, clear cell, and mucinous carcinomas. **High grade serous carcinomas** are the most common epithelial subtype. These often present at an advanced stage and have poor prognosis [60]. In contrast, **low grade serous carcinomas** are often more indolent tumors but can be more resistant to platinum-based chemotherapy regimens [61]. **Endometrioid carcinomas** are often diagnosed at an early stage and are typically low grade and chemotherapy sensitive. **Clear cell carcinomas** also often present at an early stage but have a worse prognosis compared to endometrioid carcinomas because they are less sensitive to platinum-based chemotherapy [62]. Clear cell carcinomas have been associated with East Asian populations, hypercalcemia, and vascular thrombotic events [63]. Lastly, **mucinous carcinomas** are infrequent but often present at an early stage [64].

Malignant Germ Cell Tumors

Malignant germ cell tumors are made up of dysgerminomas, immature teratomas, yolk sac tumors and mixed germ cell neoplasms. **Dysgerminomas** are the most common malignant ovarian germ cell tumor, and account for about 33% of all malignant ovarian germ cell tumors [65]. They are typically diagnosed in younger females and adolescents [66]. LDH is the most likely elevated tumor marker with dysgerminomas. **Immature teratomas** are another common type of malignant ovarian germ cell tumors, and they are typically diagnosed prior to age 30 [65]. They contain all three germ layers (endoderm, mesoderm, and ectoderm) and are distinguished from mature teratomas by the presence of immature neuroepithelium. Tumor markers that may be secreted by immature teratomas include AFP, LDH, and estradiol. **Yolk sac tumors** make up around 14% of malignant germ cell tumors and occur in younger females [65, 67]. These tumors are rapidly growing with about one-third of cases having extraovarian spread at diagnosis [68]. These tumors typically secrete AFP. **Mixed germ cell tumors** are infrequent, and account for about 5% of malignant germ cell tumors. They are typically made up of several types of ovarian germ cell tumors such as dysgerminomas and yolk sac tumors. As such, they can secrete several different tumor markers depending on the tissue types present including LDH, AFP, and hCG. Other rare types of malignant germ cell tumors include choriocarcinoma, embryonal carcinoma, and polyembryomas.

Sex Cord Stromal Tumors

Granulosa cell and Sertoli-Leydig cell tumors are the malignant sex cord stromal tumors. **Granulosa cell tumors** account for 90% of malignant sex cord stromal tumors [69]. The adult subtype occurs in women typically over the age of 50 and is much more common than the juvenile subtype, which is typically diagnosed before puberty. Granulosa cell tumors are often slow-growing and have late relapses [70]. Patients may present with signs or symptoms of excess estrogen such as endometrial hyperplasia or neoplasia [28]. Patients with granulosa cell tumors typically have elevated inhibins, AMH, and CA-125. **Sertoli-Leydig cell tumors** often present in females under age 40. At least one-third of patients present with signs of virilization or androgen excess [71]. Patients with Sertoli-Leydig cell tumors may have elevated AFP, inhibins, or rarely CA-125.

Staging

Ovarian cancer are staged surgically according to the International Federation of Gynecology and Obstetrics (FIGO) classification system (Table 20.3). Stage I tumors are limited to ovaries or fallopian tubes. Stage II tumors involves one or both ovaries or fallopian tubes with pelvic extension below the pelvic brim, or primary peritoneal cancer. Stage III disease includes

Table 20.3 Ovarian, fallopian tube, and primary peritoneal carcinoma staging

FIGO stage	Criteria
I	Tumor limited to ovaries or fallopian tubes
IA	Tumor limited to one ovary with intact capsule, or one fallopian tube
IB	Tumor limited to both ovaries with intact capsule, or both fallopian tubes
IC	Tumor limited to one or both ovaries or fallopian tubes with any of the following:
IC1	Surgical spill
IC2	Capsule rupture before surgery or tumor on ovarian or fallopian tube surface
IC3	Malignant cells in ascites or peritoneal washings
II	Tumor involves one or both ovaries or fallopian tubes with pelvic extension below the pelvic brim, or primary peritoneal cancer
IIA	Extension and/or implants on the uterus and/or fallopian tubes and/or ovaries
IIB	Extension to and/or implants on other pelvic tissues
III	Tumor involves one or both ovaries or fallopian tubes, or primary peritoneal cancer with microscopically confirmed peritoneal metastases outside of the pelvis and/or metastasis to the retroperitoneal lymph nodes
IIIA1	Positive retroperitoneal lymph nodes only
IIIA2	Microscopic extra-pelvic peritoneal involvement with or without positive retroperitoneal lymph nodes
IIIB	Macroscopic extra-pelvic peritoneal involvement 2 cm or less in greatest dimension with or without positive retroperitoneal lymph nodes
IIIC	Macroscopic extra-pelvic peritoneal involvement 2 cm or more in greatest dimension with or without positive retroperitoneal lymph nodes
IV	Distant metastasis
IVA	Pleural effusion with positive cytology
IVB	Liver or splenic parenchymal metastasis, extra-abdominal organ metastasis, transmural intestinal involvement

Adapted from [88]

peritoneal metastases outside of the pelvis and/or metastasis to the retroperitoneal lymph nodes. Stage IV disease involves distant metastases.

Treatment

The mainstay of treatment for ovarian cancer includes both surgery and chemotherapy. While surgery alone can cure most patients with early-stage disease, most patients present with advanced stage disease and will require a combination of both surgery and chemotherapy [72]. The standard chemotherapy regimen includes a combination of platinum- and taxane-based chemotherapy.

Studies have shown that maximal cytoreductive surgery, or removal of all visible tumor, is positively correlated with overall survival [73]. Historically, primary debulking surgery (PDS) followed by initiation of chemotherapy has been the standard of care for management of patients with advanced-staged ovarian cancer. However, patients may alternatively be treated with neoadjuvant chemotherapy (NACT), or administration of systemic therapy prior to surgery, followed by interval debulking surgery in select cases. These patients typically receive three to four cycles of chemotherapy prior to debulking surgery followed by additional cycles of chemotherapy after surgery [74]. The aim of NACT followed by interval debulking surgery (IDS) is to increase the likelihood of complete resection of disease, particularly for patients who have unresectable disease at diagnosis including diffuse disease of the small bowel mesentery, diffuse carcinomatosis, infiltration of the duodenum or pancreas, involvement of large vessels, lung metastases, liver parenchyma involvement, and lymph node metastases in the mediastinum [74]. Existing data have shown that NACT followed by IDS can reduce perioperative morbidity and mortality [75, 76]. Despite this, several studies have shown no significant differences in overall or progression-free survival between NACT followed by IDS versus PDS [76, 77]. In select cases patients who enter remission after primary treatment with chemotherapy and/or surgery may be offered observation or maintenance therapy with a poly (ADP-ribose) polymerase (PARP) inhibitor or bevacizumab [78].

Prognosis

Patients with early-stage disease have relatively good prognosis with 80% being recurrence-free at five years and overall survival at five years of 89% for stage I and 71% for stage II disease. However, patients with advanced stage disease have a high risk of recurrence and high mortality rates among those who recur. Five-year overall survival rates are 41% for stage III and 20% for stage IV disease [79]. Prognostic factors associated with improved outcome include low volume of residual disease after primary treatment, good performance status, younger age, and serous histology [80].

Contraception/Hormone Therapy

Rationale

Patients who undergo risk-reducing bilateral salpingo-oophorectomy (RRSO) for pathogenic variants (PV) (e.g., *BRCA1, BRCA2*) will undergo early surgical menopause. This causes an abrupt decrease in estrogen levels at a younger age (typically 35–40 years for *BRCA1* and 40–45 years for *BRCA2*) compared to the average age of menopause (51 years) which exposes younger women to low estrogen levels for a significant period of time, leading to possible detrimental effects on bone density, cardiovascular health, and quality of life [81–84]. While hormone therapy may improve menopausal side effects, there is concern for an increased risk of cancer with its use. Following risk-reducing salpingo-oophorectomy in women without breast cancer, short term use of systemic hormone therapy can be used to improve menopausal symptoms and life expectancy without impacting the risk of breast cancer development [49].

Options

In patients who undergo RRSO for PVs, a thorough discussion of options, risks, and benefits is essential. One major consideration is whether the patient has had a hysterectomy, as progesterone therapy must be used in combination with estrogen if the patient has an intact uterus to protect from development of uterine cancer. If the patient has had a hysterectomy, estrogen therapy alone may be used [85].

Contraindications

Hormone therapy is contraindicated in patients with a history of hormone-dependent breast and other cancer, as it can increase the risk of recurrence, see Chapter 6 [86].

Screening Recommendations

There are currently no effective screening strategies for ovarian cancer. Screening tools developed thus far have been unable to detect ovarian cancer at a stage early enough to reduce mortality and can lead to false positive results or unnecessary procedures.

Special Considerations

Genetic Considerations

Patients at risk for developing ovarian and fallopian tube cancer include those with pathogenic variants in *BRCA1*, *BRCA2*, *BRIP1*, *RAD51 C*, and *RAD51D* as well as patients with Lynch syndrome [82]. Risk-reducing surgery with bilateral salpingo-oophorectomy is recommended in this population to reduce the risk of ovarian and fallopian tube cancer [82], see Chapter 3.

Case Resolution

This 55-year-old postmenopausal patient with a 10 cm unilocular cyst with solid components, symptoms concerning for malignancy (abdominal fullness, early satiety), and mildly elevated CA-125 was referred to gynecologic oncology for evaluation and management. She was recommended surgery due to her postmenopausal status, intermediate-risk mass (O-RADS 4), and symptoms concerning for malignancy. She underwent diagnostic laparoscopy, bilateral salpingo-oophorectomy and removal of pelvic mass. The intraoperative frozen section revealed a benign serous cystadenoma. She recovered well postoperatively and received reassurance at her postoperative visit. She did not require further surveillance given her benign mass on final pathology. She was encouraged to follow up with her benign gynecologist for annual visits.

Take Home Points

- Adnexal masses are found in up to 35% of premenopausal patients and 17% of postmenopausal patients. In the United States, ovarian cancer is the fifth leading cause of cancer-related death in females.
- Risk factors for ovarian cancer include *BRCA1* and *BRCA2* mutations, hereditary nonpolyposis colorectal cancer (Lynch syndrome), and mutations in *BRIP1*, *RAD51C*, and *RAD51D*. Additional risk factors include nulliparity, early menarche, late menopause, primary infertility, and endometriosis.
- Common presenting symptoms of a pelvic mass include pelvic or abdominal pain, pressure, or fullness. Assessing for symptoms that may indicate an acute process (nausea, vomiting, fever) is important. Persistent bloating, generalized abdominal pain, and early satiety may be signs of malignancy.

- Initial workup of a pelvic mass includes transvaginal ultrasound and serum tumor markers (CA-125, HE-4, and others depending on mass characteristics) to assess for risk of malignancy.
- Two of the most common proposed ultrasound classification systems to determine risk for malignancy include the International Ovarian Tumor Analysis (IOTA) Simple Rules and the Ovarian-Adnexal Reporting and Data System (O-RADS).
- Management aims include identifying need for emergent surgery, identifying malignancy, managing symptoms, and preserving fertility when appropriate.
- Management options for pelvic masses include expectant management, surveillance, and surgical management. While minimally invasive surgery is often the preferred surgical approach for removal of an adnexal mass, open surgery may be required for larger masses or those concerning for malignancy.
- Ovarian cancer is the second most common gynecologic malignancy after uterine carcinoma and is the deadliest gynecologic cancer in the United States.
- Most patients have advanced stage disease at the time of ovarian cancer diagnosis.
- Most patients with advanced stage disease will require a combination of both surgery and chemotherapy. The standard chemotherapy regimen includes a combination of platinum- and taxane-based chemotherapy.
- Five-year overall ovarian cancer survival rates are 89% for stage I, 71% for stage II, 41% for stage III, and 20% for stage IV disease.

References

1. Borgfeldt C., Andolf E., Transvaginal sonographic ovarian findings in a random sample of women 25-40 years old. *Ultrasound Obstet Gynecol.* 1999;**13**(5):345–50.

2. Pavlik E. J., Ueland F. R., Miller R. W., et al., Frequency and disposition of ovarian abnormalities followed with serial transvaginal ultrasonography. *Obstet Gynecol.* 2013;**122**(2 Pt 1):210–17.

3. Timmerman D., Van Calster B., Testa A., et al., Predicting the risk of malignancy in adnexal masses based on the Simple Rules from the International Ovarian Tumor Analysis group. *Am J Obstet Gynecol.* 2016;**214**(4):424–37.

4. Roman L. D., Muderspach L. I., Stein S. M., et al., Pelvic examination, tumor marker level, and gray-scale and Doppler sonography in the prediction of pelvic cancer. *Obstet Gynecol.* 1997;**89**(4):493–500.

5. Siegel R. L., Miller K. D., Wagle N. S., et al., Cancer statistics, 2023. *CA Cancer J Clin.* 2023;**73**(1):17–48.

6. American College of Obstetrics and Gynecology ACOG Committee on Practice Bulletins-Gynecology. Practice Bulletin No. 174: Evaluation and Management of Adnexal Masses. *Obstet Gynecol.* 2016;**128**(5):e210–e226.

7. Howlader N., Noone A. M., Krapcho M., et al. *SEER cancer statistics review, 1975–2013.* 2016; http://seer.cancer.gov/csr/1975_2013.

8. Howlader N., Noone A. M., Krapcho M., et al. *SEER Cancer Statistics Review, 1975–2016.* 2019; https://seer.cancer.gov/csr/1975_2016/ based on November 2018 SEER data submission, posted to the SEER web site, April 2019.

9. Society A. C. *American Cancer Society. Cancer facts and figures 2016.* 2016; www.cancer.org/acs/groups/content/@research/documents/document/acspc-047079.pdf.

10. Hall M. J., Obeid E. I., Schwartz S. C., et al., Genetic testing for hereditary cancer predisposition: BRCA1/2, Lynch syndrome, and beyond. *Gynecol Oncol.* 2016;**140**(3):565–74.

11. Antoniou A., Pharoah P. D., Narod S., et al., Average risks of breast and ovarian cancer associated with BRCA1 or BRCA2 mutations detected in case series unselected for family history: a combined analysis of 22 studies. *Am J Hum Genet.* 2003;**72**(5):1117–30.

12. Ford D., Easton D. F., Stratton M., et al., Genetic heterogeneity and penetrance analysis of the BRCA1 and BRCA2 genes in breast cancer families. The Breast Cancer Linkage Consortium. *Am J Hum Genet.* 1998;**62**(3):676–89.

13. King M. C., Marks J. H., Mandell J. B. Breast and ovarian cancer risks due to inherited mutations in BRCA1 and BRCA2. *Science.* 2003;**302**(5645):643–6.

14. Lancaster J. M., Powell C. B., Chen L. M., et al., Society of Gynecologic Oncology statement on risk assessment for inherited gynecologic cancer predispositions. *Gynecol Oncol.* 2015;**136**(1):3–7.

15. Brinton L. A., Lamb E. J., Moghissi K. S., et al., Ovarian cancer risk associated with varying causes of infertility. *Fertil Steril.* 2004;**82**(2):405–14.

16. Wentzensen N., Poole E. M., Trabert B., et al., Ovarian cancer risk factors by histologic subtype: An analysis From the Ovarian Cancer Cohort Consortium. *J Clin Oncol.* 2016;**34**(24):2888–98.

17. Wu A. H., Pearce C. L., Tseng C. C., et al., African Americans and Hispanics Remain at Lower Risk of Ovarian Cancer Than Non-Hispanic Whites after Considering Nongenetic Risk Factors and Oophorectomy Rates. *Cancer Epidemiol Biomarkers Prev.* 2015;**24**(7):1094–100.

18. Penninkilampi R., Eslick G. D., Perineal talc use and ovarian cancer: A systematic review and meta-analysis. *Epidemiology.* 2018;**29**(1):41–9.

19. O'Brien K. M., Tworoger S. S., Harris H. R., et al., Association of powder use in the genital area with risk of ovarian cancer. *JAMA.* 2020;**323**(1):49–59.

20. Rizzuto I., Behrens R. F., Smith L. A., Risk of ovarian cancer in women treated with ovarian stimulating drugs for infertility.

Cochrane Database Syst Rev. 2013;**2013**(8): CD008215.

21. Givens V., Mitchell G. E., Harraway-Smith C., et al., Diagnosis and management of adnexal masses. *Am Fam Physician.* 2009;**80**(8):815–20.

22. Bulun S. E., Endometriosis. *N Engl J Med.* 2009;**360**(3):268–79.

23. Oltmann S. C., Fischer A., Barber R., et al., Cannot exclude torsion–a 15-year review. *J Pediatr Surg.* 2009;**44**(6):1212–6; discussion 1217.

24. Rossi B. V., Ference E. H., Zurakowski D., et al., The clinical presentation and surgical management of adnexal torsion in the pediatric and adolescent population. *J Pediatr Adolesc Gynecol.* 2012;**25**(2):109–13.

25. Landers D. V., Sweet R. L. Tubo-ovarian abscess: contemporary approach to management. *Rev Infect Dis.* 1983;5 (5):876–84.

26. Lareau S. M., Beigi R. H. Pelvic inflammatory disease and tubo-ovarian abscess. *Infect Dis Clin North Am.* 2008;**22**(4):693–708.

27. ACOG Committee Opinion No. 280. The role of the generalist obstetrician-gynecologist in the early detection of ovarian cancer. *Obstet Gynecol.* 2002;**100**(6):1413–16.

28. Schumer S. T., Cannistra S. A. Granulosa cell tumor of the ovary. *J Clin Oncol.* 2003;**21**(6):1180–9.

29. Varras M., Vasilakaki T., Skafida E., et al., Clinical, ultrasonographic, computed tomography and histopathological manifestations of ovarian steroid cell tumour, not otherwise specified: our experience of a rare case with female virilisation and review of the literature. *Gynecol Endocrinol.* 2011;**27**(6):412–18.

30. Drake J., Diagnosis and management of the adnexal mass. *Am Fam Physician.* 1998;**57**(10):2471–80.

31. Meden H., Fattahi-Meibodi A. CA 125 in benign gynecological conditions. *Int J Biol Markers.* 1998;**13**(4):231–7.

32. Hellstrom I., Hellstrom K. E. SMRP and HE4 as biomarkers for ovarian carcinoma when used alone and in combination with CA-125 and/or each other. *Adv Exp Med Biol.* 2008;**622**:15–21.

33. Bozkurt M., Yumru A. E., Aral I Evaluation of the importance of the serum levels of CA-125, CA15-3, CA-19-9, carcinoembryonic antigen and alpha fetoprotein for distinguishing benign and malignant adnexal masses and contribution of different test combinations to diagnostic accuracy. *Eur J Gynaecol Oncol.* 2013;**34**(6):540–4.

34. Dyckhoff G., Warta R., Gonnermann A., et al., Carbohydrate antigen 19-9 in saliva: possible preoperative marker of malignancy in parotid tumors. *Otolaryngol Head Neck Surg.* 2011;**145**(5):772–7.

35. Kim S., Park B. K., Seo J. H., et al., Carbohydrate antigen 19-9 elevation without evidence of malignant or pancreatobiliary diseases. *Sci Rep.* 2020;**10**(1):8820.

36. Roy S., Dasgupta A., Kar K. Comparison of urinary and serum CA 19-9 as markers of early stage urothelial carcinoma. *Int Braz J Urol.* 2013;**39**(5):631–8.

37. Bagshawe K. D. Choriocarcinoma. A model for tumour markers. *Acta Oncol.* 1992;**31**(1):99–106.

38. Boggess J. F., Soules M. R., Goff B. A., et al., Serum inhibin and disease status in women with ovarian granulosa cell tumors. *Gynecol Oncol.* 1997;**64**(1):64–9.

39. Dallenbach P., Bonnefoi H., Pelte M. F., et al., Yolk sac tumours of the ovary: An update. *Eur J Surg Oncol.* 2006;**32**(10):1063–75.

40. Pressley R. H., Muntz H. G., Falkenberry S., et al., Serum lactic dehydrogenase as a tumor marker in dysgerminoma. *Gynecol Oncol.* 1992;**44**(3):281–3.

41. Timmerman D., Ameye L., Fischerova D., et al., Simple ultrasound rules to distinguish between benign and malignant adnexal masses before surgery: Prospective validation by IOTA group. *BMJ.* 2010;**341**: c6839.

42. Kaijser J., Sayasneh A., Van Hoorde K., et al., Presurgical diagnosis of adnexal tumours using mathematical models and scoring systems: A systematic review and meta-analysis. *Hum Reprod Update.* 2014;**20**(3):449–62.

43. Andreotti R. F., Timmerman D., Benacerraf B. R., et al., Ovarian-adnexal reporting lexicon for ultrasound: A white paper of the ACR Ovarian-Adnexal Reporting and Data System Committee. *J Am Coll Radiol.* 2018;**15**(10):1415–29.

44. Basha M. A. A., Metwally M. I., Gamil S. A., et al., Comparison of O-RADS, GI-RADS, and IOTA simple rules regarding malignancy rate, validity, and reliability for diagnosis of adnexal masses. *Eur Radiol.* 2021;**31**(2):674–84.

45. Andreotti R. F., Timmerman D., Strachowski L. M., et al., O-RADS US Risk Stratification and Management System: A Consensus Guideline from the ACR Ovarian-Adnexal Reporting and Data System Committee. *Radiology.* 2020;**294**(1):168–85.

46. Ahmed S. A., Abou-Taleb H., Yehia A., et al., The accuracy of multi-detector computed tomography and laparoscopy in the prediction of peritoneal carcinomatosis index score in primary ovarian cancer. *Acad Radiol.* 2019;**26**(12):1650–8.

47. Byrom J., Widjaja E., Redman C. W., et al., Can pre-operative computed tomography predict resectability of ovarian carcinoma at primary laparotomy? *BJOG.* 2002;**109**(4):369–75.

48. Esquivel J., Chua T. C., Stojadinovic A., et al., Accuracy and clinical relevance of computed tomography scan interpretation of peritoneal cancer index in colorectal cancer peritoneal carcinomatosis: A multi-institutional study. *J Surg Oncol.* 2010;**102**(6):565–70.

49. ACOG Committee Opinion No. 477. The role of the obstetrician-gynecologist in the early detection of epithelial ovarian cancer. *Obstet Gynecol.* 2011;**117**(3):742–6.

50. Chan J. K., Kapp D. S., Shin J. Y., et al., Influence of the gynecologic oncologist on

the survival of ovarian cancer patients. *Obstet Gynecol.* 2007;**109**(6):1342–50.

51. Earle C. C., Schrag D., Neville B. A., et al., Effect of surgeon specialty on processes of care and outcomes for ovarian cancer patients. *J Natl Cancer Inst.* 2006;**98**(3):172–80.

52. Engelen M. J., Kos H. E., Willemse P. H., et al., Surgery by consultant gynecologic oncologists improves survival in patients with ovarian carcinoma. *Cancer.* 2006;**106**(3):589–98.

53. Giede K. C., Kieser K., Dodge J., et al., Who should operate on patients with ovarian cancer? An evidence-based review. *Gynecol Oncol.* 2005;**99**(2):447–61.

54. Dioun S., Huang Y., Melamed A., et al., Trends in the Use of Minimally Invasive Adnexal Surgery in the United States. *Obstet Gynecol.* 2021;**138**(5):738–46.

55. Hidlebaugh D. A., Vulgaropulos S., Orr R. K., Treating adnexal masses. Operative laparoscopy vs. laparotomy. *J Reprod Med.* 1997;**42**(9):551–8.

56. Matsuo K., Machida H., Yamagami W., et al., Intraoperative capsule rupture, postoperative chemotherapy, and survival of women with stage I epithelial ovarian cancer. *Obstet Gynecol.* 2019;**134**(5):1017–26.

57. Rhode J. M., Advincula A. P., Reynolds R. K., et al., A minimally invasive technique for management of the large adnexal mass. *J Minim Invasive Gynecol.* 2006;**13**(5):476–9.

58. Sunoo C. S., Laparoscopic removal of a large adnexal mass. *Obstet Gynecol.* 2004;**103**(5 Pt 2):1087–9.

59. Berek J. S., Renz M., Kehoe S., et al., Cancer of the ovary, fallopian tube, and peritoneum: 2021 update. *Int J Gynaecol Obstet.* 2021;**155**(Suppl 1):61–85.

60. Doherty J. A., Peres L. C., Wang C., et al., Challenges and opportunities in studying the epidemiology of ovarian cancer subtypes. *Curr Epidemiol Rep.* 2017;**4**(3):211–20.

61. Kaldawy A., Segev Y., Lavie O., et al., Low-grade serous ovarian cancer: A review. *Gynecol Oncol.* 2016;**143**(2):433–8.

62. Goff B. A., Sainz de la Cuesta R., Muntz H. G., et al., Clear cell carcinoma of the ovary: a distinct histologic type with poor prognosis and resistance to platinum-based chemotherapy in stage III disease. *Gynecol Oncol.* 1996;**60**(3):412–17.

63. Tan D. S., Kaye S. Ovarian clear cell adenocarcinoma: A continuing enigma. *J Clin Pathol.* 2007;**60**(4):355–60.

64. Hoerl H. D., Hart W. R. Primary ovarian mucinous cystadenocarcinomas: A clinicopathologic study of 49 cases with long-term follow-up. *Am J Surg Pathol.* 1998;**22**(12):1449–62.

65. Smith H. O., Berwick M., Verschraegen C. F., et al., Incidence and survival rates for female malignant germ cell tumors. *Obstet Gynecol.* 2006;**107**(5):1075–85.

66. La Vecchia C., Morris H. B., Draper G. J. Malignant ovarian tumours in childhood in Britain, 1962–78. *Br J Cancer.* 1983;**48**(3):363–74.

67. Shah J. P., Kumar S., Bryant C. S., et al., A population-based analysis of 788 cases of yolk sac tumors: A comparison of males and females. *Int J Cancer.* 2008;**123**(11):2671–5.

68. Young R. H., The yolk sac tumor: Reflections on a remarkable neoplasm and two of the many intrigued by it-Gunnar Teilum and Aleksander Talerman-and the bond it formed between them. *Int J Surg Pathol.* 2014;**22**(8):677–87.

69. Young R. H., Sex cord-stromal tumors of the ovary and testis: Their similarities and differences with consideration of selected problems. *Mod Pathol.* 2005;**18**(Suppl 2): S81–98.

70. Malmstrom H., Högberg T., Risberg B., et al., Granulosa cell tumors of the ovary: prognostic factors and outcome. *Gynecol Oncol.* 1994;**52**(1):50–5.

71. Litta P., Saccardi C., Conte L., et al., Sertoli-Leydig cell tumors: Current status of surgical management: literature review and proposal of treatment. *Gynecol Endocrinol.* 2013;**29**(5):412–17.

72. Fader A. N., Rose P. G. Role of surgery in ovarian carcinoma. *J Clin Oncol.* 2007;**25**(20):2873–83.

73. Bristow R. E., Tomacruz R. S., Armstrong D. K., et al., Survival effect of maximal cytoreductive surgery for advanced ovarian carcinoma during the platinum era: a meta-analysis. *J Clin Oncol.* 2002;**20**(5):1248–59.

74. Wright A. A., Bohlke K., Armstrong D. K., et al., Neoadjuvant chemotherapy for newly diagnosed, advanced ovarian cancer: Society of Gynecologic Oncology and American Society of Clinical Oncology Clinical Practice Guideline. *Gynecol Oncol.* 2016;**143**(1):3–15.

75. Kehoe S., Hook J., Nankivell M., et al., Primary chemotherapy versus primary surgery for newly diagnosed advanced ovarian cancer (CHORUS): an open-label, randomised, controlled, non-inferiority trial. *Lancet.* 2015;**386**(9990):249–57.

76. Vergote I., Tropé C. G., Amant F., et al., Neoadjuvant chemotherapy or primary surgery in stage IIIC or IV ovarian cancer. *N Engl J Med.* 2010;**363**(10):943–53.

77. Morrison J., Haldar K., Kehoe S. et al., Chemotherapy versus surgery for initial treatment in advanced ovarian epithelial cancer. *Cochrane Database Syst Rev.* 2012;**2012**(8):CD005343.

78. Tew W. P., Lacchetti C., Ellis A., et al., PARP inhibitors in the management of ovarian cancer: ASCO Guideline. *J Clin Oncol.* 2020;**38**(30):3468–93.

79. Torre L. A., Trabert B., DeSantis C. E., et al., Ovarian cancer statistics, 2018. *CA Cancer J Clin.* 2018;**68**(4):284–96.

80. Winter W. E., 3rd, Maxwell G. L., Tian C., et al., Prognostic factors for stage III epithelial ovarian cancer: A Gynecologic Oncology Group Study. *J Clin Oncol.* 2007;**25**(24):3621–7.

81. Jacoby V. L., Grady D., Wactawski-Wende J., et al., Oophorectomy vs ovarian conservation with hysterectomy: Cardiovascular disease, hip fracture, and cancer in the Women's Health Initiative Observational Study. *Arch Intern Med.* 2011;**171**(8):760–8.

82. Network, N.C.C. *NCCN Clinical Practice Guidelines in Oncology. Genetic/Familial High-Risk Assessment: Breast, Ovarian, and Pancreatic. Version 3.2023.* April 9, 2023.

83. Parker W. H., Broder M. S., Chang E., et al., Ovarian conservation at the time of hysterectomy and long-term health outcomes in the nurses' health study. *Obstet Gynecol.* 2009;**113**(5):1027–37.

84. Rocca W. A., Grossardt B. R., de Andrade M., et al., Survival patterns after oophorectomy in premenopausal women: A population-based cohort study. *Lancet Oncol.* 2006;**7**(10):821–8.

85. Sinno A. K., Pinkerton J., Febbraro T., et al., Hormone therapy (HT) in women with gynecologic cancer and in women at high risk for developing a gynecologic cancer: A Society of Gynecologic Oncology (SGO) clinical practice statement: This practice statement has been endorsed by The North American Menopause Society. *Gynecol Oncol.* 2020;**157**(2):303–6.

86. Holmberg L., Iversen O. E., Rudenstam C. M., et al., Increased risk of recurrence after hormone replacement therapy in breast cancer survivors. *J Natl Cancer Inst.* 2008;**100**(7):475–82.

87. Sadowski E. A., Thomassin-Naggara I., Rockall A., et al., O-RADS MRI risk stratification system: Guide for assessing adnexal lesions from the ACR O-RADS Committee. *Radiology.* 2022;**303**(1):35–47.

88. Amin M. B. *AJCC Cancer Staging Manual.* Vol. 1024. Springer; 2017.

Thyroid Cancer

Jordana Faruqi, Maryam Tetlay, and Nupur Kikani

Gynecologic Considerations of Thyroid Cancer

Case Presentation

A 33-year-old woman is referred to the endocrinology clinic for new-onset neck swelling. Six months ago, she noted swelling on the left side of her neck that has remained stable in size. She denies difficulty swallowing, shortness of breath, or neck discomfort. She denies major changes in her weight and negative history of hyperthyroidism or hypothyroidism. Medical history is notable for childhood Hodgkin Lymphoma diagnosed at age seven years for which she received vinblastine, doxorubicin, methotrexate, and prednisone (VAMP) followed by mediastinal radiation therapy (INRT). She has been attempting pregnancy for one year and is now 12 weeks of gestation by last menstrual period. On physical exam, she has a firm, one centimeter, nontender, palpable neck mass on the anterior left neck.

Ultrasound of the head and neck reveals a left solid, hypoechoic nodule in the left thyroid lobe with ill-defined margins and punctate echogenic foci measuring 1.9 x 3.0 x 2.5 cm. Metastatic appearing adenopathy is present throughout the left lateral neck. The largest neck node measures 3.9 x 2.4 x 1.1 cm. Thyroid lab testing reveals a thyroid stimulating hormone (TSH) of 1.1 mIU/L (normal range 0.5–5.0 mIU/L), free thyroxine (T4) 1.5 ng/dL (normal range 0.9–2.3 ng/dL), thyroglobulin 91.2 ng/mL (normal range 3–40 ng/mL), and thyroglobulin antibody <0.9 IU/mL (normal range <4 U/mL).

Fine needle aspiration of the left-sided thyroid nodule and the 3.9 cm left neck lymph node were consistent with papillary thyroid carcinoma. The patient is very distressed with her diagnosis. What are the next best steps?

Epidemiology of Thyroid Cancer

The incidence of thyroid cancer has risen dramatically in the last four decades worldwide [13]. In 2020, the incidence rate of thyroid cancer was 10.1 per 10,000 women and 3.1 per 100,000 men [14]. The dramatic rise in detection of thyroid cancer is in part due to the improvement in imaging modalities such as thyroid ultrasonography, CT imaging and the use of more sensitive diagnostic tools [15]. There is also a greater incidence of thyroid cancer in high and very high Human Development Index countries with a similar mortality rate globally [14]. The Human Development Index measures a country's average achievements according to the following dimensions of human development: health (life expectancy at birth), knowledge (measured as mean years of schooling) and standard of living (as measured by gross national income) [16].

In the past decade, there has been a push to reduce overdiagnosis to avoid overtreatment, as the greatest increase in incidence of thyroid cancer has been for small, localized tumors [17]. However, there has also been an increase in the incidence of aggressive thyroid cancer, and therefore careful diagnostic evaluation and surveillance should be performed on all patients. The incidence-based mortality from thyroid cancer in the United States increased 1.1% per year from 0.40 per 100,000 person-years in 1994 to 0.46 per 100,000 person-years in 2010 [18]. Worldwide, the age-standard mortality rate of thyroid cancer is 0.5 per 100,000 for women and 0.3 per 100,000 for men [14].

Less aggressive forms of thyroid cancer such as follicular thyroid cancer (FTC) and papillary thyroid cancer (PTC) are more prevalent in women, whereas more aggressive forms of thyroid cancer such as anaplastic thyroid cancer (ATC) and medullary thyroid cancer (MTC) have equivalent gender prevalence amongst men and women. Women may have more advanced disease at the time of diagnosis [13].

The rates of thyroid cancer by histologic type vary greatly. Approximately 90% of thyroid carcinomas are papillary thyroid carcinomas, 4% are follicular thyroid carcinomas, 2% are hurthle cell carcinomas, 2% are medullary thyroid carcinomas, and 1% are anaplastic thyroid carcinomas [15]. Papillary thyroid cancer typically have the best prognosis, followed by follicular cell carcinomas as these tumors are slow-growing and there are effective therapies for management. Anaplastic thyroid carcinomas have the lowest survival rate [15]. In the United States, the incidence of thyroid cancer is highest amongst the non-Hispanic White population with small, localized papillary thyroid cancer predominating. The lowest incidence of thyroid cancer has been noted in the Native American/Alaskan native and Black population. Those that identify as Asian/Pacific Islander are more likely to be diagnosed with advanced disease even after adjusting for sociodemographic factors [15].

As most thyroid cancer are indolent papillary thyroid carcinomas that can be treated surgically and with radioactive iodine, prognosis of thyroid cancer in general is excellent. In the United States, the five-year relative survival rate is as follows: 98.6% overall for thyroid cancer, 99.9% for localized disease, and 54.9% for distant metastatic disease [15]. Prognosis is much better for papillary thyroid carcinomas and follicular thyroid carcinomas compared to anaplastic thyroid carcinomas and poorly differentiated thyroid carcinomas [15].

Overview of the Thyroid

Synthesis and Secretion of Thyroid Hormones

The thyroid gland is an essential endocrine organ that is responsible for synthesizing and secreting the thyroid hormones thyroxine (T4) and triiodothyronine (T3) under the regulation of the hypothalamic-pituitary-thyroid axis (HPT), which functions as a multi-loop feedback system [1]. The hypothalamus releases thyrotropin-releasing hormone (TRH), which stimulates the anterior pituitary gland to produce and secrete thyroid-stimulating hormone (TSH). TSH then stimulates the thyroid gland to produce thyroid hormones T3 and T4 (often collectively referred to as "thyroid hormone"). The HPT axis is under negative feedback control, as T3 and T4 regulate TRH and TSH upstream. If circulating T3 and T4 are high, the production of TRH and TSH decreases. If T3 and T4 are low, TSH and TRH levels increase in response [2]. In clinical practice, unbound free T4 and TSH are measured to assess thyroid function, recognize thyroid dysfunction if present, and for adequate dose titration for patients receiving synthetic thyroid hormone.

A key component to thyroid hormone synthesis is iodine, an essential micronutrient converted into iodide during digestive processes. Within the thyroid, thyroid hormone is synthesized by the iodination of tyrosine residues of thyroglobulin homodimers to form monoiodotyrosine (MIT) and triiodothyronine (DIT). Thyroid peroxidase (TPO) then catalyzes formation of T4 and T3. T3 and T4 travel across the basolateral membrane of the thyroid follicular cells and enter circulation. The thyroid gland mostly secretes T4, the inactive form of thyroid hormone, which is converted to T3 (active form) or reverse T3 (inactive form) in the periphery [3].

Thyroid Hormone Action

Thyroid hormone (TH) is bound to thyroid-binding globulin and albumin in the circulation [4]. TH is essential for the regulation of growth, development, and metabolism, and affects most organ systems in the body.

Thyroid hormone increases heart rate, stroke volume, cardiac output and contractility through upregulation of genes responsible for cardiac contractility and ejection fraction such as upregulation of the expression of genes encoding sodium/potassium-transporting ATPases [5].

Thyroid hormone increases basal metabolic rate by increasing gene expression of Na/K ATPase which leads to increased O2 consumption, respiratory rate, and body temperature. Thyroid hormone stimulates metabolism of carbohydrates and anabolism of proteins and catabolism of proteins at high levels of thyroid hormone. Thyroid hormone can both induce lipolysis or lipid synthesis based on metabolic status. Thyroid hormone can cause increased gluconeogenesis, glycogen synthesis, glucose oxidation and glucose reabsorption [6, 7].

In childhood, thyroid hormone acts synergistically with growth hormone to stimulate bone growth by inducing chondrocytes, osteoblasts, and osteoclasts. It also helps with brain maturation via formation of the myelin sheath and axonal growth [6, 8].

Thyroid hormone exerts a significant influence on ovulation, menstruation and fertility [6, 9]. Hypothyroidism (low thyroid hormone levels) or hyperthyroidism (excess thyroid hormone levels) can disrupt the normal functioning of the reproductive system [10]. Hypothyroidism can lead to disturbances in the menstrual cycle, including anovulation or irregular ovulation, which can impact fertility by affecting the timing and quality of ovulation. Thyroid hormone is involved in the development and shedding of the uterine lining during menstruation [11]. Hypothyroidism can lead to heavy or prolonged menstrual bleeding (menorrhagia), while hyperthyroidism can cause light or infrequent menstrual periods (oligomenorrhea) or even amenorrhea (absence of menstruation) [10]. These menstrual irregularities can affect fertility by altering the timing and predictability of the menstrual cycle [12]. Hypothyroidism can disrupt the normal release of gonadotropin-releasing hormone (GnRH) from the hypothalamus, which can lead to reduced production of follicle-stimulating hormone (FSH) and luteinizing hormone (LH) from the pituitary gland [12]. This can impair follicular development, ovulation, and the ability to conceive [11].

It is worth noting that the effects of thyroid hormone on ovulation, menstruation, and fertility can vary depending on the severity of the thyroid disorder, individual differences, and other underlying factors. As discussed later in this chapter, thyroid cancer treatment often requires TSH suppression, which can cause iatrogenic hypothyroidism. This requires close monitoring for any new or worsening menstrual irregularities, and an individualized discussion on the benefits and harms of TSH suppression with levothyroxine (synthetic T4).

HPT Axis

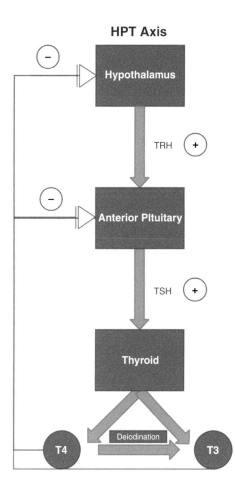

Figure 21.1 The thyroid gland is under the regulation of the hypothalamic-pituitary-thyroid axis, which functions as a multi-loop feedback system. The hypothalamus releases thyrotropin-releasing hormone (TRH), which stimulates the anterior pituitary gland to produce and secrete thyroid-stimulating hormone (TSH), which in turn stimulates the thyroid gland to produce thyroid hormones, triiodothyronine (T3) and thyroxine (T4) [15]

Evaluation of Thyroid Nodules

Thyroid cancer is the most common endocrine neoplasm encountered in clinical practice [19]. Thyroid cancer may be suspected if there is a palpable or radiologically detected thyroid nodule, a strong family history of thyroid cancer, or a new onset of compressive symptoms such as dysphagia, dysphonia or enlargement of a neck mass [15].

Thyroid nodules are defined as discrete lesions within the thyroid gland that are radiologically distinct from surrounding thyroid tissue [20]. Thyroid nodules may be palpated on clinical exam, or detected incidentally on imaging studies such as ultrasounds [20]. In general, thyroid nodules greater than 1 cm or nodules of any size with concerning features warrant further evaluation [20]. Upon discovery of a thyroid nodule, a complete history and focused exam of the thyroid gland and adjacent cervical lymph nodes is indicated.

High-resolution ultrasound can detect and evaluate thyroid nodules [20]. All patients with a suspected thyroid nodule on palpation, a nodular goiter, or incidentally discovered thyroid nodule on other imaging modalities (such as computed tomography (CT) or magnetic resonance imaging (MRI)) should obtain a diagnostic thyroid ultrasound.

Sonographic imaging will assess nodule size, characteristics, and presence of extra-thyroidal abnormalities such as cervical lymphadenopathy [20].

Diagnostic fine needle aspiration (FNA) of the thyroid nodule is recommended for the following:

Nodules greater than or equal to 1 cm in greatest dimension with an intermediate or suspicious sonographic pattern (described in detail in the following paragraph); nodules greater than or equal to 1.5 cm with a low suspicion sonographic pattern; and nodules greater than or equal to 2 cm in greatest dimension with very low suspicion sonographic pattern. Purely cystic thyroid nodules do not require FNA [20]. American Thyroid Association has published guidelines regarding risk stratification based on sonographic appearance (Table 21.1).

The American College of Radiology also has a scoring system called Thyroid Imaging Reporting and Data System (TI-RADS) (Table 21.2), which uses a scoring system to evaluate whether a nodule FNA is indicated or if observation will suffice [21]. Both scoring systems serve as a guide on when to biopsy a nodule or continue to monitor with serial ultrasounds. If fine needle aspiration is performed, the cytology is reported as outlined by the Bethesda System for Reporting Thyroid Cytopathology. The six major categories estimate risk of malignancy based on cytologic features (Table 21.3).

While ultrasound-guided FNA is highly accurate in diagnosing benign colloid nodules and classic papillary thyroid carcinoma, indeterminate results require additional diagnostic testing either with a lobectomy or molecular testing for a definitive diagnosis [23]. Thyroid molecular testing assesses DNA and RNA mutations to better evaluate indeterminate pathology. Molecular testing can help rule in thyroid cancer in indeterminate nodules that have specific genetic variants (such as *BRAF* and *RET/PTC* mutations) and may exclude thyroid cancer in certain cases [23] [24]. When available, molecular testing can help better characterize thyroid nodule cytology results.

Table 21.1 American Thyroid Association guidelines on thyroid nodules and risk of malignancy based on ultrasound characteristics

American Thyroid Association Guidelines on Thyroid Nodules

Ultrasound characteristics	Suspicion	% Risk of malignancy
Cystic, fluid – filled nodules	Benign	<1%
Spongiform, partially cystic nodules	Very low suspicion	<3%
Hyperechoic, or solid nodules with regular margins; isoechoic with regular margins; partially cystic nodules with eccentric solid areas	Low suspicion	<5–10%
Hypoechoic with solid regular margins	Intermediate-risk	10–20%
Microcalcifications, hypoechoic nodules with irregular margins; hypoechoic irregular margins; invasion into non-thyroidal structures; nodule appears taller than wide on ultrasound	High suspicion	>70–90%

Table 21.2 TI-RADS classification system to determine if fine needle aspiration is indicated

TI-RADS classification system

Composition	Echogenicity	Shape	Margin	Echogenic Foci
Cystic (0) Spongiform (0) Mixed cystic and solid (1) Solid (2)	Anechoic (0) Hyperechoic or isoechoic (1) Hypoechoic (2) Very hypoechoic (3)	Wider than tall (0) Taller than wide (3)	Smooth (0) Ill-defined (0) Lobulated or irregular (2) Extra-thyroidal extension (3)	None or large comet-tail artifacts (0) Macrocalcifications (1) Peripheral (rim) calcifications (2) Punctate echogenic foci (3)
0 points: TR1 Benign – No FNA	2 points: TR2 Not suspicious – No FNA	3 points: TR3 Mildly suspicious FNA if > 2.5 cm; follow with serial ultrasound if > 1.5 cm	4–6 points: TR4 Moderately suspicious -FNA if > 1.5 cm; follow with serial ultrasound if > 1 cm	7+ points: TR5 Highly suspicious FNA if > 1 cm; follow with serial ultrasound if > 0.5 cm

Table 21.3 Bethesda System for reporting thyroid cytopathology and risk of malignancy [20, 22]

Bethesda System for Reporting Thyroid Cytopathology	
Nondiagnostic or unsatisfactory	1–4% predicted risk of malignancy
Benign	0–3% predicted risk of malignancy
Atypia of undetermined significance	5–15% of predicted risk of malignancy
Follicular lesion of undetermined significance	5–15% of predicted risk of malignancy
Follicular neoplasm	15–30% estimated risk of malignancy
Suspicious for a follicular neoplasm	15–30% estimated risk of malignancy
Suspicious for malignancy	60–75% risk of malignancy
Malignant	97–99% predicted risk of malignancy

Pathophysiology of Thyroid Cancer

Thyroid cancer is divided into different subtypes which have varying clinical presentations, prognosis, treatment, and monitoring. Thyroid cancer can range from indolent, slow-growing asymptomatic tumors to rapidly aggressive tumors with poor prognosis. Thyroid cancer subtypes are divided into the following: Differentiated follicular-derived thyroid cancer, anaplastic thyroid cancer (undifferentiated thyroid cancer), medullary thyroid cancer, and other rare types [15].

Differentiated Thyroid Cancer

Differentiated thyroid cancer arise from thyroid follicular epithelial cells. The three main subtypes of differentiated thyroid cancer are: papillary thyroid cancer, follicular thyroid cancer, and Hurthle cell thyroid cancer [15]. There are several staging classifications used for thyroid cancer to help predict disease-specific mortality; however, they are unable to predict recurrence for individuals. For differentiated thyroid cancer, age is a critical factor regarding outcomes. According to the American Joint Committee on Cancer/Union for International Cancer Control (AJCC/UICC), all patients less than 55 years old are considered to have stage I cancer unless there is evidence of distant metastasis, in which case they are considered to have stage II disease. However, patients greater than or equal to 55 years of age are staged based on tumor characteristics, nodal involvement and distant metastatic disease [25, 26]. Table 21.4 compares general staging guidelines of differentiated thyroid cancer and anaplastic thyroid cancer.

Papillary Thyroid Cancer

Papillary thyroid cancer (PTC) is the most common form of thyroid cancer. PTC has a predisposition to metastasize to the cervical lymph nodes and less frequently to the lungs and can range from sub-centimeter indolent microcarcinomas to highly aggressive variants [15], [13]. PTC can often be readily diagnosed by fine needle aspiration which reveals the characteristic histologic findings of nuclear enlargement, overlap, irregular contours, psammoma bodies (lamellated calcification) and clear appearance of nucleoplasm [17].

Table 21.4

Differentiated Thyroid Cancer Staging (American Joint Committee on Cancer/Union for International Cancer Control)

Stage I	< 55 years old at age of diagnosis without evidence of distant metastasis
Stage II	< 55 years old at age at diagnosis with evidence of distant metastasis

Patients 55 years of age or older are staged based on tumor characteristics, nodal involvement and distant metastatic disease

Anaplastic Thyroid Cancer Staging

Stage IV	All patients diagnosed with anaplastic thyroid cancer regardless of age, resection and additional findings

Surgery is the primary treatment of papillary thyroid cancer, and the decision to perform a lobectomy versus a total thyroidectomy depends on the initial size of the cancer, presence of extrathyroidal extension or lymph node metastases. Surgery should be performed at a high-volume center to decrease risk of complications [27].

For patients who undergo total thyroidectomy, levothyroxine (synthetic thyroxine) replacement is started immediately to compensate for the loss of endogenous production of thyroid hormone. TSH suppression with levothyroxine is an important aspect of differentiated thyroid cancer care. TSH-suppressive therapy reduces the physiologic stimulation of TSH, which can stimulates the growth of cells in the thyroid bed [28].

The TSH goal for a patient is based on their risk of recurrence as determined by surgical pathology. For patients at low risk of recurrence, the initial TSH goal per the ATA guidelines is 0.5–2 mIU/L; for intermediate risk the goal is 0.1–0.5 mIU/L; and for high risk the goal is < 0.1 mIU/L. For patients who undergo only a lobectomy, TSH goal is 0.5–2 mIU/L [27].

Radioactive iodine (RAI) is a radiopharmaceutical agent that can be used for both diagnostic and therapeutic purposes in thyroid disease [29]. The sodium-iodide symporter (NIS) on differentiated thyroid cancer cells will uptake and absorb iodine physiologically. Uptake of RAI can destroy remnant thyroid tissue and cancer cells [30]. Absolute contraindications to RAI therapy include pregnancy and breastfeeding, as iodine is secreted through breastmilk [31, 32]. Women are counseled to avoid pregnancy for 6 to 12 months after receiving RAI. Breastfeeding must be stopped at least 6 weeks before administration of RAI treatment and cannot be resumed after treatment for the current child but can be safely done in future pregnancies [20]. Ceasing breastfeeding for six weeks prior to RAI is recommended to reduce the radiation dose to the breasts and the risk of milk leakage that can contaminate clothing with radioactive iodine. There is no clear evidence that RAI leads to infertility in women.

Radioactive iodine can be given to patients who have had a total thyroidectomy based on their risk stratification for recurrence [20]. At this time, the American Thyroid Association and European Thyroid Association do not provide a strong recommendation regarding radioactive iodine ablation after surgery in patients with low risk differentiated thyroid cancer. Schvartz et. al found no survival benefit of radioactive iodine ablation after surgery in patients with low-risk differentiated thyroid cancer [33]. Typically, patients with lymph node metastases, vascular invasion or aggressive histology will receive adjuvant treatment with RAI. Patients at low risk for recurrence do not routinely receive RAI [20]. TSH should be greater than 30 mIU/L prior to RAI treatment for maximum effectiveness. This may be facilitated by withholding thyroid hormone replacement for three to six weeks before RAI, or by administering recombinant human TSH (rhTSH) [27, 34]. Follow-up I-131 whole body diagnostic scan can be obtained to verify uptake [29].

For patients with *BRAF*-mutated and radioiodine refractory advanced differentiated thyroid cancer, dabrafenib (a *BRAF* inhibitor) and trametinib (selective inhibitor of MEK1/MEK2 activation and kinase activity) combination therapy is a systemic treatment option. The synergistic mechanism of dabrafenib and trametinib inhibits downstream MAPK signaling in order to lead to cell-cycle arrest [35]. However, an open-label multicenter trial evaluated dabrafenib monotherapy versus dabrafenib plus trametinib therapy, and found statistically similar response rates with monotherapy compared to combination therapy [36].

Follicular Thyroid Cancer

Follicular thyroid carcinoma (FTC) is also derived from the thyroid follicular epithelium and is able to concentrate radioactive iodine [17]. In contrast to papillary thyroid carcinoma, the onset of FTC peaks between 40 to 60 years, follows a more aggressive course, and has a higher prevalence in women [37]. Follicular thyroid cancer diagnosis requires excisional biopsy or histologic evaluation from thyroid surgery after FNA to identify key features of this malignancy [17]. On histology, characteristic findings of PTC are absent and uniform microfollicular architecture of cuboidal cells lining follicles are seen [38].

Follicular thyroid cancer is treated with surgery, thyroid hormone suppression with levothyroxine, and radioiodine therapy in high-risk patients and selected intermediate-risk patients [20].

Hürthle Cell Thyroid Cancer

Hürthle cell carcinomas were previously designated as a variant of FTC. However, research has shown that hürthle cell carcinomas have a distinct molecular profile separate from FTC [17]. These thyroid cancer are more aggressive when compared to PTC and FTC counterparts [15]. Clinically, they often present as an asymptomatic thyroid nodule. Histologically, these tumors have an increased number of atypical mitochondria. Additional characteristic findings include eosinophilic oxyphilic cells with abundant cytoplasm, round oval nuclei, and prominent nucleoli [38]. Hürthle cell carcinomas portend a poor prognosis and are challenging to treat, as they have poor iodine avidity and a higher risk of recurrence [39]. Surgery is the primary treatment for Hürthle cell tumors [40]. While radioactive iodine can be used, it is less effective as only 10% of patients with Hürthle cell carcinoma will have iodine-avid lesions. For patients with high-risk features or invasion, a FDG-PET scan is a more accurate imaging modality [41].

Poorly Differentiated Thyroid Cancer (PDTC)

Poorly differentiated thyroid cancer are rare thyroid tumors. These tumors were initially described as a distinct subtype by Carcangiu et al. [42]. Patients often have locally advanced disease on diagnosis. Diagnosis can be made with fine needle aspiration with histology demonstrating overlapping cells with a high nucleus to cytoplasm ratio and scant cytoplasm with minimal colloid [42]. Histological criteria for diagnosis includes evidence of an insular, solid or trabecular growth from a follicular-derived thyroid lesion without typical PTC nuclear features and the presence of necrosis, convoluted nuclei or mitotic activity [43]. Unfortunately, there is no standardized treatment for these cancer. Total thyroidectomy is treatment of choice. Radioactive iodine ablation has shown variable response, as older age and extranodal extension are associated with loss of radioactive iodine avidity [44] [45].

Undifferentiated Thyroid Cancer

Anaplastic Thyroid Cancer

Anaplastic thyroid cancer (ATC) accounts for less than 1% of all thyroid cancer. ATC typically presents as a rapidly growing neck mass with concomitant dysphagia and hoarseness. Anaplastic cancer can occur de novo, evolve from a differentiated thyroid cancer (PTC, FTC, Hürthle-cell carcinoma) or coexist with differentiated thyroid cancer [46]. The peak incidence of ATC is within the 60th and 70th decades of life with a slightly higher incidence in males. Historically, anaplastic thyroid cancer had a four-month median overall survival from time of diagnosis. ATC rapidly progresses to metastatic disease preferentially involving the lungs, bone, and brain. There has been significant advancement in the treatment of ATC. A recent retrospective cohort study found the median overall survival rate of anaplastic thyroid cancer was 9.5 months when stratified by stage and type of therapy [47]. Improved overall survival rates can be attributed to neoadjuvant *BRAF*-directed therapy followed by surgery [47].

ATC diagnosis requires prompt referral to a large multidisciplinary center of expertise [15]. Rapid testing for *BRAF* V600E should be obtained once anaplastic thyroid cancer is diagnosed, and all patients with anaplastic thyroid cancer are classified as stage IV, regardless of complete resection and incidental findings [48]. Further information regarding staging of thyroid cancer may be found in Table 21.4.

Histology on FNA shows the presence of spindle cells, pleomorphic and prominent nuclei with atypical mitosis or necrosis in the background [46]. Recently, treatment of *BRAF* V600E positive ATC patients with dabrafenib and trametinib has shown encouraging results. A small study evaluating the safety and efficacy of dabrafenib and trametinib combination therapy in *BRAF* V600E- mutated anaplastic cancer showed an overall response rate of 69% [49].

Medullary Thyroid Cancer

Medullary thyroid cancer (MTC) accounts for 1 to 2% of all thyroid cancer. MTC originates from the parafollicular neuroendocrine cells of the thyroid and is associated with multiple endocrine neoplasia (MEN) 2A and 2B. Approximately 25% of patients with MTC have a MEN syndrome [15]. A diagnosis of MTC should prompt surveillance for other neoplasms associated with MEN 2A and 2B.

The MEN syndromes are autosomal-dominant conditions that significantly increase the risk of multiple tumors and cancer in an individual and affected family members [50]. Both MEN 2A and MEN 2B result from pathogenic variants in the *RET* protooncogene. However, the constellation of disorders differ. Individuals with MEN 2A are predisposed to medullary thyroid cancer, pheochromocytoma, primary hyperparathyroidism, cutaneous lichen amyloidosis, and Hirschsprung disease. Those with MEN 2B commonly present with medullary thyroid cancer, pheochromocytoma, a marfanoid body habitus, ganglioneuromatosis and mucosal neuromas [50].

MTC can be diagnosed by fine-needle aspiration and immunohistochemical staining for calcitonin [51] [52]. Medullary thyroid cancer tumor markers include calcitonin and carcinoembryonic antigen (CEA) [53]. Pathogenic drivers in medullary thyroid cancer include the overexpression of tyrosine kinase inhibitors (VEGFR, EGFR, MET) [53].

Medullary thyroid cancer does not require suppressive dosing of levothyroxine, as the cells involved are not hormonally responsive to TSH. Replacement therapy is aimed at maintaining euthyroid levels [51]. All patients with presumed sporadic MTC should undergo genetic testing for a germline *RET* mutation in addition to first-degree relatives of patients [52]. Treatment includes complete surgical resection for locoregional MTC. A total thyroidectomy is the preferred surgery since bilateral or multifocal disease occurs in patients with inherited MTC and 10% of those with sporadic MTC. Recurrent or metastatic MTC warrants additional treatment which may include repeat surgical resection, external beam radiation therapy, or systemic therapies [51, 54, 55].

Vandetanib and cabozantinib are currently FDA approved for the treatment of medullary carcinoma. Recent multicenter phase III trial patients showed a median progression-free survival of 30.5 months in the vandetanib arm compared to 19.3 months in the placebo arm, and 11.2 months for the cabozantinib arm as compared to 4 months in the placebo arm [55] [54]. Development and clinical evaluation of more specific tyrosine kinase inhibitors for rare oncogenic mutations for targeted therapy is underway [28].

Non-Thyroid Origin Thyroid Malignancies

Metastasis to the Thyroid Gland

While the thyroid gland has an extensive blood supply, metastasis to the thyroid is uncommon [56]. Metastasis to the thyroid may be diagnosed in the setting of a known non-thyroidal malignancy during preoperative work-up, or incidentally on histologic examination of thyroid [56]. The overall incidence of thyroid metastasis is 2%, with the most common site of the primary tumor is the kidney, followed by lung, and gastrointestinal tract cancer [56].

Thyroid Lymphoma

Primary thyroid lymphoma accounts for less than 5% of all thyroid malignancies and less than 2% of extranodal lymphomas [57, 58] with a higher incidence in women than men [59]. Patients may present in their sixth or seventh decade of life [59]. Patients with preexisting Hashimoto's thyroiditis have a greater risk of developing primary thyroid lymphoma with a relative risk of 67 as compared to patients without thyroiditis [60]. Prognosis and treatment depend on the histology and staging of the tumor at diagnosis [59]. The most common subtype of primary thyroid lymphomas is diffuse large B-cell lymphoma, followed by mucosa-associated lymphoid tissue (MALT) [59]. Fine needle aspiration biopsy may accurately detect primary thyroid lymphoma with an accuracy rate of 80–100%. Treatment options include radiation therapy for localized, indolent disease and radiation therapy plus chemotherapy for aggressive disease with multi-agent chemotherapy [59]. For diffuse large B-cell thyroid lymphoma, five-year disease specific survival rate is 71 to 75%, and for mucosa associated lymphoid tissue lymphoma, the five-year survival rate is 96 to 100% [59].

Struma Ovarii

Struma ovarii is a rare dermoid tumor of the ovary where greater than 50% of the overall tissue type is thyroid [61]. Patients typically present with symptoms of lower abdominal pain, mass, or less commonly, ascites. Clinical or biochemical evidence of hyperthyroidism is rare in these patients. There are no distinguishing features of these tumors on ultrasound. If struma ovarii is suspected, a pelvic ultrasound should be obtained followed by a radioactive iodine uptake scan of the pelvis to confirm the presence of thyroid tissue [66].

These tumors in general have a favorable prognosis, with overall survival estimated to be 81% at 10 years and 60% at 25 years [62]. Poor prognosis is associated with tumor size greater than 10 cm and malignant struma ovarii, often characterized by extensive high-grade papillary carcinoma. Treatment for benign struma ovarii consists of an oophorectomy. In malignant struma ovarii, there is no consensus on treatment. However, treatment may involve oophorectomy followed by adjuvant RAI ablation and thyroidectomy. Due to the rarity of struma ovarii tumor, there is no standardized clinical management and management is based on published case studies [63].

Risk Factors for Thyroid Cancer

Ionizing Radiation

Childhood exposure to ionizing radiation is a well-established risk factor for thyroid cancer. This was first recognized by Duffy and Fitzergald in 1950, when they found that a large cohort of patients who had received radiation to the head or neck in childhood developed thyroid cancer [64]. It is unclear if ionizing radiation exposure in general has contributed to higher thyroid cancer levels, but it has been noted that *RET* and *PTC* chromosomal rearrangements are more prevalent in radiation-exposed regions of the world, including areas of Ukraine exposed to the Chernobyl accident, Kazakhstan and Japan [13, 65–67]. There is also an increased risk of papillary thyroid cancer [68].

Preexisting Benign Thyroid Disease

Benign thyroid disease including hyperthyroidism, hypothyroidism, thyroiditis, and benign thyroid nodules may precede thyroid cancer; however, it is unclear if these abnormalities have a causal relationship or directly influence the development or the progression of thyroid cancer [13]. Large studies show elevated risk of thyroid cancer in patients with benign thyroid nodules, goiters, hyperthyroidism, and hypothyroidism but weak associations in patients with autoimmune thyroiditis [13]. A prospective study from Denmark evaluated the risk of thyroid cancer after the diagnosis of benign thyroid disease. They found the standardized incidence ratios for differentiated thyroid cancer were significantly elevated for all benign thyroid diseases with the exception of hypothyroidism [69].

Genetic Factors

Hereditary syndromes and their associated gene mutations confer an increased risk for thyroid cancer. Table 21.5 delineates the hereditary cancer syndromes associated with thyroid cancer.

Gynecologic Factors at the Time of Diagnosis of Thyroid Cancer

Thyroid cancer is approximately three times more common in women compared to men [70]. This disparity has been well-documented in the literature across the world [70]. However, it is unclear why this stark disparity exists. In women, risk of thyroid cancer varies by age. Incidence rises sharply around menarche and peaks at approximately 40 to 49 years of age [70]. Epidemiological studies investigating the association of thyroid cancer with reproductive factors such as menarche, menopause and parity have conflicting results. It is unclear if sex hormones contribute to the striking disparity in the incidence of thyroid cancer between men and women. As thyroid nodules are more common in women, perhaps there are higher rates of detection of thyroid cancer [70]. Additional investigative studies are needed to further characterize the effect of hormonal and reproductive factors in the incidence of thyroid cancer.

Estrogen can increase proliferation in thyroid cancer cell lines. Estrogen is a potent growth factor for thyroid cells (both benign and malignant) which promotes its effects through genomic and nongenomic pathways mediated via to MAPK and PI3 K tyrosine kinase signaling pathways [71]. Estrogen is associated with an increase in adherence, migration and invasion of thyroid cancer cell lines in in vitro studies. Addition of estrogen antagonists reversed this effect [72]. In contrast, estrogen inhibited growth in anaplastic thyroid cancer cell lines [70] [72].

In vitro studies have demonstrated an association of papillary thyroid cancer proliferation and levels of estrogen; hence we must consider hormonal therapies and their association with thyroid cancer. Epidemiological studies however, have been inconclusive in demonstrating an association between thyroid cancer and hormone specific therapies. Meta-analyses of studies correlating reproductive factors such as age at menarche, age at menopause and parity with papillary thyroid cancer have conflicting results [7].

Although there is no definitive evidence on the effect of hormone therapy on thyroid cancer cell proliferation, hormone therapies may alter thyroid function. The estrogenic component of oral contraceptives can increase liver proteins including thyroid binding globulin (TBG), sex hormone-binding protein (SHBG), and coagulation factors [73]. TBG is responsible for binding to and transporting thyroid hormones with a greater affinity for T4 than T3. An increase in TBG leads to more binding and sequestration of T4, but does not affect the amount of bioactive free T4 [74]. Therefore, patients who have a preexisting thyroid condition requiring thyroid hormone replacement may require higher doses of thyroid hormone after initiating estrogen containing oral contraceptives. If the oral contraceptive is stopped, patients may subsequently require lower doses of thyroid hormone. TBG starts to increase several weeks after oral contraceptives are started. Thus, we recommend monitoring thyroid function tests six to eight weeks after initiation of oral contraceptive.

There have been few studies evaluating the treatment of thyroid cancer and subsequent reproductive function. Hirsch et al. evaluated the rates of pregnancy in patients under the age of 40 years who received radioactive iodine treatment for thyroid cancer between 2000–2020. They found that pregnancy rates for thyroid cancer survivors were statistically

Table 21.5 Hereditary cancer syndromes associated with thyroid cancer

Syndrome	Gene Affected	Clinical Manifestations
Familial Adenomatous Polyposis Syndrome	APC	• Inherited colorectal cancer/polyposis syndrome with near 100% lifetime risk for colon cancer • Papillary thyroid cancer (cribiform morular variant) • Desmoid tumors, jaw tumors, supernumerary teeth
Li-Fraumeni Syndrome	TP53	• Soft tissue sarcomas • Early-onset breast cancer • Osteosarcoma • Acute leukemia • Brain cancer • Adrenal cortical tumors • Melanoma • Wilms' tumor • Cancer of the stomach, colon, pancreas, esophagus, lung, thyroid and gonadal germ cells
Cowden Syndrome	PTEN	• Hamartomous tumors of multiple organ systems • Mucocutaneous abnormalities • Breast cancer • Benign thyroid disease and/or non-medullary thyroid cancer • Benign uterine fibroids and endometrial cancer • Renal cell carcinoma • Gastrointestinal polyps and colorectal cancer • Lhermitte-Duclose disease • Macrocephaly, autism, intellectual disability
DICER1 tumor predisposition Syndrome	DICER1	• Pleuropulmonary blastoma, lung cysts • Uterine, cervical, and bladder rhabdomyosarcoma, ovarian Sertoli-Leydig cell tumors • Childhood onset multinodular goiter or differentiated thyroid cancer
Familial non-Medullary Thyroid Cancer (Familial Papillary Thyroid Cancer)	Unknown	• Patients with 2 or more first degree relatives with non-medullary thyroid cancer

comparable when compared to age-matched controls. However, the study found that there was a higher incidence of infertility and a longer time to conceive in the thyroid cancer group, regardless of single or repeated radioactive iodine treatments [75].

Thyroid Cancer and Pregnancy

The prevalence of thyroid cancer during pregnancy is estimated to be 14.4 per 100,000 births [76]. The incidence has increased in the last few decades [76]. No difference has been reported in overall survival or disease-free survival between pregnant or nonpregnant controls with thyroid cancer [76].

Partial or total thyroidectomy is the mainstay of treatment for thyroid cancer [20]. Delaying surgery until after delivery has not been shown to affect recurrence rates among women diagnosed with differentiated thyroid cancer (DTC) during gestation [77]. According to the current American Thyroid Association (ATA) guidelines, well differentiated papillary thyroid cancer diagnosed early in pregnancy can be monitored with routine ultrasound surveillance [20]. Surgery is indicated during gestation only if aggressive features are present by 24 weeks' gestation. Aggressive features include an increase in tumor size during gestation by greater than 50% in volume and 20% in diameter or if metastatic cervical lymph nodes are present. If surgery is required during pregnancy, it is recommended in the second trimester of pregnancy [78]. For tumors that remain stable in size or if the diagnosis of thyroid cancer is made after 24 weeks' gestation, surgery can be performed after delivery [78]. The impact of pregnancy on women with medullary or anaplastic carcinoma is unknown as few studies have been performed in these populations. As the risk of progression is high in aggressive thyroid malignancies, surgery during pregnancy is the preferred treatment [77, 78].

The TSH goals for differentiated thyroid cancer discussed previously apply without modification in patients during pregnancy since suppressed TSH levels do not cause maternal or neonatal complications. TSH should be monitored every 4 weeks until 16 to 20 weeks' gestation, and at least once between 26- and 32-weeks' gestation [78].

Radioactive iodine is used frequently as adjuvant therapy in patients with iodine-avid disease. There is no clear evidence that RAI is associated with infertility in women. One study found patients exposed to radioactive iodine were more likely to undergo premature menopause and have difficulty with conception compared to the control group [79]. However, a meta-analysis reviewing the effect of RAI therapy for differentiated thyroid cancer on fertility did not show a decrease in pregnancy rates although demonstrated a significant decrease in anti-mullerian hormone levels after therapy [80]. RAI is contraindicated during pregnancy due to the risk of fetal hypothyroidism and malignancy [81, 82]. Women are counseled to avoid pregnancy for 6 to 12 months after receiving RAI. Breastfeeding must be stopped at least six weeks before administration of RAI treatment and cannot be resumed after treatment for the current child but can be safely done in future pregnancies [20].

Tyrosine kinase inhibitors (TKI) such as sorafenib, lenvatinib, and cabozantinib are used frequently in the treatment of metastatic differentiated and medullary thyroid cancer [52]. Administration of these medications during organogenesis have resulted in embryofetal toxicities in animal reproduction studies [83]. While there are no official guidelines regarding tyrosine kinase inhibitors and pregnancy, fertility and pregnancy planning should be discussed and use of these agents should be limited or avoided during pregnancy given potential teratogenic risk [84].

Even though survival is not impacted by pregnancy, pregnancy is associated with an increased risk in the progression of thyroid cancer. Human chorionic gonadotropin (HCG) can cause rapid growth of both benign and malignant thyroid tumors. The HCG molecule is homologically identical to the TSH molecule and can compete for and bind to the TSH receptor, stimulating growth. The rise in serum estrogen during pregnancy has also been associated with an increase in the size of preexisting benign thyroid nodules and an increase in the development of de novo benign thyroid nodules. A retrospective study by Vannucchi et al. demonstrated that patients who had thyroid cancer detected during pregnancy were more likely to develop recurrent and persistent disease. Up to 87.5% of patients who developed thyroid cancer during pregnancy were found to have an estrogen-receptor-positive tumor [70, 85].

Pregnancy has not shown to increase disease recurrence in women who have previously had thyroid cancer, have had excellent response to treatment, and are in remission. Thus, these patients do not require close surveillance during gestation. However, patients with known incomplete or indeterminate biochemical or structural response to therapy, may have thyroid cancer growth during pregnancy and should be monitored closely [86].

Surveillance of Thyroid Cancer

The mainstay of surveillance for differentiated thyroid cancer is maintaining TSH goals with levothyroxine therapy, thyroid ultrasound surveillance to monitor for structural evidence of disease, CT or PET imaging as needed to monitor for stability of metastases, monitoring thyroglobulin or thyroglobulin antibodies for biochemical evidence of disease, and monitoring adverse effects from treatment [20]. Patients with transient or permanent damage to their parathyroid glands during surgery will require regular monitoring and replacement of their calcium levels [20].

Thyroid cancer patients are risk re-stratified at every follow up visit based on their response to therapy. They are deemed as having excellent response to therapy if there is no evidence of clinical, biochemical, or structural disease. If they have abnormal thyroglobulin levels or rising thyroglobulin antibodies, they are designated as having a biochemically incomplete response. If they have evidence of disease on imaging, they are designated as having a structurally incomplete response; and if they have nonspecific biochemical or structural findings they are deemed as having an indeterminate response. TSH goal is then changed based on their dynamic risk [27].

For individuals with medullary thyroid carcinoma after total thyroidectomy, yearly serum calcitonin and CEA can be monitored. If there is a rise in calcitonin or CEA, repeat imaging should be performed. Imaging via CT or MRI can be pursued to assess for distant metastasis [52]. If the individual has MEN2A or MEN2B syndromes, they should undergo yearly screening to evaluate for pheochromocytomas [52]. Family members of patients with known *RET* mutations should also undergo genetic screening and counseling for hereditary cancer syndromes [52].

For anaplastic thyroid cancer, patients require active surveillance given the aggressive nature of the disease [87].

Case Resolution

Risks and benefits of thyroid surgery were carefully discussed with the patient. She opted to undergo thyroidectomy post-partum. During the remainder of her pregnancy, she underwent thyroid ultrasounds each trimester to monitor for stability in tumor size and lymph node burden. No new lymph nodes were noted and the thyroid nodule remained stable. She successfully delivered at 39 weeks gestational age without complications. She subsequently underwent a total thyroidectomy. Postoperative parathyroid hormone level was <10 pg/mL on postoperative days one, two, and three. Serum corrected calcium ranged from 7.3 to 7.7 mg/dL during this period, and she was placed on calcium supplementation postoperatively. Suppressive levothyroxine therapy was initiated with a TSH goal of 0.1–0.5 mIU/L. Final pathology revealed a classical variant of papillary thyroid cancer and 15 of 38 lymph nodes were positive for metastatic PTC. No evidence of lymphovascular invasion or extrathyroidal extension was noted on pathology. Due to her significant nodal disease, she underwent RAI therapy. She stopped breastfeeding six weeks prior to RAI treatment and was informed that she could not breastfeed her current child after treatment. She was also informed that her RAI treatment does not preclude her from breastfeeding future children. She resumed her estrogen containing oral contraceptive pills, and three months later, her levothyroxine dose was increased to maintain the appropriate TSH levels. She is now undergoing yearly surveillance with serial thyroid ultrasounds, thyroid function tests and thyroglobulin levels.

Take Home Points

- All thyroid nodules should be evaluated with a thyroid ultrasound. Those with high-risk radiologic features should be referred for fine needle aspiration.
- Papillary thyroid cancer is the most common form of thyroid cancer. Surgery, adjuvant radioactive iodine therapy, and thyroid hormone suppression are the mainstays of treatment.
- For patients with iodine-avid differentiated thyroid cancer, such as papillary thyroid cancer, at low risk of recurrence, the initial TSH goal is 0.5–2 mIU/L.
- Radioiodine treatment is contraindicated in patients during pregnancy due to the risk of fetal hypothyroidism and malignancy. For breastfeeding patients, breastfeeding should be stopped six weeks prior to RAI treatment and discontinued for the current child thereafter. RAI does not preclude women from breastfeeding future children.
- TSH should be monitored every 4 weeks during pregnancy until 16 to 20 weeks gestation, and at least once between 26- and 32-weeks' gestation in pregnant individuals with thyroid cancer.
- For patients requiring thyroid hormone therapy, dose increases may be required in hyper-estrogenic states such as pregnancy and when starting estrogen-containing products. Conversely, discontinuation of estrogen containing medications or postpartum states may require dose reduction to maintain adequate thyroid hormone levels.

References

1. Moore K., Agur A. *Clinically Oriented Anatomy.* 7th ed. Wolters Kluwer | Lippincott Williams & Wilkins; 2014.

2. Melmed S., Koenig R., Rosen C., et al. *Williams Textbook of Endocrinology.* 14th ed. Elsevier; 2019.

3. Gardener D. *Greenspan's Basic & Clinical Endocrinology*: McGraw Hill; 2011.

4. Bartalena L., Robbins J. Thyroid hormone transport proteins. *Clin Lab Med.* 1993;**13**(3): 583–98.

5. Yamakawa H., Kato T. S., Noh J. Y., et al. Thyroid hormone plays an important role in cardiac function: From bench to bedside. *Front Physiol.* 2021;**12**:606931.

6. Shahid M. A., Ashraf M. A., Sharma S. *Physiology, Thyroid Hormone.* StatPearls; 2022.

7. Mullur R., Liu Y. Y., Brent G. A. Thyroid hormone regulation of metabolism. *Physiol Rev.* 2014;**94**(2):355–82.

8. Mughal B. B., Fini J. B., Demeneix B. A. Thyroid-disrupting chemicals and brain development: An update. *Endocr Connect.* 2018;**7**(4):R160–R86.

9. Maruo T., Katayama K., Barnea E. R., Mochizuki M. A role for thyroid hormone in the induction of ovulation and corpus luteum function. *Horm Res.* 1992;**37** (Suppl 1):12–18.

10. Poppe K., Velkeniers B., Glinoer D. The role of thyroid autoimmunity in fertility and pregnancy. *Nat Clin Pract Endocrinol Metab.* 2008;**4**(7):394–405.

11. Krassas G. E., Poppe K., Glinoer D. Thyroid function and human reproductive health. *Endocr Rev.* 2010;**31**(5):702–55.

12. Unuane D., Tournaye H., Velkeniers B., Poppe K. Endocrine disorders & female infertility. *Best Pract Res Clin Endocrinol Metab.* 2011;**25**(6):861–73.

13. Kitahara C. M., Schneider A. B. Epidemiology of thyroid cancer. *Cancer Epidemiol Biomarkers Prev.* 2022;**31**(7):1284–97.

14. Pizzato M., Li M., Vignat J., et al. The epidemiological landscape of thyroid cancer worldwide: GLOBOCAN estimates for incidence and mortality rates in 2020. *Lancet Diabetes Endocrinol.* 2022;**10**(4):264–72.

15. Cabanillas M. E., McFadden D. G., Durante C. Thyroid cancer. *Lancet.* 2016;**388**(10061):2783–95.

16. Human Development Index. www .who.int/data/nutrition/nlis/info/human-development-index.

17. Daniels G. H. Follicular thyroid carcinoma: A perspective. *Thyroid.* 2018;**28**(10):1229–42.

18. Lim H., Devesa S. S., Sosa J. A., Check D., Kitahara C. M. Trends in thyroid cancer incidence and mortality in the United States, 1974–2013. *JAMA.* 2017;**317**(13):1338–48.

19. Nguyen Q. T., Lee E. J., Huang M. G., et al. Diagnosis and treatment of patients with thyroid cancer. *Am Health Drug Benefits.* 2015;**8**(1):30–40.

20. Haugen B. R. 2015 American Thyroid Association Management Guidelines for adult patients with thyroid nodules and differentiated thyroid cancer: What is new and what has changed? *Cancer.* 2017;**123**(3):372–81.

21. Tessler F. N., Middleton W. D., Grant E. G., et al. ACR Thyroid Imaging, Reporting and Data System (TI-RADS): White Paper of the ACR TI-RADS Committee. *J Am Coll Radiol.* 2017;**14**(5):587–95.

22. Liu X., Medici M., Kwong N., et al. Bethesda categorization of thyroid nodule cytology and prediction of thyroid cancer type and prognosis. *Thyroid.* 2016;**26**(2):256–61.

23. Roth M. Y., Witt R. L., Steward D. L. Molecular testing for thyroid nodules: Review and current state. *Cancer.* 2018;**124**(5):888–98.

24. Gong L., Liu Y., Guo X., et al. BRAF p. V600E genetic testing based on ultrasound-guided fine-needle biopsy improves the malignancy rate in thyroid surgery: Our single-center experience in the past 10 years. *J Cancer Res Clin Oncol.* 2022:1–9.

25. Nixon I. J., Wang L. Y., Migliacci J. C., et al. An international multi-institutional validation of age 55 years as a cutoff for risk stratification in the AJCC/UICC staging system for well-differentiated thyroid cancer. *Thyroid.* 2016;**26**(3):373–80.

26. Thyroid Cancer Stages. www.cancer.org/cancer/thyroid-cancer/detection-diagnosis-staging/staging.html.

27. Haugen B. R., Alexander E. K., Bible K. C., et al. 2015 American Thyroid Association Management Guidelines for Adult Patients with Thyroid Nodules and Differentiated Thyroid Cancer: The American Thyroid Association Guidelines Task Force on

Thyroid Nodules and Differentiated Thyroid Cancer. *Thyroid*. 2016;**26**(1):1–133.

28. Sherman S. I. Evolution of targeted therapies for thyroid carcinoma. *Trans Am Clin Climatol Assoc*. 2019;**130**:255–65.

29. Palot Manzil F. F., Kaur H. *Radioactive Iodine For Thyroid Malignancies*. StatPearls; 2023.

30. Ravera S., Reyna-Neyra A., Ferrandino G., Amzel L. M., Carrasco N. The sodium/iodide symporter (NIS): Molecular physiology and preclinical and clinical applications. *Annu Rev Physiol*. 2017;**79**:261–89.

31. Padda I. S., Nguyen M. *Radioactive Iodine Therapy*. StatPearls; 2023.

32. Luster M., Clarke S. E., Dietlein M., et al. Guidelines for radioiodine therapy of differentiated thyroid cancer. *Eur J Nucl Med Mol Imaging*. 2008;**35**(10):1941–59.

33. Schvartz C., Bonnetain F., Dabakuyo S., et al. Impact on overall survival of radioactive iodine in low-risk differentiated thyroid cancer patients. *J Clin Endocrinol Metab*. 2012;**97**(5):1526–35.

34. Ladenson P. W. Recombinant thyrotropin versus thyroid hormone withdrawal in evaluating patients with thyroid carcinoma. *Semin Nucl Med*. 2000;**30**(2):98–106.

35. Khunger A., Khunger M., Velcheti V. Dabrafenib in combination with trametinib in the treatment of patients with BRAF V600-positive advanced or metastatic non-small cell lung cancer: Clinical evidence and experience. *Ther Adv Respir Dis*. 2018;**12**:1753466618767611.

36. Busaidy N. L., Konda B., Wei L., et al. Dabrafenib versus dabrafenib + trametinib in BRAF-mutated radioactive iodine refractory differentiated thyroid cancer: Results of a randomized, phase 2, open-label multicenter trial. *Thyroid*. 2022;**32**(10):1184–92.

37. United States Cancer Statistics: Data Visualizations. https://gis.cdc.gov/Cancer/USCS/#/Demographics/.

38. Fariduddin M, Syed W. Hurthle Cell Thyroid Carcinoma. [Updated February 13, 2023]. In: StatPearls [Internet]. Treasure Island (FL): StatPearls Publishing; 2023.

39. Lee K., Anastasopoulou C., Chandran C., et al. *Thyroid Cancer*. [Updated May 1, 2021]. In: StatPearls [Internet]. StatPearls Publishing; 2021.

40. Sanders L. E., Silverman M. Follicular and Hurthle cell carcinoma: Predicting outcome and directing therapy. *Surgery*. 1998;**124**(6):967–74.

41. Pryma D. A., Schoder H., Gonen M., et al. Diagnostic accuracy and prognostic value of 18 F-FDG PET in Hurthle cell thyroid cancer patients. *J Nucl Med*. 2006;**47**(8):1260–6.

42. Carcangiu M. L., Zampi G., Rosai J. Poorly differentiated ("insular") thyroid carcinoma. A reinterpretation of Langhans' "wuchernde Struma."*Am J Surg Pathol*. 1984;**8**(9):655–68.

43. Volante M., Collini P., Nikiforov Y. E., et al. Poorly differentiated thyroid carcinoma: The Turin proposal for the use of uniform diagnostic criteria and an algorithmic diagnostic approach. *Am J Surg Pathol*. 2007;**31**(8):1256–64.

44. Nishida T., Katayama S., Tsujimoto M., Nakamura J., Matsuda H. Clinicopathological significance of poorly differentiated thyroid carcinoma. *Am J Surg Pathol*. 1999;**23**(2):205–11.

45. Ibrahimpasic T., Ghossein R., Shah J. P., Ganly I. Poorly differentiated carcinoma of the thyroid gland: Current status and future prospects. *Thyroid*. 2019;**29**(3):311–21.

46. Pizzimenti C., Fiorentino V., Ieni A., et al. Aggressive variants of follicular cell-derived thyroid carcinoma: An overview. *Endocrine*. 2022;**78**(1):1–12.

47. Maniakas A., Dadu R., Busaidy N. L., et al. Evaluation of overall survival in patients with anaplastic thyroid carcinoma, 2000–2019. *JAMA Oncol*. 2020;**6**(9):1397–404.

48. Shonka D. C., Jr., Ho A., Chintakuntlawar A. V., et al. American

Head and Neck Society Endocrine Surgery Section and International Thyroid Oncology Group consensus statement on mutational testing in thyroid cancer: Defining advanced thyroid cancer and its targeted treatment. *Head Neck.* 2022;**44**(6):1277–300.

49. Subbiah V., Kreitman R. J., Wainberg Z. A., et al. Dabrafenib and trametinib treatment in patients with locally advanced or metastatic BRAF V600-mutant anaplastic thyroid cancer. *J Clin Oncol.* 2018;**36**(1):7–13.

50. Callender G. G., Rich T. A., Perrier N. D. Multiple endocrine neoplasia syndromes. *Surg Clin North Am.* 2008;**88**(4):863–95, viii.

51. Kim M., Kim B. H. Current guidelines for management of medullary thyroid carcinoma. *Endocrinol Metab (Seoul).* 2021;**36**(3):514–24.

52. Wells S. A., Jr., Asa S. L., Dralle H., et al. Revised American Thyroid Association guidelines for the management of medullary thyroid carcinoma. *Thyroid.* 2015;**25**(6):567–610.

53. Jaber T., Dadu R., Hu M. I. Medullary thyroid carcinoma. *Curr Opin Endocrinol Diabetes Obes.* 2021;**28**(5):540–6.

54. Wells S. A., Jr., Robinson B. G., Gagel R. F., et al. Vandetanib in patients with locally advanced or metastatic medullary thyroid cancer: A randomized, double-blind phase III trial. *J Clin Oncol.* 2012;**30**(2):134–41.

55. Elisei R., Schlumberger M. J., Muller S. P., et al. Cabozantinib in progressive medullary thyroid cancer. *J Clin Oncol.* 2013;**31**(29):3639–46.

56. Nixon I. J., Coca-Pelaz A., Kaleva A. I., et al. Metastasis to the thyroid gland: A critical review. *Ann Surg Oncol.* 2017;**24**(6):1533–9.

57. Freeman C., Berg J. W., Cutler S. J. Occurrence and prognosis of extranodal lymphomas. *Cancer.* 1972;**29**(1):252–60.

58. Thieblemont C., Mayer A., Dumontet C., et al. Primary thyroid lymphoma is a heterogeneous disease. *J Clin Endocrinol Metab.* 2002;**87**(1):105–11.

59. Stein S. A., Wartofsky L. Primary thyroid lymphoma: A clinical review. *J Clin Endocrinol Metab.* 2013;**98**(8):3131–8.

60. Holm L. E., Blomgren H., Lowhagen T. Cancer risks in patients with chronic lymphocytic thyroiditis. *N Engl J Med.* 1985;**312**(10):601–4.

61. Yoo S. C., Chang K. H., Lyu M. O., et al. Clinical characteristics of struma ovarii. *J Gynecol Oncol.* 2008;**19**(2):135–8.

62. Robboy S. J., Shaco-Levy R., Peng R. Y., et al. Malignant struma ovarii: An analysis of 88 cases, including 27 with extraovarian spread. *Int J Gynecol Pathol.* 2009;**28**(5):405–22.

63. Smith L. P., Brubaker L. W., Wolsky R. J. It does exist! Diagnosis and management of thyroid carcinomas originating in struma ovarii. *Surg Pathol Clin.* 2023;**16**(1):75–86.

64. Werner & Ingbar's *The Thyroid A Fundamental and Clinical Text.* 10th ed. Wolters Kluwer | Lippincott Williams & Wilkins; 2013.

65. Drozd V., Saenko V., Branovan D. I., et al. A search for causes of rising incidence of differentiated thyroid cancer in children and adolescents after Chernobyl and Fukushima: Comparison of the clinical features and their relevance for treatment and prognosis. *Int J Environ Res Public Health.* 2021;**18**(7):3444.

66. Jargin S. Thyroid cancer after Chernobyl: Re-evaluation needed. *Turk Patoloji Derg.* 2021;**37**(1):1–6.

67. Gilbert E. S., Land C. E, Simon S. L. Health effects from fallout. *Health Phys.* 2002;**82**(5):726–35.

68. Lebbink C. A., Waguespack S. G., van Santen H. M. Thyroid dysfunction and thyroid cancer in childhood cancer survivors: Prevalence, surveillance and management. *Front Horm Res.* 2021;**54**:140–53.

69. Kitahara C. M., K Rmendiné Farkas D., Jorgensen J. O. L., Cronin-Fenton D., Sorensen H. T. Benign thyroid diseases and risk of thyroid cancer: A nationwide cohort study. *J Clin Endocrinol Metab.* 2018;**103**(6):2216–24.

70. Rahbari R., Zhang L., Kebebew E. Thyroid cancer gender disparity. *Future Oncol.* 2010;**6**(11):1771–9.

71. Derwahl M., Nicula D. Estrogen and its role in thyroid cancer. *Endocr Relat Cancer.* 2014;**21**(5):T273–83.

72. Rajoria S., Suriano R., Shanmugam A., et al. Metastatic phenotype is regulated by estrogen in thyroid cells. *Thyroid.* 2010;**20**(1):33–41.

73. Torre F., Calogero A. E., Condorelli R. A., et al. Effects of oral contraceptives on thyroid function and vice versa. *J Endocrinol Invest.* 2020;**43**(9):1181–8.

74. Chakravarthy V., Ejaz S. *Thyroxine-Binding Globulin Deficiency.* StatPearls Publishing; 2022.

75. Hirsch D., Yackobovitch-Gavan M., Lazar L. Infertility and pregnancy rates in female thyroid cancer survivors: A retrospective cohort study using health care administrative data from Israel. *Thyroid.* 2023;**33**(4):456–63.

76. Sullivan S. A. Thyroid nodules and thyroid cancer in pregnancy. *Clin Obstet Gynecol.* 2019;**62**(2):365–72.

77. Gibelli B., Zamperini P., Proh M., Giugliano G. Management and follow-up of thyroid cancer in pregnant women. *Acta Otorhinolaryngol Ital.* 2011;**31**(6):358–65.

78. Alexander E. K., Pearce E. N., Brent G. A., et al. 2017 Guidelines of the American Thyroid Association for the Diagnosis and Management of Thyroid Disease During Pregnancy and the Postpartum. *Thyroid.* 2017;**27**(3):315–89.

79. Navarro P., Rocher S., Miro-Martinez P., Oltra-Crespo S. Radioactive iodine and female fertility. *Sci Rep.* 2022;**12**(1):3704.

80. Piek M. W., Postma E. L., van Leeuwaarde R., et al. The effect of radioactive iodine therapy on ovarian function and fertility in female thyroid cancer patients: A systematic review and meta-analysis. *Thyroid.* 2021;**31**(4):658–68.

81. Kim H. O., Lee K., Lee S. M., Seo G. H. Association between pregnancy outcomes and radioactive iodine treatment after thyroidectomy among women with thyroid cancer. *JAMA Intern Med.* 2020;**180**(1):54–61.

82. Kurtoglu S., Akin M. A., Daar G., et al. Congenital hypothyroidism due to maternal radioactive iodine exposure during pregnancy. *J Clin Res Pediatr Endocrinol.* 2012;**4**(2):111–13.

83. Abruzzese E., Trawinska M. M., Perrotti A. P., De Fabritiis P. Tyrosine kinase inhibitors and pregnancy. *Mediterr J Hematol Infect Dis.* 2014;**6**(1):e2014028.

84. Abruzzese E., Mauro M., Apperley J., Chelysheva E. Tyrosine kinase inhibitors and pregnancy in chronic myeloid leukemia: Opinion, evidence, and recommendations. *Ther Adv Hematol.* 2020;**11**:2040620720966120.

85. Vannucchi G., Perrino M., Rossi S., et al. Clinical and molecular features of differentiated thyroid cancer diagnosed during pregnancy. *Eur J Endocrinol.* 2010;**162**(1):145–51.

86. Rakhlin L., Fish S., Tuttle R. M. Response to therapy status is an excellent predictor of pregnancy-associated structural disease progression in patients previously treated for differentiated thyroid cancer. *Thyroid.* 2017;**27**(3):396–401.

87. Poisson T., Deandreis D., Leboulleux S., et al. 18F-fluorodeoxyglucose positron emission tomography and computed tomography in anaplastic thyroid cancer. *Eur J Nucl Med Mol Imaging.* 2010;**37**(12):2277–85.

Chapter 22

Vulvar Melanoma

Ana M. Ciurea

Case Presentation

A 50-year-old Caucasian woman with a history of severe photodamage, multiple non-melanoma skin cancer and no significant past medical history presents for evaluation in the dermatology clinic for an atypical hyperpigmented patch on the external genitalia. The lesion has been present for an unknown duration and was identified during a routine physical examination performed by her gynecologist. Patient denies bleeding, fever, fatigue, weight loss, headache, or dyspnea. Family history is unremarkable. On physical examination, the patient was noted to have a 3.5 cm, irregularly shaped, multicolored patch with a 4 mm dark brown to black papule within it, involving the right labia minora, majora, and clitoris (Figure 22.1). Palpation of bilateral cervical, supraclavicular, axillary, and inguinal lymph nodes shows no lymphadenopathy. Two skin biopsies of the right labia demonstrate atypical intraepidermal melanocytic proliferation, consistent with melanoma in situ and present at peripheral tissue edges. What are the next diagnostic steps and what is the recommended management?

Epidemiology

Incidence and Long-Term Prognosis

Vulvar melanomas (VMs) are aggressive malignant tumors of the female genital tract, which develop from melanocytes with a high incidence of metastatic spread. VM typically arises de novo, in the absence of a preexisting melanocytic neoplasm. Although VMs are rare tumors, melanoma is the second most common primary malignancy of the vulva in women, after squamous cell carcinoma [1, 2]. VMs account for 1% of all melanomas in women and 5% of all vulvar malignancies [3]. The incidence of vulvar and vaginal melanoma are 0.108 and $0.026/10^5$ per year based on 15 years' experience of population-based registries that represent approximately 10% of the United States population [4].

The majority of VMs occur in Caucasian, postmenopausal women in the fifth to eighth decade of life, although they may occur at any age. Only a handful of cases have been reported in pediatric patients, usually in association with lichen sclerosus [5, 6]. Gynecologic tract melanomas are typically aggressive with the vulva as the most common site (70%) [7]. The prognosis is poor, due primarily to depth of invasion (Breslow thickness, measured from the top of the tumor to the deepest tumor cells) at the time of diagnosis.

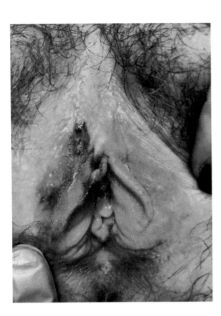

Figure 22.1 Case presentation

While the overall mortality of cutaneous melanoma has decreased by 7% annually during the last seven years, unfortunately this does not apply for VMs. The five-year overall survival rate for cutaneous melanoma is 92%, compared with only 47% for VM; and sadly, there has been no significant improvement over time [3, 8, 9]. A recent US population-based study of 1863 women has shown that 30% of women have advanced disease at the time of diagnosis. Vaginal involvement and/or distant metastasis are often present, with mean size of the primary tumor of 31 mm and more than 46% have a Breslow's thickness greater than 2 mm at time of presentation. This study suggests 52–63% of initially nonmetastatic patients will eventually develop distant metastasis [8]. Survival at five years is higher in women ≤60 years of age compared with ≥ 60 years of age (61.9% versus 39.7%) [7].

An analysis of the Dutch Cancer Registry has shown that even if matched for sex, age, tumor ulceration status, Breslow thickness, lymph node status, and distant metastases, VMs have a slightly worse prognosis compared with cutaneous melanoma. This could be explained by a different tumor biology, variable treatment approach or lack of specific treatment guidelines for vulvar melanomas [10].

Etiology and Risk Factors

The cause of vulvar melanoma is complex and multifactorial, remaining largely unknown. Chronic inflammation, such as from lichen sclerosis, has been linked to vulvar melanoma, however this mechanism is debated and warrants validation in larger prospective studies [11, 12]. Infection with HPV subtypes has also been implicated with melanoma, but its role in the pathogenesis remains unclear [13]. Unlike most cutaneous melanomas, ultraviolet radiation does not appear to play a significant causal role in the pathogenesis of vulvar melanoma. However, a vulvar melanoma with a Breslow thickness of 5.4 mm arising in a 25-year-old woman with extended indoor tanning bed use has been reported [14].

Pathogenesis

Molecular characterization of VMs may shed more light on the carcinogenesis. From a molecular genetic perspective, vulvar melanomas more closely resemble acral lentiginous melanoma (melanoma occurring on the hands and feet) rather than cutaneous melanoma. VMs have a different tumor biology with frequent *c-KIT* mutations which provides a therapeutic target. Dysregulation of *c-KIT* affects cell proliferation, tumor growth, and metastasis. *c-KIT* mutations are detected in up to 21.6% of VMs [3, 15, 16]. The high rate of *c-KIT* mutations appears to be characteristic for VMs, which also distinguishes them from vaginal melanomas (27% versus 8%, respectively) [17].

More rarely, *NRAS* and *BRAF* mutations have also been described. *NRAS* mutations occur in 10.2% of VMs, which is less common than in cutaneous and vaginal melanomas [18]. It appears that *NRAS* mutations are more frequent in patients with nodular melanomas, which accounts for a smaller portion of the VMs and are more common in vaginal melanomas [19]. *BRAF* mutations are found in only 8.2% of VMs. In contrast, *BRAF* mutations are common in typical and atypical nevi of the vulva [20].

Diagnosis and Workup

Physical Examination

Vulvar melanomas may present as macules, papules or nodules (Table 22.1) of irregular coloration, with asymmetric borders, a diameter often larger than 6 mm in size, with a mean size of 3 cm (standard deviation ± 4 cm). There are often accompanying nonspecific symptoms such as vulvar bleeding, pruritus, discharge, irritation, or lymphadenopathy [35]. Melanomas can arise throughout the genital tract, including the cervix and the vagina as well as any site on the vulva. Primary vulvar melanomas most frequently develop on the labia majora, followed by the labia minora and clitoral hood. Roughly 50% of vulvar melanomas arise on the mucosa, 38% on the hairy–glabrous (nonhairy) skin junction, and 13% on the skin of the external genitalia [35].

Amelanotic melanoma is an aggressive type of skin cancer that does not produce the pigment melanin, which gives most melanomas their dark appearance. They account for only 2% of VMs, yet in a 25-year study of 219 Swedish females, amelanotic reddish polyps were the most frequently observed clinical manifestations of vulvar melanoma [35].

Table 22.1 Common dermatologic terms

Macules: flat, nonpalpable lesions	<10 mm in diameter
Papules: elevated, palpable lesions usually	<10 mm in diameter
Patch: palpable lesions	>10 mm in diameter, elevated or depressed compared to skin surface. May be flat topped or rounded
Nodules: firm papules or lesions that extend into the dermis and/or subcutaneous tissue	

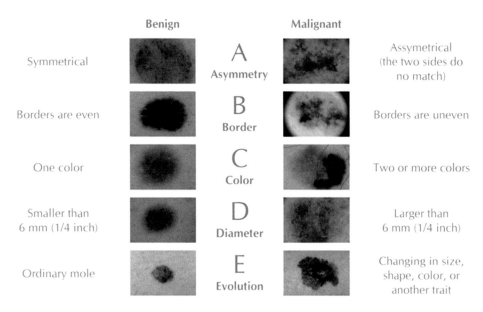

Figure 22.2 ABCDEs of melanoma

Differential Diagnosis

For macular lesions (flat nonpalpable lesions < 10 mm), the major differential includes melanotic macule of the external genitalia, melanocytic nevi, vulvar melanosis, postinflammatory hyperpigmentation, and low-grade and high-grade vulvar intraepithelial neoplasia. Palpable pigmented lesions must be distinguished from atypical appearing seborrheic keratosis and melanocytic nevi. Melanotic melanoma may initially be diagnosed as hemorrhoids.

The ABCDE rule (Figure 22.2) is a simple guide for first assessment of pigmented lesions: "A" stands for asymmetry and most melanomas are asymmetrical; "B" stands for border as melanomas typically exhibit an irregular border, while nevi typically have a smoother border; "C" stands for color. While benign moles are often a unique color of brown, multiple colors including different shades of brown, black, blue, white, or red are typically a sign for malignancy. "D" stands for diameter and lesions greater than 6 mm should raise awareness. "E" stands for elevation or evolving, and any change of shape, size, structure, color, or symptom is a potential indicator for malignancy [36].

Diagnostic Tests

Dermoscopy and In-Vivo Reflectance Confocal Microscopy

Dermoscopy or skin surface microscopy is a noninvasive, in-vivo diagnostic tool used by trained dermatologists in evaluation of suspicious skin lesions. Dermoscopy allows the visualization of subsurface skin structures in the epidermis, at the dermoepidermal junction, and in the upper dermis. Dermoscopy may facilitate the early identification of vulvar melanoma. It can help identify and differentiate melanomas from melanocytic lesions, dysplastic nevi, basal cell carcinomas, and squamous cell carcinomas among other skin lesions [37].

In-vivo reflectance confocal microscopy (RCM) is an emerging technique that allows for noninvasive high-resolution imaging of the skin and the mucosa which may be used in the detection of vulvar and other mucosal melanomas. The characteristics of mucosal melanomas include: [1] architectural atypia, consisting of a high density of dendritic cells, pagetoid cells, and melanocytes arranged in sheets and nests and [2] cytologic atypia, characterized by large, pleomorphic shape, bright cytoplasm and a hyper reflective nucleus [38].

Although studies have reported using dermoscopy and RCM of pigmented lesions of the vulvar region, this can be a difficult area to examine. Specialized equipment and appropriate hygienic measures may be required, such as use of an antibacterial translucent wrap overlying the window of the instruments.

In women of any age, associated pruritus, bleeding, discharge, discomfort, lymphadenopathy, or vulvar ulceration should raise concern for possible melanoma. There is a significant overlap between benign and malignant lesions and a biopsy should be performed in all suspicious lesions for a definitive diagnosis. A biopsy specimen that includes as much of the lesion as possible, ensuring adequate depth for staging purposes, is warranted. The biopsy may be performed using a Keyes punch instrument or a shave biopsy with a scalpel under local anesthesia. Lidocaine 1–2% solution is preferred. The actual injection should be performed with the smallest needle possible (e.g., 27- or 30-gauge). Choice of instrument is generally determined by provider preference, the level of experience and instrument availability. In general, 3–8 mm punch biopsies are preferred for pigmented lesions of the vulva. For tumors thicker than 1 mm, examination of lymph nodes is generally recommended.

Computed tomography is limited in the evaluation of VMs. MRI is most commonly used, given its superior soft tissue contrast resolution. At PET/CT, VMs usually show high FDG (radiotracer) uptake.

Histopathology

Historically, cutaneous melanoma has been classified into subtypes based on the tissue from which the primary tumor arises. The main subtypes are cutaneous melanoma (CM), which arises in non-glabrous (hairy) skin; acral melanoma (AM), a distinct form that originates in the glabrous (nonhairy) skin of the palms, soles, and nail beds; mucosal melanoma (MM), the rarest subtype, which arises from melanocytes in the mucosal lining of internal tissues; and uveal melanoma (UM) which develops from melanocytes in the uveal tract of the eye. Lentiginous refers to the initial origin of these tumors as a macular (flat) brown spot, resembling a benign lentigo (freckle).

Mucosal lentiginous melanoma is the most frequent histologic type of melanoma of the genital skin but can also be of superficial spreading or nodular subtypes, particularly on keratinized surfaces. Superficial spreading and nodular melanomas however occur less frequently.

Atypical melanocytes arranged as confluent nests and sheets, with prominent pagetoid spread and absent dermal maturation are typically seen microscopically. Ulceration, cell necrosis and abundant reticular dermal mitoses are also often present. Mucosal lentiginous melanoma exhibits many histologic similarities to acral lentiginous melanoma. As with cutaneous melanoma, prognosis is determined by tumor thickness at presentation.

Prognosis, Staging and Management

VMs are often diagnosed late and have a poor prognosis. In one study, the five-year overall survival rate was only 46.6% compared with 92% in cutaneous melanoma [8]. Previous studies suggest that Breslow thickness, ulceration, older age, ethnicity (African Americans), stage at diagnosis, histologic subtype, mitotic rate, ulceration, lymphovascular invasion, perineural invasion, and microscopic satellitosis are negative predictors for outcome [9]. The international multicenter VULvar CANcer study involved 100 international centers and found that tumor size and American Joint Committee on Cancer (AJCC) stage (Table 22.2) were the only independent prognostic factors associated with local and distant recurrence of vulvar melanoma [41].

Treatment is largely surgical. In patients with localized disease, there appears to be no significant difference in tumor specific survival among those undergoing a radical vulvectomy compared with more conservative surgery such as a wide local excision. Sentinel lymph node biopsy should be offered to all women with VM and clinically unsuspicious nodes if the AJCC stage is greater than IA or in the presence of ulceration [3].

Imiquimod is a topical immune response modulator that has both antiviral and antitumor activity which has been used in the treatment of vulvar melanoma/melanoma in situ when surgical resection is not feasible [39]. While studies have shown that tyrosine kinase inhibitors are ineffective in unselected cases of advanced melanoma, it may be considered in those patients harboring a *c-KIT* mutation [3]. Cutaneous melanoma treatment has been

Table 22.2 American Joint Committee on Cancer 2017 prognostic stage group for cutaneous melanoma

Stage	T	N	M
0	Tis	N0	M0
IA	T1a	N0	M0
IB	T1b, T2a	N0	M0
IIA	T2b, T3a	N0	M0
IIB	T3b, T4a	N0	M0
IIC	T4b	N0	M0
IIIA	T1a/b-T2a	N1, N2a	M0
IIIB	T0	N1b, N1 c	M0
	T1a/b-T2a	N1b/c, N2b	M0
	T2b/T3a	N1a-N2b	M0
IIIC	T0	N2b/c, N3b/c	M0
	T1a-T3a	N2 c, N3	M0
	T3b/T4a	Any N ≥N1	M0
	T4b	N1a-N2 c	M0
IIID	T4b	N3	M0
IV	Any T, Tis	Any N	M1

revolutionized by the approval of immune checkpoint inhibitors (e.g. nivolumab and pembrolizumab), BRAF inhibitors (ex. vemurafenib and dabrafenib) and MEK inhibitors (ex. trametinib and cobimetinib). With the advent of these targeted agents and immunotherapy, there exists promising new treatment modalities that may improve care and outcomes of patients with vulvar melanoma.

Reproductive Considerations

Oncofertility counseling by a physician specialized in reproductive medicine should be offered to all patients of reproductive age who have not completed family-building [21, 22]. Fertility concerns may impact treatment adherence and therapy decisions. Reliable contraception should be used during and for at least five months after completion of melanoma therapy [23, 24].

The reproductive impact of novel anticancer drugs utilized for vulvar melanoma are unknown. Based on general toxicity studies and in the absence of dedicated animal studies on fertility, a fertility–lowering effect of the BRAF-MEK inhibitors cannot be excluded. Programmed cell death-1 (PD-1) and the programmed death-ligand 1 (PD-L1) are expressed at very low levels in the ovary; however, because of the lack of preclinical data in regard to fertility, the effect of inhibition of these ligands is unknown [25, 26, 27].

Treatment-related side effects may also impact fertility. Common side effects of BRAF/MEK inhibition as well as immune checkpoint inhibitors include, but are not limited to, fever and gastrointestinal adverse events [31, 32, 33]. For the BRAF-MEK inhibitor combinations, the side effects are usually reversible and include pruritus, dryness, acneiform eruption, photosensitivity, hair loss, fever, arthralgias, fatigue, and nausea [29, 30]. Immune checkpoint inhibitor (ICI) therapy can impair fertility directly or indirectly by altering endocrine function. ICI associated hypophysitis can occur in up to 13% of patients with combination therapy, however, can usually be reversed by appropriate hormone replacement.

Consideration of fertility preservation is recommended for reproductive aged patients with a new diagnosis of vulvar melanoma, regardless of the type of planned therapy. Options include use of a gonadotropin–releasing hormone agonist (GnRH) during gonadotoxic therapy, ovarian stimulation with cryopreservation of oocytes or embryos, and cryopreservation of ovarian tissue [34].

Regarding pregnancy, BRAF and/or MEK inhibitors may impact fetal and embryonic growth and infant development through MAPK pathway signaling inhibition. PD-L1 is highly expressed in the placenta, and administration of PDL-1 inhibitors appears to increase miscarriage rates in murine models. Unfavorable effects on embryofetal development including teratogenic effects of anti-BRAF and anti-MEK inhibitors in melanoma therapy cannot be excluded [28].

Adjuvant melanoma therapy with immune checkpoint or MAPK inhibitors, should be avoided in pregnancy. In advanced stages of disease, treatment with BRAF and MEK inhibitors during pregnancy may be considered when the potential benefit for the pregnant patient outweighs the potential risk for the fetus. An interdisciplinary tumor board should be consulted to aid in decision making and therapeutic alternatives should be discussed [33, 34].

Importantly, BRAF inhibitors may reduce the efficacy of oral or systemic hormonal contraceptives. Therefore, an additional effective nonhormonal contraceptive method (such as IUD, barrier methods, partner vasectomy) should be used during BRAF/MEK inhibition. A reliable contraceptive in female patients is required for patients undergoing immune checkpoint inhibitor therapy (dual contraceptive method). Contraception for four to five months after treatment discontinuation is recommended [33].

Surveillance/Screening Recommendations

It is important that a dermatologist evaluate the vulvar region during routine skin cancer screening examinations, inquire about any new or changing lesions, and instruct the patient to undergo regular gynecologic surveillance [40]. The most effective strategy to reduce vulvar cancer incidence is the opportune treatment of predisposing and preneoplastic lesions associated with its development.

Conclusion

Pigmented lesions of the vulva can pose a diagnostic challenge. Understanding the distinct epidemiology, clinical and histopathologic characteristics of vulvar melanomas can facilitate appropriate patient treatment. Although the risk of transformation of benign lesions into melanoma is low, maintaining a high level of suspicion is necessary given the aggressive clinical course of vulvar melanoma. The early detection of VM requires awareness of health professionals of this rare disease, as well as patient education on self-examination of the genital tract, with a handheld mirror if necessary, and detection of all atypical pigmented lesions and local recurrences.

Case Resolution

After the diagnosis of melanoma in situ was confirmed, the patient underwent a wide-local excision which demonstrated melanoma in situ, present at the peripheral tissue edges. Treatment with imiquimod 5% cream applied three times a week for 16 weeks led to complete disease resolution. Three years after the initial presentation, she developed a local recurrence and underwent surgical resection with negative margins. She has been without evidence of disease since.

Take Home Points

1. Vulvar melanomas are rare, aggressive tumors of the female genital tract with high metastatic potential and dismal prognosis, likely due to delay in diagnosis, different tumor biology, unclear treatment strategies, and treatment response.
2. Histopathological evaluation and immunohistochemical analysis are paramount to confirm the diagnosis.
3. Close monitoring, patient education regarding self-skin examination, with handheld mirror if necessary, and screening are necessary for all atypical lesions and to identify local recurrences.
4. Treatment requires a multidisciplinary approach. Vulvar melanomas have frequent *c-KIT* mutations, which provides an additional therapeutic target in recurrent disease.
5. Novel treatment modalities for cutaneous melanomas include checkpoint inhibitors and targeted therapies, with recent evidence demonstrating efficacy in vulvar melanomas.

References

1. Muzarku E. C., Peunn L. A., Hale C., Pomeranz M. K., Polsky D. Vulvar nevi, melanosis and melanoma: An epidemiologic, clinical, and histopathologic review. *J Am Acad Dermatol.* 2014;**71**(6):1241–9.

2. Moxley K. M., Fader A. N., Rose P. G., et al. Malignant melanoma of the vulva: An extension of cutaneous melanoma? *Gynecol Oncol.* 2011;**122**:612–17.

3. Wolmuth C., Wolmuth-Wieser I. Vulvar melanoma: Molecular characteristics, diagnosis, surgical management, and medical treatment. *Am J Clin Dermatol.* 2021;**22**:639–51.

4. Weinstock M. A. Malignant melanoma of the vulva and vagina in the United States: Patterns of incidence and population-based estimates of survival. *AM J Obst Gybecol.* 1994;**171**:1225–30.

5. Li K. P., Ajebo E. M., Diamond D., Powell M., Belcher M. Primary vulvar melanoma in an adolescent patient. *Pediatr Dermatol.* 2023. doi: 10.1111/pde.15296

6. La Spina M., Meli M. C., De Pasquale R., et al. Vulvar melanoma associated with lichen sclerosus in a child: Case report and literature review. *Pediatr Dermatol.* 2016;**33**(3):e190–e194.

7. Erickson M. K., Pontes D., Memon R., Schlosser, B. J. 16835 A US population-based epidemiologic study of vulvar melanoma from the Surveillance, Epidemiology, and End Results (SEER) database. *J Am Acad Dermatol.* 2020;**83**(6):AB72

8. Siegel R. L., Miller K. D., Jemal A. Cancer statistics, 2020. *CA Cancer J Clin.* 2020;**70**(1):7–30. doi: 10.3322/caac.21590. Epub 2020 Jan 8.

9. Wohlmuth C., Wohlmuth-Wieser I., May T., Vicus D., Gien L. T., Laframboise S. Malignant melanoma of the vulva and vagina: A US population-based study of 1863 patients. *Am J Clin Dermatol.* 2020;**21**(2):285–95. doi: 10.1007/s40257-019-00487-x.

10. Pleunis N., Schuurman M. S., Van Rossum M. M., et al. Rare vulvar malignancies; incidence, treatment and survival in the Netherlands. *Gynecol Oncol.* 2016;**142**(3):440–5.

11. Rosamilia L. L., Schwartz J. L., Lowe L., et al. Vulvar melanoma in a 10-year-old girl in association with lichen sclerosus. *J Am Acad Dermatol.* 2006;**54** (Suppl):S52–S53.

12. Schaffer J. V., Orlow S. J. Melanocytic proliferations in the setting of vulvar lichen sclerosus: Diagnostic considerations. *Pediatr Dermatol.* 2005;**22**:276–8.

13. Rohwedder A., Slominski A., Wolff M., Kredentser D., Carlson J. A. Epidermodysplasia verruciformis and cutaneous human papillomavirus DNA, but not genital human papillomavirus DNAs, are frequently detected in vulvar and vaginal melanoma. *Am J Dermatopathol.* 2007;**29**:13–17.

14. Pawelec M., Karmowski A., Karmowski M. Where the sun does not shine: Is sunshine protective against melanoma of the vulva? *J Photochem Photobiol B.* 2010;**101**:179–83.

15. Curtin J. A., Busam K., Pinkel D., Bastian B. C. Somatic activation of KIT in distinct subtypes of melanoma. *J Clin Oncol.* 2006;**24**:4340–6.

16. Willmore-Payne C., Holden J. A., Tripp S., Layfeld L. J. Human malignant melanoma: Detection of BRAF- and c-kit-activating mutations by high-resolution amplicon melting analysis. *Hum Pathol.* 2005;**36**:486–93.

17. Pleunis N., Schuurman M. S., Van Rossum M. M., et al. Rare vulvar malignancies: Incidence, treatment and survival in the Netherlands. *Gynecol Oncol.* 2016;**142**:440–5.

18. Hou J. Y., Baptiste C., Hombalegowda R. B., et al. Vulvar and vaginal melanoma: A unique subclass of mucosal melanoma based on a comprehensive molecular analysis of 51 cases compared with 2253 cases of nongynecologic melanoma. *Cancer.* 2017;**123**:1333–44.

19. Grill C., Larue L. NRAS, NRAS, which mutation is fairest of them all? *J Invest Dermatol.* 2016;**136**:1936–8.

20. Gray-Schopfer V., Wellbrock C., Marais R. Melanoma biology and new targeted therapy. *Nature.* 2007;**445**:851–7.

21. Hassel J. C., Livingstone E., Allam J. P., et al. Fertility preservation and management of pregnancy in melanoma patients requiring systemic therapy. *ESMO Open.* 2021;**6**(5):100248.

22. Filippi F., Serra N., Vigano P., et al. Fertility preservation for patients with melanoma. *Melanoma Res.* 2022;**32**(5):303–8.

23. Scott A. R., Stoltzfus K. C., Tchelebi L. T., et al. Trends in cancer incidence in US adolescents and young adults, 1973–2015. *JAMA Netw Open.* 2020;**3**(12):e2027738.

24. van der Meer D. J., Karim-Kos H. E., van der Mark M., et al. Incidence, survival, and mortality trends of cancer diagnosed in adolescents and young adults (15-39 years): A population-based study in the Netherlands 1990-2016. *Cancer (Basel).* 2020;**12**(11):3421.

25. ESHRE Guideline Group on Female Fertility Preservation, Anderson R. A., Amant F., et al. ESHRE guideline: female fertility preservation. *Hum Reprod Open.* 2020;**2020**(4):hoaa052.

26. European Medicines Agency ICH guideline S9 on nonclinical evaluation for anticancer pharmaceuticals (EMA/CHMP/ICH/ 646107/2008, May 2010). www.ema.europa .eu/en/documents/scientific-guideline/ich-g uideline-s9-non-clinical-evaluation-antican cer-pharmaceuticals-step-5_en.pdf.

27. Bonelli M., Di Giuseppe F., Beken S. Impact analysis of ICH S9 on non-clinical development of anticancer drugs. *Regul Toxicol Pharmacol.* 2015;**73**(1):361–6.

28. Poulet F. M., Wolf J. J., Herzyk D. J., DeGeorge J. J. An evaluation of the impact of PD-1 pathway blockade on reproductive safety of therapeutic PD-1 inhibitors. *Birth Defects Res B Dev Reprod Toxicol.* 2016;**107**(2):108–19.

29. Eigentler T. K., Hassel J. C., Berking C., et al. Diagnosis, monitoring and management of immune-related adverse drug reactions of anti-PD-1 antibody therapy. *Cancer Treat Rev.* 2016;**45**:7–18.

30. Hassel J. C., Heinzerling L., Aberle J., et al. Combined immune checkpoint blockade (anti-PD-1/anti-CTLA-4): Evaluation and management of adverse drug reactions. *Cancer Treat Rev.* 2017;**57**:36–49.

31. Menzer C., Beedgen B., Rom J., et al. Immunotherapy with ipilimumab plus nivolumab in a stage IV melanoma patient during pregnancy. *Ur J Cancer.* 2018;**104**:239–42.

32. Azim H. A. Jr, Peccatori F. A., Pavlidis N. Treatment of the pregnant mother with cancer: A systematic review on the use of cytotoxic, endocrine, targeted agents and immunotherapy during pregnancy. *Part I: Solid tumors. Cancer Treat Rev.* 201;**36**(2):101–9.

33. Practice Committee of the American Society for Reproductive Medicine. Electronic address: asrm@asrm.org. Fertility preservation in patients undergoing gonadotoxic therapy or gonadectomy: a committee opinion. *Fertil Steril.* 2019;**112**(6):1022–33.

34. Dolmans M. M., Taylor H. S., Rodriguez-Wallberg K. A., et al. Utility of gonadotropin-releasing hormone agonists for fertility preservation in women receiving chemotherapy: Pros and cons. *Fertil Steril.* 2020;**114**(4):725–38.

35. Ragnarsson-Olding B. K., Kanter-Lewensohn L. R., Lagerlöf B., Nilsson B. R., Ringborg U. K. Malignant melanoma of the vulva in a nationwide, 25-year study of 219 Swedish females: Clinical observations and histopathologic features. *Cancer.* 1999;**86**:1273–84.

36. Liu W., Hill D., Gibbs A. F., et al. What features do patients notice that help to distinguish between benign pigmented lesions and melanomas?: The ABCD(E) rule versus the seven-point checklist. *Melanoma Res.* 2005;**15**(6):549–54.

37. Vaccari S., Barisani A., Salvini C., et al. Thin vulvar melanoma: A challenging diagnosis. Dermoscopic features of a case

series. *Clin Exp Dermatol.*
2020;**45**(2):187–93.

38. Theillac C., Cinotti E., Malvehy J., et al. Evaluation of large clinically atypical vulvar pigmentation with RCM: Atypical melanosis or early melanoma? *J Eur Acad Dermatol Venereol.* 2019;**33**(1):84–92.

39. Fuchs E., Khanijow A., Garcia R. L., Goff B. A. Imiquimod treatment of vulvar melanoma in situ invading the urethra. *Gynecol Oncol Rep.* 2021;3;**38**:100875.

40. Omari M., Zaimi A., Kacem H. H., Afqir S. Vulvar melanoma: A diagnostic challenge for young women – a case report. *Ann Med Surg (Lond).* 2022;**25**(81):104473.

41. Iacoponi S., Rubio P., Garcia E., Oehler M. K., Diez J . (VULCAN Study collaborative group). Prognostic factors of recurrence and survival in vulvar melanoma: Subgroup analysis of the VULvar CANcer Study. *Int J Gynecol Cancer.* 2016;**26**(7):1307–12.

Index

Please note: page numbers in *italic type* indicate illustrations or tables

Printed in the United States
by Baker & Taylor Publisher Services